The Blair Supremacy

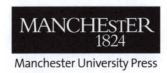
MANCHESTER
1824

Manchester University Press

The Blair Supremacy

A study in the politics of Labour's party management

LEWIS MINKIN

Manchester University Press

Manchester and New York

distributed in the United States exclusively by Palgrave Macmillan

Published by Manchester University Press
Oxford Road, Manchester M13 9NR, UK
and Room 400, 175 Fifth Avenue, New York, NY 10010, USA
www.manchesteruniversitypress.co.uk

Distributed in the United States exclusively by
Palgrave Macmillan, 175 Fifth Avenue, New York,
NY 10010, USA

Distributed in Canada exclusively by
UBC Press, University of British Columbia, 2029 West Mall,
Vancouver, BC, Canada V6T 1Z2

British Library Cataloguing-in-Publication Data
A catalogue record for this book is available from the British Library

Library of Congress Cataloging-in-Publication Data applied for

ISBN   978 0 7190 7379 3 hardback
ISBN   978 0 7190 7380 9 paperback

First published 2014

Typeset in 10/12pt Sabon
by Graphicraft Limited, Hong Kong
Printed in Great Britain
by TJ International Ltd, Padstow

By the strength of our common endeavour we achieve more than we achieve alone.
Clause IV, Labour Party Rulebook, 1995.

When we created New Labour it was about taking the Labour Party out of smoke-filled rooms and away from machine politics.
James Purnell, Minister for Culture, BBC *Newsnight*, September 2006.

I've never led this party by calculation.
Tony Blair, Labour Party Conference, 30 September 2003.

Oh what scoundrels we would be if we did for ourselves what we stand ready to do for Italy.
Cavour.

Contents

Preface: Origins, roles, methods and sources ... ix
Abbreviations ... xiv

Introduction ... 1

Part I: Antecedents ... 9

1 The tradition of party management and the road to
   destabilisation ... 11
2 Revolt and restoration ... 42
3 Contentious alliance, OMOV and the management of
   democratic renewal ... 82

Part II: Forging 'New Labour' management ... 115

4 'New Labour' and the culture of party management ... 117
5 The Leader, the machine and party management ... 146
6 Transforming fundamentals and laying new foundations ... 176
7 Creating 'the Party into Power' project ... 200
8 Managing the changing NEC: partnership and shifting
   power ... 229
9 Managing policy relations with business and unions ... 266
10 Managing new policy institutions ... 303
11 Managing the party conference ... 333
12 Managing candidate selection ... 369
13 Managing the Parliamentary Labour Party (PLP) ... 401
14 Employment relations, representation and party
   management ... 435

Part III: Crisis and control ... 461

15 The crisis of party management ... 463
16 Distrust, management and the long road to Iraq ... 503
17 New challenges and management on the road to Warwick ... 557
18 Managing for legacy ... 609

Part IV: Appraisal   661

19 Summary: analysis and characterisation   663
20 Evaluation and perspectives   707
21 Epilogue: Brown, management inheritance and
    new moves to reform   734

    Index   781

Preface: Origins, roles, methods and sources

This study is highly unusual, not only in its content but in its origins and in the mixture of roles, working methods and procedural values from which it grew. These built up in continuation of the combination of academic and advisory roles, which deepened following my writing Neil Kinnock's 1983 speech on the organisational reform of the defeated Labour Party. That marked one starting point in the history of this book. But I now date the origins of the present study from a long interview with Tony Blair in 1989 at his home. I sought then to understand his views on the future of the party and the unions and I also gained a glimpse of a major difference between us over the conduct of Labour's internal politics (disclosed in Chapter 2, p. 77 and n. 76).

The very favourable academic and party reception for *The Contentious Alliance*, published in 1991,[1] led to my appointment in 1992 as advisor to the National Executive Committee (NEC) review group on relations between the party and the trade unions. Blair and I had some strong and open disagreements there. In 1996, I also became an advisor to the NEC Party into Power discussions, which reviewed relations between the party and a future government. Some of my critical perspective on leadership, manipulation and distrust under Blair's leadership, which are further developed here, were vigorously argued and contested at times in those discussions.

What happened next said something healthy about Blair and the fluidity of relations around him, and tells something about my own role-playing and the rules I developed for myself over time. I had turned down a shadow ministerial post under Kinnock in 1983 and subsequently did not ask for or encourage positions, favours or honours. I did not want to be drawn too deeply into implicit obligations, seductions and dangers to the trust of others. As advisor on the two controversial major review committees I had worked without any public comment. I became known as somebody whose discretion could be trusted, and whose independent and creative judgement was expressed from a deep understanding of Labour politics.

Perhaps because of this, in spite of the battles over the Party into Power, I was asked by Jon Cruddas, Blair's Deputy Political Secretary in 1997, to act in independent liaison between Cruddas and the unions whilst preserving my own position on the union-party relationship. Later, in 2000–1, with what became Blair's tacit approval, following what I had thought (mistakenly, see Chapter 15, particularly p. 472) was the beginning of his more sensitive relationship with the party, I became involved in a similar dialogue with other Political Office aides, covering a wider Labour Party procedural agenda, again in line with the values I had pursued as advisor to the two major reviews. In 2005–6 that dialogue with No. 10 eventually petered out over, amongst other things, disagreement about the management of the implementation of what became known as the Warwick Agreement with the unions.

All the way through it was my practice to interweave into the advisory and liaison work the role of lone scholar, digging away at the existing literature, documentation and cuttings, interviewing and discussing, seeking my own interpretation, noticing features that others did not and observing patterns or their absence. I could feed in and draw upon an understanding of, and contrasts with, past Labour procedures, practices and politics, and decades of observational pattern-making.

Since 1967, I have been an investigator and private discussant in innumerable Labour Party meetings of different kinds and at different levels, and interviewed most major managerial figures and many leading politicians in connection with my studies.

It was around 2002, I think, when the idea that I was preparing a future book took clearer shape. Though a continuing critic, I disclosed that aim to No. 10 and to any other regular interviewees who asked. I persevered with the interviews and multiple selective follow-up discussions over long periods with party officials, union leaders and officials, ministers and their aides, MPs' internal party representatives, and key activists. Some of this continued during 2005–6 but with much weaker contact with No. 10, and more spasmodically with others after 2007. From June 1990 when the last interview took place for *The Contentious Alliance*, until October 2012, I had interviewed and often taken part in repeated follow-up sessions with 133 different people, and discussed with many hundreds more.

All the digging, the talking, the observations and the comparisons convinced me of the importance, for the party and the public, of pulling together, analysing and presenting what had emerged. I renewed the view that the academic in politics, especially one playing dual and triple roles, has the responsibility to assist in seeking to ensure that people in politics act with their eyes open. As Goethe said, 'Unless you use your eyes to see, you end up using them to cry with'.

Sources and acknowledgements

I have followed here the normal practice of stipulating printed sources in what became over 2,000 Notes, but ideas and information in the many verbal sources in the dialogue and interviews which often enabled me to give meaning to printed sources had problems of attribution. This has always been the case with the evidence used in my work, an element of which derived from or was supported by information from confidential sources. In this study these sources were more pervasive because the project involved a much greater intrusion at a higher level into a wide range of normally undisclosed behaviour. Without that confidentiality this study could never have been satisfactorily attempted.

To a lesser degree, the problems of attribution arose also from my personal method of conducting interviews and conversations, especially those repeated many times over the years. I regard research as both a rigorous investigation and a creative art. Some interviewing and discussions had long developed into a mixed form: formal interrogative but also opening up, comparing and sharing elements of interpretation useful to both of us.[2] This was often followed later by my attempts to connect the information to other past and present developments. Confirmation or adjustment was constantly assessed in the light of other evidence and, where necessary, led to further investigation and many discussions. The insight and authenticity of the product of this combination of methods have been attested to in the past reception for my work both within the party and in the academic community.[3]

The long-term sharing involved in co-creative interviewing meant I owe a huge debt to the very many people who have, over forty years, enhanced my education and understanding. And it has also meant that on occasions there was a lack of clarity about who introduced what information, and what obligations were involved in recognising their contribution in part or in whole. Confidentiality was a dominating general consideration. For all these reasons, although with permission I have named some limited exceptional assistance below, and, again with permission, some, on rare occasions, are cited in the Notes, I have heavily restricted the naming of sources. Having made these points here I have also dispensed with the occasional academic practice of giving in Notes long lists of unspecified 'private sources'.

I would particularly like to thank the many people around the Leader and central party organisation, in official and ex-official positions, who took part. There were repetitive discussions with some whose trust and willingness to talk deepened over the years, despite some strong differences of opinion. I hope that I have done them, their work and the important subject, justice. I am noting here, with permission, some special debts incurred over a very long period drawing from the knowledge, understanding and insight of particular veteran senior party and ex-party officials, namely: Alan Haworth, Secretary of the Parliamentary Labour Party (PLP) from 1992 to 2005, Andrew Sharp, Regional Director, North and Yorkshire Labour Party from 1993 to 1999 then Group Head of Party Services at Millbank to 2002, Mike Watts, Labour Party Director of Personnel and Finance, 1987 to 1993, and Larry Whitty, Labour Party General Secretary from 1985 to 1994. I must also make special mention of two very senior

Labour Party politicians and ex-Secretaries of State after 1997, David Blunkett MP and Clare Short MP, and my veteran local councillor, MP and ex-minister John Battle; they did not always agree with me or each other but over the years they provided (within discreet limits) a knowledge-able and stimulating discussion of the party and the practice of politics.

Staff of the Trades Union Congress (TUC) have always given scrupulous assistance over many years of my research and continue to do so. Close cooperation also came from the changing staff of the Trade Union and Labour Party Liaison Organisation (TULO), which became an increasingly significant entity in the party. Byron Taylor, the National Officer of TULO after 2002, provided a valuable new input by drawing from his experience of the culture of party management as a party official and fusing it with his understanding of the difficult union experience of being on the receiv-ing end of managerial behaviour.

I am grateful for years of high-level academic analysis of the Labour Party and for comments on this study by David Howell and Eric Shaw. I also thank Cesca Gaines for helpful comments on early chapters and Arthur Lipow for his provocative encouragement. Thanks are also due to Kevin Theakston who gave me an improved understanding of some relevant aspects of British government, and Peter Nolan who corrected some eco-nomic misconceptions. Keith Ewing did the same for some sections on labour law. There was at times also private assistance from the staff of polling agencies IpsosMORI, YouGov, PoliticsHome, Populus and ICM. Tony Mason from Manchester University Press showed praiseworthy patience and gave much good advice and editorial assistance.

Family assistance in some of the tasks along the way came in various forms from Daniel and Natalie Minkin, and Tom and Stella St David Smith, in administration from Daniel Furniss, in comments on public attitudes to honesty by Judge Chris Furniss and in computing operation from Andy Wood. I thank profusely Paul McHale-Webster who helped me in years of dealing with recalcitrant technology and other problems covered by his multiple expertises. Liz Minkin edited my English, questioned my explana-tions and deserves a medal for putting up with me and this huge work.

None of the individuals or organisations named in this preface is person-ally responsible for any of the judgements in this study and, MUP aside near completion, none knew what they all were.

Notes

1 Lewis Minkin, *The Contentious Alliance*, Edinburgh University Press, Edinburgh, 1991, and 1992 pbk edn with epilogue.

2 See on this 'The Interview as Joint Enquiry' and 'The Interview as Creative Dialogue', in Lewis Minkin, *Political Research as a Creative Art*, SHU Press, Sheffield, 1997, Chapter 5, pp. 144–50. This study, reviewed in the *Times Higher Educational Supplement*, 3 October 1997, as a 'godsend to a generation of

research scholars', led to a government commission, The National Council for Creative and Cultural Education, and I became its Vice-Chair.

3 See particularly Eric Shaw, 'Lewis Minkin and the Party-Union Link', in John T. Callaghan, Steven Fielding, and Steve Ludlam, *Interpreting the Labour Party: Approaches to Labour Politics and History*, Manchester University Press, Manchester, 2003, pp. 166–81.

Abbreviations

ACAS	Advisory Conciliation and Arbitration Service
AEEU	Amalgamated Engineering and Electrical Union
ASLEF	Associated Society of Locomotive Engineers and Firemen
BERR	Department of Business Enterprise and Regulatory Reform
BJPIR	*British Journal of Politics & International Relations*
CAC	Conference Arrangements Committee (standing orders committee)
CBI	Confederation of British Industry
CDS	Campaign for Democratic Socialism
CLP	Constituency Labour Party
CLPD	Campaign for Labour Party Democracy
CWU	Communications Workers Union
EDM	Early Day Motion
EEPTU	Electrical, Electronic, Telecommunications and Plumbing Union
EPLP	European Parliamentary Labour Party
ERA	Employment Relations Act
FBU	Fire Brigades Union
GMC	General Management Committee of the CLP – later General Committee (GC)
GMWU	General and Municipal Workers Union (later the GMB)
GPMU	Graphical, Paper and Media Union
GRA	Grassroots Alliance
IPPR	Institute for Public Policy Research
ISTC	Iron and Steel Trades Confederation
JPC	Joint Policy Committee
LCC	Labour Co-ordinating Committee
LPCR	Labour Party Conference Report
LWAC	Labour Women's Action Committee
MEP	Member of the European Parliament
MSF	Manufacturing, Science and Finance Union
NCC	National Constitutional Committee
NCU	National Communications Union
NEC	National Executive Committee

NPF   National Policy Forum
NULO   National Union of Labour Organisers
NUM   National Union of Mineworkers
NUPE   National Union of Public Employees
NUR   National Union of Railwaymen
OECD   Organisation for Economic Cooperation and Development
OMOV   One Member One Vote
PFI   Private Finance Initiative
PIP   Partnership in Power
PLP   Parliamentary Labour Party
RFMC   Rank and File Mobilising Committee
RMT   National Union of Rail, Maritime and Transport Workers
SCA   Shadow Communications Agency
SERA   Socialist Environment and Resources Association
SOGAT   Society of Graphical and Allied Trades
TGWU   Transport and General Workers Union
TSSA   Transport Salaried Staffs' Association
TUC   Trades Union Congress
TUFL   Trade Unionists for Labour
TULO   Trade Union and Labour Party Liaison Organisation
TULV   Trade Unions for a Labour Victory
UCATT   Union of Construction, Allied Trades and Technicians
UCW   Union of Communication Workers
USDAW   Union of Shop, Distributive and Allied Workers

Introduction

The dynamic leader

There can be no doubt about the huge impact that Tony Blair had on the Labour Party. A dynamic Leader, he piloted and drove the organisation through a ferment of new developments. At every annual party conference, he was the recipient of huge acclaim, reflecting what appeared to be not just a pre-eminence but an unusual and unshakeable supremacy over the party that he and his allies Gordon Brown, Peter Mandelson, Alastair Campbell and Philip Gould now renamed 'New Labour'.* As the process and his methods of producing change and consolidating power are examined and reassessed here, the major focus is on three fundamental questions around which a wide range of other issues are raised. How was it all achieved? Was it really, as projected, a supremacy? Why did it end in the controversial way that it did? The answers to these and many other questions are sought in a probing interrogation of the distinctive character, mechanisms and development of Blair's party management.

Party management

By party management I clarify here that I do not mean the administration of the party's organisational apparatus as it carried out its various functions, although, where relevant, that will be an element in the study. I mean what the managers, past and present, themselves often talked of as 'management': the attempt to control problem-causing activities, issues and developments in order to ensure that outcomes were produced which the managers considered to be in the party's best interests. How the best interests were understood was usually closely related to advancing the aims and objectives established by the party leadership. Management of this kind was and is not a specific office. It was and remains an important function, carried out, either regularly or spasmodically, and often covertly,

---

* 'New Labour' retains its quotation marks in the text to signify a movement of ideas and organisation as well as a contested and time limited title for a particular version of the Labour Party.

by usually a coalition of officials and internally elected representatives alongside their other work.

Anybody familiar with my work over the years will become aware that this focus on illuminating party management and its methods is a development of elements of my past studies. *The Labour Party Conference* revealed for the first time the covert liaison, agenda-setting and procedural devices in the old management of Labour Party policy-making.[1] *The Contentious Alliance* explored for the first time the largely unwritten regulation of relations between the union and parliamentary leaderships, and its effects on party management.[2] But party management has been moved to a central position here because that was what happened in the party. The organisation and culture of its operation under Blair had some important and distinctive new features. It became a greatly expanded yet hitherto under-examined dimension of activity. Here I have focused on many (although, of necessity, not all) of the major tasks and controversial changes of the 'New Labour' era. And though this study is not primarily biographical, consequences will be drawn from the fact that party management was Blair's academy of higher education and his regular training ground in practising the arts and crafts of politics.

Investigation of this activity, in an attempt to put together a new understanding, takes us at times into subterranean processes, and into a multi-faceted and interwoven analysis across time and the different dimensions and forums of party activity. The examination here includes features that were often hidden and unacknowledged. It unveils many new discoveries and insights and not a few surprises. What will become apparent is that without a detailed examination of this management, its origins, form and distinctiveness, much that is significant about key developments in the Labour Party's internal politics during the Blair years would be missed. It gives a new view of the building and maintenance of 'New Labour'.

'New Labour' and the history of party management

A satisfactory analysis has to begin before Blair became Leader, setting out important historical features of Labour's organisation and the traditional model of management of the party. Through this examination can be found various mechanisms which later influenced Blair's own management, but also experiences under Kinnock and Smith against which Blair and his allies strongly reacted in ways that later shaped their distinctiveness. There is an important detailed focus on the battle over one-member-one-vote (OMOV) under the leadership of Smith where Blair was heavily involved, and his agenda of organisational separation from the unions came to the fore. The analysis challenges common views of the origins and process of that battle and suggests that the victory was not what it seemed to be. Some consequences for him as Leader were helpful but also, as will be shown, others were deeply problematic for his management aspirations.

After he became Leader, Blair and his allies brought with them a new pessimism about the electoral predicament, linked with a comprehensive critique of the deficiencies of the party which was diagnosed as in need of a party revolution.[3] That presented considerable and urgent management problems. The analysis explores what these problems were, and what attitudes and organisation were brought to bear in managerial behaviour. What emerged as the culture of Blair's party management was at the heart of party life and its development. The questions that begin here in examining the culture and organisation of party management continue throughout the study, and involve not only asking what the managerial skills and assets were but what were the vulnerabilities and limitations that arose in and from the managerial process and behaviour. The values, perspectives and codes of conduct within this management culture tell us much that is important about the character of 'New Labour' and its Leader. Important portents of the future, including the later remarkable change in Blair's reputation and the developing intensity of the battles within the leadership, are revealed here.

Blair's attempt to manage the reform of fundamentals and foundations of the party was a continuing feature, and over the reform of Clause IV was presented as a complete leadership triumph, with the NEC circumvented, the union opposition crushed and the radical purposes secured. But like so much else of Blairite management it had another face. This involved a more important union role than has been presented hitherto. It included a mysterious change in the union-related content of the new clause, an important and welcomed but hidden NEC and union input into the change, and a major limitation of the triumph. How these happened points to some important features of 'New Labour' management and also some problematic side effects. *The Road to the Manifesto* plebiscite was held to be another triumph, with all purposes secured, but here there were some major unanticipated misadventures, with purposes not achieved. And the crucial backdoor politics around the initiative involved an episode extraordinarily telling about Blair's attitude towards winning, even though generating distrust.

Seeking to subordinate the unions, and introducing an unprecedented attempt to move closer to the increasingly valued business community, whilst still expecting the unions to play a traditional supportive role, was an extraordinary task. Probing how this was managed within the party and in relations with the Trades Union Congress (TUC) leads to major questions of whether or not this was now 'more or less a business party'[4] or 'Labour Party PLC.'[5] A more interesting, complicated and changing reality is revealed though various chapters. At different points, the enquiry also moves into union responses to their treatment and their relations with party management. In the patterns of their behaviour did they still play to the circumscribed roles and mainly conventional 'rules' which constrained their behaviour in the traditional relationship? Did the new relations mean – as so often predicted – that there was a movement apart towards the ending of the party's structural link with affiliated organisations? There is a very big surprise here, explored and explained.

The Party into Power

Through the procedure known as *The Party into Power* came the formulation of new arrangements covering relations between the party and a Labour government. The internal politics of arriving at a conception of a new 'partnership' is investigated to question what influences were brought into play by the Leader, his managers, the unions and other actors. How did they operate and at what stage? Were the limitations on partnership in practice an unanticipated product of its complexity and problematic operation or was it a continuation of the original managerial perspective?

In subsequent chapters, the implementation of these plans for partnership will then be followed through in detail, integrated into a study of the managerial role in all the major institutions and processes at national level of the party, new and old, keeping an eye on resistances, reactions and constraints as well as managerial successes. All the institutions incited new managerial concerns about control. What remained of the significance of the party conference and the National Executive Committee (NEC) and new institutions, the National Policy Forum (NPF) and the Joint Policy Committee (JPC)? Myths and common misconceptions are cleared up. A significant element of the partnership understanding was that the general election manifesto would be the consensual means by which the party would participate in establishing the policy for the second and possibly third terms. In that light, what happened in practice to the gestation of the manifesto? How was that managed and with what consequences?

Backstairs in the Parliamentary Labour Party

Alongside examining the different institutional managements, and noting the new managerial powers, highlighted here is the generally unexpected response to managing the Parliamentary Labour Party (PLP). The PLP was often characterised in this first term as in various states of docility – a view already qualified by Cowley's studies of parliamentary revolts.[6] But when the focus moves away from voting behaviour in the Commons to a broader canvas of behaviour within the party, much more is revealed. Attention is drawn to the extraordinarily prickly secret backstairs relations between the PLP management and the management at the party centre, and the differences between the management cultures. This examination allows us to delve into an often unexplored question: how was it was that the PLP, an institution where dissent was, apparently, threatened with a severe disciplinary regime under Blair, secured so much freedom from sanctions?

Coupled with this, there is a case study of the politics of government implementation of the policy on union recognition and employment relations. Here, what can be seen is the highly unusual role of some of Blair's managers linking in unexpected ways with a new union assertiveness and a new role for the PLP. Seen also is the way that different government managers played in relations with the Confederation of British Industry (CBI). More than is generally understood this had an effect on implementation and the changing balance of forces around the unions and business, with some lasting political consequences.

Managerial vulnerability and 'the end of control freakery'

By the turn of the millennium, the managerial solutions to the problems met by 'New Labour' in 1994 had become themselves seen to be deeply problematic in ways that confounded managerial expectations. Candidate selection became subject to new arrangements and more heavily pressurised management. The special concern here, as elsewhere, is with the role and methods of the Leader and his managers in influencing the procedures and outcomes. But what emerged also were the problems that this management caused for the party's public reputation as addicted to 'control freakery' and the pressure this then produced for a reform of management on the one hand and the defence of Blair on the other.

In this situation, 'Can you adapt and change?', a question hurled regularly at the party by its leadership since 1994, now became posed for the Leader himself in dealing with its own management and control. Could they and did they? The questions became all the more pressing in the light of increasingly hostile public attitudes towards 'control freakery' and political manipulation. It was all the more difficult because the drive to overcome the reputation for 'control freakery' also coincided in practice with a new attempt by Blair to win more freedom of action for his own bold leadership. How the difficult conjunction of problems was dealt with is uncovered, revealing a series of developments, actions and reactions, some of them very clever indeed in a politics of the misleading and the surreptitious. It even tells us something generally unrecognised about the link between party management and the intensifying battle between Blair and Brown.

The extensive managerial operations will continue to be examined in each of the major institutions, enabling a comparison of management across time frames and contexts. What differences developed, what continuities remained, and why? In the light of the evidence here but also in other spheres of the study, a very quizzical eye will be cast on what was said to be 'the end of control freakery' as it was presented to the party and the public. Here as elsewhere the fine academic analysis by Russell which concludes that 'the building of New Labour' was 'of necessity negotiated'[7] will be strongly challenged. With that in mind, there will be a focus on the way that management of the build-up of the wider party and union

voice over Iraq was conducted and then what happened to party accountability over it. Contrasting with this experience a peculiarity in the second
term needs delving into: why was a leadership, obsessed from the first
with control and managed party unity, involved in a pattern of ministerial
public deviance from collective cabinet responsibility?

New pressures and new union leaders

In the second term the management and its behaviour became a further
test for the management of the unions and a test of traditional union
obedience to the priority of their industrial role, their supportive solidarity
in the party and their refusal to use sanctions against the party leadership.
One not untypical view offered was that 'union money no longer buys
votes that make a difference so it is used by being made contingent on
policy delivery'.[8] The reality will be explored through various sensitive
developments including a crisis over party finance where two of the unions
adopted, it seemed, a new threatening position in relation to finance. It
was a crisis that appeared about to shake the Labour Party but ended with
the unions supporting an unpublicised union rescue plan without policy
implications. Why?

Problems intensified when major changes taking place at leadership level
in the unions brought to office a new generation from the left of the unions
who had deep reservations about playing along with the old managerial
game at all. In the final stages of the second term it looked as though there
would be an open and cataclysmic pre-election confrontation. Yet, to general surprise, out of the struggle came the Warwick Agreement of 2004,
an agreement which, for a while, took on iconic significance as a 'peace
in our time'. How did this unexpected agreement come about and was it
linked, as diagnosed, to union finance? What role did party management
play in all this? And what happened to the new peace?

Centralism uniformity and pluralism

This analysis links us to another enquiry. Labour has always been a party
which embodied a high degree of internal pluralism, based on its internal
factions and tendencies, its federal relations with affiliated organisations,
its divided central authority, and its changing amalgam of leadership and
democratic internal arrangements. Under Blair, however, there was a new
centralising managerial impetus behind the search to make 'New Labour'
a united and effective political force and in doing so to undermine other
centres of internal power. It was generally expected, therefore, that in
creating and reinforcing the leader's supremacy there would be a uniform-
ity and homogeneity to managerial activities on his behalf. Did that happen?
The strong leadership of Kinnock had obscured a subdued dissent and
a pluralism with a variety of sources.[9] That forewarns the observer to

question what happened to Labour's internal dissent and pluralism under Blair and how management dealt with them. This is another area where what is discovered challenges some widely accepted assumptions. All here was also not what it was presented to be.

Culmination and departure

The General Election result of 2005 left Blair with a reduced majority still seeking to push through controversial legacy legislation which was to the right of the Labour Party mainstream, and still attempting also to change party and union representation. In September 2006 there occurred what was described by Peter Mandelson as a 'moment of madness',[10] as Blair became the first Labour Prime Minister to be forced into a time-limited notice by a revolt in his own party. It was a fascinating and instructive period in Labour history which requires a broad analysis of problems, discontents and revolts proliferating across the party. From examining the Blair style of leadership and party management, there are good reasons to doubt whether 'the moment of madness' was such an irrational outburst. And what has been found here drives a reassessment of why it was that what had often been regarded as an unshakable supremacy, bolstered, as shown, by extensive management, was overcome by the party giving him his notice.

Appraisal

In the final section of this study there are two interrelated chapters of appraisal. In the Summary and Analysis, the many detailed new findings are summarised in differentiated time frames noting patterns of management, major variabilities and exceptions, interspersed with analytical comment. This facilitates assessment in relation to challenging common assumptions and various empirical and theoretical positions. Various characterisations of the mode of politics and the power relations between leader, party and government are examined in the light of the complex and often cloaked realities, uncovered by the study. The Evaluation and Perspectives then engages critically with the narrative of managerial success bringing into the evaluation a range of events and developments often unnoticed but uncovered in this study. In this, critical evaluation is made of the major consequences of party management for party democracy, trust, ethical renewal, 'the contentious alliance' with the unions, party cohesion, party reputation and, more generally, British political life. 'The Blair supremacy', such as it was, is presented as an important example of highly motivated and focused political skills but it is also evaluated as an education in broader and longer term collateral and consequential damage.

The study ends with an epilogue where the party management of the new Leader, Brown is examined in the light of the inheritance from Blair, including the problems exacerbated before an election result that became recognised as 'the end of New Labour'. The concluding section covers the movement of the Labour Party into the deep political trouble which had to be faced after the 2010 general election. It offers a final view of the development of problems and party management under Miliband and briefly raises questions over the developing and future character of Labour Party politics.

Notes

1 Lewis Minkin, *The Labour Party Conference: a Study in the Politics of Intra-party Democracy*, Allen Lane, London, 1978 and Manchester University Press, Manchester, 1980.
2 Lewis Minkin, *The Contentious Alliance*, Edinburgh University Press, Edinburgh, 1991, particularly Part 1, Foundations, pp. 1–104.
3 Philip Gould, *The Unfinished Revolution: How the Modernisers Saved the Labour Party*, Little Brown, London, 1998.
4 Colin Crouch, 'Coping with Post-democracy', Fabian Ideas 598, Fabian Society, London, 2000.
5 David Osler, *Labour Party PLC: New Labour as a Party of Business*, Mainstream Publishing, London 2002.
6 Philip Cowley, *Revolts and Rebellions: Parliamentary Voting under Blair*, Politicos, London, 2002; and Philip Cowley, *The Rebels: How Blair Mislaid his Majority*, Politicos, London, 2005.
7 Meg Russell, *Building New Labour: the Politics of Party Organisation*, Palgrave Macmillan, Basingstoke, 2005, p. 8.
8 Thomas Quinn, *Modernising the Labour Party: Organisational Change since 1983*, Palgrave Macmillan, Basingstoke, 2004, p. 189.
9 Minkin, *Contentious Alliance*, p. 630 and p. 643, note 30.
10 BBC News Channel, 7 September 2006.

PART I

Antecedents

1

The tradition of party management and the road to destabilisation

The distinctiveness of what happened in the governance of the Labour Party under Blair can only be fully understood in relation to the heritage of the party's organisational form, its democratic culture and the traditional pattern of party management. Blair, his allies and his managers were politically born into this heritage and they drew from its character, attitudes and practices some useful lessons for the future but they also noted what they regarded as its inadequacies and unacceptable obligations. This, as will be shown, was to lead Blair into some crucially important organisational and cultural departures. The foundations of the original managerial tradition and its history are presented here as a compressed, complex but essential historical analysis, preliminary to the developments leading eventually to the Blair experience itself.

Party history, the pattern of organisation and the culture of management

The party was created in 1900 as a confederal alliance of affiliated independent organisations – mainly trade unions but also socialist societies, the Independent Labour Party, briefly the Social Democratic Federation, and then the Fabian Society. On to this was built after 1918 a unitary structure of individual membership. These different extra-parliamentary organisations were the basic units of what was, by convention, a conference-delegate democracy with multiple chains of mandated democratic representation stretching upwards to the annual party conference – recognised as the sovereign body.* From the party in parliament came the leadership of the party as whole. This had special discretion through various formulae but it was a natural extension of the principles of conference delegate democracy that the parliamentary arm of the Labour Party should have an obligation to implement party policy based on the decisions of the conference and the general election manifesto.

---

* The party conference was sometimes referred to in the party simply as 'conference'. That practice is not used here except in the quotations from party sources. Capitalisation also differs here from those used in the quotations.

The democratic process also embodied what appeared to be complete union dominance. In 1918, after a reform of the constitution which established a national system of constituency parties (CLPs), at the party conference, the unions cast 2,471,000 votes, the CLPs 115,000, and the socialist societies 48,000. The unions controlled also a majority of the seats on the NEC elected from the extra-parliamentary units. In addition, the unions, by affiliation fees and donations, provided substantial finance for the upkeep of the organisation the party. They sponsored a substantial section of Labour MPs and provided extra financial resources for the expenses of fighting general elections. All of this created the possibility that working through these democratic and financial arrangements the parliamentary leadership would be subordinate to the extra-parliamentary party, and the unions through finance and votes would be the dominant power as they imposed themselves on the parliamentary public representatives.

Party leadership

In practice, to the repetitive disappointment of sections of the local parties, the unions, and some backbench MPs, neither the formal democratic arrangements nor the appearance of trade union dominance gave anything like an accurate characterisation of Labour's internal power relations. When the party grew as an electoral force, becoming first the official opposition and then forming two short-lived minority governments in 1924 and 1929, a major change took place in the distribution of power. It became skewed towards the party's parliamentary leadership with Ramsay MacDonald instituting the role of Leader as a pre-eminent figure. This was a pattern familiar to scholars of political parties after the study by Robert Michels,[1] and, later, in the British context Robert Mackenzie.[2]

Although the spirit of intra-party democracy continued to be an element in the elections and some internal procedures within the PLP, and at times led to attempts to revive party influence, acting as the Cabinet and Shadow Cabinet the leadership were not subject to policy control from below. Working within the historic grain of parliamentary and executive-dominated government, the normality was of a hierarchical relationship with the primary responsibility of the PLP being to support the policies formulated by a leadership. Added to the pressures of electoral competition and public representation, these influences contributed to the ascendancy of the party's leading parliamentary figures.

The unions: roles, 'rules' and management relations

What was most unusual and consistently important about the cultural environment underpinning the ascendancy of the parliamentary leaders over the output of policies was a system of mainly unwritten regulation of relations with the unions. Often overlooked by observers, this system added a special element to the forces which sustained a high degree of influence by the leading politicians over the outcome of policy-making. The fundamental grounding was the mutual acceptance by the union and parliamentary leaders of different spheres and functions – the political and the industrial – each with its own roles, responsibilities and autonomy. On this basis, over time there evolved or was instituted a range of mainly unwritten 'rules' and protocols underwriting the mutuality and ethos of 'the movement' and dealing with its major potential conflicts. They were based on shared values of unity, solidarity, democracy and freedom, and a working principle of adherence to priorities; and in observance together they reinforced cohesion.

These roles 'rules' and protocols were later detailed in full in Minkin's *The Contentious Alliance*[3] and are too extensive to be fully laid down here, but the most important elements relative to party management are registered below. Although the regulation had a mutuality of restraint and protected the industrial freedom of the unions, the jealously guarded autonomy of individual unions and the independence of the Trades Union Congress – which continued to speak for all the unions regardless of party affiliation – and though the rule guaranteed political access, advance information and consultation to the unions, the most significant feature was the extent to which they restricted the unions. On the face of it union leaders with the backing of their organisations were free to use their formal position in terms of votes and finance to at least co-determine party policy and to control its political leaders in their implementation. Yet within the regulatory arrangements they were more constrained than the politicians and it was the political leadership which gained regular supportive mechanisms in party management. Since the Wertheimer analysis of 1929,[4] which puzzled over the difference between government policy and that of the TUC, this difference of role and the rule-governed union restraint have frequently confused observers as well as being subject to continuous crude misrepresentation about the behaviour of 'union barons' and 'party paymasters'.

Key to it was that within these mainly conventional arrangements, the union leaders and their representatives who formed a distinct group within the PLP and on Labour's NEC were generally understanding of the need for party management. Their own internal union experience usually involved such activities and the factional alignment of the loyalist right in the party corresponded and overlapped with that in the unions. In addition, the rules and protocols reflected highly motivating allegiance and values. In spite of recurrent tensions (see below) there was a continuous and at times an emotional sense of solidarity of the unions with the Labour Party – 'our party' – and a Labour government – 'our government' – together in 'this great movement of ours'. It was a protective loyalty that continued to operate in spite of disappointments. Protectiveness also extended to the party's organisational health, its financial stability, its developing boundaries of membership and its changing electoral needs. Solidarity led the

majority of unions to seek a supportive role acting as ballast to the parliamentary leadership in debates and votes within the various forums of
the party. A collectivist view of party democracy and freedom also reinforced the management of party discipline. There was a strong emphasis
on loyalty to majority decisions rather than furtherance of minority rights.

Union-favoured policies, as they emerged annually through their internal
processes, could cover a wide range of territory, and each union had its
own traditions and interests and a distinctive mix of policy positions, but
normally the priority policy issues were on economic-industrial concerns,
especially on union territorial areas, widened to welfare issues and exceptionally to major political issues judged as close to the immediate concerns
of the members.[5] These needs and the assertion of priority workers' interests, whether general to unions or of an individual union, could also be
pursued in terms of a justice which dovetailed into the party's social values.
They could also act as territorial shields of the industrial sphere against
interference by the politicians. Nevertheless, the most striking feature was
of a division of responsibilities whereby political initiative and detailed
policy-making on the wide policy agenda was generally understood to be
a matter for the politicians.

Leadership, the NEC and party management

The parliamentary leadership also became pre-eminent in influencing the
NEC. Though it was accountable to the conference and obliged to carry
out conference policy, the NEC had the constitutional authority to propose
to the conference amendments to the constitution and resolutions and
declarations affecting the programme, principles and policy of the party.[6]
At the annual conference it had important procedural rights and advantages
including initiating major statements of policy and making a final judgement of the acceptability of resolutions initiated within the party before a
vote was taken.[†] Through these facilities it became in effect a joint leading
policy body as well as the ruling administrative authority.

On the NEC, a majority of seats were held or controlled by the unions,
but members of the TUC General Council were prohibited from membership. These NEC members were heavily committed to a politics of what
was seen as moderation and common sense rooted in practicalities of
working-class life. Operating as the NEC trade union group, their role
definition emphasised their limited involvement in strategy and policy and
acceptance that the politicians should be 'left to get on with their job'.[7]

[†] Within the party, motions to conference were termed 'resolutions' both before
and after conference decisions because they were generally considered to be part
of a chain of decisions from the local parties or affiliated organisations. I have
continued that practice here. Resolutions on the same subject were often mixed
together and referred to as a 'composite resolution', or just 'a composite'.

There developed a crucial prohibition against the use of organisational or financial measures on the committee against deviant actions of the Labour governments or in pursuit of policy claims. 'Rules' of reciprocity governed union voting for membership of the NEC, ensuring representation by size and various other criteria. These reinforced the continuity of the NEC role and behaviour. A similar pattern governed the operation of the elected Conference Arrangements Committee (CAC), also at times known as the standing orders committee, the body formally responsible for organising the party conference. It had a loyalist majority drawn by size and tradition from the unions and was in practice very responsive to the leadership and the collective party interest.

Management intervention

Adding to the resources of loyal support, anticipating the potential for political problems and finding ways of producing outcomes that were in the party's best interest became a regular managerial activity in party forums. With the resources of party organisation and the growing authority and skills of those playing leading roles, especially the long-serving Party Secretary (later termed the General Secretary) Arthur Henderson, the extra-parliamentary party was managed in a way which was conducive to producing outcomes which the leadership considered to be in the party's best interests. By 1914 'leading performers were turning conference management into a fine art'.[8]

As the party grew in its public representation, it became a permanent priority for the senior party officials in alliance with the NEC and especially those who played leading roles, to manage procedures in various ways which dealt with the potential clash between the responsibilities and practicalities of this public representation and the conduct and outcomes of internal party democracy. This had a formal character through the powers of the NEC to initiate rule-making and lead in ensuring policy coherence. Successful party management also drew from the NEC's general supervision of a party organisation and the rules under which it operated. It drew also from the increasing authority of the leader represented on the committee and from the general prestige, expertise, charisma and communicational skills of leading figures. Management could organise support for the leader preparing the ground for his performances. In turn, backing from the leader and the NEC reinforced the authority of management.

Where sometimes the conference management arrangements failed to produce a policy outcome which suited the parliamentary leadership, the parliamentary leaders had considerable discretion in implementation. Various historic discretionary procedural formulae, including giving effect 'as far as may be practicable',[9] could on occasions legitimately be used to filter, delay or even partially reconstruct the decisions of the conference without openly flouting its authority. The PLP remained an autonomous body with its own internal rules and its own managers, and the conference could not interfere in those arrangements. Under Clause V of the constitution, a joint committee of the NEC and the Parliamentary Committee (usually read to mean the Shadow Cabinet or the Cabinet when Labour was in office) decided what items should go into the manifesto. And when it formed the government, the parliamentary leadership had a high degree of autonomy in carrying out the manifesto and in pursuit of what it defined as the national interest.

Interests, ideology and factions

Growing individual membership and activism in the CLPs was encouraged as a sign of the health of the party, and a major organisational advantage in connecting with the Labour electorate. But at the same time they, like the affiliated socialist organisations, were also thought of as a management problem. The normal assumption was that whilst the unions were practical, loyalist and dependable – strong holds of the loyalist Labour right – the CLPs and the socialist organisations were idealistic, unrealistic and unreliable – middle-class strongholds of the critical Labour left. It was a clash of stereotypes which distorted the extent of the working-class composition of the individual membership and the strength of left-wing currents amongst them. But it had enough accuracy to influence management views for many years. The unions with their clear sense of priorities and their normally right-wing moderate majority were seen as the natural safe base.

Making for particular management problems was that the left in the unions was a highly active and organised minority, and with the backing of the Communist Party was able to gather wider union support on some priority policy issues. In the period of industrial militancy leading to the General Strike of 1926, there was left-wing push for industrial action for political purposes. The left in the unions were also more sceptical of 'rules' and protocols which limited union policy influence. They held a more open view of the boundaries of party membership and were more critical of disciplinary codes. In their support for more radical socialist positions this left were often regarded by the leadership and on the right as 'vanguardist' rather than democratic, seeking not to represent the people and particularly the working class as they were but as the left hoped that they would be with their socialist consciousness raised.

Union policy-making, block votes and management

In formal terms union members made policy through elected delegates to sovereign union conferences held annually or biennially. Their mandates bound the union's executive committee, its officials and delegates to the party conference. Federated unions – the mineworkers and the textile workers – occasionally split their votes, and the Amalgamated Society of

Woodworkers did regularly. But the normality was that each union's votes were cast as blocks which did not register minority opinion. Ironically the historic origins of this block voting had been as a management coup at the 1894 TUC by Lib-Labs in an attempt to forestall the birth of a Labour Party.[10] In the party, it continued to be an important management device.

The concentration of blocks of votes amongst a small number of large unions and a concentration of power at the senior levels of those unions were arrangements which had the advantage of presenting a limited set of relationships with which to liaise in order to manage party requirements. This offered to the majority of union leaders aligned with the traditional right of the party, the assistance of party managers in the choices offered at the party conference. From this perspective, for the leadership and managers the more concentrated the block vote the better.

Within the unions, although the senior official – usually but not always the General Secretary – and the central executive committee had much greater authority and power than formal arrangements suggested, it was by no means all managed control from above. The input of the unions had a long-term impact on domestic policy development. Mandating of the union representatives, on the basis of prior organisational policy decisions, helped produce a culture of responsiveness and accountability within those organisations especially on issues of immediate priority concern to the members. But it was at times a clumsy and constricting procedure.

Tied to sometimes dated policies which bound delegates and union officials, it could constrain the dialogue. At other times it was a flexible and sensitive process that carried union leaders with movements of opinion which ran counter to that desired by the party leadership. In both cases that limited the role of party managerial influence. The politics of successful conference management was often about using the procedures to try to create choices in a way which best fitted the favourable alignment of mandates, or, if the mandates were undesirably critical or constraining, finding the choice of wording which gave sympathetic union leaders an opportunity to get off the hook and in that way help produce the desired voting outcome.

Government crisis and the union response

The solidarity role of unions in managerial support and the dominance of the loyalist majority against the left were never strong enough to overcome completely the points of substantial conflict in the unions' relationship with Labour's political leaders. The changing composition of the PLP with the rise of new professionals produced new tensions with the manual worker unions. More immediately, the need to make a broader socio-political appeal to the electorate and the pursuit of a national interest by the 1924 and 1929 Labour governments sometime brought conflict with both general and particular union claims – especially when industrial disputes were involved. Tension reached crisis point in 1931 over the attempt to cut unemployment benefit when the Labour Prime Minister MacDonald together with four other Labour Cabinet members formed a National Government with the party's opponents and was expelled.

This became a major test of the relationship and of its traditions of behaviour. The unions following the lead of Ernest Bevin who, working with Walter Citrine of the TUC and carrying arguments from the TUC research department, now moved for a period to a more assertive general supervision of Labour politics and economic policy but still playing the role with restraint. He and the unions did not attempt a new constitutional imposition of their own power over the parliamentary leadership nor did they seek to give the party conference more detailed control, or interfere with the PLP autonomy. These were considered impractical and unwise arrangements. There were, however, continuing tensions over the ILP's assertion of its autonomy and in 1932 that organisation disaffiliated. The left made some attempts to strengthen CLP representation and reform the union block vote. But these were fought off and no significant constitutional changes affected party democracy with the exception that in 1937 a rank-and-file reform movement forced the formation of a section of the NEC elected by the CLPs. The unions chose another way of managing the movement's problems. They re-launched a forum of regular dialogue between the party and the TUC, the National Joint Council (later National Council of Labour).

This built coordination of the political and industrial leaderships with close links so as to avoid major divisions over policy, yet the unions still treated the relationship with the political leadership as a partnership that protected the different roles and responsibilities. Within the party there was a renewal of the obligation by the parliamentary leadership to ensure regular consultation in opposition or in government, to refrain from compromising the party's independence and more generally not to offend the basic concerns and priorities of the Labour movement. This was integrated without a binding rule change, through a renewed leadership commitment to a majoritarian intra-party democracy expressed within conference sovereignty.

Only indirectly connected with this came new obligations on the union side. Conscious of the proprieties involved in parliamentary democracy they came to accept further constraint in the use of finance in political influence in candidate selection. The Hastings Agreement of 1933 restricted the level of union financial sponsorship and, in the *Memorandum on the Selection of Candidates*, unions were not allowed to mention finance in selections. Increasingly also in term of sponsorship there was a tendency to respect the norms of parliamentary life with regard to the rights and freedoms of members, guarded by the House authorities. All these reinforced the growing prohibition against any threat of sanctions in pursuit of union policy interests within the party.[11]

As the TUC and party leadership moved closer together by the mid-1930s they consolidated their agreement over policy after the pacifist Lansbury had resigned as Labour Leader in 1935. Increased internal management over CLPs was deepened in dealing with various movements on the left seeking unity with the Communists in the fight against fascism. They were met by new attempts to defend Labour boundaries with a conference decision in 1936 which prohibited activity with the Communists. A series of disciplinary measures included proscription of the left-wing Socialist League in 1937 and the expulsion of, amongst others, Aneurin Bevan and Stafford Cripps in 1939 over advocacy of a popular front.

The political alliance and management unity at leadership level grew stronger but at the same time, alongside union affiliation to the party, there developed further a duality of union representation which would become a central and complicating element in future union politics. The TUC had since the General Strike increasingly also sought a better relationship with employers and independent regularised access to government whichever party was in power. It played a central role in relations with the wartime coalition over national economic, industrial and social policy-making and in building new tripartite corporate relationships with subsequent governments and employers' organisations.

Party management consolidation and control

Consolidation and management

In 1945, as Samuel Beer pointed out, 'to an extent unprecedented in British political history the legislation of a Government was dictated by a party programme'.[12] The Labour government carried into office in 1945 a manifesto drafted initially by a NEC campaign committee.[13] It drew heavily from long-term policy commitments agreed by the party. It then implemented the bulk of the policies. Relations of the party and the unions with the government generally worked in accordance with the understandings reached in the early 1930s. Although there were tensions with the unions over wage regulation and wage restraint, what is striking about this period – even more so in the light of what was to follow under subsequent Labour governments – was the deep loyalty which this government evoked from the union majority. Across the party but particularly on the right there was a sense of achievement in the government's respect for the movement's priorities and that evoked a deep commitment in return. This was commensurate with support amongst the party's working class supporters and reflected in the huge rise in individual membership which had risen from 487,000 in 1945 to 629,000 in 1948. It then leaped to over a million by 1952.

Gratitude felt towards the government and a Cold War fever which reinforced factional alignment of right and left, together with a shared perception of the need for political consolidation, united the senior

ministerial figures, the leaders of the major trade unions and their representatives on the NEC. The new cohesion of the traditional right factions
of party and unions became also a consolidation of the party management
process, affecting all the major national party forums as well as the regions.
After 1948, with the exception of one minor defeat in 1950 which was
covered by discretionary formulae, not one defeat was suffered by the
leadership at the party conference until 1960. With the political leadership
operating in accordance with 'not only the moral responsibility but the
concrete responsibility of implementing Labour Party policy as determined
by Annual Conference',[14] this conference authority was integral to party
management, legitimising strong central leadership and actions against
organised dissent.

On some issues, particularly defence policy, the Labour Government had
met strong criticism from a minority on the left of the PLP. That broadened
in 1951 following the resignation from the Cabinet of Aneurin Bevan and
Harold Wilson and a minister, John Freeman, over the issue of prescription
charges. As what became known as the Bevanites, they joined with Barbara
Castle, Richard Crossman, Tom Driberg and Ian Mikardo, strengthening
the left-wing dissent in the PLP, albeit with different degrees of leftism.
The major parliamentary revolt of 57 Bevanites in March 1952 over the
defence white paper led to a fierce loyalist response and long battles over
party discipline which produced their own legacy of grievance. From the
right it was against what was regarded as disloyalty, irresponsibility and
the divisive dangers of 'a party within a party'. From the Bevanites and
the left generally, it was against unrepresentative factional control over
the parliamentary committee, authoritarian management, and what was
regarded as a danger to a vibrant energetic party.

The initial reaction from the majority of the PLP was the re-imposition
of new PLP standing orders. Voting against a three-line whip was banned
and the PLP was empowered to withdraw the whip which meant exclusion
from the PLP and, if it chose, to recommend to the NEC expulsion from
the party.[15] But the moderate centre of the PLP refused to support draco-
nian action against individual rebels. The shock of the Bevanite revolt
in the Commons was repeated over the NEC election results. In 1950, of
the seven CLP positions only three were held by the left. After the 1952
elections held at the party conference the six leading Bevanites were all
elected to the NEC accompanied by centrist Jim Griffiths. Major influential
party managerial figures from the leadership, Hugh Dalton and Herbert
Morrison, were thrown off. That and the robust left-wing temper evident
amongst the CLP delegates gave a huge lift to the Bevanites, but it greatly
alarmed the party's leaders and it produced a particularly belligerent
response from right-wing union leaders. Later that year, on the prompting
of the Shadow Cabinet the PLP voted to call for the abandonment of all
group organisations in the House other than those officially recognised.
The Bevanite group, angry at what they regarded as authoritarianism, was
forced to disband.

Saving the party and the block vote as hero

Strengthening loyal support

This set the scene for a long struggle over who should be the future Leader, years of factional conflict in one form or another, and a party management aiming to ensure, as far as possible, harmony behind the parliamentary leadership. Even though the CLP membership had shot up during the Labour government and reached over a million in 1952, the unions' five million votes were still preponderant and the concentration of these votes into the hands of a small number of large unions made the management of the conference heavily focused on links with a small group of leaders of the General and Municipal Workers Union (GMWU and later known as the GMB), the National Union of Mineworkers (NUM) and the Transport and General Workers Union (TGWU). In 1953 the mechanism for casting votes at the conference whereby a union leader held up a card to be counted, was changed to ballot boxes which made the card votes more secret. A system of multiple voting cards supplied for the whole delegation reinforced the sense of collective representation by making it impracticable for a union to claim separate cards for individual delegates.

In the PLP, at the core of the loyal support were the sponsored MPs from the major manual-worker trade unions. Their class collectivism and concern for group unity and loyalty could always be drawn upon in defence of the leadership. In 1954 the collective organisation of sponsored trade unionists known as the PLP trade union group of MPs, which had declined following the more integrated role of the TUC within Government advisory and consultative arrangements, was suddenly revived at the instigation of the TUC. To some extent this was a move to protect the principle of free collective bargaining from both unofficial movements and the politicians, but the covert agenda was the use of the group to protect the political leadership against Bevan and the Left.[16]

On the NEC, where it was still the case that the right was in the overwhelming majority, there developed a bitterly charged atmosphere stoked also from the outside by union leaders. The majority on the committee, including the organised unity of the NEC trade union group, were as always generally supportive of the party management and of disciplinary efforts to secure party unity behind the leadership. They saw their role as essential for party stability and leadership effectiveness. Through NEC seniority, union representatives often became chairs of committees and played managerial roles working closely with senior politicians and the party's officials. This coalition based on a common political outlook and immediate priorities also shared a core culture of procedural values in upholding and administrating the rules and protecting the discipline of the party behind majority decisions.

In their administrative role, it was integral to their self-image and sense of propriety that party officials considered themselves party civil servants. In that role differentiating the official roles from any formal factional alignment was deemed essential to the party's integrity and healthy functioning. But they were also election campaigners seeking to maximise unity and energy and defend the party's borders. They understood the problematic judgements necessary to the role of leadership and the importance of having supportive allies. As conference managers they were covertly part of a network of communication which responded to the needs of the political leadership whilst working through the CAC under a coordinating theme of seeking 'a good conference'.[17] In all this the officials shared a political outlook with a majority on the NEC which in Shaw's summation of this period 'used its powers to promote the factional cause of the dominant right'.[18]

Reinforcing this perspective was a unity on the historic 'problem of the left'. Whilst recognising the existence of a loyalist left they saw themselves in the great chain of those who had fought to protect the party and Labour governments against damaging left-wing activities. In this they drew on the history and folklore of ILP activity in the Commons, acting as 'a party within a party' faction during the 1929–31 Labour government. Now, in the Cold War period, with factionalism again the target, it was the Bevanites through Tribune Brains Trusts and later, Victory for Socialism, whose activity was seen as drawing out public concern about disunity.

The small but hugely energetic Trotskyist groups, who had entered or operated within the Labour Party, were particularly viewed as an alien and duplicitous covert threat to the organisational and ideological integrity of the party. In campaigns and in the union factional battles the left often acted with a degree of unity, whilst in response party officials, senior politicians and leading trade union figures bracketed the left collectively in terms of dealing with the party management problem of those who were anti-leadership. Bevanites, together with Communists in the unions and Trotskyists in the party were often seen as part of the same problem. In those battles saving the party became a *raison d'être* for the existence of the factional right and also of the party officials working with them.

However, there continued to be less than complete unity on disciplinary actions. Leadership and managerial initiative, at any one time, was conditional on a calculation of the likely degree of opposition and also adverse political costs entailed for the party. If it appeared as clumsy overreaction and an offensive initiative, it might further stoke trouble exacerbating disunity and provoke further sympathetic unrest. As had happened in the PLP, mediated by the moderate centre and centre right, this consideration carried into managing behaviour an element of restraint and constraint on the NEC. On 18 February 1953, Tribune Brains Trusts were subject to what appeared to be a ban. Then in the face of criticism from the centre right as well as the left, this was reinterpreted as 'not a ban' by the General Secretary.[19] An article in *Tribune* on 22 October 1954 critical of the TGWU leader Arthur Deakin was condemned by the NEC and was followed by hints of expulsion. In the face of a widely critical response, the NEC was forced to withdraw. An attempt to expel Aneurin Bevan, on 23 March 1955, failed by one vote after Clement Attlee had advocated that the matter be passed to a sub-committee interview.

In 1955, in a further move to strengthen the leadership against the Bevanites, there was a sudden retroactive raising of affiliation by the Transport and General Workers and the General and Municipal Workers unions, giving an extra 350,000 conference votes to the loyalist cause. The big three now cast 2,328,000 votes out of a total union vote of 5,606,000 and a total conference vote of 6,500,000. If the union block vote was, for the critical left, a tyranny, for the loyalist right it now became even more synonymous with the loyalty of moderate, sensible union leaders working together to defend the priorities of working people. Media criticism of the union role at this time was low-key or non-existent. With this supportive base, procedural management at the conference was also based on rule interpretation, agenda devices and constructed choices, which facilitated situations which were likely to produce the desired outcomes.[20]

Although there was a subordinate but not insignificant cross-pressure of internal considerations and pressures from within the dominant coalition, overall, at the conference as on the NEC, on major issues support was normally assured. Future leaders would look back at the supportive fortress of this period and its backing for party management with some wistfulness – although without enjoyment of any union industrial policy influence that limited the operation of the politicians in that area. Policy statements by the NEC provided the most authoritative output of the conference and (with the exception of a carefully supervised experiment in 1953) these were not subject to amendments by the delegates. The loyalist majority in the unions was also accompanied by a large if sometimes minority vote from the CLPs.

In difficult circumstances, last-minute persuasion by skilled managers could produce victory out of certain defeat – the vote on German rearmament in 1954 was a result of a mysterious sudden lunch-time conversion of the woodworkers' union to support for the leadership, in spite of its mandate. Through procedural controls and the skills of their use in liaison with the loyalists, union leaders could obscure union mandates. This was marked following the election of Gaitskell as a revisionist Leader in 1955 by many devices of management used in securing long-term changes in public ownership policy.[21] Nevertheless, in 1959/60, his open attempt to change the socialist Clause IV of the party's constitution met deep resistance and effectively had to be sidelined.

The managerial framework and the rules

Party management was only one of a wide range of tasks of party officials and of senior NEC members. These tasks, most of them consensual and essential for the party, gained legitimacy, trust and confidence within the party which carried over into the authority which was sometimes an asset in party management activities. Management was also assisted by deep reserves of traditional working-class loyalty in the CLPs as well as the unions – with its deference to 'our leaders' and 'our party officials'. The rulebook, within which was the constitution of the party, had been subject only to a moderate conservative adjustment over time. Strict obedience to its rules as interpreted by the NEC and party officials was assisted by that longevity and a reverence shown towards it as a symbol of the party's history and identity. Together with the pervasive codes of conventional 'rules' and protocols, the reverence for the rulebook reinforced a general respect for rule-governed obedience. It was also a primary means by which the party defended itself against fragmentation and disruption. Reinforcing central authority in this management were also a range of constitutional powers. Authority was further built up by huge and repetitive majorities registered at the conference over the years behind rule changes proposed by the party officials and the leadership.

Candidate selection

One important, and sometimes controversial, area of management was concerned with candidate selection. A major feature here was the alliance at regional level which followed the historic development of the party in linking the trade unions to the formation of the party at that level. Close relations of unions and party officials that included regular attendance at regional and national party meetings, a commitment to 'the movement', a shared perspective in defence of the leadership and affinity with the factional right provided the basis for common working understandings and joint action. The localised strength of trade unions and the operation of candidate selection from meetings of the General Management Committee of the CLPs, later known as the General Committee (GC) which included groups of union delegates, also made it easier for the regional party machine and the regional union leadership to manage outcomes in concert.

Although local constituency parties had a numerous and vocal membership on the left, the linkage of regional union and party officials also connected to the local right of the parties who were particularly strong in safe Labour seats. They could act as allies in support of recommended candidates, and in defence of loyal MPs occasionally threatened with de-selection. If that failed the national centre could and did declare it improper to de-select on grounds of policy disagreements with the MPs views in the PLP.[22]

Although as Shaw found in his illuminating study, discreet communication did express some unobtrusive individual preferences, the close working relations with the regional unions made direct central control less necessary in influencing selections.[23] The colonisation of particular seats by individual unions were amongst the features which limited that control.

The centre was in Shaw's words 'inevitably restrained' not only by the this 'jealous defence of trade union prerogatives' but by such things as 'the scarcity of organisational resources, the reliance on voluntary electoral labour in single member constituencies and the strength of particularistic sentiment in the provinces' resenting London interference.[24] Central party management had to operate within the practical limitations of the party's finances and an organisation described by Wilson in a report in 1955 as at 'the penny-farthing stage'. There was not at this stage even a central management list of party members. At local level, as well as at the centre a calculation had to be made about reaction and future reputation. There were always the constraints and inhibitions of pressures to legitimate the system and avoid creating major public rows in the party. Ideally, wide respect for the role of officials and for the rulebook had to be sustained.

Nevertheless, regional staff like national officials tried to operate a restrained 'political' role. Organisers provided advice to would-be candidates and networked over their own judgements in giving guidance on suitability for short-listing. Shaw notes that acting as custodian of the rules afforded 'a certain latitude' in interpreting and applying rules in ways that could advance the organisers' goals.[25] Research revealed that in candidate selection regional organisers 'varied in both their willingness and their ability to engage in . . . procedural management' in connection with candidate selection.[26]

Austen Ranney cites the view of a leading regional official, Jim Cattermole, regarding any organiser who did not keep anti-leadership candidates off short lists as 'not doing the job properly'.[27] That contrasts with the view of senior party officials that in candidate selection the accusations from the left of deliberate exclusion against them were greatly overstated.[28] In connection with the B List of parliamentary candidates, which became in 1959 the Approved List, Shaw's research found that though there appeared to be evidence of political vetting, the numbers of those rejected or deferred was small.[29] For the Approved List, most of those rejected were again from the left but most left-wingers and supporters of the Campaign for Nuclear Disarmament were accepted.[30] In exercising the NEC's power of non-endorsement a similar pattern emerges. There were exclusions of only a small number on the left on grounds of their beliefs, especially those with what was alleged to be Trotskyist associations.[31]

The role of officials, the legitimacy of factionalism and the attempt at central management using 'the machine' was tested from another angle after the formation of the Gaitskell-supporting Campaign for Democratic Socialism (CDS) in April 1960. It fought for various policy objectives against the left and then tried to ensure the success of Gaitskellite candidates in selections. Sympathetic regional organisers led by Jim Cattermole were also involved; the National Organiser Sara Barker was reported by Patrick

Seyd, drawing from CDS documentation, as having strong reservations about CDS and had to be persuaded by Gaitskell not to raise the issue at the NEC.[32] Regular meetings over candidate selection at which the Leader and the CDS secretary W. T. Rodgers were present, but not Sara Barker, were organised not from party headquarters but usually from the office of Chief Whip.[33]

Given action taken regularly against factional group activity on the left and the differentiation of party officials from factions, Barker's view was not surprising. Taking the behaviour of CDS to the NEC would have strengthened the representation of officials as civil servants of the party whilst close association with CDS threatened their legitimacy. It says something about the cross pressures involved that only seven of twelve regional organisers were specified by Seyd as taking part and even that figure was later judged by Reg Underhill as an exaggeration.[34] Examining this managerial episode, Patterson judged from candidates selected that it was the left that was largely successful.[35]

It was later confirmed by national officials of this period that there were central political filters determining who had the right attitudes to be allowed to advance as party officials through the party machine. Yet these were not politically rigid or effective enough to fully prevent the emergence of a more liberal element. In 1967 in Yorkshire, Joyce Gould, then on the centre left, found Assistant National Agent Sara Barker blocking her promotion because of her politics.[36] Barker was unsuccessful and Gould eventually became an Assistant National Agent, then Director of Organisation under a new regime. The Southern Regional Organiser, Ron Hayward, was agreed to be a very capable and job-focused regional official although having some leftist views. In 1969 he became an innovative National Agent and a significant figure in a new regime.

Destabilization

Significance

This traditional model of party management based on the dominant right-wing-led unions provided a regular firm base and culture supporting the leadership and its attempts at discipline and control. So much so, that it was generally regarded as endemic and unshakeable except perhaps in partial and very brief spasms. Even as late as 1967 it was being diagnosed by a leading industrial correspondent and author that, 'The Party's organisational and administrative machine is irrevocably under the control of the right and centre'.[37] What happened and why after this seemingly irrevocable structure went into crisis was viewed years later by 'New Labour' as a warning of what to avoid. There was no one simple cause. New vulnerabilities and sources of change of different kinds began to appear in the 1960s and their complex interconnection over time within and between institutions, including some important delayed reactions and fortuitous accompanying shifts, produced a crucial historical rupture. It was to lead to a weakened and then fragmented management, a huge long-term internal revolt and a new pattern of power by 1979.

Change in the TGWU

Given the diverse sources and the long period of development, the analysis of those crucial and complex interactive developments could begin in different places. The most obvious and important new feature to which attention will be paid below was in the mid-1960s, relating the electoral strategy of the Leader to the implications for, and response of, the unions. But it could be said to start earlier with the change in the hitherto rock-solid TGWU leadership as far back as 1956. This followed the replacement of the retiring General Secretary Arthur Deakin very briefly by Jock Tiffin who died, and then unexpectedly a left-wing General Secretary, Frank Cousins. His election involved recognition of his personal ability but was also in the eyes of a body of union opinion a reaction to the pull from Deakin's party role too far to the right. That had been internally divisive and diminished the union's industrial role.[38] However, with Cousins constrained by union mandates, customs and personnel inherited from Deakin, the change did not have immediate consequences for party conference voting and its management.[39] For the moment a new unity was marked amongst the political leaders bringing in the ex-Bevanites. Bevan, shortly before his death in 1960, in a new move towards intra-party liberalism, secured in 1959 a suspension of the PLP standing orders.

However, another Labour election defeat in 1959 was followed by a more assertive revisionism by Gaitskell, and the TGWU was part of the opposition when the Leader was forced to retreat over changing Clause IV. With Cousins to the fore Gaitskell was defeated over unilateral nuclear disarmament in 1960. The TGWU clearly had now changed its past role in what was considered by a respected historical authority, Allan Flanders, to be a violation of the conventional 'rules' of the relationship.[40] Gaitskell's rejection of conference authority over its decision on nuclear weapons was then a break with the conventional understandings reached after 1931. Together they introduced a new uncertainty about the 'rules' of the union-party relationship, and Gaitskell's action had reduced the long-term effectiveness of the conference as an instrument of collective discipline and party management.

In the short term, with concessionary qualifications, the unilateralist defence policy was reversed the following year in a move supported strongly by an alliance of major union leaders. That produced the basis for a more powerful leadership working with a new loyalist block vote of the right. That leadership was able to exert a more aggressive disciplinarian party management in the face of deviant PLP voting involving five MPs, amongst them Michael Foot. They had the whip withdrawn and in December 1961 there was a reimposition of the standing orders. The old regime appeared to have been replenished but the TGWU role had become unstable as an instrument of leadership support.

Expulsion of the veterans

Meanwhile, linked to this reinvigorated disciplinarian politics, in another area of the party, a second early turning point had occurred in relation to management change. In the eyes of the managers the character of their activities on behalf of the party since 1918 had been specially legitimised by repetitive substantial conference majorities on proposed rule changes proposed by the leadership. Now in 1962, came the cause célèbre to which Shaw draws attention.[41] This was an attempt to expel four veteran Labour Party members, including the eminent philosopher Bertrand Russell, and a leading social scientist, Barbara Wooton, plus Canon Collins and Lord Chorley. George Brown, chair of the Organisation sub-committee and new 'overlord' of headquarters, backed by newly promoted National Agent Sara Barker, moved to use the list of proscribed organisations in relation to the four members accepting an invitation to a peace conference in Moscow. It appeared to them to be a routine management activity in relation to Communist front activity. Yet these were widely respected and very independent-minded veteran Labour members. Expulsion was challenged by Wooton on the grounds that it applied only to membership of organisations; there was no legal basis for using the proscribed list for this purpose.[42]

According to Gaitskell's official biographer Philip Williams, the Leader was opposed to their expulsion.[43] All the more surprising then was that, after a brief retreat in the face of Wooton's challenge, a rule change was prepared – an 'associated with' clause – by which Brown and Barker attempted to provide new grounds.[44] It was supported on the NEC by 17 votes to 8.[45] But outside, a wide range of hostile opinion in the party including respected figures on the Labour right, moved against what was seen as a development with McCarthyite connotations. But the moderate right could not exercise the usual background restraint, leaving Brown to drive himself into a corner.

The case he made at the conference was described by journalist and author Geoffrey Goodman as 'sheepish and self-conscious'[46] and the supportive contribution of MP Charles Pannell was described in *Tribune* as 'met by loud laughter'.[47] Philip Williams in an abbreviated account refers to the proponents as 'retreating amid ridicule'.[48] In an unprecedented response to an NEC rule proposal – especially significant over a party management issue – the proposal was referred back in a private session by 3,497,000 votes to 2,793,000. The loyalist block vote split and it was estimated that as many as 95 to 98 per cent of the CLPs voted against.[49] The scale of that helped to discredit the device of proscription,[50] and it raised a more general problem for the legitimacy of hard-line management. The full significance of all this was heightened by what followed. Most of the ex-Bevanites, particularly Crossman, had been fierce critics of the whole episode.[51] Within a few months, Gaitskell had died suddenly, Brown was rejected in the contest that followed, and, in 1963, Harold Wilson, from a tradition with more liberal attitudes towards management, became the Leader.

New leadership, new forces and party modernisation

New personnel

There was much continuity to Wilson's strategic leadership. He resumed Gaitskell's electoral search for a new social coalition in recognition of the decline of the manual working class. In 1962, under Gaitskell, the party's rules on party decision-making had been changed so that only Labour Party individual members could be union delegates to the party conference. Under Wilson in 1965 this was extended to union delegates attending constituency party meetings – a move that had some weakening effect on the union role in candidate selections. There was also a repetition of strong management control at the party conferences before and after the 1964 General Election victory in which Labour gained a very narrow majority. The factional alignment of the TGWU leadership was temporarily neutralised by bringing Cousins into the Labour Government as a minister.

Wilson also established that he favoured a clearer separation of party and government roles – an old Bevanite position. The party could not instruct the government and he would not interfere in internal party matters issues – that was a responsibility of the NEC. At this stage it was still firmly controlled by the loyalist right generally supportive of the old management system. Yet his hands-off stance was itself a signal of change in approach to party management and, in a significant indicator of a new NEC openness to change, in 1966 a critique of the Approved List of candidates by Mikardo as a procedure 'shallow and time consuming' was accepted by the NEC. It reverted to being simply a list of available candidates.[52]

With a second general election victory secured in 1966, Wilson participated in some longer-term initiatives of major importance through the appointment of Richard Crossman. An old Bevanite ally of Wilson and a long-time member of the NEC, he was a known critic of oligarchic control. He was also a believer that too much power was dangerously concentrated in the hands of the Prime Minister.[53] From that view of what he saw as the modernisation of the party, it may be doubted how much of Crossman's approach to party reform had Wilson's full – as opposed to temporarily expedient – support.[54] Nevertheless, Wilson made Crossman President of the Council in the government and then also gave him the position of chairing a liaison committee to prevent the party becoming estranged from the government. From these positions, Crossman's initiatives over party management provided a framework which years later still had a resonance in the arguments about party management under Blair.

In Crossman's view, as he had described it to the NEC as early as June 1963, of central importance to the modern party was an emphasis on 'the confidence, morale and democratic nature of the Party' and the importance of political education for trained cadres of party workers.[55] He thought it integral to social democracy that people should be given a chance to decide for themselves, and that precept included the party.[56] In the lead up to the 1966 conference, he gained Wilson's approval for the party to develop an independent long-term policy role for the next election manifesto.[57]

At this time also, Wilson asked Crossman to join with the Chief Whip John Silkin to work for parliamentary reform and to make sure that the rank and file felt linked to the leadership.[58] Party management in the Commons was already being undermined by changing attitudes towards dissent and reform. Manual-working-class representatives, with their traditional collectivist attitudes of solidarity and loyalty, were being replaced by higher-education professionals who were more prepared to defend the individual rights of MPs. The traditionally loyalist PLP trade union group had diminished in importance with its functions replaced in part by more direct links to the Labour Government.[59]

Crossman and Silkin recognised this change as bringing with it a robust assertiveness which would not necessarily be confined to the left. A new liberal interpretation of the PLP standing orders was introduced in which organised group activity was allowed. Wilson also saw the significance of the compositional changes and the dangers of a crude authoritarian reaction.[60] Although his own reaction to dissent became verbally more intemperate, as Shaw pointed out, Wilson whenever he had to choose took the liberal side in internal PLP battles. Although a new and slightly more hard-line code of conduct was re-introduced in the PLP in 1968, and in April 1969 Silkin was replaced by Bob Mellish, a man regarded as a tough disciplinarian, in spite of major revolts, in great measure, the liberal regime survived.

It did not help in overcoming dissent and division that the Leader had become, as Crossman described it, 'de-partyd' in his focus.[61] Wilson's policies and, at times, his style of governing, estranged the party from the government on some major policies, including those closest to the interests of loyal trade unionists. In the face of adverse conference decisions from 1966, he had enunciated the doctrine of 'the Government must govern' to defend its absolute independence. But the government could not govern without support of the PLP and lacking an assured majoritarian base at an authoritative party conference, imposing PLP discipline was very difficult. An attempt at heavy sanctions made splitting the party more likely.[62]

Meanwhile, a *Manifesto Plan for an Efficient Party* had been launched in 1965 by four editors of Labour journals. The instigator was Jim Northcott, ex-Chairman of the Transport House Staff Council. The Plan's informed strictures contributed to further undermining the authority of the old managing regime, adding to the growing criticism of its illiberalism, a castigation of conservatism in the face of decline. In the next decade, new attitudes towards management were fed also by changes in the social composition of the membership which involved an infusion of young higher-educated professionals who had a less deferential approach to those in power and reacted against old methods of managerial control. Crossman's role in the PLP with its determined shift to liberalism as a sign of modernisation became a leading force encouraging other reforming forces unleashed after the 1966 election. Pressure for an inquiry into party organisation pushed by Crossman, by Tony Benn (then a modernising centrist on the NEC) and by Ian Mikardo, met great resistance from the senior officials and NEC allies.[63] The inquiry was authorised in 1966 with Crossman as a member although not its Chairman. His proposal for a reinforced political General Secretary as a second focus of power in the party added to the push for more pluralism and was accepted in the report although it was never fully acted upon.

In a move pushed for by his own constituency party but also consistent with his view of the need for the NEC to be less subject to ministerial domination,[64] Crossman announced that he would not be standing for election to the NEC in 1967. His absence may have weakened the party's role in the making of the 1970 manifesto but in any case his influence was limited in reshaping the party's role via the NEC by his past clumsy criticism of the abilities of trade-union-sponsored MPs. As it happened also it would have faced a major problem with his leadership colleagues. Cabinet discussions on the manifesto left Crossman and Crosland in a minority looking for more radical egalitarian policies.[65]

Nevertheless, in 1967, with Callaghan elected to the post of treasurer, this left room on the NEC for two new CLP representatives. Frank Allaun and Joan Lester represented the defence of public expenditure against cuts but also the defence of intra-party democracy particularly in the active role of Allaun. Thus began the long shift to the left on the NEC and the strengthening of the reassertion of conference authority. At that 1967 conference some of the fringe discussion focused on the clear signs of a new left leadership coming to power in the unions. On the NEC as well as in the party machine, this unprecedented development in the unions was seen as heralding a new order and that fed into an anticipation of management change further encouraging some in the machine to adjust their own attitudes.

The retirement of two long-serving officials – Len Williams as General Secretary in 1968, and Sara Barker as National Agent in 1969 – might have been followed by a Leader's nominee and another traditional party official in those positions, but pressed by the unions a unifying official of the TGWU, Harry Nicholas, became General Secretary. More significant, an innovative regional official Ron Hayward became the new National Agent and then General Secretary in 1972. In his interview for the National Agent's post Hayward had made clear that he would be a new organisational broom and a carrier of more liberal perspective on party management. His appointment by a still right-wing-dominated NEC in a contest with an official associated with older attitudes, was another indication of a new receptivity to change.[66]

Hayward believed, with Crossman, that 'too rigid an insistence on imposing rules, too obtrusive a presence, inflamed feelings and sharpened differences'.[67] He also emphasised the neutrality of the party machine – servants of the party, independent of the leadership and of faction. This move to affirm the civil-servant role was followed by a liberalisation of the party machine. It included the abolition of the list of proscribed organisations. As Shaw has shown, the old management was also falling foul of a more interventionist judiciary over issues of natural justice.[68] The NEC here responded to the judgement of Reg Underhill, a respected moderate who had become the new National Agent in 1972, that the proscribed organisations measure was 'unnecessary, impracticable and even counterproductive'.[69]

Attacks on the managing regime as 'out-of-date' fitted a political era when liberalism and critics of old power structures were widely on the offensive. New attitudes developing on the NEC meant that in by-elections as well as other candidate selections the NEC would now only intervene if there were an irregularity in the procedures and the same applied to an MP threatened with de-selection. Political protection was ended and partisan political interventions at regional level were increasingly disapproved of. Not even the most staunch PLP loyalists were guaranteed assistance from the managers in the event of a threat of de-selection.[70]

Labour modernisation and problems with the unions

Meanwhile, major changes in the union leadership had taken effect at the party conference, contributing visibly to the sense of a new order. Frank Cousins had resigned from the Government in July 1966 – a critic of its union-related policies but also crucially a man who had lost trust in the word of the Prime Minister.[71] Cousins was determined to see Jack Jones from the left as his successor in the TGWU. The election of a new left-wing leader Hugh Scanlon as President of the AEEU in 1968 coincided with the passage of the leadership of the TGWU to Jones and the election of other left-wing union leaders in the NUM and (briefly) the shopworkers' union, USDAW. The end of what was called 'Carron's Law', autocratic support for the party leadership from the AEEU leader, in the context of a change in the dominant issues, added to a new configuration of power on the floor of the 1968 party conference. That year there were an unprecedented five defeats for the platform. The change also slowly produced new patterns of union voting for the NEC increasing the strength of the left. These new union leaders gave general support to the growing re-assertion of intra-party democracy and conference authority helping unleash forces which would burst to the fore after they had departed.

It was not unusual for a Labour government to have major disagreements with the unions, but now unifying links between the government and the unions were also harmed by the increasing loss of social affinity between the two leadership groups and the lack of the kind of close and trusting personal relationships which had held it together in the past. The conflicts were exacerbated by Wilson's version of a modernising electoral strategy. This emphasised that it was 'a people's party' aiming to maximise new support amongst the middle class and attempting to distance itself from the manual-worker cloth-cap image carried by the trade unions. The Leader sought to capture and retain the centre ground of British politics making Labour, not the Conservatives, the natural party of government. It became more pragmatic and less ideological the longer it was in office. Wilson appeared at times to be making a positive virtue of its willingness to court unpopularity with the traditional labour movement as the government also became unpopular with the electorate.

That had increasing managerial consequences in the PLP. From 1966 to 1970 the values of the manual-worker trade unionists in the House were cross-pressured by government policy towards the unions and the electoral strategy of which it was a part. Rigid discipline was not compatible with the extent of PLP antipathy to the Government's industrial relations policies. In the White Paper, *In Place of Strife*, the Government sought to regulate collective bargaining and penalise offending unions and unionists. The proposal had to be withdrawn under pressure from the NEC and the PLP. This was to be remembered by future Labour leaders as a retreat which they must never replicate because it damaged them electorally. Yet this was a cultivated myth.

There was no evidence that that episode damaged the party at the 1970 General Election.[72] In contrast, the electoral strategy and the decline of intra-party democracy had discernible political costs. There was a decline in manual-worker support for the Labour Party – the beginning of what became known as class de-alignment – and there was evidence of a marked decline in local union affiliation. At the same time there was a haemorrhage of party members and a huge decline in party activism.[73] In the light of later research on the influence of constituency campaigning in elections, and the potential importance of word-of-mouth communication, we may judge that that decline limited the effect of Labour's campaign organisation in a way that did significant damage.

Democratic party management and reform: alternative approaches
After 1970, the mood of British politics changed in ways unanticipated by Labour's leadership. There was new industrial militancy amongst the miners, the dockers, and the engineers, which gained wide Labour-movement support. At the same time there was a realisation that party membership and activity and its trade union support had been damaged by the leadership's policy priorities and tactics. This, and the attempt to seek unity against

a new right-wing Conservative Government under Edward Heath, which had brought in a legal framework for industrial relations, produced a move for closer union-party relations. In the PLP the trade union group was once again revived but working closely with the front bench in defence of the trade unions and collectivism with a new interest in rebuilding the party's electoral support from its traditional base. In this atmosphere, there was now more contrition by MPs and receptivity also to a party conference that moved to the left with a resurgence of support for targeted public ownership.

Two radical approaches now emerged seeking to manage relations with the leadership. In 1970 a composite resolution deploring the refusal of the Parliamentary Labour Party to act on party conference decisions was, led by Allaun on the NEC, forced onto the agenda and supported by the conference card vote.[74] In 1973 a new rank-and-file organisation, the Campaign for Labour Party Democracy (CLPD), took off with proposals for mandatory re-selection of MPs and then, later, election of the Leader by the whole of the party. Although CLPD did not talk in such terms, the party would be managed through its extra-parliamentary institutions controlling the leadership and attuned to the pressures unleashed from below.

Second, following this, in a move that challenged a crude view of union power within the Labour Party, there was an attempt from the unions to change the relationship with the PLP leadership in a more consensual way. Although Jones and Scanlon both gave their support to the re-establishment of intra-party democracy and the authority of the party conference, they did not support changing the mode of election of the Leader. As a priority, Jack Jones (following the precedent after the disaster of 1931) sought in 1971, the relaunching of machinery of coordination with the PLP leadership. This would in effect be management through a partnership. A tripartite Liaison Committee was set up in 1972 to link the PLP, the NEC and the TUC. Alongside the formal procedure was a new trusting, working linkage of Jones, Michael Foot the Shadow Minister of Labour and Harold Wilson. This did much to repair the damage done to the relationship. The committee became the major policy forum dealing with the detail of Conservative industrial-relations policy, binding the parliamentary leadership to a clear repeal commitment. This was honoured in government after they had jointly agreed the outlines of what became the general election manifesto of February 1974.

Contrasting forces and the complications of management breakdown

Labour regained office at that election, carried on during a national miners' strike in confrontation with the Heath Conservative Government. The Labour victory in this 'who rules?' election in February, and in a second election in October, reinforced (for the moment) a turn-around in attitudes towards the importance of the electoral role of the trade unions. The Liaison Committee and the axis of cooperation that bound Jones, Foot and Wilson, continued in government with Foot as Secretary of State for Employment, then after 1976 as Deputy Leader. The cooperation was consolidated and paralleled by similar links between Len Murray at the TUC with Dennis Healey, Chancellor of the Exchequer, and Jim Callaghan, Prime Minister after Wilson resigned in 1976. The abolition of the Industrial Relations Act, the delivery of a range of new industrial rights, protection for the low-paid, job-creation measures and the strengthening or creation of tripartite institutions were amongst measures which reinforced the unity and, in the early years, a sense of achievement.

Relations between the government, the party and the unions now became extraordinarily complex. Some in the right-wing press portrayed this relationship as the unions and the TUC 'running the country', led by 'Jack Jones – Prime Minister'. It was an image which did some electoral damage, even though Jones could not achieve implementation of the measures of industrial democracy and wealth tax he had assiduously pushed. And despite the image, in 1975, it was Jones who led a rescue of the Labour government supporting – against a lifetime of arguing for free collective bargaining – a tight policy of voluntary wage restraint which in various forms lasted for the life of the government. That solidarity continued through the strict economic measures adopted in response to a 1976 IMF loan. As Callaghan noted, 'The Government received more support and understanding from the trade unions at this period than it did from some National Executive members'.[75]

Direct relations with the NEC had a different dynamic as a product of the difference between political leftism and trade unionism. Aided by movements to the left in the voting of unions and CLPs since 1967 and some fortuitous factors, including the chance effect of some of the 'rules' of union representation, including 'Buggins' turn', reciprocal arrangements, representation by size and traditional occupancy, and the new representation of Labour Youth and of Labour Clubs, there was a slow long-term adjustment in the political composition of the NEC resulting in a left-wing majority by 1975. After this, for the first time in the party's history, a Labour government faced an NEC which was controlled by the left and, crucially, also led by a dissident member of the Cabinet – Tony Benn.

But all was not as might be read from that advance. Although this NEC left-wing majority was kept in power by the conference votes of the unions, relations between the NEC left and the union leaders on the Liaison Committee deteriorated over government policies. The unions disliked the tone and scale of NEC opposition to the government and gave more priority than the NEC left to showing solidarity. NEC representatives gave much more priority to pressure from the conference and the wider party. At the conference, with unions as well as CLPs responding to their mandates, the

NEC was pressurised by 15 defeats in 1975 and 1976. Yet on the government's economic and incomes policies, statements by the tripartite Liaison Committee supported by union representatives were used as management devices to gain conference support until 1978.

Dissent and management in the PLP

Although dissenting votes by Labour backbenchers grew each session[76] and most of the 23 defeats for the Government came from Labour MPs joining the opposition lobby[77] only six were attributable to the Tribune Group left.[78] Here was the extraordinary range of dissent anticipated by Crossman. At the same time the composition of the PLP Liaison Committee moved back to the right after 1975 but without that change leading to a renewal of sanctions from the old disciplinary code, because there was no obvious solution which did not make the disciplinary situation worse. The inter-party and intra-party parliamentary battle became fierce as the Labour whips' office sought to keep the Conservatives out of office. Walter Harrison, his Deputy Chief Whip, became renowned for his committed role and dragooning methods.

Nevertheless, Norton points to the successful operation of the government whips and business managers not through their disciplinary powers but their powers of persuasion and organisation.[79] Callaghan was concerned to establish better relations with the PLP through its departmental committees, although this had varying results (see Chapter 13, p. 47). The Deputy Leader Foot became a bulwark of stability for the government, holding together with conviction the traditional alliance with the unions, appealing for loyalty to save the government but remaining a committed defender of the rights of MPs.[80]

Another important feature of the politics was that at the same time as the NEC and the party at Head Office were shifting to the left and consolidating the new liberalisation of the extra-parliamentary party, a different perspective was beginning to affect the politics of the PLP. Resentment grew amongst loyalists in the PLP because the NEC no longer extended political protection in the de-selection of loyalists and they feared both the constitutional extension of that procedure and the taking away of their sole right to elect the Leader and Deputy Leader. These potent fears led to new support for one-member-one-vote procedures in selections and elections as a means of outflanking the left-wing activists, and it led some to see a black future for the party. There was a sense of being at bay in the face of what appeared to them to be growing party hostility to parliamentarians, combined now with a subversion of party staff.

The left and party staff

The rise of the left on the NEC had led to a new politicisation of party staff who had in the past been dominated by the culture of the traditional right. Sometimes the calls from the staff left for organisational reforms were well ahead of the NEC. Meanwhile, within the regional party machinery and the National Union of Labour Organisers – the party officials' union – there was another current on the right who believed that the wrong people were in control of the NEC, politicising administrative decisions and making their job harder.[81] They were accused of facilitating the development of the influence of the Militant Tendency – a front for the Trotskyist group, the Revolutionary Socialist League, operating together with the new militant higher-educated radicals, often working in the public sector who took up the cause of intra-party democracy.

The issue was taken up vociferously in the mass media after the de-selection of the minister Reg Prentice in 1975. After the NEC had agreed that the National Agent Reg Underhill should prepare a report, it emerged as *Entryist Activities* with information drawn from a Militant internal document on its separate organisation, tactics and objectives. As its contents became known, most of the party's regional organising staff, and some of the national officials, wanted the NEC to take action against the organisation.

The NEC left, on the other hand, thought of the party as a broad church that did not take formal disciplinary measures to penalise people for what they believed. They were resistant to what was seen as a politically motivated attack from the right and there were also residual doubts about the intolerance of sections of the party organisation, given the folklore of the Sara Barker years. It made them discount for some time the truth of, and danger from, Militant's secret organisation. The issue burst into the public domain in 1976 after Militant supporter Andy Bevan was appointed as National Youth Officer. This was by a two to one majority (consisting of a right-wing NEC member and the General Secretary[82]) on the 3-person appointing committee. This decision was confirmed by the NEC by 15 votes to 12.[83] The left united against what they saw as a witch hunt whilst Labour's youth organisation was increasingly taken over by followers of Militant.

Organisational regeneration

At that time a concern for other priorities drove a new push from some of the unions, led by the General and Municipal Workers' union (later renamed the GMB), to get a regeneration of the party organisation. This was seen by the NEC left as a factional manoeuvre directed against them. It was a suspicion with some substance but the primary motivation of the union was the party's viability. Later, in 1979, the GMB was central to the formation of Trade Unions for a Labour Victory (TULV), which aimed to give the party organisational and financial support and to encourage organisational reform. That pushed it into NEC territory and initially, in relation to pensions, also duplicated the TUC's collective policy voice. It was not a heavily publicised birth but it was to have major long-term political significance through five Labour Leaders.

Party policy-making, the winter of discontent and the second-term manifesto
There was an extensive system of NEC sub-committee working under independent party auspices to prepare policies for the next election manifesto. This was a project first proposed by Crossman and supported by Wilson a decade earlier, but now the NEC was led from the left with Tony Benn, a member of the Callaghan Cabinet, heavily involved in the production of the policies on which the manifesto was based. Meetings of the NEC with Callaghan became at times very abrasive as he faced regular critical scrutiny of government policies. Years later, whenever the Blairites of the 1990s looked nervously for the problems that they might face in government, this image of a Leader at bay regularly emerged.

At the 1978 conference, the government's 5 per cent pay policy was defeated in the absence of agreement and a statement from the Liaison Committee. The government had ignored warning from allies in the unions that the pay norm was now too low and too rigid; it would produce grassroots industrial trouble. That came from an outbreak of pent-up militancy from lower-paid workers in the public sector in 'the winter of discontent', after Callaghan had postponed the expected election in October 1978. By the time that industrial action had ended, there had been a decline in the attachment of Labour voters to the party. Not only that, but it generated a strong public reaction against militant trade unions and its rights and some of Labour's core values and policies. The 'winter of discontent' became a defining event influencing the later management policies of Kinnock, Blair and Brown. Benefiting from it all was the new right-wing Conservative Leader Margaret Thatcher at a time when Labour's press support had weakened and the former *Daily Herald*, for years the Labour movement's own paper, had become the *Sun*, a right-wing tabloid owned by Rupert Murdoch's News International.

But for the moment, in the party the crucial event became what happened in the writing of the manifesto. Specific party policies initiated by the NEC had minimal influence over the draft. There were a series of disagreements because, it was said by the party side, the Government was unwilling 'to concede to the Party any real measure of joint determination'.[84] Eventually a new draft was prepared in No. 10 Downing Street in which the Prime Minister still refused to accept the most contentious party proposals. This provoked a fierce reaction inside the party led by party officials and the NEC, giving a further boost to the clamour for more party control over the Leadership.

Management fragmentation and the growing insurgency

Public, party and academic attention now focused heavily on the series of conflicts in the Labour Party, driven on both sides by a highly combustible mix of idealism and resurgent factional interest. Behind all that, however, was the important fact that the traditional model of party management and the system of supportive alliances, controls and cultural norms which had marked the party for most of its history were now severely undermined. The character of the breakdown of management, and the problems of the insurrection that accompanied and followed it, became embedded in the folklore and fears of restoration reformers and of Blairite management years later.

Notes

1 Robert Michels, *Political Parties: A Sociological Study of the Oligarchical Tendencies of Modern Democracy*, Hearst's International Library Co., 1915.
2 Robert McKenzie, *British Political Parties: the Distribution of Power within the Conservative and Labour Parties*, Mercury Books, London, 1955.
3 Minkin, *Contentious Alliance*, particularly Chapter 2, pp. 25–53.
4 Egon Wertheimer, *Portrait of the Labour Party*, London, 1929. See also Minkin, *Contentious Alliance*, pp. 5–7 for 'Wertheimer's puzzle'.
5 These priority issues are dealt with in detail in Minkin, *Contentious Alliance*, Chapter 2, pp. 40–5 and explored also in later chapters of that study.
6 Constitution and Standing Orders of the Labour Party (hereafter 'Rulebook'), Rule VIII2f.
7 Alan Bullock, *The Life and Times of Ernest Bevin*. Vol. 1, *Trade union leader, 1881–1940*, Heinemann, London, 1960, p. 286.
8 David Howell, *British Social Democracy: a Study in Development and Decay*, Croom Helm, London, 1976, p. 13.
9 Rulebook, 1918 Party Objects, Rule 3(d).
10 Lewis Minkin, 'Politics of the Block Vote', *New Socialist*, Vol. 1, September/October 1981.
11 Minkin, *Contentious Alliance*, pp. 33–4.
12 Samuel. H. Beer, *Modern British Politics*, Faber & Faber, London 1965, p. 179.
13 Ibid. p. 176.
14 NEC Minutes, 25 February 1948.
15 Eric Shaw, *Discipline and Discord in the Labour Party*, Manchester University Press, Manchester, 1988, p. 33.
16 Martin Harrison, *Trade Unions and the Labour Party since 1945*, Allen & Unwin, London, 1960, pp. 136–45 and p. 150. Also Irvine Richter, *Political Purpose in Trade Unions*, George Allen & Unwin, London, 1973, pp. 146–50.
17 Detailed in Minkin, *Party Conference*, pp. 63–76.
18 Shaw, *Discipline and Discord*, p. 293.
19 Ibid. p. 37.
20 Minkin, *Party Conference*, pp. 15–16.
21 Ibid. pp. 324–6.
22 Shaw, *Discipline and Discord*, pp. 95–6.
23 Ibid. p. 113.
24 Ibid. p. 295.
25 Ibid. p. 107.
26 Ibid.
27 Austen Ranney, *Pathways to Parliament*, Macmillan, London, 1965, pp. 159–60, first cited in Shaw, *Discipline and Discord*, p. 108.

28 Interviews with Sara Barker, Joyce Gould and Reg Underhill between 1969 and 1974.
29 Shaw, *Discipline and Discord*, pp. 90–1.
30 Ibid. p. 97.
31 Ibid. p. 91.
32 Ibid. p. 114 and n. 126 citing Patrick Seyd, 'Factionalism in the Labour Party: A Case Study of the Campaign for Democratic Socialism', Unpublished M/Phil dissertation. Southampton University, p. 209. It drew from access to CDS documentation.
33 Peter Patterson, *The Selectorate: the Case for Primary Elections in Britain*, MacGibon and Kee, London, 1967, p. 62. Shaw, *Discipline and Discord*, p. 114.
34 Shaw, *Discipline and Discord*, p. 331, n. 150.
35 Patterson, *Selectorate*, pp. 65–6.
36 Interviews with Joyce Gould 2006 and October 2009.
37 Patterson, *Selectorate*, p. 57.
38 Geoffrey Goodman, *The Awkward Warrior, Frank Cousins: His Life and Times*, Davis-Poynter, London, 1979, p. 105.
39 Minkin, *Party Conference*, pp. 166–7.
40 Allan Flanders, *Management and Unions: the Theory and Reform of Industrial Relations*, Faber, London, 1970, pp. 36–7.
41 Shaw, *Discipline and Discord*, pp. 61–4.
42 *Tribune*, 3 August 1962, and Shaw, *Discipline and Discord*, p. 63.
43 Philip M. Williams, *Hugh Gaitskell: A Political Biography*, Jonathan Cape, London, 1979, p. 950, n. 174.
44 *Tribune*, 3 August 1962.
45 Shaw, *Discipline and Discord*, p. 316, n. 74, citing NEC minutes, 25 July 1962.
46 Goodman, *Awkward Warrior*, p. 339.
47 *Tribune*, conference report, 5 October 1962.
48 Williams, *Gaitskell*, p. 690.
49 *Tribune*, 5 October 1962.
50 Shaw, *Discipline and Discord*, p. 66.
51 *Tribune*, 2 August 1962.
52 Shaw, *Discipline and Discord*, p. 104.
53 Richard Crossman, Introduction to new paperback edn of Bagehot, *The English Constitution*, Collins/Fontana, London, 1963.
54 Anthony Howard, *Crossman: The Pursuit of Power*, Jonathan Cape, London, 1990, p. 265.
55 Janet Morgan (ed.), *The Backbench Diaries of Richard Crossman*, Hamish Hamilton and Jonathan Cape, London, 1981, entry 26 June 1963, pp. 1008–9.
56 Richard Crossman, *The Diaries of a Cabinet Minister*, ed. Janet Morgan, Vol. II, Hamish Hamilton and Jonathan Cape, London 1976, entry 24 September 1966, p. 50.
57 Ibid. entry 1 October 1966, p. 58.
58 Ibid. entry 10 August 1966, p. 608.
59 Harrison, *Trade Unions and Labour Party*, p. 264 and p. 295.
60 Howard, *Crossman*, p. 284.
61 Richard Crossman, *The Diaries of a Cabinet Minister*, ed. Janet Morgan, Vol. III, Hamish Hamilton and Jonathan Cape, London, 1977, entry 4 September 1968, p. 180.

62 Crossman, *Diaries*, III, entry 15 July 1968, p. 138.
63 NEC Minutes, 24 November 1965: Tony Benn, *Out of the Wilderness: Diaries 1963–7*, Arrow, 1988, p. 340.
64 Howard, *Crossman*, p. 285.
65 *Crossman Diaries*, III, entry 8 March 1979, pp. 848–52.
66 Shaw, *Discipline and Discord*, p. 172
67 Ibid. p. 171.
68 Ibid. pp. 170–1.
69 Ibid. p. 174.
70 Ibid. pp. 296–7.
71 Goodman, *Awkward Warrior*, p. 485 and p. 489.
72 Minkin, *Contentious Alliance*, p. 117, and notes 31–4, p. 150.
73 Patrick Seyd and Lewis Minkin, 'The Labour Party and its Members', *New Society*, 20 September 1979.
74 Composite resolution No 16 carried by 3,085,000 to 2,801,000.
75 James Callaghan, *Time and Chance*, Collins, London, 1987, p. 459.
76 Philip Norton, 'Parliament', in Anthony Seldon and Kevin Hickson (eds), *New Labour Old Labour: the Wilson and Callaghan Governments*, Routledge, London 2004, p. 197.
77 Ibid. p. 192.
78 Ibid. p. 195.
79 Ibid. p. 199.
80 Interview with Michael Foot, the Leader of Labour Party in 1981.
81 Shaw, *Discipline and Discord*, pp. 215–16.
82 Ibid. p. 220 and footnote 15.
83 Ibid. p. 220.
84 Geoff Bish (Labour Party Head of Research), 'Drafting the Manifesto', in Ken Coates (ed.), *What went Wrong*, Spokesman, Nottingham, 1979, p. 201. Also, interviews with Bish, and headquarters and No. 10 staff of that period.

2

Revolt and restoration

The open rebellion

Rebellion and the management trauma

No Labour Leader had moved into Opposition in circumstances like those faced by Callaghan in 1979 after his defeat by Margaret Thatcher. The revolt which involved an attempt to exert new controls over the PLP and its leadership had been built upon grievances over policies which deviated from those of the party under two different periods of Labour government. Now it moved much more into the open and became definitive of the politics of the period. Whether the failure to follow party policy was diagnosed in terms of lack of will, of commitment or of the pressures from other countervailing powers around government, the answer was seen as reinforcing respect for the party and its conference decisions through constitutional change. That, it was thought, would enable the party's ideological and policy case to be put and implemented with conviction and energy arousing public enthusiasm.

Previous attempts at constitutional change had been seen after the fall of a Labour government, although never with this scope, breadth of grassroots organisation or the planning of the Campaign for Labour Party Democracy (CLPD). This was later integrated into the Rank and File Mobilising Committee (RFMC) which was an unusually unified temporary alliance of a wide range of groups on the left. The Trotskyist group, Militant Tendency, was also accepted into the committee. Crucially, in the past, the major mechanisms of party management had enabled the leadership to confront, filter and neutralise such challenges, but now the leadership was divided and management was exceptionally weak.

In the past, managers worked through the NEC backed by a strong degree of union support. But this NEC under the control of a left majority became motivators and facilitators of revolt, and union support was much more unstable. Again unprecedented, the most senior official of the party, Ron Hayward, the General Secretary took a rebellious public line at the post-election conference, 'Why was there a winter of discontent? The reason was that, for good or ill, the Cabinet supported by MPs ignored Congress and Conference decisions. It is as simple as that.'[1]

Within the parliamentary leadership and on the right of the party and unions there were acute tactical divisions on how to respond: compromise or fight back, and on what basis? Where once the observer might marvel at the skills, tactical dexterity and at times effrontery of managers working to the Parliamentary leadership, now it was the insurgents' own managers, constantly networking with CLPs and unions, who adroitly gained the ascendancy – sometimes using the union delegates to push the union leaders past where they wanted to be, often successfully challenging and pressurising the CAC which still had a loyalist union majority.

The activist organisation CLPD, and then RFMC, organised and campaigned around the wording of key resolutions which were planned early enough to be fed into the unions and CLPs and to secure favourable mandates. At the party conference fringe the CLPD meetings operated as a form of open conspiracy. Speeches were interwoven with briefings, and floor contributions became a dialogue on conference tactics and counter-tactics. Out of all this came a coordination which, working with their NEC allies, seized the initiative and could take advantage of the various limitations and cock-ups of their opponents.

Even the limited management secured for the Parliamentary leaders through the CAC via the backdoor authority of the leader was undermined after 1979 by the intervention of the NEC and by changes in attitude of senior party and union officials. The influence of CLPD spread into the headquarters and its in-house trade unions. Together with the research and political officers of the unions they provided for a time an important auxiliary network interwoven within the revolt. Overall, within the limitations noted below, it was an extraordinarily successful movement. In response, membership of and attendances at the local parties shot up. To many participating in the upheaval they were days of hope and a new adventure in rank-and-file activism. Years later, however, these events would come to provide justification for a stronger leadership and a managerial renaissance.

NEC leadership role and party management

Where in the past the loyalist right had caucused before the NEC and often worked through the trade union group to give support to the leader, the NEC left now caucused as the dominant group to steer the committee and determine its main output. With left-wing leaders Tony Benn and Eric Heffer chairing the then Home Policy Committee and the Organisation Committee, they were able to push forward their policy and constitutional agenda. In the period from 1979 to 1982 they produced their own distinctive combination of leadership via the traditional procedures of the NEC together with efforts made to engage with the movements of opinion and policy submissions from below. There was an alliance of the NEC left with the CLPD and later with the RFMC and a network of sympathisers from the left. With the tide running to the left in the party on various key policy issues, the NEC was able to draw from a variety of radical groups and experts and authorise major changes in policy.

Staff appointments under the control of the NEC continued to move in a left-wing direction and, to the irritation of the traditional right and leadership supporters,[2] policy staff working to the NEC committees were now an important influence in assisting the left-led NEC where once they had worked to a right-led committee. Geoff Bish, the Research Director, was a key figure in preparing the ground for the NEC to move into the post-election role as supporter of the constitutional revolt, although later he became one of the first to acknowledge its problems.

At different levels of the party machine, old and new cultures clashed. The NEC continued to be suspicious of the politics of the regional staff. In some of the regions, criticism of the NEC political and organisational inadequacies mounted discreetly. For much of the time the NEC gave little attention to administering the party. Headquarters' trade union branches by contrast became sources of left-wing initiatives calling for their version of constructive reorganisation of the party and of the Head Office.

There was a new opening up of NEC procedures after an initiative from the left to heighten the knowledge of the increasingly militant activists about what was being done by the governing body and to encourage its accountability. In 1980 the minutes of the NEC meetings were published, and voting on the NEC began to be recorded when requested by an NEC member. To open up constitutional issues to regular debate, at the recommendation of the NEC the 'three year rule', whereby resolutions could not be repeated for three years – a procedure which had in the past been used by the CAC to hold off the campaign for reform – was waived by the NEC in 1979 in connection with mandatory re-selection[3] and the election of the Leader[4] and then for a time abolished.[5]

Working to the tide in the party, from the NEC, non-amendable documents were used to gain conference support against the old parliamentary leadership positions. The NEC statement *Peace Jobs and Freedom*, which developed both defence policy and attitudes towards the EEC, was put before a special conference in 1980. It was the same with subsequent NEC documents in 1981, *Nuclear Weapons and the Arms Race* and *Withdrawal from the EEC*, which changed defence policy and policy on Europe. The NEC was able to ensure firm conference commitments.

Constitutional issues

Nevertheless, the revolt had weaknesses and limitations which were to prove crucial. In spite of the apparent momentum of support for reform, the two major constitutional reform issues already raised – mandatory re-selection, and election of the Leader by the whole party – still proved to be highly contested at the party conference. In 1979, mandatory re-selection was carried but not overwhelmingly: 4,008,000 votes to 3,039,000, and proposals for widening the electorate for the Leader and Deputy Leader were defeated by 4,009,000 votes to 3,033,000. A third constitutional proposal, that the NEC alone would be the final arbiter of the manifesto, rather than the long-established joint meeting, was supported by the NEC, on the eve of the 1979 conference, and then carried at the conference by 3,936,000 votes to 3,008,000. With momentum apparently shifting to the reformers but neither side able to claim broad-based success, these votes were a recipe for unresolved conflict.

Callaghan attempted to seek a compromise which would come to terms with the revolt and then move away from the constitutional conflicts. In 1980, having failed in their attempt to persuade the NEC to drop all proposals for constitutional change the union-instigated Commission of Enquiry into Party Organisation produced a compromise on electing the Leader which Callaghan accepted: voting for the Leader would move to an electoral college but the PLP would have 50 per cent; the affiliated organisations and the CLPs 25 per cent each. But with a minority of leading figures seeing the situation as ripe for a new politics and considering defection, the atmosphere in the PLP and the Shadow Cabinet was such that the compromise was rejected.

Union leaders and party management

This period was especially revealing about clashing union motivations and behaviour. The revolt over constitutional reform and over policy issues was often portrayed as the trade union leaders asserting their political power, most notably by Ben Pimlott, showing 'How Labour went unilateral'.[6] It was a damaging image, lazily and sometimes misleadingly deployed in the media.[7] But insofar as the union leaders were attempting political management, their priority was to assist in securing an organisationally and financially viable Labour Party. That was what they spent most of their time on in the organisation Trade Unions for a Labour Victory (TULV) and during a union-instigated Commission of Enquiry.

As for the controversial constitutional issues, the unions had not initiated the constitutional conflict, although some of the unions had acted as 'the bomb' triggered by CLP activists and later the NEC. Acting within their organisational mandates and delegation opinion the unions were split almost 50–50 on the three key constitutional issues. Acting collectively through TULV and the Commission, the union leaders sought to manage the party crisis by an orderly process of discussion, gaining consensus on the key reforms then bringing the whole constitutional argument to a close as soon as possible. This they saw as the traditional union role of coming to the aid of the party, but it was an uncomfortable experience as they became bogged down in detailed proposals within the party environment.

The Commission also proposed some formal changes in the procedure of party management. The CAC was for the first time to have one independently elected CLP representative. This was widely welcomed.[8] More crucially, the Commission recommended reinstatement of the three-year rule for constitutional changes, thus impeding a continuation of the battle. At the conference the NEC was defeated by overwhelming union votes in its recommendation to oppose this reversal.[9] This kind of political intervention provoked internal controversy in the unions incited by both left and right.

On the left there were those who saw the TULV and Commission role as part of a right-wing plot to undermine the NEC, thwart the left and the constitutional revolution. On the union right it was seen by some as an obstacle to a full-scale fightback against the advance of the left. The most contentious issue highlighting the tensions between the union leaders and the NEC in party management was the decision of the NEC to support a constitutional provision that the manifesto be produced under NEC control. Significantly, this action was generally regarded with great scepticism by most of the union leadership. Access, partnership and continuous dialogue were seen as more practical and more legitimate than the search for complete and sole party control which would be unworkable. The manifesto must remain a joint product with the parliamentary leadership. The union leaders made an attempt to secure this as part of a stabilising settlement through a new National Council of Labour which would embrace the unions and the PLP leadership as well as the NEC, but this failed to win union support or political agreement by the politicians. The NEC's own pro-reform position backing the RFMC proposal at the 1980 party conference was defeated, although mandatory re-selection was again narrowly carried.

Extraordinary disarray in the PLP was also exhibited in the lack of tactical coordination amongst union loyalists. In the boilermakers' delegation vote at the 1980 Conference on electing the Leader, the union's leaders who were opposed to change left the pro-change delegation to its own devices at the crucial time,[10] thus giving room for the delegation to swing the entire conference vote behind the principle of an electoral college. For the implementing special conference held in Wembley in January 1981, complicated tactical decisions from within the engineers' union produced a formula of 40:30:30, giving the affiliated organisations more votes than the PLP/MEPs and the CLPs.[11] This engineers' position was taken advantage of by supporters of reducing the influence of the PLP leadership. Enough other union votes were pulled behind it, and so the outcome unwanted by most union leaders became the policy and they and the party were stuck with it.

PLP reform and division

The battles spread to the politics and management of the PLP. On its left there was a reform movement which sought to integrate the PLP into the party constitution as a means of reinforcing the authority of the conference. On the right and centre of the PLP this was seen as creating a new democratic centralism which would be exercised by the NEC on behalf of the conference, compromising MPs' independence in parliament. There was already a deep concern on the right over the impact of deselection[12] and of an 'unrepresentative' NEC considered to be unwilling to take on its political and organisational responsibilities. The right-wing Manifesto Group looked to an NEC reform in which ordinary party members, local government and the PLP should be represented,[13] what was later to become the Blair agenda in 1997.

But the leadership had other problems now with the management of the PLP because of a more broadly supported reform movement concerned with its internal procedures. This included proposals to strengthen the PLP meeting as a decision-making body with its own agenda and powers of scrutiny and ratification. There should be a diminution of the patronage power of the whips particularly in choosing Labour representatives on the parliamentary select committees. There should also be elections for the Cabinet as well as the Shadow Cabinet.

Although the whips and the leadership were temporarily forced to retreat after a clumsy rejection, a new working party set up by Callaghan recommended that the 'informality' of PLP proceedings in recent years be continued and rejected a number of proposals for more formal arrangements. Proceeding by voting, it was said, would always create the problem of what action is to be taken against the minority. The arguments were couched in liberal terms, drawing attention to the atmosphere in the late 1940s and the 1950s with its less tolerant spirit represented in the PLP. Adherence to informality won out. As for the role of the whips, there should be extensive advance discussion but the whips would retain their power over committee appointments. The drive to elect a Labour Cabinet was also sidelined but with a limited change – the elected Shadow Cabinet was to become the Cabinet in the Government's first year – thereafter it was to be a matter for the Prime Minister.

Later, a second working party considering the role of the PLP in formulating the general election manifesto made the recommendation that the Liaison Committee linking the PLP and the Cabinet when there was a Labour Government be renamed the Parliamentary Committee, a nod towards more PLP participation but without immediate substantive consequences. This proposal was lost to history till 2001 and then was found to have unforeseen consequences for participation in the Clause V meeting of the NEC and the Parliamentary Committee.

After this, there was a deepening reluctance to use the party's constitution to pursue proposals which might be seen as threatening parliamentary autonomy, and there was also increasing recognition from most of the left of the PLP that the moment had passed. Amongst union leaders, even those on the left, there was particular hostility to this attempt to impose parliamentary procedures from the outside. At the 1981 Party Conference a resolution to 'fully incorporate the Parliamentary Labour Party's standing orders into the Party Constitution'[14] was remitted at the request of the

NEC and a constitutional amendment on similar lines was declared to have fallen.[15] No vote was allowed also on a resolution which supported the constitutional amendments which had been submitted on this theme in 1980.[16] All this conference management manoeuvring appears to have been by a tacit agreement between the CAC and the NEC Chairman Alec Kitson of the TGWU and the Chair of the NEC Organisation Sub-committee, Eric Heffer – two supporters of the Campaign for Labour Party Democracy.

At the same conference, the NEC won a temporary victory on authorisation of the manifesto,[17] only for the constitutional amendment to be defeated,[18] by what was said to be an unfortunate error – a misplaced vote by the leadership of the union USDAW. Some doubt must be raised over this explanation, given that it came from a traditional-right union whose leaders thought that the Labour government had 'not done too badly' and had great concern about this change.

Foot as Leader: defection and counter attack

The victory of Michael Foot in the election for Leader in October 1980 added momentum to a movement on the right of the PLP towards a split from the party. Dissatisfaction reached a peak in early 1981 after the vote at the special conference took the election of a future Leader out of the hands of the PLP alone. A new organisation, Solidarity, was formed to organise the fightback. But for some in the PLP that was all too late. The management of the issue of electing the Leader was judged to be 'a dirty shabby surrender'.[19] It was regarded as the last straw – the final instalment of what was regarded, in melodramatic terms, as the irretrievable loss of the Labour Party to the trade unions and the ultra-left. A small but significant section of the PLP defected in January 1981 to form the Social Democratic Party. From them would come a new influence upon the Labour Party via electoral pressure from outside and, much later, a small but also significant infusion into what became the Blairites.

Throughout 1980, Labour had been well ahead in the polls in spite of (or maybe at that stage because of) the revolt. But in 1981, with a consistent and unrestrained media message that the Labour Party was in the pockets of 'the union bosses' and under the influence of left-wing 'loonies', the polls moved strongly away. The special conference vote in 1981 became a gift to the new SDP and all who wanted to typify the union leaders as power-hungry barons. Faced with huge problems in attempting to keep the party together and defend policy agreed by conference, Michael Foot's ratings as Leader were poor. The SDP leaders by contrast became media heroes and the government's unpopularity over unemployment was now benefiting the defectors, not the Labour Party.

At this point Tony Benn decided to challenge for the post of Deputy Leader, against the advice of a majority of his close supporters who were in effect bounced by his public announcement of candidature. The resulting controversy on the left became a deep fracture that led to a split from the Tribune Group of MPs – and the formation of the more Bennite, Socialist Campaign Group which later became labelled as 'the hard left'. Neil Kinnock emerged as an alternative leader of what became known as the 'soft left'.

Benn's campaign stimulated hugely enthusiastic meetings (and enormous media antipathy) and Benn was only narrowly defeated. But the NUPE vote after a ballot revealed that Benn and the reform movement had been driving forwards from a narrow and precarious base, which was weakening further as the battle continued. Association of the reform revolt with the left gave it organisational vigour but also a limiting image. In the unions, support for the procedural reform agenda from the 'rank and file' was based on the priorities of a minority. Even in those CLPs fully committed to the three reforms, CLPs acting as candidate selectors continued to take electoral opinion into account in their selections[20] and there was growing concern in the party at its weak electoral position.

The NEC union restraint and recapture

The strength of the movement to the left had been facilitated by the leadership of the NEC and its influential role in relation to the mechanics of party management. For years afterwards some on the left continued to think of the future in term of this potential role. Yet the rise to the power of the NEC left always had some shallow and contingent features. Some of these gave a significant conservative advantage to the incumbents but it was a position always vulnerable to a determined and united counter-attack.

Also, whilst the NEC was increasing its immediate influence over policy, union leaders were seeking to manage the longer-term transformation taking place in the facilities available to the PLP front bench but not to the NEC for policy-making. The Short Money – assistance granted by the state to the Opposition for policy-making – was now available to the leadership in parliament. With additional financial assistance from the trade union leadership there were now resources for the creation of an alternative policy advisory staff and independent policy-making machinery in the PLP. Crucial here was that the NEC's attempt to ensure that they captured sole control over these resources was repulsed by the so-called union 'bosses'.

Collective union counter-attacks

Amongst the membership of the unions there was a growing unease and then vocal dissatisfaction against what appeared to be the over-concentration of their leaders on internal political actions within the Labour Party at a time of rising mass unemployment. It produced a renewed concern amongst union leaders to stop the conflict. This spread to headquarters trade unionists and union political and research officers. Wiser heads in the CLPD, particularly its leading figure Vladimir Derer, also recognised that support for the campaign had peaked in 1980[21] and CLPD voices now spoke of the constitutional revolt having for the moment run its course with what had happened at Wembley probably unrepeatable.[22]

Union leaders from the traditional right of the party watched the behaviour of the NEC Left with a growing anger as many of their cherished political positions and roles were challenged. In a reversal of the position taken in the 1960s when the right controlled the NEC, they found many failings in the behaviour of the NEC. Financial management was one target. The NEC's acceptance of a broad church, seen as an irresponsible abdication of the responsibility for boundary maintenance protecting the party against Trotskyist entryism, was another. Conflicts over the 'rules' and protocols of the relationship between the unions and the party exacerbated the tensions.

The NEC in February 1980 gave a commitment for the complete repeal of trade union legislation, a move not requested by the TUC who were sensitive to the polling data on the changing opinion of union members on postal ballots before strikes, the prohibition of secondary picketing and taxation of social security payments to strikers' families.[23] The most significant conflict took place over the sacking by British Leyland of left-wing shop steward Derek Robinson, 'Red Robbo', a move strongly opposed in solidarity by the NEC. This brought a group of unions, particularly the AEU, into an angry response to NEC interference into industrial activities which broke a long-established 'rule' of non-intervention by politicians.

The right in the unions had been working since 1975 to change the NEC back to its loyalist majority but were held up by poor liaison, internal conflicts and the difficulties of counter-organising union votes which were often linked to role-governed exchanges of support which had lasted many years. Frustrated in 1980, they came back in 1981 much more organised and in ruthless mood as the St Ermin's Group.[24] They were determined to recapture control, in order – as they saw it – 'to save the party'. In 1981, when the revolt of the campaign for party democracy and the Bennite movement appeared at their peak they recaptured five seats. A sign of the times was the astonishing failure of the AEU to vote for its own nominee, the sitting tenant of the Treasurer's post, left-wing MP Norman Atkinson.[25]

Meanwhile, the broader collective of TULV senior union leaders which had a different centre of political gravity now sought with increasing desperation to call a halt to the entire internal constitutional war, also in order to save the party. A meeting of TULV leaders and the NEC, held at Bishop's Stortford on 5 and 6 January 1982 to discuss party organisational and financial support, was turned into an argument over the political conflict, and an agreement was reached to call a halt to any further constitutional changes or challenges for leadership positions. This implied also a quid pro quo of no reversal of the changes made on reselection and the procedure for electing the leadership. With united backing in the unions this peace over constitutional change was, in effect, imposed on the party by the union leaders and generally adhered to by both sides.[26]

However, there was no let-up in the internal war for control over the NEC. Jim Mortimer's appointment in 1982 as new General Secretary was seen as a victory for the centre left, but at the party conference in another sweep the traditional right organised though the St Ermin's Group won a further three positions and regained control of the NEC. In one case, Sid Weighall, the NUR General Secretary, failed to cast his vote for the NUM candidate and sitting tenant, the left-winger Eric Clarke, after giving a pledge to do so and following an NUR conference decision. The 'rules' of union representation were thus broken again but at the cost to Weighall of his job.[27]

Foot, the Soft Left and intimations of re-control

Labour's wilting electoral position was becoming more urgent in the context of constant accusations that the Labour Party was becoming a party of the extreme left. With the defeat of Tony Benn in October 1981 and a partial shift to the right on the NEC, Foot had begun a reappraisal of his past attitude towards the growing problem of the Militant Tendency and to consider more interventionist party management to deal with it. The NEC was asked to set up an inquiry into its activities – the Hughes-Hayward inquiry. Its report found, as had the Underhill Report of 1975, that Militant was an organised group with its own programme, policy and organisation. The report proposed a register of recognised groups which only allowed groups found to be compatible with the constitution. This was supported by the 1982 party conference.

Although what became called the 'soft left' still fought 'the Trots' in organisational rather than ideological terms and was still constrained by views of the party as a pluralistic broad church with rights of dissent, this marked the first significant break in the united left-influenced NEC position. Concern over Militant and defence of the party's boundaries now began to subordinate fear of the return of the old authoritarianism. In November 1982, the strengthened right took control over all the NEC committees, removing Benn and Heffer from their committee chairs. Although the major policy changes remained for the moment entrenched and under the protection of Foot, the organisation sub-committee could now be used to target entryism. In December 1982, in a major management change, Militant was proscribed by the NEC.

The election and the legacy

The Falklands War consolidated a transformation of Margaret Thatcher's electoral position, making her Government virtually unbeatable in the general election of 1983. Constrained by Foot and the need to regain some unity, plus a confident belief that the left programme was about to be discredited, the Labour right made little attempt in 1983 to change the major policies which had emerged from the left ascendancy. Callaghan and Healey, contravening their own years of appeals for party unity, made damaging attacks on unilateral nuclear disarmament during the campaign, thereby giving ammunition to the party's opponents. The Labour campaign was disastrously organised. The SDP only just failed to replace Labour as the second party but it split the anti-Tory vote; and Labour, in losing three million supporters since 1979, received only 27.6 per cent of the vote – its lowest since 1918. The outcome was a Conservative majority of 144.

The policies in the manifesto, cleverly labelled 'the longest suicide note in history' by the right-wing Labour MP Gerald Kaufman, took much of the odium of the defeat, although as Heffernan and Marquesee later pointed out, other than on unilateral establishment of a non-nuclear defence policy, the policies had more public support than appeared to be the case.[28] But there was always going to be a problem of leaders failing to forcefully advocate policies of which they vehemently disapproved.

The legacy of this defeat and what led up to it shaped a vivid memory and sometimes a caricature of what went wrong and why, what to avoid and what to replicate. On the right and for leaders all the way down to Blair and Brown, it was an experience that should never be repeated. More broadly in the party, even on the left over time, the events of 1979 to 1983 came to be seen by many of those involved as a political dead-end, involving the party in chaotic and divisive in-fighting which gave ammunition to its enemies. But for the moment, the whole experience provided a huge incentive for unity and self-discipline and a restoration of elements of past party management with new initiatives which would later feed into the forces strengthening around Blair.

Reassertion of leadership and management

Election disaster and Thatcherism

In an election for Leader and Deputy Leader, based on the procedures and enlarged electorate forged in 1981, Neil Kinnock defeated Roy Hattersley, but together they formed what was regarded as a 'dream ticket' which would unite soft left and right and help produce new party stability. It was to be a stability forged in a continuing adverse political climate as under Thatcher, the Conservative Party victory in 1983 was to be followed by a further move rightward, a subsequent victory in 1987 and a further victory under John Major in 1992.

Thatcherism wove together economic liberalism, a strong state with social authoritarianism and individual responsibility. That shifted the agenda of British politics to the right on a range of policy areas, including privatisation, labour law, the welfare state, education and council-house ownership. It prioritised fighting inflation with a policy of sound money but establishing no responsibility for the level of employment. Thatcher's radicalism involved bold statecraft working not just for continuing Conservative victory but for a ruthlessly comprehensive shift of British political life, especially in the position of the Labour Party and the unions.

The cooperative social partnership assumptions of British political life since the Second World War were rejected. The unions were seen as coercive bodies subversive of the market and politically dangerous in confronting government. Over three terms, her labour-law reforms strengthened some union internal democratic procedures but also reasserted the power of employers and weakened the unions.

Changing the Labour Party and creating a new party management

Kinnock, reacting to Foot's low-key style but also influenced by Thatcher's model of strong leadership, immediately also took on a more commanding persona in relations with his colleagues and sought to strengthen management from the Leader's office. In a speech at Stoke on 12 September 1983, Labour's new Leader strongly committed himself to a programme of organisational reform. Within weeks, some of the specific commitments were implemented, including a new Campaign Strategy Committee, significantly made answerable directly to the Leader. The financial resources of the Short money supplemented by the unions gave individuals on the front bench more capacity for independent policy-making and facilitated the establishment of a strengthened office under Dick Clements and Charles Clarke with Patricia Hewitt as Press Secretary. The staff was expanded using the new public provision of opposition finance. In effect, what was now constituted was an executive office of the Leader with Clarke acting as its chief of staff. That laid the basis of a new concentration of power but it was not one that Kinnock was able to use without constraints and inhibitions.

The immediate constraints on him were indicated by the failure to secure a swift change in General Secretary and a restructuring of Head Office. Kinnock and his organisational reform agenda also met opposition from the left group on the NEC including Benn, Skinner and future General Secretary Tom Sawyer. Benn and Skinner tended to downplay the significance of the state of party organisation and to see all reform as a guise behind which there would be a redistribution of power to the parliamentary leadership and the enhancement of the leadership's political management of the party. If they were short-sighted about the desperate state of the party organisation they were perceptive about what was to come in terms of the strengthening of party management and the enhanced role of the leadership in relation to the party.

Kinnock emphasised moving out of the election disaster zone and the argument that you could only help the poor by gaining governmental power, and you could only do that by gaining the support of the better-off as well as the poor. This was a new expression of the importance of broadening the party's appeal from its traditional base. The priority of avoiding the open loud disunity of the past in not giving ammunition to the Tories was attuned to a growing party mood. Many who had been energetic CLPD supporting activists looked in dismay at some of the new problems, then adopted new priorities and accepted some positions they had previously shunned. Their sense of urgency now switched to establishing organisational forms and supportive mechanisms which would assist in producing a Labour government and sustaining it in office.

Management allies

There was still a strong enough left in 1983 to envisage a Kinnock-led leadership uniting soft and hard left in ways which would still dominate NEC politics. After the NEC election results that year, the balance on the committee was still uncertain. But it was the traditional right which moved into a comfortable political role on that committee and a closer relationship with Kinnock. Some union leaders from the right had joined with union leaders on the soft left and already committed themselves to him as a man who prioritised the party's recovery. In terms of both the operation of the St Ermin's Group and their activities on the NEC, they were better organised, and more cohesive than the left. Working through the trade union group of the NEC, they were more attuned to the traditional stability role behind the Leader as well as active defence against the Trotskyists. And with the calling by Arthur Scargill, without a ballot, of a national miners' strike in March 1984, the union right were more consistently attuned to the Leader's political management problems.

Constitutional reform and OMOV

One by-product of the years of constitutional revolt was the undermining of what had been a moderately conservative culture in relation to institutional forms and procedures.[29] What that now opened up was an opportunity to manage a radical counter-reformation under the theme of modernisation. The electoral college to elect the Leader had given him a broad party base of authority, so that was not touched. Central to the changes sought was support for one-member-one-vote (OMOV) in CLP representation. The idea of broadening internal party participation directly to all the members rather than the CLP General Committee (GC) had the advantage of taking the fight on to a higher moral ground. In focusing on all the members at the grass roots, it had a managerial purpose in limiting the influence of the activists who were believed to be less in touch with Labour voters. It also gave the traditional right, who had favoured this procedural position since the late 1970s, a sense of principled purpose after being on the defensive for so long.

It became a left–right issue rather than a unions versus the CLPs alignment. Many on the left shared in principle the concern to expand the electorate but the bulk of the CLPD and Bennite left initially feared a procedural device which indirectly enhanced the influence of the mass media and, in that, prevented a level playing field. In its most traditional commitment the left saw OMOV as a weakening of the collectivism which held the party together, and saw the potential use of this reform as a means of dividing the party from the unions. Above all, it saw practical difficulties of ensuring accountability under new OMOV arrangements and saw the GC monthly meetings with the MP as the best location for that account-ability. In making those concerns paramount, it at times exemplified a new and uncomfortable form of activist elitism. This was gradually outflanked at the grass roots by the strengthening democratic commitment to OMOV in most – although not all – election procedures.

When this agenda was first adopted as a proposal by the Leader in 1984 with the backing of the NEC, it was focused on using one-member-one-vote ballots in mandatory reselection. This would act as a means of protecting MPs from activists on General Committees and also be a reduc-tion in union influence. Why this issue was chosen as the first item for reform of the union-party relationship as compared, for example, with the union vote at the conference, is explicable in terms of this being an area where the Leader and his advisors thought that they could more easily win a public victory and media applause without immediate disadvantages for national party management.

But when it came to the conference vote in October a promised delivery of TGWU backing was overturned by the left in the delegation by two votes. That caused a narrow conference defeat for the leadership by 3,592,000 votes to 3.041,000. Given the huge union predominance at the party conference and the fact that OMOV would undermine union influ-ence in selections, it became part of the common sense of the time that constitutional change was 'defeated by the unions',[30] who were regarded by leading modernisers as 'the source of organisational rigidity'.[31] Yet it was a misreading which became part of the mythology. The individual unions had divided ten against ten in the vote, with the five largest unions also split. The AEEU, GMB and USDAW voted in favour. NUPE joined TGWU against. The split was also a feature of union internal politics. The leadership of NUPE and that of the National Union of Railwaymen (NUR), both of which favoured change, were overturned by their executive com-mittees. The defeat was a shock for Kinnock. From this point on, OMOV in candidate selection became to Kinnock and the media the touchstone issue of successful management and the Leader's authority.

Defeat of the miners

Meanwhile, the miners were heading for a major defeat. The Thatcher government was organised and determined to reverse the defeat Heath had suffered in 1974 and eventually, after a year, the striking miners went back to work with no settlement. This was seen as a defeat for 'the unions' and industrial militancy, and that now changed important influences on Labour's internal politics. There was a slow realignment in the party away from the hard left, influenced by a realism over the miners' strike and the conjecture of Eric Hobsbawm that the 'Forward March of Labour' may have been halted.[32] The weakening of trade unionism and decline of the manual working class and its traditional lifestyles, together with a range of social and economic developments, pointed to the need for new political adjust-ments to build wider electoral support.

In this new context, policy gradually moved on radically from the 1983 Manifesto, beginning with managing the ending of the commitment to withdrawal from the EEC and ending opposition also to council-house sales. Assisted by changes in policy attitudes in the unions following the adverse experience of rationalisation in the public sector, there was also an adjustment of support away from a general public-ownership policy, although still retaining a commitment to reacquisition of the areas privatised.

Managing the attack on 'the Trots'

There had been expulsions of some key figures from Militant in 1983, but this only touched the surface of their organisation. Their activities had alienated union leaders and some on the soft left who had been unsupportive of strong central action. In the party conference they had become adept at pushing themselves and their message to the fore. In response more attention was now paid by the managers and their allies to how the conference might be organised to give the major voice to the party mainstream. Added also were the influences of the new communication team in seeking to build up the Leader, his image and messages and to limit media damage. That had the best possible lift-off in Kinnock's powerful 1985 conference assault on the behaviour of the Militant Tendency in the Liverpool Labour Party, together with Eric Heffer's dramatic walk-out.

This sharpening of political lines over Militant also brought further important changes on the NEC, over time strengthening the 'soft left' whilst the Campaign Group support was slowly weakened. Tom Sawyer, a NUPE official and an ex-Bennite, within a short period from 1985 to 1987 became a pivotal loyalist ally of the Leader as Chair of the Home Policy Committee. The soft left, which at one stage included eight shadow cabinet members, was not regarded as collectively reliable by the Leader and not encouraged by Kinnock or Sawyer to act as a cohesive group. Instead a growing mutual appreciation had united Kinnock with the mainly right-wing trade union group, who responded by delivering for the Leader in a disciplined way on the crucial issues. From the Leader's office the team became much more adept and aggressive in their management liaison with the NEC indicating, at times heavily, 'what Neil wants'. Kinnock himself was a very hands-on committee Leader pushing, persuasive and, at times, domineering. To take counter pressures off NEC members, the provision for recorded voting on the NEC was dropped in November 1985.

Marketing, spin and new party management

Reorganisation

With Jim Mortimer replaced by Kinnock's candidate LarryWhitty, in 1985 the headquarters was restructured with a new and heavy emphasis on campaigning. The ten-headed management structure was reduced to three

Directors, Campaign and Communication, Party Organisation and Policy Development. The office of the General Secretary was strengthened and a campaigns unit was separated from the organisation department. After this, a recruit from television, Peter Mandelson, was appointed as the new Director of Communications.

The later narrative of the modernisers who were to become the core of 'New Labour' emphasised the opposition to them and their role as the new communication pioneers. Yet by this time in 1985 there was already a body of opinion which had developed a new perspective on the kind of campaigning talents now required. It was there in Kinnock's Stoke speech. It was there in the unions' new interest in modern campaigns and communications, which was to serve them well in winning all the 1985 political-fund ballots forced on them by the Thatcher government.[33] At the Greater London Council there were developments in the same direction.[34] The sophisticated new party communication management under Mandelson arrived at party headquarters after the two years of discussion and a reorganisation which had helped prepare the ground and in a climate at least partly conducive to change.

The organisation and form of the new communication management itself caused problems. A Shadow Communications Agency (SCA) led by Philip Gould and Deborah Mattinson was brought in by Mandelson to advise. In December 1985, out of a communications review by Gould,[35] came a perspective that influenced the Kinnock management and later, with fewer reservations, that of Blair. It introduced a comprehensive emphasis on the methods of political marketing, already operated in the Conservative Party.[36] The persistent problem was that the prescriptions of method, objectives and process for communications became in effect an alternative organisational formula with major implications for power and management, party democracy, and relations with the unions.

The central SCA diagnosis was that the party was too associated with old-fashioned images. In ensuring the necessary changes, there must be 'decisiveness, toughness and direction' from strong leadership. There should also be greater coordination of operations and messages with clearer job descriptions and ultimate responsibility for running the campaign unambiguously held by one person, the Director of Campaigns and Communication, who would coordinate the campaigning role. In shaping this role there was an awareness of competing with the methods of the powerful Bernard Ingham working closely with Margaret Thatcher as Chief Press Officer and expanding his domain of influence.

What specially irked some on the NEC was that Mandelson, in a style which he made his own, acted in a covert way that broke with NEC accountability. He developed a semi-independent position with its own empire and initiatives. Also, the recommendation by the SCA for a shift of focus from CLP grass-roots local communication to influencing communication through the mass media, adding to the political agenda which sought a move away from the influence of the 'unrepresentative activists', was thought by critics likely to weaken the party in its electoral campaigning, as it did.

Media management

Mandelson's supreme success was that, drawing from his experience of television and political journalism, he was able to contest dominance of an overwhelmingly hostile media in its relationship with the party. There had always been a problem in handling the Conservative-owned and hostile press – a situation which had become more adverse in the period leading up to the 1979 General Election with the defection of the Labour-supporting *Daily Herald* now the *Sun*. It was widely recognised in 1983 that the Labour Party lagged far behind the Conservatives in its communicational expertise and in coping with a partisan press working with the Conservative Central Office. Dealing with these problems was to become a central priority of the new leadership and the legitimation of much of Mandelson's personal media management.

He became the impressively creative and influential model of a modern spin doctor – a term brought over from the USA. At its simplest, 'spin' as an aspect of the communications strategy was as old as political rhetoric – putting a targeted case in the best possible light and using the best language to influence public perception. Facing a media which often held views of Labour's inadequacy which Mandelson himself largely shared,[37] he sought to put over the good story of what Kinnock was doing to change the party. Their joint approach involved a special concern with damage limitation, especially from actions or words from the left and the unions whose every misdemeanour was publicised, some invented and many exaggerated.

Mandelson seized the agenda, engaged journalists with the party's message, and stayed with that message, repeating it simply and clearly. He also became an expert in the form and timing of leaks and in the focused background briefing. Two sympathetic commentators noted his interpersonal skills as 'he wheedled cajoled flattered and pestered'.[38] Drawing indirectly from the observations of the academic media specialist Jay Blumler in 1983, he made aggressive complaining a fine art in a way that at times strenuously pressurised the journalists, and in that activity turned the tables on them.[39]

The party was widely and heavily affected. Everything was to be organised so that a coherent message was sustained. The theme and layout of a party conference, its agenda and timing, its background symbols, the membership of the platform and the role of major speakers were all part of the communicational strategy. This also affected the public standing of the Leader in relation to the NEC and the ascendancy of the leadership over dissent. 'Blood on the floor' was an attention-seeking tactic said to be the brainchild of Mandelson, in which advance publicity heightened the sense of confrontation with the unions, the left or the activists, in order to lodge

in the mind of the recipient the subservience of the targets and the dominance of the Leader.

Presidency

The party Leader became a media hero as he took on the Militant Tendency
for their behaviour in the Liverpool party. In this, as Foley puts it, 'he had
made the party look as leader-led as the Conservatives'.[40] Yet though he
was tough and had the rhetorical skills, the enlarged office staffing and the
push from there, it was not so easy to keep him 'presidential' because
Kinnock himself, steeped in Labour tribal history, was never fully comfortable playing up to that role. His verbose and at times uncertain presentation had some repetitive faults that aroused doubt about him in the Prime
Minister role. The nearest he got to a wider public acceptance of this
projection after his brief 'he's a hero' moment, was through a film made
for the election campaign in 1987: 'Kinnock the Movie' – as it became
known – which featured an impressive public projection of his leadership
role. Even here the prominent and powerful 'first in a 1,000 generations
of Kinnocks' speech was about what a collective Labour movement 'platform' had given him.

But that collectivity was also being partially undermined by the interaction of his management and the media. The party leadership was set tasks
by the media and set themselves tasks that friendly journalists and loyalist
supporters could take up in relation to what was portrayed as a problematic party. In a highly publicised argument over proposals for black sections
in the party and what the Leader regarded as separatism, the candidate
for Nottingham East, Sharon Atkin, made some intemperate public remarks
about Kinnock and 'the racist Labour Party' and was replaced as candidate
by the NEC. The harsh removal was conceived as a defence of the Leader
and a reassurance to the electorate via the media that action was being
taken against 'the loony left'.[41]

Mandelson's politics of presentation stretched into building up talented
political allies and advising them. The image of rising stars Tony Blair and
Gordon Brown were boosted, but competitors in leading positions were
disadvantaged or even undermined. Yet in spite of all that, Mandelson was
never quite as influential as his reputation suggested. He was never as close
to Kinnock as was Clarke and never fully in the inner loop on policy-
making. Mandelson had some strong distrustful critics in headquarters and
on the Shadow Cabinet, and not a few castigators of what was regarded
as the Machiavellian and self-satisfied arrogance with which he played his
political role.

New leadership and the new policy management

After 1985, with media responses constantly in mind, Kinnock moved to
change the processes of policy-making in ways which became more formally inclusive of the PLP leadership and moved away from the potential

tensions of two policy centres. Kinnock had committed himself to this kind of joint policy-making in a campaigning speech for the leadership. NEC trade union responses here were important. They had in the past favoured institutions of coordination rather than mechanism of control over the leadership. Now their trust in Kinnock eased a change whereby NEC policy committees became seven joint policy committees of the NEC and the PLP Front bench, sharing financial resources.

In practice, though trade unionists from the NEC took the chairs of the Home and International Policy Committees, as before, they rarely took independent policy initiatives, and the frontbench Chairs of the subject committees took control over policy, sometimes moving outside the joint process for economic policy and other issues not covered within it. Generally after 1985 the NEC was a supportive accommodating body at times in difficult circumstances. There was only one reverse at the NEC in 1986 over nuclear energy and possibly another over the appointment of a new Campaigns and Communication Director in 1990, but otherwise all the Leader's proposals went through. Nevertheless policy still had to be processed and sometimes negotiated through an NEC which was procedure- and rule-conscious and could be sticky about its own role. The committee had a fair sprinkling of barrack-room lawyers.

Setting the scene for policy, procedural change and the Blairite future

Following the disappointing General Election result in 1987, in which defeating the Liberal-SDP Alliance was the primary achievement, there was an acceleration of the momentum of change in policy and process. Kinnock initiated a 'Labour listens' series of activities and a comprehensive review covering every aspect of policy. Behind the theme of 'Labour listens' was a continuation of the long-term electoral pressures directly from the Conservatives and also mediated through the alliance of Social Democrats and the Liberals, which became the Liberal Democrats.

Electoral pressures were crucially mediated internally through the SCA. In an investigation of 'Labour and Britain in the 1990s' reported to the NEC in November 1987, the agency's conclusions were that virtually all the social conditions and attitudes which people associated with Labour were declining. What was emphasised had major party implications. The public movement was said to be towards individualism and away from collective provision. The party was too associated with the past, the unions and the poor. The main reasons for not voting Labour were given as its extremism and internal division, its lack of strong leadership, its domination by the trade unions and its policies towards defence and tax. Within this was also a distrust of its economic competence. The study reported that Labour's policies no longer matched people's personal and family aspirations.

It appeared to be an overwhelming case and was a strong influence around Kinnock, providing a platform for important policy changes. In that respect, the review was a success and it further strengthened the Leader. Closer links were built between the directorates and the Leader's office, which at this stage of further electoral insecurity took to itself a more commanding position over policy-formulation managed so as to ensure no major deviation from the planned movement away from past positions. Only in the case of Michael Meacher, front-bench spokesperson on employment, whose position favouring limited union secondary action was slowly undermined by the spin attack on him, was there a major management problem.

However, that management control began increasingly to be seen in the wider party as a developing problem. It did not add much to the quality of intra-party discussion and made little contribution to a revival of party morale. Participation by the membership had been very limited. Policy was still being made through the usual unamendable documents. Complaints about the review, however, did lead to some later new thinking by Whitty and Sawyer about what mechanism might give the party a greater sense of involvement.

A contrasting response came from 'the modernisers', a term adopted around this time for a new tendency on the right of the PLP.[42] From the circle of Tony Blair, Gordon Brown, Peter Mandelson, Philip Gould and Patricia Hewitt, a critique pointed in the direction which would eventually be taken much further by Blair and 'New Labour'. It was argued that there was not enough management and therefore not enough pressure on the party to be radical. Particularly for Patricia Hewitt, now acting as the policy coordinator, the review-group process was not tight enough in giving attention to the electoral exigencies, picking out the priorities of vote-winning policies and developing persuasive themes attuned to likely public acceptance.

Hewitt's attempts to intervene in the policy-review group operating from the Campaign Strategy Committee had been constrained by some practical difficulties of breaking in. And there were reservations, even by loyalists, that the policy destination should be derived from values and could not be determined primarily by input from focus groups. There was also a persistent distrust, which embraced allies as well as opponents and lasted well into Blair's years as Leader, that from the Gould stable came focus-group findings which were influenced by the intervention of Gould himself. Later, there was academic support for this criticism.[43] Even Blair, who used Gould's findings extensively, noted with amusement in his autobiography, 'how extraordinary' was the confluence between Gould's own thoughts and what the groups seemed to say.[44]

The shared perspectives of Gould, Hewitt and Mandelson (who, as a parliamentary candidate moved more on the outside after 1990) as they worked closely with Blair and Brown left an influential legacy on the linkage of party and media management. They held that the policy-making processes should be more tightly integrated with marketing goals. Both should be closely supervised by the media managers working in and to the Leader's office. The Leader should be closely involved in the detail of driving the change.[45] In policy-making, intra-party democracy of the members had to take second place to those focused on media presentational objectives and the electoral problems that had to be anticipated. With entrenched traditionalist opposition, radicals would have to be tough.

The NEC composition was viewed as unsuitable for the new tasks. It should be reformed and further subordinated as a policy body. In their own activity some radicals also felt strongly that they should not be held back by long-established protocols. Mandelson particularly felt only a limited obligation to be bound by traditional definitions of role responsibilities. He saw himself as working to the Leader's office and also on behalf of the party's future (not always the same thing) rather than as an employee supervised by the NEC. In pursuit of more influence at the party centre, in 1989 he secured the candidature of the safe seat of Hartlepool with Blair's active support and through the influence of GMB union official Tom Burlison. But Mandelson was judged in Kinnock's office as leaving the Leader in the lurch, and relations deteriorated. An attempt to keep the national post whilst acting as a candidate was turned down by Kinnock, as was any role in the election campaign. Working with Blair and Brown and like-minded allies, he was still assiduously courting and being courted by journalists, and remained an influential figure. His interpretation of the primary responsibilities of party officials as being more closely attuned to the Leader's preferences rather than democratic hierarchies became an influence also passed down after 1994 into Blair's party management.

Unions and management

In the process of gaining approval from the party conference for policies which moved the party away from some of its past positions, there was a further development of the machinery of party management. A profusion of links between the General Secretary as chief manager, the organisation directorate, the policy directorate and the Conference Arrangements Committee were operating in planning the agenda. Yet behind the scenes also the politics of party management at the conference was even more dependent on liaison with a few large unions.

Though the CLP vote was kept artificially inflated, giving every CLP a minimum vote of 1,000 each, the unions were casting around 90 per cent of the votes at each conference in the period of Kinnock's leadership. At this time also, as unions amalgamated, fewer were affiliated and the larger unions cast a higher percentage of the votes. By 1990 34 unions were casting an affiliated vote of 5,347,000 of which 3,258,000 were held by four unions. This was a boon to management if these unions could be consistently won, and there was some hope that the old loyalist block vote would now be re-established, with its regular steamroller of votes. At this time there was also a reorganisation of the right-wing factional organisation

Labour First with Roger Godsiff and John Spellar as organisers.[46] It was flexible in form and with no clear membership but it fed an additional organisational assistance behind the Leader which continued all the way to Blair.

But support for Kinnock's party management from the unions was never as solid as it had been in the old days of the classic party management model. The most striking deviance from the past heyday of the loyalist block vote was that Kinnock's acknowledged ascendancy went alongside continuing unpublicised reverses at the party conference. At the four conferences from 1983 to 1986 there were 26 defeats for the platform. At the five conferences from 1987 to 1991 there were 23 defeats. They were a further aggravation for the advocates of a strengthened management.

However, where necessary these reverses were ignored or filtered and, crucially, this second period of Kinnock's leadership involved a series of major changes, even the securing of a majority on a new Statement of Aims and Values which clearly embraced the value of markets. In votes on key policy issues, including a fundamental change in defence policy away from unilateral nuclear disarmament and a historic change in attitudes towards rights rather than immunities in labour law, Kinnock gained important successes. With this went also a consolidation of the movement away from planning, public ownership and the producer, moving towards more diverse forms of social ownership coupled with a new acceptance of the importance of consumers and users. An important new theme from Hattersley was emphasised as the distinctive combination of social justice with economic efficiency.

The unions were also generally highly supportive of the Leader's constitutional, organisational and financial changes, and were themselves prominent in pushing some key aspects of headquarters' financial and organisational reform. All NEC statements were accepted, as was the reorganisation of head office, even where union members' interests were directly involved, and the major innovation of a National Constitutional Court. As the election came near a combination of union cooperation and adroit management meant that at the party conference of 1991 there were no defeats other than on the localised industrial dispute at Pergamon Press.

The unions: distance and contact

All national Labour politics was conducted with an eye on the Conservative enemy and their media allies. The legislation for Political Fund ballots of 1985–6 appeared initially to be a watershed in Labour politics, providing a way for union members to vote themselves out of political finances and therefore out of the party. But the case for a political voice and a political fund was strong, whatever views there were about the connection with Labour which, as it happened, had a more stable core support than was thought.[47] Powerfully presented, the case was accepted overwhelmingly

in one union after another, and over the years to follow in all Political Fund ballots. Following this the TULV organisation was changed into Trade Unionists for Labour (TUFL) which, to allay factional suspicions, on left and right, was specifically prohibited 'under any circumstances' from becoming involved in policy matters of the Party. From that union campaign came a strong indication of the fruitfulness of an organisation of communication which emphasised a two-step flow to the shop floor 'campaign contacts' and from them to the members.[48]

It was a message that was applicable to electoral as well as intra-union decision-making, but lessons from the unions were not being listened to at this stage because the direct battle with the media took all the attention and the unions were a central feature of the diagnosis of the SCA which favoured changing 'everything'.[49] An understandable preoccupation with the direct influence of the mass media meant that the modernising advisors played down the importance of the two-step, word-of-mouth flow of communication through active supporters. In the National Agents department, Joyce Gould at times despaired at the way that Phillip Gould and the SCA talked down the electoral importance of the local parties, activists and links to the unions.[50]

For his part after the NUM strike, Kinnock was conscious of the electoral dangers which would arise from being seen to be in the pockets of the unions or advocating a full return to the laws which governed industrial relations during the period of the winter of discontent. One view in the Leader's office was that unionisation would in future be less important as an electoral benefit, and any improvement in union power was likely to be a liability to the party.[51] Most of the political leadership sought to keep some public distance from the TUC and to put over the message of an independent Labour Party, free to make its own political decisions. Though the Liaison Committee remained in being till 1990 it never reclaimed its old importance. Instead the focus turned to the smaller and more discreet Contact Group with TUC leaders.

The TUC had never been happy with the role of the NEC left from 1979 to 1983, and became now generally content with the parliamentary leadership back in the driving seat. Under the Thatcher Government there had been a dramatic decline in trade union membership as well as industrial power – a consequence of mass unemployment changing occupational patterns, and remorselessly cumulative legal regulation. The loss of neo-corporatist arrangements with the government, and the diminution of access and status, hit the TUC particularly hard. They were constantly seeking ways to rebuild that position. Good cooperative relations with the Labour leadership and a future Labour Government seemed by far the best way forward.

The TUC administrators and leaders were very sensitive to public opinion on the unions and labour law and to the increased importance of the consumer. In these circumstances it accepted that a future Labour

Government must adjust but would keep up the close cooperative links with the unions, and in pursuing fairness would do its best for organised labour, working people and their social priorities. A common agenda was forged around European conceptions of social partnership in which the unions would be involved in a national economic-industrial dialogue with employers' organisations and the government. In that shift was the union belief that European social partnership legislation could advance labour interests and help protect British workers from Tory policies.

There were regular and close office contacts particularly between Charles Clarke, head of Kinnock's office, and John Monks, head of the organisation department and later the Deputy General Secretary of the TUC. Whilst preserving its public autonomy the TUC, anticipating and influencing the build-up of union mandates for the party conference, was able to play a back-door role in encouraging union policy in the right direction, accepting union balloting laws and limits on secondary action and secondary picketing, and acting as path-makers in assisting a shift in the party towards greater acceptance of Britain's place in Europe. These shared perspectives and the trust and cooperation at office level provided an extra underpinning of party management.

Over union support for the closed shop, in December 1989 the background links between Tony Blair, who was the Shadow Secretary of State for Employment, and John Monks eased acceptance of Blair's declaration of support for the outlawing of the closed shop and his determination to carry it through. The move received backing also from union general secretaries Ron Todd and John Edmonds, but the NEC's People at Work policy group, which includes print-union representatives Gordon Colling and Tony Dubbins, were not consulted.[52] For them this was a bounce with an implicit dare to publicly challenge it, which they did not take up. The circumventing of NEC union representation was to have longer-term repercussions, provoking a call later for affiliated unions to have their own collective representation on policy, independent of the TUC. That would ultimately have a significant effect on controversial developments in the Labour Party under Blair.

Still, the general new receptivity of the unions was shown at the 1990 TUC Congress, when a strong combined push of the TUC and the Labour leadership produced a historic shift in labour-law policy away from supporting collective freedom and legal immunities to acceptance of a legislative framework of rights based on 'fairness not favours'. This involved a major adjustment of the conventional 'rule' of the relationship which prohibited legal or political interventions in industrial relations. Accompanied by a new emphasis on individual employees' rights rather than institutional rights, it was followed by similar policies at the party conferences of 1990 and 1991. Now legal rights, it was thought, would be fundamental in potential gains over union recognition, rights of union-membership protection against victimisation, acceptance of a statutory minimum wage and also of the European Social Charter. But that shift to rights as social justice left open some tricky disagreements over the enforcement of the legal framework and the content of the rights.

Whilst these changes were taking place, moving the Labour Party towards what Blair after Smith would eventually inherit, many of the old 'rules' and protocols of the relationship reinforcing trust and common purpose were still upheld from both wings. Advance consultation was the norm. The rules and protocols of territorial areas continued to distinguish the independent political role of the TUC, as well as protecting the political autonomy of the party from the TUC. They also still protected the autonomy of individual unions from political interference.

The unions exerted no financial sanctions and even in order to assist an appeal from the party went so far as to change the terms of their financial engagement, holding up the level of their affiliation, sometimes artificially, and as usual with no policy payoff. It was a practice which in some unions had the affect of further distorting the link with the number of levy payers. The unions in 1988, encouraged by Whitty, also sought to end the traditional 'begging bowl' arrangement for the general election fund and base it on regular subventions from affiliation fees.[53] Through this they sought both assured income for the party and the avoidance of accusations of union control. Ad hoc financial support for the frontbench politicians and the Leader's office also had an insulating wall placed there by the unions for the same reason.

Through the commission of enquiry into party organisation in 1980, the unions had accepted then that the party had been over-reliance on unions' funds and called both for state financing of political parties and a new attempt at diversification of income. In 1988, that was taken further. The unions initiated and supported the Whitty-Mainwaring business plan which underwrote attempts to secure a wider base of individual donors. It was on these foundations that there would come later, under Blair, very large high-value donor contributions. Gala dinners were held to raise money from the wealthy. As for the party members, the unions also proposed and helped finance a national membership system established in 1990 from which fundraising would be easier. At the time it was not clear how far this would in future centralise and intensify party management.

Return to the OMOV agenda

However, attempts at constitutional change involving the party position of the unions continued to be problematic as well as divisive within the unions. In 1987 Kinnock had proposed an electoral college which would introduce OMOV in the CLP section, but with the affiliated organisation section casting a maximum of 40 per cent of the vote in the established way. This carried the conference, yet Kinnock himself began to have doubts about it. The college proved controversial in drawing attention to union branches which were often not in healthy activity, and to the weak linkage between union affiliation and political commitment. They included, as before, levy-paying by union members who were not even party supporters. On the other hand, the criticism of union-branch life was challenged with a survey by Martin Upham and Tom Wilson which showed the vast majority of affiliated branches made their decision at a branch meeting after looking at written details.[54] This strengthened the defence of the electoral college on grounds of inclusivity in a party losing its manual-working-class representation in the PLP and in the CLPs. Keeping the linkage of a broad section of otherwise politically uninvolved working-class opinion became an important element in the wider argument over the union-party relationship.

Party management: new controls and old limitations

After an investigation, the NEC pushed by Kinnock supported expulsions against Militant members of the Liverpool District Labour Party, and moves later to expel members of another Trotskyist group, Socialist Organiser. The fact that organisations worked behind the newspaper subterfuge from what was regarded as an alien ideological and moral tradition hardened the Leader's stance. But the task of dealing with so many expulsions involved attendance by the leadership at the NEC in time-consuming activity. Disciplinary functions carried out by the NEC were producing increasing problems in the face of an interventionist judiciary determined to uphold natural justice.

In response, the party redrafted its disciplinary code so that its judicial functions were passed after 1986 to a new institution with eleven members, the National Constitutional Committee acting as a final court of appeal, elected annually by procedures which, like the conference, involved a trade union majority of seven members. Under the new rules, rights of appeal to the party conference over expulsions were narrowed.[55] NCC activities were generally not reported in the press and in term of publicity that whole area of management became a silent zone. The NEC still had powers to discipline Labour Party organisations which did not conform to the rules. It retained various rights in terms of candidate selection including the right to withhold endorsement.[56] It also created the new offence of a sustained course of conduct prejudicial to the party.

There was also a shift towards more central control of by-election candidates after the loss of the Greenwich by-election in 1987 and Glasgow Govan in 1988. Both candidates had been from the left and both were assailed mercilessly by the 'loony-left' chasing press. In 1989, the NEC was now given the power through a by-elections panel to determine the short-list. It involved testing a candidate's capacity to meet the various challenges of a high-profile election but over the years it also became a means of political sifting, keeping off the unacceptable. After 1988, in the Leader's office, new staff member Neil Stewart took on responsibility for the political management of by-elections, the NEC, the Conference and Militant. This also extended to playing a discreet role in relation to candidate selection.

Nevertheless, in the light of the later development of party management under Blair, it is important to note that, as Shaw pointed out, the principles and practices of the liberal regime were not all reversed.[57] The headquarters staff generally limited managerial interventions. They drew an important line between attitudes towards the mainstream party left and to the Trotskyists, although at times this was a loose and pejorative term. Larry Whitty, National Organiser Joyce Gould and Deputy National Organiser Jean Corston still generally adhered to the Ron Hayward code of impartiality. They resisted pressure from elsewhere within the machine for a change of behaviour, and at times intervened to assert their perspective against party officials working to the older interventionist code. Their view, shared by Kinnock, was that although the party's civil service was not something detached from the party and always bore in mind consideration of the party interest, it was vital to emphasise sustaining trust and respect for rules.

Yet after 1989 the Leader's office did discreetly work to arrangements with regional allies in the unions, seeking to ensure that in political as well as capability terms there was a good spread of candidates, women as well as men. But the fear that personal support from the Leader would rebound if the favoured prospective candidate was not selected was always an inhibition on obviously placing a candidate. Kinnock was still uncomfortable in being seen to abandon his differentiation from the political reputation of what was regarded in the past as the machinations of the authoritarian right. In these circumstances loyalist union leaders in some of the regions, particularly the north-east, sometimes took their own sympathetic initiative in seeking to organise parliamentary support for the Leader.

Although officials privately reported that as the 1992 General Election approached a new desperation led to some cutting of corners, here, as in other areas, management intervention was restricted in its form and extent, part of a complicated politics with fine lines to walk and awareness of potentially significant political costs. That applied also to the composition of the machine. The officials still had a strong National Union of Labour Organisers, which in sentiment and values was close to the loyalist traditional right. But it could lay down lines of protection of its own members. The attempt by the Leader, in 1990, to get rid of the London organiser Terry Ashton failed in the face of coordinated opposition from that union.

Party management and the PLP

In the PLP, after the miners strike ended in 1985 and the PLP moved into a new era of emphasis on the priority of winning the general election, there were new developments which strengthened the Leader. The front bench was expanded during this period from around 40 to more than 60 by

1987,[58] and the Shadow Cabinet, which had 12 members for a long time, had risen to 18 by 1989.[59] Under the increasing dominance of the Leader, the Shadow Cabinet elections also moved to the right. In 1989 critics Brian Gould and Meacher came off. Blair and Brown who had become MPs and Kinnock loyalists in 1983, but developing their own perspectives, came on. Their alliance with Mandelson became more central to future party developments as Brown and Mandelson became mentors to Blair over the politics of the party, its organisation and its media presentation.

With the Leader seeking room for manoeuvre in industrial-relations policies and a rapidly changing social composition of the PLP and of trade union representatives themselves, the PLP trade union group activities went into decline. The now loyalist Tribune Group had lost its *raison d'être*, and under the influence of Blair and Brown and other Kinnock loyalists it was allowed to become moribund. Still, Kinnock seriously engaged with the PLP meetings, behaving as he did in the pressurised NEC meetings, arguing, exhorting, intervening continually, returning to the point, and arguing again. He preferred that oratorical mode of political operation amongst colleagues, and as a past parliamentary rebel himself remained a strong supporter of the Crossman-Silkin tradition of management, seeing it as integral to the process of generating self-discipline.

According to Nick Brown, a later Chief Whip under Blair, Kinnock had 'repeatedly encouraged the whips' office to adopt a more open, more cooperative and less coercive approach to the question of party management'.[60] There was no PLP disciplinary action for deviant voting behaviour in the House even though, when it happened, he reacted with an anger which some saw as bullying. Around the Leader, no obvious discussion of an extension of sanctions took place. Only Ron Brown was subject to suspension and that was for an extravagant demonstrative incident with the mace for which he refused to apologise.

Contests and insulation of the leadership

The Campaign Group of Labour MPs, heir to the Bennite tradition and renamed the Socialist Campaign Group, was weakened by a series of de-alignments away from their version of the left. Continuing frustration that they were unable to stop Kinnock moving away from past positions led eventually in 1988 to the Campaign Group initiating a leadership election with Benn and Heffer as candidates for Leader and Deputy Leader Their defeat was overwhelming. They received only 11.37 per cent for the Leader and 9.483 per cent for the Deputy. Prescott, who also stood independently as Deputy, emphasised the importance of the party, building its membership and the morale of activists. It was to become his big project all the way through to Blair's election but he could not make headway in a left v leadership contest and gained only 23.7 per cent of the vote.

Predictably the defeat of the left further strengthened Kinnock and Hattersley. What this protracted contest also indicated to many in the union leadership as well as in the PLP was that such contests should be rare and if possible avoided. There was little opposition when the rules were changed to raise the threshold for nominations from 10 to 20 per cent, thereby further adding to the management constraints in launching a challenge. After this major defeat the Campaign Group shared in an increasingly self-disciplined avoidance of public conflict which made party management easier.

Leadership, party activists and the new constitutional radicalism

The voting in this leadership election revealed some important differences in the voting patterns of activists and members. The overwhelming evidence was that the wider the franchise in the CLPs, the more likely the parties were to vote for Kinnock and Hattersley.[61] That information gave a further push towards OMOV of the party members, added to a downgrading of the role of the activists and stimulating an emboldened new modernising radical movement prodding the Leader. The formally independent Institute for Public Policy Research created in 1989 by Lord Hollick and Patricia Hewitt, with Hewitt as Deputy Director, in practice worked in close and discreet cooperation with the Leader. It took on the role of a platform for serious outriders for new policy initiatives, new political relationships and various initiatives, in Hewitt's description 'to get ahead of the game', in the electoral war.[62] Hewitt with Philip Gould later moved into the central management of the 1992 election campaign.

The activist Labour Coordinating Committee, though it had been founded by the left in 1978, had by 1987 became the home of a new realism about socio-political change and the policies needed to deal with it. It became a vehicle for attitudes and ideas which fed into what later became 'New Labour'. At its most constructive, the organisation could look self-critically and honestly at the culture of the left and the condition of the party, seeking to open up the local parties and to raise the level of membership participation as part of radical modernisation. At its least constructive it became the vehicle of a careless modernising rhetoric from which leading members thrilled to their own apostasy, sometimes without much questioning of the political costs. That also would feed into the groundwork of 'New Labour'. It did not have the grass-roots activist organisation that CLPD had had at its height, but it had drive and dynamism and it had close links to the Labour front bench including Blair, who was himself a member of the LCC as was Cherie Booth (Blair). Though it continued as a pressure group it also became a friendly agency of party management through which was initiated a range of proposals for reform including OMOV which LCC had opposed in 1984.

Bottom-up pressure and top-down management

At this stage also, in 1988, the regular instigation of party conference resolutions from sympathisers was re-established in a more organised form in party headquarters. In 1989, the acceptance of a management-influenced composite and omnibus resolution, Composite 3, moved by the modernising union leader Edmonds for the GMB and backed by LCC, called on the NEC to consult widely and report to the 1990 Conference on a range of policy-making reforms. This now enabled Kinnock to re-engage with the issue of OMOV. In the CLP support for the principle of OMOV was spreading but it was not a uniform movement. It varied in support according to the institutional focus of the reform and the procedural choices available. OMOV reform became a mix of top-down and bottom-up forces and the mix was at its most top-down over the issue of election of the NEC.

The CLP section of the NEC had never been as consistently oppositional in its representation as its left-wing reputation suggested. There had been a regular loyalist representation and always a celebrity, personality and publicity factor in voting and with them a spread of non-factional votes. Nevertheless, this was the section where in the past the party had registered publicly its changing political alignments in the glare of the publicity covering the party conference, where the annual results were announced. From seats on the NEC, alternative left-wing leaders could lay down public markers and make a distinctive stand which drew party attention. Changing the NEC election procedures to give the Leader what was thought would be more assured CLP support became a priority as the General Election drew near.

But on this it was found that there was not the reform enthusiasm in the CLPs as had been evoked by OMOV in leadership elections or in candidate selection procedure.[63] In the consultation of 1990 on NEC elections, only nineteen CLPs responded, and the interpretation of the result was contested (depending on whether branch responses were given equal status to that of General Committee responses[64]). Proposing the change for the NEC, Richard Rosser made no mention of the consultation. Nevertheless with strong union support, organised by the trade union right through Godsiff and Spellar, the proposed rule change making it a mandatory requirement for CLPs to conduct local OMOV ballots to decide how their NEC votes would be cast went through by 4,341,000 votes to 551,000. This was Kinnock's first victory over OMOV. (For a similar victory in 1993 in relation to the form of voting for the NEC, see Chapter 3, pp. 99–100.) Its initial effects on NEC voting seemed to confirm a loyalist advantage from the change in that in 1991 right-winger Gerald Kaufman came on to replace left-winger Jo Richardson, and Benn's vote declined, but the pattern was not clear cut. The vote of left-wing activist hero Dennis Skinner's rose.

Yet on proposals for reform of the NEC composition to make it more representative of a range of party identities and collectivities, Kinnock and his managers were themselves unenthusiastic, given his increasing robust personal support in the union group. In 1989 the otherwise influential 1989 composite 3 from the GMB, accepted by the platform, included reforming the NEC composition, but this was ignored. The suggestion that there should also be election of local party officers and delegates to the party conference by ballots of members were not proceeded with because of practical problems which produced local resistance. These included financial costs, communicating knowledge of the candidates, the organisational time factor and also the difficulty of involving local affiliated organisations or of excluding them.

Women's representation

A movement for positive discrimination in women's representation eventually and crucially fed into Blair's party management. It began as a genuine bottom-up exercise pushed first by the Labour Women's Action Committee (LWAC), created in 1983 by the Campaign for Labour Party Democracy. Their proposals for the NEC women's section to be elected by the women's conference and for one woman on every parliamentary short list were read and opposed by the Kinnock leadership as an attempt to strengthen the left. Yet that was only a part of an agenda which increasingly gained non-factional women's support in all sections of the party.

By 1988 the NEC was forced to submit and gain conference authority for a rule change supporting the one woman on every parliamentary short list. Another proposal also from LWAC for a measure of all-women short lists in selections after an MP's retirement and in by-elections, met initial intra-party opposition and again leadership opposition but also gained increasing support. Electoral pressures, and international examples of quota representation, now began to coalesce with managerial moves to counter the influence of the left through the women's organisation. A reformed women's conference in 1989 called for 40 per cent quotas for women at local and national levels of the party. This was brought into the party's rules at the 1991 party conference. Phased changes began to radically improve NEC and conference representation of women and the changes had important managerial effects at the conference under Blair, as will be shown.

The unions: reform and management agendas

Block vote: the unions as radicals

Both in terms of reducing the unions' voting preponderance and facilitating the splitting of union votes, reforming the block vote had been a part of the background agenda of reform of the party conference for many years. Much attention was paid to the inadequacies of the unions' own internal democratic processes and how they linked with that of the party. There were question marks also about the accuracy of the affiliation system, the political sensitivity of the mandating system and the degree to which votes cast in the Labour Party policy process reflected up-to-date views of the general body of union members. This scrutiny and criticism were most acute when union votes were cast against the views of the leadership. Much less attention was given to the regular important management efforts to win the unions away from their mandates and commitments when they stood in the way, whether supported from below or not.

In a context of new awareness of Labour's need to adjust its electoral appeal and encourage CLP membership, a movement for reform had built up by 1988 such that amongst union leaders a consensus had grown that this was the time for reform. The Leader and his aides were not convinced that that would assist the immediate priorities of party management. In 1989, in a card vote the block vote was used to defeat composite 4 which was against abolition of the block vote.[65]

The trajectory of reform opinion seemed to be moved towards a partnership of 50:50 affiliated organisation and CLPs, although there was a second and growing body of opinion that it might be better moved to a re-composition of the conference bringing in the PLP. In the 1990 NEC consultation the 40 (affiliated organisations): 30 (CLPs): 30 (PLP) option received the largest body of CLP organisational support. That seemed to be the option which would gain most consensual support on speedy reform, with the advantage of bringing the PLP and the conference into a closer interaction, enhancement of the policy role of the PLP yet also boosting the significance of conference decisions.

However, change here was again held up more by the uncertainty of the Leader than the resistance of the unions. In discussions between the union leaders, the General Secretary and the Leader it was agreed that reform would come by stages after the General Election. Meanwhile, a proposal that the union vote be reduced from around 90 per cent to 70 per cent was agreed by the NEC on 25 April 1990 with trade union group backing, and then was supported by the conference.

Governing with the party

A development that was to move to central importance in the party under Smith and then Blair, as what later became known as Partnership in Power, also emerged at this time but with varied purposes envisaged. In discussion between Kinnock, Whitty, Clarke and Stewart of the problems of past Labour governments, the concern grew that there would again emerge a gulf between party policy and that of the government with a damaging display of disunity that would attract media attention. The union role was central to this concern. With only weak consultative mechanisms there would be no way to avoid the build-up of antagonistic mandates. So the search was on for those mechanisms which might be more participatory but also more effective party management and media management devices.

The possibility of a radical reform was helped here by a broad agreement that the present policy-making procedures were utterly inadequate, particularly when compared with what the party and trade union leaders had seen of the continental social-democratic processes. Out of this discussion came the idea of a rolling party programme building on the work of a new institution, a national policy forum together with standing policy commissions, which would give new opportunities for a joint policy-making dialogue with the members.

The policy process envisaged was complicated and so was the process of producing it. On 7–8 April 1990, at Northern College, Larry Whitty chaired a small informal seminar on his new proposals attended by NEC members, Margaret Beckett, Diana Jeuda and Clare Short, and also Lewis Minkin.[66] It worked through the details and the possible problems before proposals went to the NEC. In an important development, the initial outline was seen at that meeting as an over-centralised version. This led to an argument over how far the deliberative policy process leading up to a conference would result in a consensual or contested policy and what opportunities there could be for amendment and a late stage of submissions. No firm conclusions were reached,[67] but, following other soundings, a document prepared by Whitty, *Democracy and Policymaking for the 1990s*, which agreed the new process in principle, did include the commitment to 'options and where appropriate minority reports' coming from the National Policy Forum. This would become a feature heavily contended and managed later under Blair.

Presentation of the proposed new arrangements at the party conferences of 1990 and 1991 was marked by some grandiose claims of a future transformation in the role of the ordinary party members. Tom Sawyer, winding up the debate for the NEC in 1990 said, 'there will be a dominant role in the policy forum and the policy commissions for you, not for the platform'.[68] The Campaign for Labour Party Democracy, on the other hand, diagnosed a potentially dangerous subversion of traditional party democracy. In the GMB and the TGWU, both unions sympathetic to the proposals, there was a determination that the NEC should not be sidelined and its accountability to the party conference should be protected. Pressure on this resulted in the document being hardened up as it went through the NEC. In view of what happened later, under Blair, special note should be made that at the conference, Whitty was emphatic that 'The policymaking structure would be entirely run by the National Executive Committee which would retain its constitutional authority'.[69] There was no mention at this stage of a Joint Policy Committee created later under Smith and through which Blair eventually took over the NEC policy role.

What the Whitty plan would have been like in practice as a participatory or managerial exercise is not clear. Plans for the constitutional changes became ever more complex. Kinnock himself developed doubts about their workability, and by 1992 with increased tensions affecting relations with the GMB Leader (see p. 77) he was beginning to have deeper doubts about a process which potentially tied the Labour Government into detailed party-union discussions which might challenge the primacy of the government. The positive scenario of cooperative working relations with the unions became superseded by one that was more negative and beset by distrust. Eventually the whole thing was put to one side until after the General Election.

Getting ahead of the game

The distrust arose because although the trade union question had been of marginal observable significance in Labour's 1987 defeat,[70] at the edges of the policy review, new questions were now being raised about the future of the relationship. The belief that the interests of capital and labour were no longer in conflict led to a view amongst modernising radicals that Labour Party association with the unions was inappropriate for its future electoral identity. Around Blair, Brown and Mandelson, it was not the enhanced power of the Leader and the unprecedented expansion of his office that was emphasised – as it was generally amongst observers. The radicals focused on the exceptions, qualifications and limitations to that power, especially those produced by the unions. That, to them, was the real story.

Any defeat at all was seen as a public disadvantage. Any uncircumscribed powers could become a potential problem. Any problem not under control could be a media embarrassment. Any protracted consultation was an attrition of leadership energy. Any inhibitive traditional rules and customs were an obstacle to effective executive power. Power relations in the party still involved an element of pluralism and the constitution of the party could not be changed without a union majority. Watching as a shadow minister, Blair was developing a determination to secure wholesale change,[71] with a particular emphasis on dealing with the union role.[72]

Challenging that relationship in its entirety was not an easy task and amongst many Labour loyalists it was not considered sensible. Not only were the unions part of the collective movement that had given 'a thousand years of Kinnocks' their platform, but they had been a practical source of party unity and stability and on the NEC the base of his management. To the party they still gave a permanent supportive electoral base and with it means of communication, organisation and financial support. It was the normality of the politics of administering the Labour Party that if they had any special difficulties, organisational, communicational or financial, they could turn to the unions for assistance. This they did in dozens of small ways.

Nevertheless personal relations of some of the senior union leaders, particularly with Charles Clarke, were often difficult and marked on occasions by mutual disrespect. On some policy issues the unions induced a long struggle, on the environment for example, and over union balloting or defence expenditure. On the issue of a bill of rights, divisions amongst the politicians and opposition from the unions to the enhanced role of the judiciary pulled that to a shuddering halt. Further, in supporting industrial disputes, the NEC – though careful in its statements – sometimes went further than the parliamentary leadership preferred. There was a regular concern over the electoral costs of disputes sometimes linked by the press to the stigma of the winter of discontent regardless of the level of public support. Over an industrial dispute at News International, a boycott was declared by the NEC which the Leader felt obliged to support, although it caused him trouble in his relations with the media, and added to the repetitive charge that the union affiliation indicated Labour's subservience now and when the party formed a government.

On the Labour Coordinating Committee, within IPPR, in the party's campaigns and communication department, and around the SCA, those in discussions about the unions were often looking to clean up all the problems in order 'to get ahead of the game' in electoral tactics and methods. Outriders, spinners and friendly columnists ran with the issue of a 'parting of the ways'.[73] This leading critic asserted that 'the defensible bits' amounted to 'only money and power'.[74] Out of the medley of criticism, the radical aim became firmed up as the ending of collective affiliation but seeking to expand the role of party links to trade unionists as individual members. Moderniser radicals tended not to see the extent of potential internal party opposition nor to register the immediate damage to the party that breaking affiliation might cause. They greatly underestimated the consequential political costs it would incur.

New attempts had also already been made to build better links to business. Friendly allies, led by banker Jon Norton, sought to organise business support. Smith's 'prawn cocktail campaign' to the City sought to take the edge off the City's critique of Labour's economic competence and to show a new receptivity in not restricting enterprise and in encouraging business growth. No commitments were made, although the 1992 manifesto went as far as referring to a future Labour Government 'with which business can do business'. From the fringes, however, there were much more ambitious moves. The old established Labour Finance and Industry Group, now paralleled and rivalled by the new Industry Forum, made attempts 'to open up the people's party' in bringing more business representatives to the party conference. On the outer ring of the Forum there was even a small movement of opinion towards the affiliation of business organisations to the party.

New separatism and Kinnock's response

Heavily preoccupied with focus-group findings about adverse electoral perceptions of union power and also with their own future organisational plans, the Kinnock office veered uncertainly between seeing the unions as welcome and essential allies in the search for solutions or seeing them as the big problem they had to face, especially under the next Labour government. Aware of, and feeding into, that mix of feelings around the Leader, modernising radicals began to attempt to publicise their new agenda using their command of the skills of spin. The lead-up to the 1989 party conference and its fringe contributions were heavily influenced by a stirred-up media conjecture about separation from the unions. At this conference, the LCC held a meeting under the title 'Labour and the Unions – the end of the road?' In a private conversation at that conference, a senior official from the campaigns and communications department said privately, and with complete confidence, 'Our next step is getting rid of the unions'.[75]

These noises-off produced a damaging dilemma for those in the unions generally sympathetic to reform, including Edmonds, leader of the GMB. Were the particular reforms being proposed by the Leader to be treated on their merits or received with suspicion as the thin end of the wedge? Tony Blair ignored private warnings that disavowal of separatist spin was potentially disastrous; the call for ending collective affiliation would ignite distrust in the unions and rebound against consensual plans for reform.[76] Nor was Blair much troubled by the immediate electoral response; at this time, between 1988 and 1990, the percentage of voters who thought that the unions had 'too much say in the Labour Party' had declined from 54 to 50 per cent.[77] In spite of that, he knew where the party needed to go. His conviction of the urgency and rationality of his case, a gross misreading of reactions within the party and the unions and a damaging overconfidence that media spinning skills were bound to pay off with public and party, led him and his allies astray. They now caused Kinnock huge difficulties and created a problem that would be damaging to the party and themselves for years to come.

The spin bites back

By 1990, Kinnock's office thought that he now had a majority for OMOV on the candidate-selection issue, only to be told by Edmonds that he could no longer deliver his union because of new internal pressure. In reality this was a tactical response on his part. He had become convinced that the Kinnock office was part of a network who were involved in a covert agenda of breaking with the unions.[78] Thus, two years before the huge post-election conflict, this was where Edmonds drew a 'line in the sand' and signalled his response to those playing with separation. In the meantime, the NEC's consultations over voting arrangements in 1990 produced just one CLP (out of 144 responding) favouring the unions having no vote at the Conference. Yet that blindingly obvious message was still discounted by Blair and those around him confident of their case and the ability to spin their way forward.

Meanwhile, Kinnock and Clarke at first reacted with fury at Edmonds's lack of cooperation. But warnings that the voices of separation were undermining the reformist position and reinforcing conservatism now began to be taken seriously by Kinnock, who was not himself in favour of their position.[79] Some people close to his office were guided off the separationist line they had been outriding. But it was too little, too late. The coalition for reform had been broken by the spin. There was now an impasse over reform of candidate selection. In the 1990 consultation 80 per cent of CLPs favoured ending the electoral college in selections but 91 per cent were in favour of affiliated organisations' right to nominate and to participate in the selection.[80] The conference agreed in 1990 that the final selection in the next round should be by OMOV but that 'further consideration be given to the best means of involving members of affiliated union and socialist societies in the selection process'.[81]

Edmonds, by nature a reforming radical leading a union long associated with the party's traditional right, continued to support other procedural reforms which did not directly threaten the unions' position and he went along with most of the managerial concerns. That included the beginning of a significant change in mandatory re-selection. In 1990 and 1991 the conference agreed, following a consultation, that a full re-selection contest would be triggered only after a ballot to decide whether members were satisfied with the sitting MP. It was a move with (at the time) 'the widest franchise possible'[82] which addressed the reality that three-quarters of Labour MPs had been reselected on a short list of one in the last parliament, and that most CLPs found the process unnecessary, time-consuming and costly. But it was also a move away from the general committee oversight that in the view of CLPD best sustained accountability.

The reconciliation of positions on candidate-selection reform was then pushed to one side to be reviewed after the election against the background of potentially a much deeper conflict over the identity of the party. John Prescott[83] gave a private warning, which senior party officials and union leaders were also picking up from their own sources, of the signs of a post-election assault on the unions expected from the Blair-Brown-Mandelson stable. In response, one proposal that emerged was that in the pre-election period in 1992, backed by the major unions, a discussion of 'The Contentious Alliance' should be the focus of a pre-emptive conference on reform within support of the union-party relationship. This was called off, at Minkin's suggestion, because it would give the right-wing media an eve of election gift which could be further exploited by separationists to launch their campaign. Calling it off, as it turned out, was a wrong decision. The modernisers' crusade was going ahead regardless.

Notes

1 LPCR 1979, p. 189. The annual verbatim conference report underwent changes of name over the years. It is here referred to throughout by the abbreviation LPCR.
2 Dianne Hayter, *Fightback!: Labour's Traditional Right in the 1970s and 1980s*, Manchester University Press, 2005, pp. 116–17.
3 LPCR 1979, pp. 263 and 271.
4 LPCR 1979, pp. 260–2.
5 LPCR 1979, pp. 310 and 312.
6 *New Statesman*, 8 October 1982.

7 This is discussed at length in Minkin, *Contentious Alliance*, pp. 192–3 and pp. 195–6.

8 LPCR 1979, p. 214.

9 Minkin, *Contentious Alliance*, p. 496 and LPCR 1980, p. 210.

10 Minkin, *Contentious Alliance*, p. 201.

11 This is described in more detail in Minkin, *Contentious Alliance*, p. 202.

12 Haytor, *Fightback*, p. 229.

13 Ibid. p. 91 and p. 136.

14 Composite resolution no. 34, LPCR 1981, p. 199.

15 Minkin, *Contentious Alliance*, p. 202.

16 Composite resolution no. 35, LPCR 1981, p. 205.

17 LPCR 1981, p. 206 and p. 210.

18 LPCR 1981, p. 210 and p. 212.

19 John Grant MP, member of Labour Solidarity campaign before defecting to the SDP, *Guardian*, 3 March 1981.

20 John Bochel and David Denver, 'Candidate Selection and the Labour Party: What the Selectors Seek', *British Journal of Political Science*, 13(1), 1983, p. 58.

21 Interview with Vladimir Derer, 1981.

22 Leo Panitch and Colin Leys, *The End of Parliamentary Socialism: From New Left to New Labour*, Verso, London, 1997, p. 195, quoting leading activist Jon Lansman.

23 MORI polling February 1979, during the winter of discontent, had shown huge majorities amongst trade unionists for these changes.

24 John Golding, *Hammer of the Left: Defeating Tony Benn, Eric Heffer and Militant in the Battle for the Labour Party*, Politico's, London, 2003; Dianne Hayter, *Fightback!*, also 'The Fightback of the Traditional Right in the Labour Party', PhD, University of London, 2005, especially pp. 98–162.

25 Minkin, *Contentious Alliance*, pp. 324–8.

26 Ibid. pp. 202–5.

27 Ibid. pp. 328–30.

28 Richard Heffernan and Mike Marquesee, *Defeat from the Jaws of Victory: Inside Kinnock's Labour Party*, Verso, London, 1992, p. 27.

29 Minkin, *Conference*, p. 335.

30 Hayter, 'Fightback', PhD, p. 48.

31 Philip Gould, *The Unfinished Revolution: How the Modernisers Changed the Labour Party*, Little Brown, London, 1998, p. 25.

32 Eric Hobsbawm, 'Forward March of Labour Halted?', Marx Memorial Lecture, 1978 reproduced in *Marxism Today*, September 1978.

33 Lewis Minkin, 'Against the Tide', in Ivor Crewe and Martin Harrop, *Political Communications: the General Election Campaign of 1983*, Cambridge University Press, Cambridge, 1986, pp. 190–206.

34 Nita Clarke, responsible for public relations at the GLC, was only narrowly defeated for the post of Communications Director in 1985.

35 Philip Gould and Associates, *Communications Review*, 20 December 1985.

36 Jennifer Lees-Marshment, *Political Marketing and British Political Parties: the Party's Just Begun*, Manchester University Press, 2001, pp. 134–80 for the sections on Kinnock.

37 Peter Mandelson, *The Third Man: Life at the Heart of New Labour*, Harper, London, 2010, p. 83.
38 Colin Hughes and Patrick Wintour, *Labour Rebuilt: The New Model Party*, Fourth Estate, London, 1990, p. 183.
39 I relayed the Blumler observations and their significance to Mandelson at the 1985 conference.
40 Michael Foley, *The British Presidency: Tony Blair and the Politics of Public Leadership*, Manchester University Press, Manchester, 2000, p. 79.
41 Heffernan and Marquesee, *Defeat from Victory*, pp. 75–8.
42 John Rentoul, *Tony Blair: Prime Minister*, Little Brown, London, 2001, pp. 171–3.
43 Heather Savigny, 'Focus Groups and Political Marketing: Science and Democracy as Axiomatic?', *BJPIR*, 9(1), February, 2007, pp. 122–37.
44 Tony Blair, *A Journey*, Hutchinson, London, 2010, p. 298.
45 Peter Mandelson and Roger Liddle, *The Blair Revolution: Can New Labour Deliver?* Faber & Faber, London, 1996, pp. 104–7 and p. 114.
46 Hayter, *Fightback!*, p. 97.
47 Minkin, *Contentious Alliance*, pp. 566–9.
48 Lewis Minkin, 'Mobilisation and Distance: The Role of Trade Unions in the 1987 General Election Campaign', in Ivor Crewe and Martin Harrop (eds), *Political Communications: The General Election Campaign of 1987*, Cambridge University Press, Cambridge, 1989, pp. 261–74. Also Minkin, *Contentious Alliance*, Chapter 17, pp. 544–61.
49 Deborah Mattinson, *Talking to a Brick Wall: How New Labour Stopped Listening to the Voter and Why We Need a New Politics*, Backbite, London, 2010, p. 36.
50 Interview in 1989 with Joyce Gould, then Director of Organisation, who had been National Agent of the Labour Party during the successful Political Fund Ballot campaigns.
51 John Eatwell, Economic adviser to the Labour Leader, Memo PD 1205, December 1987.
52 Martin Westlake, *Kinnock, The Biography*, Little, Brown and Company, London, 2001, p. 336.
53 Minkin, *Contentious Alliance*, p. 537.
54 *Tribune*, 6 June 1990.
55 Shaw, *Discipline and Discord*, p. 283.
56 Ibid. pp. 280–1.
57 Ibid. p. 301.
58 Andy McSmith, *Faces of Labour: The Inside Story*, Verso, London, 1996, p. 20.
59 Ibid. p. 25.
60 Nick Brown, *Fabian Review*, August/September, 1996.
61 Hughes and Wintour, *Labour Rebuilt*, p. 92, from figures compiled by Jeannette Gould.
62 Interview with Patricia Hewitt, 1993.
63 Confirmed to me by Larry Whitty, October 2006.
64 Conference edition, *Campaign for Labour Party Democracy*, October 1990.
65 Minkin, *Contentious Alliance*, p. 365.

66 Meg Russell's meticulous study *Building New Labour: the Politics of Party Organisation*, Palgrave Macmillan, Basingstoke, 2005, p. 33, note 18, is unusually misinformed about those who took part in this meeting. It was significant that there was nobody there from, or representing, the Leader's office; Clarke and Sawyer were not there. Nobody 'facilitated' the occasionally heated discussions; as head of the host college, Bob Fryer provided the hospitality facilities.

67 Diary, and my own observations.

68 Tom Sawyer, LPCR 1990, p. 119.

69 Larry Whitty, LPCR 1991, p. 101.

70 Ivor Crewe, *Guardian*, 16 June 1987 and Gallop Political Index, July 1987, Table 72.

71 Mandelson and Liddle, *The Blair Revolution*, p. 39.

72 Derived from comments in interview with Tony Blair, 21 August 1989.

73 The most influential and thoroughly argued case was presented by John Lloyd, in *Marxism Today*, March 1998.

74 Ibid. p. 39.

75 Meeting with me at the rear of the conference hall.

76 This point was made very strongly to Blair in my interview on 21 August 1989. Unusually for a man normally anxious to persuade, he did not engage with my criticism of media management damage. I was left with the impression that he thought that he could spin his way to victory.

77 *Gallop/Daily Telegraph*, 4 September 1988 and 3 March 1989, Gallop Political Index, August 1990.

78 Interview with John Edmonds, 10 November 2003.

79 Both Kinnock and Charles Clarke were very supportive of the reformist view taken in the Contentious Alliance. Kinnock made a point of ensuring that a representative of his office attended the launch.

80 John Evans (NEC), LPCR 1990, p. 11.

81 Ibid.

82 Tom Burlison (NEC), LPCR 1991, p. 12.

83 Discussion after the launch of *The Contentious Alliance*, 3 October 1991.

3

Contentious alliance, OMOV and the management of democratic renewal

Smith, Party management and 'the unions'

Trauma

The 1992 General Election result was a profound disappointment to the Labour Party and for some it was a trauma. Since the devastating defeat of 1983 the position had improved under Kinnock, but only from 27.6 per cent of the vote to 34.4 per cent of the vote. He immediately resigned and, in elections for his successor, John Smith and Margaret Beckett became Leader and Deputy Leader. There was enormous gratitude for what Kinnock had done towards the recovery, but Smith was widely welcomed as potentially a more electorally effective Leader. His ethical concerns were impressive and his personal presentation was reassuringly professional without being flamboyant. However, to the increasingly prominent and coherently focused political force on Labour's right led by Blair, Brown, Mandelson, Hewitt and Philip Gould, who now more openly took to themselves the label of 'the modernisers', Smith lacked the urgency and radicalism demanded by Labour's deeper predicament, beginning with 'the union problem' arising from the contentious alliance.

The modernisers and transformation

The union problem and modernisation objectives

The public advocacy of Smith as Leader by some of the union leaders had elicited a strong reaction from modernisers and their press allies which focused on the failure of union leaders to consult their members before announcing their support. Criticism then moved on to the power that the union leaders held within the party. Though the explosion of concern about relations with the unions had an element of spontaneity born out of the depressed 'where can we go now' mood, it was also a pre-planned assault. To this was added an element of deflection protecting Kinnock and the managers from criticisms of the failed campaign in which Gould and Hewitt especially had worked with a high degree of independence of the party's institutions.

What was unusual about the 1992 modernising tendency was that although they were essentially centrists with a yearning for electoral success, they developed an unusually Bolshevik attitude to their historic role and an attraction to the virtue of fundamental party change.[1] The immediate focus was on one-member-one-vote in candidate selection and leadership elections and a radical reform of the block vote of the unions at the Party Conference. But complicating all dealings with the unions, and what made the resultant crisis so deep, were the repetitive signals that the calls for OMOV should lead as quickly as possible to the greater objective which would involve a total organisational transformation based on one-member-one-vote, shedding collective affiliated membership entirely.

Amongst those who moved towards the idea of an organisational separation, there were different views on the stages and methods of its development. Leading modernisers were generally more publicly circumspect than some of their supporters or the media spin about their objectives. Nevertheless, as noted, the separatist aim had been privately clarified and this message had passed outwards. The party should build up this individual membership (as Blair was doing in his own constituency of Sedgefield) to make it representative of the community, and this would include many individual union members.

Epitomising a weakness that would accompany later reform proposals under Blair's leadership, their attraction to the idea of dealing with the union problem by ending collective affiliation was at the expense of a sensitive analysis of its collateral damage and its consequences. As the spin-driven campaign by advocates of a separation went into confident overdrive convinced that it spoke for the party or soon would do so, it undermined the trust that was essential for the more evolutionary changes which Smith proposed.

Reform and party management

The overwhelming character of the crisis forced Smith to make the union issue more of a priority than he initially preferred. He became fully persuaded of the need for OMOV in candidate selection and at this stage considered that future leadership elections must involve only a one-member-one-vote ballot of party members plus the representation of MPs. The unions would have to come out of the arrangement. But this was not a dogmatic position and he saw advantages in the evidence of enthusiastic participation he had encountered in his own election of the wider franchise. His main preoccupation was with winning on the central issue of OMOV in candidate selection, managing an honourable and viable settlement overall and then encouraging the closing down of constitutional argument. After that he and the party could concentrate on policy and campaigning.

He saw himself as pro-union in the sense that he accepted that they were 'an estate of the realm' and for a time he visualised a future Labour Government reintroducing a national economic forum in which the unions would be full partners. Although there was no high-profile TUC-Labour Party Liaison Committee after 1992, the Contact Group was kept in operation, linking the political and industrial leadership. Smith would probably have lived within the 'rules' and protocols of traditional party-union relations. He was very well schooled in the historic union ballast role and personally he had always had a good relationship with the union leaders whom he regarded as 'friends'. On that basis, and with an emphasis on being straight and securing mutual respect, he believed that he could persuade the union leaders to accept the specific changes. But he hardened his responses as his position came to be severely challenged by some of the union leaders as well as the modernisers.

Smith saw no attraction in a new presidentialism and was uninterested in plebiscitarian leadership. As for spin, glamour and glitz, he recognised the importance of modern communications and went along with the basics of what was necessary to project the party as a professionally competent organisation. But he did not encourage a cult of the personality nor was he enamoured of a heavy influential role of communications staff advisers and consultants in policy-making decisions. In general, as he said later, he 'did not like the black arts of public relations that's taken over politics'.[2] The Shadow Communications Agency was wound up and with it the focus-group routines. A new low-profile advertising agency was brought in to advise. Peter Mandelson, Philip Gould and his co-worker Deborah Mattinson found themselves out in the cold.

Smith recognised that leadership involved the responsibility to initiate and commit in public as well as in private, but he also saw the value of his own low-key style epitomising managerial competence and trust, encouraging collegiate cohesion and keeping different groups on board. That was to be a central element in the management of the party at the top as well as in the wider party. In relations with his senior colleagues he took for granted the need to organise some leadership balance between left and right and to make tactical accommodations in achieving party cohesion.

In this search for cohesion, as Leader he was not averse to modernising changes in policy. Although Blair and Brown were sometimes in a minority of the Shadow Cabinet, they had relative freedom to operate. With their new agenda, their energy and their media contacts they drove some policy initiatives accepted by Smith to counter Labour's public negatives, especially on what was thought to be the party's instinctive proclivity for 'tax and spend', and on crime and its causes, where Blair as Shadow Home Secretary was making an effective impact. Brown the Shadow Chancellor sought to move the economic policy away from both high taxation and 'job killing regulation'[3] and shift the emphasis towards a new aggressive concern with job creation and financial services.[4]

But when it came to party reform, Smith held to his own views of the practicable. In the game of politics he had a strong sense of tactics and did not shy away from past routines and techniques of traditional management to achieve the best outcomes. But, as he made clear to Whitty, he was not drawn to detailed regular personal intervention in such management nor to extending the range of machine controls. He accepted an agenda of plans for a growing and more active party which were being developed with some enthusiasm under the NEC finance working party, set up under his leadership. The limitations of this approach were increasingly frustrating to the modernisers. Kinnock, it was said, had done nothing to change the culture of the party,[5] whilst Smith was now missing an opportunity for 'a real symbolic break with Labour's past.'[6] He was characterised as having a 'one more heave' approach to electoral success, although this was not a sentiment Smith ever expressed.[7] As for party management, Blair saw Smith's views as 'unsophisticated' and 'twenty-five years out of date',[8] and an 'abdication of responsibility'.[9]

Frustration was increased for the modernisers because their confident talent, including their media skills, gave them assurance about their ability to create the tide towards radical reform which would move past traditional affiliations and positions whilst Smith, it was said, dragged his feet. For his part, Smith was critical of this enthusiasm for large-scale and apparently perpetual organisational change. It was at odds with much of the traditional Labour right's practical reformism, which appreciated the potential costs of change as much as the benefits and understood the wisdom of settling immediate difficult problems before you plunged into others. In this regard he and many union leaders shared the same view – that it was 'the modernisers' who were unsophisticated.

The spin campaign and goodbye to the unions

The spin campaign focused on ending the link with the unions was relentless and widely supported in sections of the mass media. It seemed, in this phase, the dominant voice in many public and private meetings, accompanied by a head-nodding pessimism. Particularly on the London dinner-party circuit, it appeared that everybody was saying the same thing. You could reasonably gain the impression that there was 'a consensus in the Labour Party that the time had come for one member one vote pure and simple'.[10]

This drive was fed by research commissioned by Philip Gould, examining the views of those Conservative voters who had considered voting Labour. Some of the data was produced during the prolonged pessimistic public assault on the party, and when the question of separation had already been launched and become a major talking point. The conclusion drawn from this research was that it proved that Labour had lost because 'the process of modernisation had been too slow'.[11] According to Gould, when the polling data was privately shown to Blair the latter became 'manic', saying 'you must get it out'.[12] The research was then leaked by Gould to the *Sunday Times*.[13] Another press report of the polling by Peter Kellner was given a more specific media focus. The polling, it was reported, 'revealed' that the unions were the reason that the party had lost the election. 'Labour', the heading on the article said, should 'bid goodbye to the unions'[14].

The fit between polling results and where Blair and the modernisers wanted to go has to be seen against specialist academic studies. A central theme of the electoral diagnosis by Heath, Jowell and Curtice was that the voters did not trust Labour's economic competence and its ability to deliver on promises over education and health.[15] Butler and Kavanagh also focused on the 'credibility gap' about delivery.[16] Westlake's later biography of Kinnock reviewing the causes of the 1992 defeat makes no specific reference to the unions.[17] Neither did Mark Stuart's more substantial review of causes in his biography of Smith.[18] Survey data showed that 'the trade unions' were very low down in the reasons given by electors for making the decision of which party to vote for.[19]

The unions' response and political action

It became part of the common sense of the attack on the unions to label them as conservative organisations resisting reform because of their unshakable fear of change. Philip Gould's more developed thesis on the Labour Party, 'born a conservative party',[20] included the role of the unions as a source of organisational rigidity.[21] Certainly as industrial organisations, they were more used to the defensive than the offensive role and they were as addicted as are most organisations to familiar and stable arrangements. From the Gould analysis it could never be imagined that, as Whitty described later, 'most of the changes in the party's decision-making, campaigning, communication and administration introduced in recent years have been led and in many cases supported financially by the trade unions'.[22]

Before the General Election of 1992 it was reasonable to judge that notwithstanding the continuing argument about candidate selection, a major programme of internal constitutional reform which changed the position of the unions and the procedures of the relationship was now both desirable and possible – providing that there was trust and a sense of common purpose. A majority of union leaders were won to a dialogue on such an agenda, and in terms of moving on block-vote reform, as we have seen, were ahead of the Leader. But trust and common purpose were notably diminished in the atmosphere generated by the leading modernisers following the General Election. Though many union leaders had been expecting something like this, the sheer intensity of the campaign to push their organisations out of the party took them aback. They saw themselves the scapegoats for the failure of the politicians and their advisers. Their defensive reaction was 'no way are we being pushed out'. A new 'Keep the Link' campaign emerged from the unions. On this fundamental issue they were virtually united.

As for detailed reforms of the union position in the party, there was no homogeneity of union positions of the kind that had been implied in the Gould diagnosis of their conservatism. The different union labourisms were reflected in varying attitudes to specific reforms as well as to policies. As

Table 3.1 Affiliated unions with over 10,000 affiliated members and their conference votes 1993

Transport and General Workers Union (TGWU)	1,076,000
GMB	859,000
National Union of Public Employees (NUPE)	530,000
Amalgamated Engineering and Electrical Union (AEEU)	471,000
Union of Shop, Distributive and Allied Workers (USDAW)	312,000
Manufacturing Science Finance (MSF)	304,000
Confederation of Health Service Employees (COHSE)	190,000
Union of Communication Workers (UCW)	182,000
National Communications Union (NCU)	121,000
Graphical Paper and Media Union-Sogat 82 (GPMU)	117,000
National Union of Rail, Maritime and Transport Workers (RMT)	113,000
Union of Construction, Allied Trades and Technicians (UCATT)	80,000
Iron and Steel Trades Confederation (ISTC)	53,000
Knitwear, Footwear and Apparel Trades (KFAT)	45,000
National Union of Mineworkers (NUM)	41,000
Transport Salaried Staffs' Association ((TSSA)	32,000
Bakers Food and Allied Workers Union (BFAW)	26,000
Ceramic and Allied Trades Union	25,000
Fire Brigades Union (FBU)	20,000
Association of Locomotive Engineers and Firemen (ASLEF)	19,000
Musicians Union (MU)	11,000
A further five unions had 2,000 or fewer affiliated	7,000
Total	4,645,993

usual, these divisions were historically associated with the political traditions of the right and left but they also involved varied individual union positions. It was characteristic of the union relationship that the Leader of the party could almost always find some base of support for a version of reform and change on the right of the unions and it was true here over OMOV for candidate selection. As for voting in leadership elections, there had only ever been a small majority for reform of the existing procedure and at this stage there were still influential union voices quietly favouring pulling out of the arrangements, with the AEEU its strongest advocate.

But in the face of the unrestrained assault they now faced, major union leaders reacted in 1992 as they had done in 1979 when an avalanche of constitutional reform proposals was coming from the left. It forced their attention more on reform but their immediate concern was to stabilise the situation and to manage an orderly framework for the discussion and coordination of whatever coherent changes were required in order to move to a workable settlement. This in their view was not conservatism, just practical politics with a century of wisdom behind it. The priority was to hold off the calls for divorce or separation which they believed (correctly) were very unrepresentative and were supported outside the party by the same social and political forces which had been trying to break the Labour Party since it was founded. With the political atmosphere surrounding the union-party relationship deteriorating by the week, on a proposal from the NUPE representative Tom Sawyer, it was agreed by the NEC that a Trade Union Review Group (as it became known) would be established by the NEC to consider the relationship between Labour and the unions, 'in the round and not on a piecemeal basis'[23].

Party democracy and party management

The deep passions attached to this argument over the unions were reflected in a vivid public clash over what should be the form of the party's democratic order. Major issues of representation emerged, direct versus delegatist, individual versus collective. On democratic grounds there was a case both for and against the traditional union connection. A view from the radical modernisers that the party electorate should ideally consist only of the individual party members in one-member-one-vote arrangements had the appeal of being straightforward with clear boundaries to the party, no multiple roles and simple majorities easily arrived at. On the other hand a union conception of an inclusive collective democracy, in which the political levy payers as well as individual party members operated within a federal structure, produced a much larger electorate, and a base which guaranteed a manual-working-class component at a time when amongst individual Labour members, representatives in the PLP and the whole of British political life it was declining far in excess of the real social change.

Behind this clash of ideals and perspectives there was a more practical and power-oriented argument going on about the positives and negatives of 'the link', with the issue of future party management a rumbling background concern. This was at its most agonising on the traditional right of the NEC including its trade union group. They had, they thought, 'saved the party' in their battles with the Bennite left as had their forefathers done in battles with the left long gone. They had acted as a praetorian guard for Kinnock and saw the unions still as an essential stabilising element working in a rule-governed and loyal relationship with the Leader. Pushing the unions out struck them as showing a deep ignorance of the party and a lack of understanding about politics. How did the moderniser-separatists think that the party would be managed? Who would play the traditional union role as party ballast? Who would keep the party's feet on the ground? The questions were in part an assertive call to get real, in part a despairing call for the novice would-be political leaders to appreciate union solidarity.

There was no clear united public response on party management issues at this stage from Blair and the modernisers. Their perspective was apparently dominated only by a principled crusade for the spread of 'a process of change whereby we are going to have one-member-one-vote coming into many of the decisions of the Labour Party'.[24] However, there was from those around Blair an assumption growing in significance that management could be helped by the institution of new plebiscitarian procedures involving the individual members which could circumvent the unrepresentative activists and the unions. Another view which was occasionally privately imparted to trade union officials was that the union ballast was best exercised by individual trade unionists joining the party and operating as groups of individuals. Blair made this point later publicly at an early stage as Leader of the Party.[25] Independently, but feeding in later, Larry Whitty played with various ideas of building a new stable regional underpinning of the party leadership. But for the moment the focus was on the immediate procedural battle.

Review group: composition and agenda

Before the Trade Union Review Group had its first meeting, on 20 July 1992, it was plunged into deep controversy about its composition. In response to criticism of its alleged union domination a further MP and an MEP were added to the committee, and the General Secretaries of the GMB and TGWU passed the responsibility to other officials of their unions. This absence of the senior union leaders was later to work to the tactical advantage of the leadership. It comprised five NEC trade union section members – Tom Burlison GMB, Tony Clarke UCW, Gordon Colling GPMU, Nigel Harris AEEU, and Tom Sawyer NUPE, one union official from the NEC Women's Section – Diana Jeuda USDAW – and a senior official of the TGWU, Margaret Prosser.

The parliamentarians included Margaret Beckett, Robin Cook, Bryan Gould, John Prescott and Clare Short, the Leader of the EPLP, Glyn Ford and the ex-MP and Political Secretary of the National Union of Labour and Socialist Clubs, John Evans. In addition, the General Secretary Larry Whitty, Director of Organisation Joyce Gould and academic Lewis Minkin were also members of the committee. In October 1992 Bryan Gould resigned and went to New Zealand. He was replaced in November by Tony Blair who with Gordon Brown had just been elected to the NEC in a contest where left-wing MP Dennis Skinner was rejected. In 1993 Joyce Gould resigned as Director of Organisation and was replaced by Peter Coleman. Party officials Tony Mainwaring and Jon Cruddas also attended the committee meetings.

The review provoked further controversy over the May 1992 NEC Organisation sub-committee's acceptance of Kinnock's proposal that 'the final vote to choose the Parliamentary candidate shall be by one member one vote ballot of the individual members'[26] That had been confirmed by the NEC later that month. At its June meeting however, the NEC accepted by 13 votes to 8 a motion from Robin Cook that the NEC reaffirmed its decision on candidate selection but that its implementation be referred to the review group.[27]

The working process

The major source of initiative for the main documents was the General Secretary Larry Whitty, but throughout the process other committee members initiated proposals. There were some important immediate decisions, but otherwise it was a slow explorative, consultative and adjustive process, aiming for a final report to the 1993 conference, but awaiting interplay with the big union conferences and the CLPs. Smith and his office staff kept clear of concerted steering from the outside but Murray Elder, head of his office, and to an increasing extent Smith, privately participated in a variety of informal bilateral discussions seeking to probe areas of potential agreement and of support for Smith's position.

Trade union attitudes towards reform

The progressive general reaction of the union representatives on the committee is best understood within the *Framework of Working Principles, Themes and Values* presented by Minkin to the group in September 1992.[28] Building on changing attitudes in the unions, it argued that the party-union connection guaranteed the manual-working-class component of the party's broad social composition, linked the party to the problems of people at work, maintained an important channel of communication to some of the party's core voters and also provided ballast – ensuring the party's stability and unity in a crisis. However, there had to be an openness to new identities and social forces at the expense of its labourist identity.

Since its foundation the party's formal procedures had been based on union majorities in all conferences at regional and national level. It was now proposed that there should be a new power-sharing partnership between the affiliated membership and the individual membership. No union representative opposed this. 'There should be in principle' said the review group's interim report later, in a historic passage, 'a move to a figure where trade unions do not on their own hold a majority of the vote'.[29] The logic of this was carried into every party procedure including leadership elections where even supporters of continuing union involvement agreed that the unions should have a reduced representation. Another key objective in the framework was that the party's procedures should embody a new fusion of democratic traditions with a changed balance of individual and collective representation in the different areas and forums of the relationship. No union representative openly contested this either.

Unions and contrasting radicalism

The modernisers' regular critique of conservative trade unions sits oddly with their response to this document and their representatives' behaviour, unless of course rejection of total change is the only measure of conservatism. Some key initiatives on the review group divided the unions into different but radical camps. The AEEU, a fierce advocate of OMOV for the NEC and candidate selection, was not far away from the position of moderate modernisers who were prepared to accept the permanence of a formal union-party relationship although not its present form. They also favoured a conference reform in which the unions would have only 30 per cent of the votes. Union delegates would be elected by ballot, with votes proportionate to the unions' individual Labour Party membership.

Another union, the GMB, which was to loom large as apparently the iron opponent of OMOV reform in candidate selection, had been in favour of it before 1990 and at the earliest stage of these discussions now was in favour of the unions coming out of elections for the Leader. But in the group discussions the GMB and the NUPE representative proposed different versions of a registered supporters' (sometimes called associate members) scheme for candidate selection. This preserved the involvement of those trade-union political levy payers who were prepared to register their individual support and were in principle eligible to join the party, and they would participate as part of the affiliated organisations section of an electoral college.

There was a strong momentum behind these proposals when Blair joined the group in November 1992. A vociferous Nigel Harris of the AEEU was his only publicly committed ally in support of OMOV but, as has been shown in Chapter 2, on the NEC there was a fluidity of opinion on candidate selection procedures and there were important sub-currents on the review group. Colling and Evans, amongst others, had expressed critical reservations at the registered supporters scheme although, because this scheme appeared to be approaching a unifying position, there was not the wider open criticism there might have been.

Blair was immediately forthright and evangelical over introducing OMOV across the field of Labour Party decision-making. He introduced an open scepticism about the existing two categories of membership implicitly opposing the idea of affiliated members. His intervention impressive in its boldness gave both quiet waverers and critics of registered supporters a psychological boost and created a new opportunity for OMOV over candidate selection. However, the decisive turning point came not from Blair, nor from Smith, nor from the review group. It came at a private meeting of the NEC trade union group on 25 November 1992, dominated by the traditional right. The key figures here were Gordon Colling (who instigated the meeting) and Evans, working to a background paper done by John Spellar from AEEU.

Some at that meeting favoured OMOV, but the main thrust was the range of problems inherent in the counterproposals. The GMB and NUPE advocates of the registered supporters proposal found themselves on the defensive and with potential allies absent or moving away. The two unions then found it very difficult to respond because they could not agree a common position on the mechanics of the scheme. The Northern Region of the GMB then prioritised levy payers becoming individual members of the party and their public view was seen as a GMB split.[30] Thereafter, the registered supporters proposals lost momentum and as a result became simply an option in the interim report, rather than the recommendation of the review group.

Smith's position and the review group

That report, with a proposed consultative document, was put to the NEC on 22 February 1993. It focused mainly on the options for the three controversial areas. At this meeting John Smith made clear to the NEC his own preferences. They were very much in accord with the broad preferences he had given – at press insistence – during his election campaign. For the election of the Leader he had favoured a ballot of the individual party members and the MPs/MEPs with each section having 50 per cent of the vote. He also supported a reduction in the proportion of the trade union vote at the conference dependent on increases in the individual party membership, with the union votes cast by individual delegates. On selection of parliamentary candidates his preference was for OMOV in selections for the next election, and whereas he was quietly flexible on elements of the other two issues, on candidate selection he was adamant. This reform would remain a touchstone of his leadership.

Unhappy modernisers

Meanwhile, Philip Gould tells us that Blair and Brown were very unhappy with the way things were going, indeed at the end of their tether with frustration about the slow pace of change.[31] In January 1993 Blair spoke publicly in favour of ending two classes of membership.[32] That month, yet more research had been privately presented to the Shadow Cabinet showing that 'most floating voters still regarded Labour as a party of the past'.[33] In spite of an injunction that it must not be leaked, the modernisers were determined to push Smith into more radical changes; Mandelson, given the document by Blair and Brown, leaked it via Patrick Wintour in the Guardian.[34] Then, on 6 January 1993, Mandelson in a letter to the Guardian underlined that the party must go through more far reaching changes than Smith had in mind. These tactics were described by Macintyre as 'a classic Mandelson operation'.[35]

The modernisers were very adept at this kind of operation, but there were some deep problems that they continued to be very slow to appreciate. Their undoubted skills – working with the tide of bias in the right-wing press on anything connected with the unions, and in the context of fashionable London views – led them into extravagant anticipations of where the party was prepared to go. At times they seemed totally lacking in awareness of the damage they were doing to themselves, perpetually mistaking the sound of their own noise for the voice of the party – an old ultra-left vanguardist trait. Yet, blindingly obvious was that in none of the 33 resolutions submitted to the 1992 party conference on constitutional issues was there clear support for the objective of separation, or even the gradual phasing out of collective affiliation.

Shifting CLP opinion on candidate selection

That tide of opinion not only moved against the separatists, it moved against Smith's position. Back in 1990 in a consultation, support for the abolition of the electoral college and preference for OMOV from the CLPs had been 87 per cent.[36] At the time of Smith's election, optimistic supporters of OMOV put CLP support at around 80 per cent. But when the consultation results came in June 1993 only 35 per cent of CLPs who replied were committed to OMOV, with a further 15 per cent favouring what was known as 'levy-plus' (see below). The majority of constituency returns 'favoured some form of continuing union involvement'.[37]

There were various contributions to this turnround of opinion against OMOV. Some of it was undoubtedly affected by suspicions of the separationist agenda and some of that was deliberately stoked from the anti-OMOV side. But they did not need to stoke. Trade union leaders were hearing it privately, and informed journalists were reporting, as the minuscule but well-positioned network of separationists kept publicly resurrecting the objective. At a conference on 'Organising for Recovery' sponsored by the New Statesman and Society and New Times held at the TUC Congress House on 22 May, just prior to the union conference of MSF, enthusiastic support for separation or divorce, expressed by speakers in the session on 'Unions and Parties', was noted with alarm by union representatives.[38]

As the argument went on and on and on, the case that the unions were the party's fundamental problem lost ground to another view – that the preoccupation with 'the union problem' was engulfing the party, demoralising it and becoming electorally counterproductive in focusing attention away from the essentials of economic and social policy. The alliance of the three big union leaders also seemed strengthened by this growing mood to the detriment of personal relations between Edmonds and Smith. The union leader had seen Kinnock's intervention over candidate selection in 1992, as he had in 1990, as closely linked to the voices off-stage advocating separation. This reinforced his view that this was a line-in-the-sand issue with those voices likely at some point to influence the Leader. Smith found this suspicious attitude towards himself, by somebody he had regarded as a friend, deeply unreasonable. Morris was seen by Smith as much easier to relate to but unable to deliver. Bickerstaffe was regarded by Smith as the friendliest and the one most willing under the right circumstances to play the role of peacemaker. But for the moment they all appeared immovable.

The tide

From spring to summer in 1993 the tide had blown strongly through the conferences of key unions beginning with USDAW (where Diana Jeuda was a key player). This union, always regarded as a weathercock, went against OMOV and was followed by UCW and MSF, where in each case the party leadership hoped for support for OMOV in candidate selection but the union's executive body was defeated. The initiative held by the GMB, TGWU and NUPE was reinforced when, on the 17th May, they released polling by MORI showing the extent to which Labour-identifying levy payers favoured retaining a say in candidate selection (66 per cent) as well as leadership elections (62 per cent). Their leaders were winning the argument.

In the summer of 1993, Smith appeared to be in deep trouble. Those who sought the means to produce an overall agreement could only see the likelihood that he would go down to overwhelming defeat as a majority of the major unions were committed against OMOV in candidate selection. To overcome this majority opposition would require something remarkable. And yet the victory did happen, through union restraint and a complex series of party management manoeuvres.

Management operations and the basis of the Smith victory

Union restraint

As already illustrated and thoroughly explored in *The Contentious Alliance*, the union role within the Labour Party had generally involved a high degree of restraint in relations with the political leaders. The conflict of 1992/93 stretched this restraint to its limits, given that for some the relationship itself was now at stake. The behaviour of the GMB (historically *the* loyalist union) in pushing its opposition to the Leader's rule change right down to the wire of the vote at the party conference was a source of astonishment to many in the party – perhaps even to the GMB itself.

Nevertheless, the major unions still played this hand within self-imposed constraints that, in retrospect, can be seen to have facilitated the victory of the political leadership. It was a feature which few people understood and to this day virtually all commentators and academics writing on the conflict simply fail to register it. The key example was over reform of the balance of voting at the party conference. It might well be expected that the big unions, on the defensive in general but specifically over OMOV in candidate selection, might have been concerned to maximise their votes at the decisive Conference of 1993. The implication behind much of the critique of 'union bosses' was that in their opposition to change, they were addicted to power maximisation.

Yet, at the first review group meeting on 20 July 1992, union representatives, including those from the GMB, NUPE, and TGWU had strongly supported the immediate reduction of the union vote from approximately 90 per cent to 70 per cent as a way of showing good faith and a willingness to be flexible (as they had done at various conferences over reform of the block vote). It became the basis of voting at the 1993 party conference when the other controversial rule changes were to be taken. Had the decision been held off for a year with these other reforms, the balance of voting on the constitutional changes would have been different and the Leader would probably have been defeated over the rule change on candidate selection.

Then there was also the unions' financial restraint. This was in marked contrast to the public image of the 'No Say No Pay' campaign, said in the press to have been launched by the NUPE leadership at their conference.[39] In truth, there was never such a campaign, and no reference to any financial sanctions in the NUPE Executive Council statement nor in any speeches in their conference. Nor was there, as journalist Alastair Campbell alleged, 'a crude threat that the unions will pull the plug on Labour's finances unless the block vote is retained'.[40] This pull-the-plug fiction was built upon a clumsy private briefing by Sawyer related to the financial consequences of a complete divorce of the unions by the party, and the result of the unions having no say at all,[41] a point already made by others.

Indeed, what was striking to anybody who looked closely at it was the failure to use any other financial leverage. At this time also there were discussions on the executive committee of TUFL of the need for financial stringency in TUFL's use of its funds but this was not applied to the existing provision for the Leader's Office. In the many months of formal and informal meetings of the review group, there was not a breath of mention of sanctions linking union funding and the reforms.

Union divisions change

One of the problems facing the registered supporters scheme had been that the TGWU was committed to union branch participation in a reformed electoral college for selections, and the furthest that its Executive would move involved balloting individual levy payers. Eventually, in an endeavour to produce a more closely aligned union position, in May 1993 the GMB moved towards the position of the TGWU, thus for the moment shedding the registered supporters scheme for the next round of selections. In doing so it more clearly left space for another union to take its traditional place closer to the Leader's position. With NUPE leader Rodney Bickerstaffe increasingly finding Smith a man he could have a trusting dialogue with about many things and receiving a commitment that the constitutional issues under discussion would be the end of the fundamental reform agenda before the next election, that union's position began discreetly to help Smith. Bickerstaffe did not particularly want the move to OMOV but saw the opportunity for more influence on industrial issues – particularly the minimum wage. Sawyer, who also sought to recover his own prominent

NEC insider position under the new Leader, then brought his range of tactical skills to bear in assisting the Leader's office.

There was thus very little coordination secured by the highly publicised 'private' meetings of the large unions which began on 12 May 1993 and continued up to the party conference. Leaders in some unions, including UCW and RMT, kept attending even though their leaders were sympathetic to OMOV and not in tune with their union's stances. At a later stage the GMB moved back towards the registered supporters scheme in an attempt to construct a new alignment which would keep the wavering NUPE in the opposition camp. It failed, as we shall see. The opposition to OMOV in the unions never came up with a united alternative platform.

Leadership skills and tactical initiatives

The huge majority for Smith in his election and the sense of urgency behind the drive for a Labour Government were always an asset for Smith. He had been, and remained, the first choice of most union officials as Leader. It was crucial also that he conveyed that he was not a separationist but somebody who saw the party-union relationship in evolutionary terms and sought to manage a practicable settlement which would leave the party as a more effective force. He retained a large amount of trust which was always an asset to him, in spite of growing criticism including a critique of the performance of the front bench launched by GMB leader John Edmonds at his union conference in June.

In coupling a defence of union participation within the party with an attack on the oppositional incompetence and cautious economic policy of Labour's leaders, Edmonds was saying publicly what some others in the party were saying privately. But it so raised the stakes as to make compromise on the procedural issues less likely. Smith could easily foresee that the government and his media critics would have a field day with the allegation that he was weak and had been 'defeated by Edmonds'.[42] It says much about Smith's dogged position that he was prepared to take the decision back to the NEC and the conference if he lost at the conference. It is also significant that Edmonds was ready to move a motion of confidence in Smith if Smith lost. Such were the complexities of this battle.

Without doing major damage to his authority as the Leader, Smith would not and could not retreat on candidate selection but drawing from his authority and trust he could take unilateral initiatives which added to his resources of persuasion. There were three such key initiatives. The first was that when it became clear that OMOV for candidate selection was losing ground in the CLPs, and that continuing participation had support amongst union Labour identifiers, Smith, in a first initiative on 19 May, came forward in support of a new version of what was known as levy-plus in which trade unionists who paid the political levy could pay a small additional sum per year and gain full membership and voting rights.

Various people had been involved in this initiative. Sawyer of UNISON, backed by Bickerstaffe, had already begun to move in favour of the levy-plus proposal. It had an older parentage. It could be dated back to a proposal from Gordon Brown in the mid-1980s. Prescott had supported it in 1989 and supported it now. Its significance in this context was that what emerged from the final review group report also described the levy-plus payers as registered supporters. It thus established two different conceptions of registered supporters. There was the original GMB/NUPE proposal which preserved their involvement as union representatives with OMOV votes in the affiliated societies section, and there was this individual-member involvement – both now described as registered supporters. This gave some union leaders sympathetic to Smith a new opportunity for flexibility in the application of their union mandates on registered supporters.

On this basis, after much negotiation, NUPE moved into full but discreet support and gave Smith a new position to take into discussions with some of the wavering union leaders. With this agreement in the bag, on 14 July Smith took a second major initiative. At the final meeting of the review group unexpectedly he just walked in, insisted that this was 'decision time' and asserted the case for OMOV and levy-plus in candidate selection linking it with the idea of registered supporters. He was helped by the atmosphere of crisis and the crying need for agreement but also by the consensus that had emerged on the other reforms. He may also have been helped by the tactical story spread around that there had already been a private agreement with the union leaders.

In any case, it drew on the fact that, confirming previous sub-currents, there was more hidden cooperation from the union representatives than might be gathered from their leaders' stance. Aware that the recommendation to the NEC would give a crucial party momentum, and anxious not to damage the Leader, the union representatives from the GMB and TGWU, particularly the latter, expressed some low-key reservations in the light of their union policy but expressed no outright opposition and did not call for a vote. The sense of the meeting was taken as its decision. At the end of this meeting, members of the group were asked to stay in place whilst only Smith talked to the press. He announced to the journalists that there had been an agreement. The announcement was met much later by consternation from the GMB and TGWU leaders who were put on the back foot by being kept in ignorance of the outcome of the meeting until they heard or read the spin. 'Brutal but all part of the game', as Smith later described it.[43]

Given what was seen as the authoritative support of the review group, Smith gained the support of the NEC for the proposals at its next meeting on 19 July. The NEC also had the right to give its views to the party conference on the basis of that decision. This sense of a major movement taking place now gave sympathetic union leaders a new argument for attempting to persuade their unions to shift. This was, it was said, the 'agreed' position. However, it did leave some resentment over the tactics, and the 'agreement' was far from signed and sealed with the union leaders. For the moment with some of them, it even exacerbated their resentment and the sense of impasse.

Indeed by September, at the TUC, the general opinion was that the Leader had still dug himself 'into a hole'. Still facing a wall of majority union opposition, and a growing clamour that he must change, Smith took a third major initiative in choosing to shift the agenda. His TUC speech, in both style and content, provided a powerful reinforcement of his value to the unions as the Leader. It did much to satisfy union unease at the development of the party's employment and employment rights policy – the priority union agenda.

He announced a charter of rights for all workers giving basic employment rights, coming into force on the first day of employment, including the right to join a trade union and have recognition from employers, support for the signing of the European social chapter and guaranteeing a national minimum wage. This was coupled with re-commitment to restoring full employment using all instruments of macro economic management. It was also accompanied by a fierce criticism of the policy of privatisation and of Conservative Government attempts to water down the rights of workers achieved through European legislation. In adopting this platform with such clarity Smith gave added justification for allies to argue in their unions that he must not be defeated. However, the promises made to unions were seen by Blair, Brown and the modernisers as a threat to their economic and political credibility, and they increased their pressure on Smith.

Procedural management and the mobilisation of allies

Yet the vote at the party conference where the unions held 70 per cent of the votes had still to be won. TGWU, GMB, RMT, MSF, NUPE, USDAW and UCW were all mandated in favour of positions which were not in accord with what the Leader wanted. On the face of it the Smith position was lost. However, behind the apparently unshakable opposition was a new level of activity by allies working discreetly with the Leader's office and headquarters party managers. Some of these were won to the idea of levy plus/OMOV as a reasonable alternative, others simply wanted the war to end without a humiliating defeat for the Leader and with the party intact.

Indeed, by the time of the party conference, there was now a growing belief that defeat for Smith on this issue would be a disaster for the party. It would damage the party's electoral standing, it would undermine (perhaps even destroy) a Leader who shared fundamental values with the unions, it would give new ammunition to the separationists, and it would plunge the party into internal war. The personal regard for Smith himself was also a growing element at this stage. Shifts took place and support grew, open and covert, enthusiastic and reluctant, in the unions and in the head-quarters' management. The latter became a crucial asset for the Leader linking closely to the politics of procedural management at the conference.

This was particularly true of Whitty the General Secretary, whose commitment to the union link was unquestionable. Indeed, it had caused some deep friction with Blair which was to outlast the Review Group. He had also been involved in some detailed disagreements with Smith. But, as he told the NEC at the July meeting which supported the Review Group recommendations, he was convinced that Smith must not be defeated. He encouraged his managerial staff accordingly. At this stage the elected managers of the Conference Arrangements Committee and their Secretary, party official Sally Morgan, became a crucial element determining the outcome in liaison with Elder from the Leader's office.

Tactics of management

The resolutions submitted by the big three unions appeared to consolidate the chance of a defeat for the Leader over candidate selection. But what the managers knew, had seen in the past and would face again many times in the Blair years, was that it all depended on the specific wording of the choices placed before the delegates and which choice was judged the most authoritative. The union delegations would normally (but not invariably) be expected to respond favourably to the initiative of their senior official. The latter could be assisted by the choices offered by the composited resolutions and, crucially, the exact wording of the rule-change amendment proposed by the NEC. The primary aim of the managers was to get the rule change accepted regardless of the votes on the resolutions. Elder worked closely with supportive union leaders and officials to focus and spread votes in the way most conducive to victory. The overall scenario of the tactics was not as clear at the time it was being put together as it later became in retrospect.

One consistent ally of Smith all the way through on OMOV had been the AEEU. Before the conference the union quietly agreed to allow its own resolution (a straight commitment to OMOV in candidate selection) to stand alone and (in effect) be defeated so that the leadership could gain a better chance of victory on a more cleverly ambiguous composite of resolutions from the RMT and NUPE on the rule change. The AEEU representative on the CAC needed a lot of convincing, including an intervention by the union President, to get this agreement set up. But, eventually, that is what happened.

It must also be noted that the AEEU leader who had long pushed the OMOV case at the NEC may well have received some solace by the surprising NEC constitutional amendment that emerged without warning embodying the introduction of individual postal balloting for the CLP section of the NEC, the Women's Section, the Treasurer, the Conference Arrangements Committee, the auditors and the National Constitutional

Committee. In line with the past managed outcome of reform proposals concerning OMOV for the NEC in 1990, the support from below was uncertain. There had been no party consultation on this and it was not discussed on the trade union review group which covered the whole agenda of party reform. In the voting on this rule change, over 30 per cent of the potential vote abstained,[44] but it went through.

The RMT/NUPE composite resolution, which was prepared by the managers after helpful discussions between Murray Elder and Tom Sawyer from NUPE, both mentioned levy-plus and also registered levy-paying members participating 'on a fairly agreed basis'. That had a high degree of ambiguity. In agreeing this composite, the leaders of these two unions, Jimmy Knapp (RMT), and Rodney Bickerstaffe and Tom Sawyer, used the idea of registered supporters and levy-plus to legitimise their support and then gave crucial assistance to the Leader by failing to vote for the GMB-backed resolution on registered supporters.

The rule change prepared by party officials and proposed on behalf of the NEC was the real prize embodying the detail of the new OMOV arrangements. Opponents of the rule change in the unions did not keep their eyes on its wording. Drafted by David Gardner, with Whitty's agreement and at the suggestion of Sally Morgan, it linked the acceptance of OMOV in candidate selection with the acceptance of all-women short lists in candidate selection. It was initially an attempt to win more support in the CLPs, involving an educated guestimate that the tactical move would gain more votes than it lost there.[45] This change, together with the emphasis on levy-plus payers as registered supporters, had by the Sunday evening with the help of sympathetic union leaders secured the votes of NUPE, USDAW and UCW behind the rule change, in spite of difficulties with union conference mandates opposed to OMOV. But other unions, notably MSF, failed to move and the vote still looked lost.

Not only that, but new problems were emerging in the CLP section now holding 30 per cent of the votes. It was evident that there was a lot of uncertainty. Where the issue was seen as a step towards separation the reaction was hostile; where it was seen simply as democratic reform there was considerable support. At the suggestion of Sally Morgan there emerged the first systematic development of CLP mobilisation – a coordinated campaign aimed at CLP delegates, organised from the office of the Leader's PPS Hilary Armstrong. With the reluctant assent of Whitty, who feared establishing a precedent, the national and regional party officials as well as loyalist MPs were used to bolster this campaign. By contrast, the anti-OMOV unions were hardly organised at all in this final internal phase. Only the Campaign for Labour Party Democracy was active on that side.

Yet, in spite of the pressure on CLP delegates, there was still insufficient support there to guarantee victory on OMOV in candidate selection. Every vote became vital. At one point in the morning's debate a very effective speech by Bill Morris and then in another twist in the story, a surprisingly belligerent speech critical of the two other major unions from the NUPE delegate Maggie Jones, appeared to turn the mood in the hall against the Smith position. One well-informed private speculation was that on advice from within the hierarchy of NUPE, Jones's performance was an ambitious version of the Mandelsonian 'let them see the blood on the floor', to draw attention to the new loyalists. But it badly misfired. Both Elder and Morgan took the view that after these speeches Smith might be facing defeat.[46] Communications Officer David Hill noted that support 'appeared to be slipping'.[47] Late on Wednesday morning Elder and Morgan cast around for somebody who might turn the debate. Morgan came up with the idea of John Prescott, a supporter of levy-plus and Smith and also a known strong supporter of the broad constitutional relationship with the unions.

But before the final speeches and the vote came a crucial development in the MSF union which swung the outcome. It had postponed its decision on the Sunday evening. In a final lunch-break vote on the day of the debate, the delegation (which had at an earlier meeting agreed to follow its mandate by supporting the TGWU position, yet assisted the Leader by agreeing to vote against the GMB's resolution) now made its decision on the crucial rule change. It agreed – by 19 votes to 17 – to abstain on the grounds that the issue of ending union involvement (which the union opposed) had been amalgamated with the issue of all-women short lists (which the union supported), thus giving the delegation contradictory mandates. MSF official Ann Gibson, following what had been discussed in other delegations, argued for abstention on the grounds that the two positions were incompatible. By this means the rule change was saved at the eleventh hour, although most of the people in the hall were unaware of it.

Candidate selection: the result

When it came to what became the famous Prescott finale, he produced an extraordinarily powerful and subtle speech urging trust in Smith. This may have affected and legitimised the actions of some of the waverers in the CLPs who did not want the unions excluded but also did not want Smith (and the rule change) defeated either. It may have produced more support for the RMT/NUPE composite. But more importantly, his withering comments on those who 'did us no favour' by throwing doubt on 'the unity and solidarity of the movement', combined with his full-hearted repudiation of the idea of separation: 'we as an NEC have had your instruction to strengthen those links', gave a definitive view of the meaning of the candidate selection result.[48] To that extent, it was a major setback for Blair, Brown, Mandelson and Gould and their supporters.

The rule change involving OMOV plus registered members plus a commitment to increase numbers of women candidates, backed by the NEC, went through by 47.509 per cent to 44.388 per cent, and the supportive if ambiguous RMT/NUPE levy-plus composite, also backed by the NEC, went through by 48.926 per cent to 48.127 per cent. The CLPs were said by party officials to have voted approximately 60:40 in favour.[49] In another crucial bonus for the leadership, the composite backed by the GMB supporting union involvement through registered supporters went down by 53.114 per cent to 44.017 per cent. Yet just how procedurally engineered this victory was can be gauged by the votes on two other composite resolutions. The straight and unambiguous OMOV position from the AEEU, recommended by the NEC, was lost by 70.857 per cent to 26.003 per cent – a huge defeat, and the electoral-college resolution of the TGWU (which in effect rejected OMOV) was victorious by 48.645 percent to 48.454 per cent.

Nevertheless, to the chagrin of the TGWU, the vote on the complicated rule change took precedence. It was a famous victory but one heavy with ambiguity. This was initially fought as a crusade over an unqualified commitment to OMOV. Yet that position was in the end sent down to overwhelming defeat in order to win the tactical battle. It might well be argued therefore that this was the victory that never was. Yet later, in practice, the declared victory proved to be a triumph. It gave a basis for those who now just wanted to call a halt to do so, and it even encouraged some of those who had strongly opposed OMOV in candidate selection to go quiet, an acknowledgment that on this the battle was lost.

The block vote and the end of the union preponderance

The obsessive focus on candidate selection tended to obscure the importance of the rest of the reform agenda. Arguably, the historic and most important long-term change secured by the review group was the agreement by the unions to accept in principle the ending of the huge preponderance in conference votes that they had held since the party was founded.

The solution to reducing that preponderance which had been initially mentioned as a possibility by the NEC in a document to the 1990 Conference – the bringing in of the Parliamentary Labour Party as a third force in the Conference[50] – had drawn a range of cross-factional adherents including a significant body of support in the CLPs. Bringing it in could bring voting at the conference more into line with voting in the electoral college for the leadership, and it would extend integration and participation to an important sector of the party which felt excluded. It would give them a new sense of ownership and it would give the conference a broader legitimacy.[51]

But by 1992 various new movements of opinion had taken place. Unusually, possibly to bury it, the issue was passed by the Trade Union Review Group to a subcommittee – Tony Blair, Lewis Minkin and Clare Short, with the Secretary Tony Mainwaring. They could not reach agreement, but in the discussion and after it, it became clear that the view of the PLP leaders was that this would produce significant new party management problems. Some union representatives on the right now responded to these concerns. Gordon Colling argued that this would place enormous pressure on MPs and MEPs to cast their votes in line with their sponsoring organisation.[52] Others did not think that the unions should concede such an immediate weakening of their own position. Following this, and a loss of support from the CLP in the consultations, the proposal was sidelined. Under Blair later, bringing PLP representatives into NEC membership was seen instead as a further means of managing the NEC.

Opinion in the unions, and in the party generally, was hardening behind acceptance of the principle of conference parity between affiliated organisations and the CLPs. That felt like equality between unions and CLPs, although in effect it gave the unions minority status as smaller affiliated organisations would be casting a vote of up to 1 per cent. It had the strength of being a defensible position as the only workable basis for a partnership. It also became another variant of the line in the sand. Only the AEEU leadership, which in 1992 had supported 30 per cent, quietly held that position, coming into line only in 1996.

But old considerations led the majority of the committee to an evolutionary change beginning only when the membership reached 300,000 (the 1993 figure was 260,000.) There was still a concern, particularly on the traditional right, about avoiding destabilisation to the leadership's capacity for party management which they thought the unions would supply. As for the voting process, the old bloc-vote procedure inherited from the TUC and reinforced by the party which allocated to an organisation just one voting card (which might be worth many hundreds of thousands of votes) was abolished. There would be individual delegate voting cards with the results of the vote expressed in percentage terms.[53] This followed the procedural reforms pioneered in 1988 at the Labour Women's Conference. It did not preclude mandating of delegates in line with union rules where there was a clear policy decision.

This was a position acknowledged even in the AEEU proposals in which delegates would have a free vote as individuals where there was no union policy. Individual delegate representation at the conference was highly favourable to the CLPs. In the 1993 rulebook they had one delegate per first 500 members or part thereof and then one per 250. The affiliated organisations had one delegate per 5,000 members or part thereof.[54] It was anticipated that hand votes would come to be the norm. These proposals went through the final review group meeting with little dispute and were agreed by an overwhelming majority at the conference. What was arguably the most important constitutional change affecting the conference since the party was founded went through on a vote of 64.262 per cent to 28.011 per cent.

Leadership elections

Ironically, the procedure for the election of the party's Leader (which had been the focal point of so much post-election resentment against union involvement) came to be the greatest source of consensus and a modernising fusion of individual and collective traditions. From the first, a strong body of union opinion saw the need for reform of the proportions within the procedure. These had not been the consensual first choice of most union leaders even in 1981. Smith's initial position favoured a 50:50 arrangement which excluded the unions, but he was also influenced – as was the review group – by the results of the consultation in which support for the union staying in leadership elections had strengthened in the CLPs as well as the unions during the months of argument.

On the review group, over several discussions, the movement towards reduction of the affiliated organisations vote in elections for the leadership from 40 per cent, and making the electoral college proportions a third/third/third, was generally agreed. That option, correspondingly increasing the vote of the MPs and the CLPs, was also favoured in the consultation. From being the largest entity in the college the trade union vote (which was not the total of the affiliated organisations) was now to be the smallest.

There was an important feed here from the discussions going on over candidate selection, registered supporters and a possible individualisation of union voting within the electoral college. The procedures for electing the Leader were now to involve the complete eradication of forms of block representation within the affiliated organisations section of the electoral college. Voting would take place under the managerial organisation of each affiliated organisation which could recommend the way a vote could be cast and would choose and finance the counting agency with votes reported back to the individual union. That preserved the federal collective element. But as in the CLPs votes were allocated on an individual basis and the normality would involve individual postal balloting apart from in the miners' union, the NUM, which would have pit-head individual balloting.

Those voting had to be political levy payers, and the document which went to the NEC for its meeting on 19 July also involved an additional qualification that they 'declared their support for the party' and the stipulation that 'no voter can be a member of any other political party or expelled or excluded from the Labour Party'.[55] This version became subject to later argument because of possible voters' uncertainty about who was excluded from the Labour Party; from the TGWU it met opposition against 'bans and proscriptions'. A pared-down version became part of each ballot paper in 1994. Voters must declare themselves political levy payers and supporters of the Labour Party. (Two unions, the NUM and UCATT, failed to accept this rule in 1994 and were excluded.) At the final review group meeting Smith had not responded to energetic signals from Blair that, on the procedure for electing the Leader, Smith should propose further changes.

Again, the proposal went through the conference supported by a huge majority, 65.419 to 31.606 per cent.[56]

Issues of party management

Much else was going on in and around these major decisions. Additional decisions, developments and thwarted moves, often unnoticed by commentators and subsequent studies, had long lasting consequences. Four in particular can be traced in the outcomes.

Rights of the party

The rights of the party were extended into trade union territory in two significant new areas. The obligation of trade union membership for individual members of the party, established historically by the unions, was made more flexible by the insertion of the words 'if applicable',[57] The way this was interpreted by 'New Labour' later meant that there was no obligation on the self-employed, retired or non-employed, or those working in an occupation or workplace which was non-unionised and where no active attempt was being made to establish a union.[58] As well, in future it would not only be the TUC which, by its acceptance of union affiliation, had the right to decide whether an organisation was a bona fide trade union, but under party rules the NEC could also make that decision.[59]

Another expression of this focus on the rights of the party concerned joint procedures. Hitherto there had been a clear though unwritten rule in the relationship which prevented the party regulating those trade union procedures which interfaced with the party. This had been deemed to be a matter of union autonomy, subject to each union's own rule book. On the review group however, it was generally agreed that the party should in the future attempt to share a joint regulatory role in laying down and managing agreed democratic standards at the interface of the relationship.

New liaison

It was clear throughout the review group discussion that some of the trade union representatives had not been happy with the party management of vital trade union policy issues, especially the links between the Leader's office and the TUC in Kinnock's period as Leader. That relationship was seen as not sensitive enough to the role of the affiliated unions and on occasions was held to be a means of 'stitching up' the affiliated unions prior to party policy-making. There was a concern, expressed particularly by Gordon Colling of the print union SOGAT, that though the unions should act as ballast for the leadership, the existing policy interaction was not geared up to reflecting the views of the affiliated unions. There was also a concern that the union voice be heard on constitutional and organisational issues in advance of another stampede.

TUFL had been constitutionally prohibited by its rules from any policy role, in order to protect it from political factionalism. Now the review group supported a proposal from Colling for the creation of a new committee with a wider remit which would meet with the Parliamentary leadership three or four times a year. In the text of the report, special reference was made to 'the policy strategy' and 'immediate policy concerns' of the unions over campaigning issues including over privatisation, but the summary of recommendations said simply 'to discuss all issues'. This little-noticed organisational renewal was eventually agreed by Smith and accepted with much obstruction and qualification later by Blair. It was, however, eventually to have some very significant and controversial effects on the union role in policy-making through a new liaison organisation, TULO, under Blair. (See in Chapter 9, pp. 271–2 and in Chapter 17, p. 593.)

Plebiscitary leadership and the Blairite agenda

Blair's most singular contribution to the review group had potentially major implications for union involvement in the party, for its internal democracy and for the form of party management. His support for a new plebiscitarian mechanism was a special source of tensions within the group. Twice Blair had raised the referendum proposal, linking it to members' approval of the party's programme but also to the dangers arising from union amalgamations, which would produce an ever greater concentration of union votes in the hands of fewer unions at the conference. However, the rest of the committee was thinking now in terms of steadily reducing the combined union vote at the conference, and the proposal had major practical problems including the problem of costs.

It also indicated a potential threat. A plebiscite on party policy which could be justified as a modern empowerment of members also fitted too comfortably into the centrally driven party led by a strong Leader appealing over the heads of activist intermediaries and circumventing the unions and the delegate conference. Trade union representatives with some knowledge of the Webbs' famous book on *Industrial Democracy* had long before anticipated the dangers of this kind of procedure failing to ensure popular assent.[60] Those concerned with management also noted that a ballot over the programme held just before an election would be tantamount to a vote of confidence. It would be very hard to reject but if such a rejection did take place it would be a total disaster.

Each time he introduced the issue it received no support on the committee, not even from his senior parliamentary colleagues nor from the AEEU representative. Finally, after another long discussion on 1 January 1993, he insisted that it be put to a vote – the only vote taken on the committee. He received support this time from the General Secretary, who saw some value in the proposal and for party management reasons was also anxious not to leave Blair isolated. But everybody else voted against it. Blair was never happy with this defeat and would return to the issue of the national ballot as Leader in 1995 and 1996.

Leadership challenge

As the *Contentious Alliance* study had pointed out, the costs and lengthy process of the leadership electoral college had made challenges to the leader highly problematic and thereby reduced accountability.[61] That procedure had already created a high degree of security for the Leader, which had increased after reforms on the number of nominations required for eligibility to stand were raised under Kinnock. The new obligatory OMOV procedures within the unions now threatened to further inhibit challenges, whatever the circumstances.

In the group discussions, Minkin proposed that there needed to be a special emergency procedure to deal with a Leader who was clearly shown (to précis, crudely now) to be exceptionally bad or exceptionally mad. However, the party had not been prone to seek to remove the Leader and the unions did not regard it as their function to make it easier. Some could see the glaring media story now to be that the unions wanted to take more power. From the parliamentary representatives, who included not a few who had leadership pretensions, including Blair, there was some hostility. There was also a worry that such a procedure might cause management problems allowing intrepid oppositionists to mount regular well-publicised public divisions. Whitty was later quoted by Paul Anderson as saying at the time that he would 'make it impossible'.[62] The proposal was left to lie on the table. But by 2006, when Blair's eviction was in central focus and the problems mounted, Whitty had radically changed his view.

Settlement

Overall, the results in 1993 were an impressive collective achievement. They had provided a basis for a new unity between the industrial and political wings of the party. The long battle and the way it was ended did generate some fears of prolonged internal upheaval; it left its scars, particularly on those around Smith angry at Edmonds. The TGWU had a particular sense of being cheated after their victory on their resolution. Yet there was also some general relief in the unions that the battle was over, and in most unions, on reflection, no great sense that something vital had been lost over candidate selection. Privately, Bill Morris had a sophisticated mixture of grievance combined with an acceptance that this was probably the best political outcome.

In practice, things calmed very quickly. Smith conducted himself in such a way as to help repair various relationships, helped by the fact that he made clear that he had no inclination to launch a new fratricidal upheaval on the scale of 1992. There had always been a strong undercurrent in the unions that they could work with Smith, a view still shared by Edmonds who also accepted the result. With reform out of the way there was renewed optimism that under Smith the next election was winnable. In effect, the arrangements covering the three most contentious constitutional areas had become recognised as a 'settlement'. Eventually, even Blair, who still nursed ambitions for more radical change, formally came into line with this.[63]

The GMB and the TGWU caused some problems in reducing their affiliations to the party, suggested later as being 'a price' of the Smith victory.[64] In fact, this was a development foreshadowed in the long discussions which had been taking place since the raising of affiliation fees and in the light of declining union membership since 1979. Though probably not entirely unaffected by the blast of anti-union propaganda in 1992, negotiations had, in Whitty's words, taken place 'on a separate plane to that of the argument over the OMOV vote' and without reference to it.[65] Although the general proposals for raising affiliation fees were discussed on the Review Group it was at no stage linked to organisational changes. Under Edmonds' leadership GMB affiliation had run ahead of the levy-paying membership in order to help the party. They had reduced affiliation in 1987–1992 by only 1 per cent; by contrast, the loyalist AEEU/EEPTU had reduced by 42 per cent.[66] Edmonds regarded this post-OMOV reduction of affiliation as a rectifying adjustment having no penalty implications.[67] The TGWU simply continued its past practice of reduction.

The settlement had some paradoxical consequences. The outcome on candidate selection was a victory for Neil Kinnock, the trade union right and a variety of union and CLP supporters of OMOV in candidate selection. In that victory, Blair had played a significant part on the review group. On the total package, it was said by one of Brown's biographers that 'Brown and his allies had scored a famous victory'.[68] But Blair, Brown and their closest moderniser allies had little to do with the scope and delivery of the overall package. This had been a victory for the selective gradualism of Smith, the reformers in the unions and years of party pressures for change.

It was also in effect a huge rebuff for Blair, Brown and the modernising separationist spinners, although the addiction to spin with hints of future separation was undiminished. The review group consultation had shown minuscule support for excluding the unions from the party conference.[69] The package now involved a major historical change in union linkage with the party in a way that fused two traditions – in accordance with the agreed Framework of Working Principles, Themes and Values. It was not accepted by the party conference as a de-federalisation but to protect and further legitimise the federal relationship, although it could have become the thin end of a wedge.

Perhaps more important still was the sign from the intensity of the conflict that the pursuit of such a move could split the party from top to bottom in a prolonged internal war. Whatever the frustration, there was no painless surgical way. The crucial question after this for those who still thought in terms of organisational separation was not just 'is it desirable?' but 'how would you do it?' It was not surprising that in the period immediately following the 1993 Conference Prescott gained new prestige. Blair and Brown took the last two places in the NEC elections, although a rise in Blair's vote and a big drop in that of Brown was a pointer to their changing individual status. Under the new system with a one-woman quota, Harman came on, replacing Benn whose vote dropped substantially.

The sense of settlement was consolidated by public reactions. Ironically, given the massive media focus and the doom-laden warnings over the electoral costs of a failure to reform, for 69 per cent of the electorate this made little difference to their voting intention one way or another.[70] There was little public support for a new agenda of union reform. For 53 per cent of the public the reform package was 'about right' and 7 per cent thought they had gone too far, but only 16 per cent thought that it had not gone far enough.[71] Amongst trade unionists in a poll the following year, a similar result emerged, with 62 per cent agreeing that the Kinnock-Smith reforms were 'about right' and only 26 per cent saying that they 'did not go far enough'.[72] Perhaps, as Anthony King noted, this might well have been 'the end of an era'[73] if Smith had lived. Certainly the polls by the spring of 1994 gave Labour a comfortable lead in the polls with Smith's ratings better than Major's.[74]

Smith leadership and party cohesion

The Joint Policy Committee and the National Policy Forum 1992–4
One final mechanism helped to produce a better feeling, new unity and another dimension of democratic renewal. Assisting in stabilisation during and after all the turbulence was the management by Smith and Whitty of other policy-making changes. A joint policy committee was never mentioned in the documents agreed in 1990 and 1991, and in the discussions of future policy institutions on the trade union review group in 1992–3, there had been no reference to it. It was created under Smith on 30 November 1993 and originally conceived and authorised in terms of a coordination and liaison between the NEC and the Shadow Cabinet, a process seen as finding out the major internal problem areas and then generally moving along the same path. It had the responsibility of 'overseeing the preparation and clearing of all policy documents'.[75] But in the light of what happened later under Blair, it is important to note that this was not a rejection of the authoritative NEC role. It was accepted that 'The JPC reports to the NEC which, apart from Conference, is the primary policymaking body of the Party.'[76]

Because of anxieties on the NEC that this might in practice mean a curtailing of their policy role, they made various responses to check it. At the insistence of senior figures on the NEC, there were no non-NEC frontbenchers on it and the committee was staffed by headquarters officials.

Though it was up to the JPC to decide which should be the key policy areas, this was subject to confirmation by the NEC.[77] It was also clarified later that policy documents were the property of the NEC.[78] There continued to be a separate NEC Domestic and International Policy Committee established on amalgamation in 1992.

In practice the regular cycle of mainly monthly meetings of the JPC did take over a great deal of the agenda of the NEC, and there was also often an element of duplication. Over time there was a decline of the work of the Domestic and International Policy Committee of the NEC. But the NEC continued to keep a sensitive eye on the propriety of policy-making procedures and its own final say. At one point a policy proposal from the Shadow Education Secretary, Anne Taylor, on graduate taxation and university fees was challenged by the NEC and quietly dropped. A problem of procedural propriety also emerged over an important and path-breaking document prepared by Gordon Brown, Robin Cook and John Prescott for a conference of the Labour Finance and Industry Group – about promoting partnerships between public and private finance. It eventually went through the agreed policy-making channels beginning with the Economic Commission but only after disquiet at the way it was authorised – a matter which was taken up at the next JPC and NEC.[79]

National Policy Forum and the move to deliberative politics

One of the responsibilities of the NEC agreed under Smith in 1992 was 'To set up and oversee a National Policy Forum and policy standing commissions in areas of policy to help the NEC produce a draft Rolling Programme for submission to Annual Conference'.[80] Facing the usual post-election financial stringency, 'an interim version'[81] of the Forum was introduced with arrangements which did not interfere with resolution submissions to the party conference. The composition of 81 (with a minimum of 41 women) was important in its breadth of representation from the party outside the leading institutions. CLPs through the regions, trade unions, socialist societies and coops, women's organisations, councillors, Black and Asian members and youth and student members, plus the PLP and EPLP were all represented, but not the Shadow Cabinet, the NEC or the JPC. Two representatives elected by the NPF were to be included in each standing policy commission. The unions nationally constituted only about a quarter of the total but with regional representation still to be decided.

The launching of the NPF was backed enthusiastically by Smith and Deputy Leader Margaret Beckett. Its first meeting, chaired by NEC Policy Chairman Tom Sawyer, was held in London on 7–8 May 1993. At the next NPF meeting at Leeds in November, John Smith sat in the audience throughout and took notes. His was a deeply impressive unpresidential presence. Such was the cooperative atmosphere and the level of general support for the policies as they emerged under Smith that there was little problem in the NEC accepting the policies that the NPF had agreed.

Smith thereafter gave strong backing to further innovative developments. The initial format of the forum involved plenary sessions and discussions held in workshops that were fairly traditional in form. It had become clear from the reactions of party representatives and their response to a questionnaire, that although the meeting had been generally judged a success the discussion process required more direction if it was to be effective. Also there should be a clear process of amending the documents coming to the NPF from the NEC. From this came a crucial push on to major innovation.

The specific form of the new procedures and culture surrounding them were initiated by policy officials under the Policy Director, Roland Wales, a left-of-centre ex-Bank of England official, who had strong procedural values. He was influenced by ideas from the trade union political officers drawing from an old TUC tradition and by work in the party on small study circles in political education. The officials worked with the tide of NPF opinion in creating a vigorous new deliberative institution which it was hoped would embed a view of two-way political education built upon effective participation.

Work groups and the deliberative culture

Smith died suddenly on 12 May 1994. At Birmingham two months later, with Margaret Beckett as acting Leader, the new format which was to give the NPF its distinctive culture was introduced and remained the same until 1997. After a plenary session and speeches by frontbench spokespeople who were in charge of the policy areas being covered by the three or four documents under discussion, the NPF then split into groups which examined one document at a time. The composition of the groups was normally balanced in terms of representation of CLPs and trade unions, regions, occupations and other expertise. Each group had a facilitator to encourage focused discussion. And there was a note-taker whose job it was to report on the views of the workshop. Later these reports were amalgamated by the facilitators and they provided a statement which was presented to a plenary session. This session could question and seek correction of the statement. Voting, though permitted, was discouraged. Both in the work groups and in the plenary session, where collective decisions were taken on amendments, the aim was to achieve consensus.

The most novel and attractive feature was that group members worked through each document offering comment, advice and criticism. The draft documents allowed more space for a detailed exchange of perspectives and knowledge offered with more tentativeness and less confrontation. It also allowed, in theory at least, more space for creative transformation as well as consensual accommodation. The groups were hard-working and discussions were generally thoughtful as members attempted to engage with each other. The privacy of the process (apart from a few observers) with no media representation and no verbatim reports, lessened the propensity to make gallery-playing performances. There were short visits to groups from front-bench MPs and policy advisors but they acted in a very unobtrusive way, offering comments only when asked. After the Birmingham meeting the NEC accepted everything except a resolution on provision for nursery education for all 3- to 4-year-olds.

The development of this deliberative element was in marked contrast to the traditional adversarial and resolution-based politics of the Labour movement, and in particularly stark contrast to the politics of the battle over OMOV. The working groups were a source of enthusiasm and satisfaction to those who attended. It was not unrealistic at that stage to visualise a modern politics managed through mutual education with diminished manipulation and a growth of trust – except that there was a warning signal from Blair's failure even to pay a visit to the National Policy Forum meeting during his campaign for the leadership.

The Blair ascendancy

Blair was elected as Leader after a broad and deep surge of support from within the party. The composition of the electorate and procedures in a form which Blair had not completely favoured, became – helped by an admiring media – a huge advantage to him whilst diminishing the role of the union leadership. Collective representation with individualised voting broadened the base of his leadership and ensured that Blair was elected by the largest and most socially representative electorate of any political party: 68 per cent of individual members, 61 per cent of MPs and MEPs, even 52 per cent of affiliated members voted for him. In terms of participatory democracy it was an impressive exercise and in terms of the range of his support, astonishing. John Prescott was elected Deputy Leader but the reality was that from a position of being outsiders to the 1993 settlement, arising from Smith's sudden death had come a new ascendancy of Blair and 'the modernisers'.

Notes

1 Philip Gould, *The Unfinished Revolution: How the Modernisers Changed the Labour Party*, Little Brown, London, 1998, p. 186.
2 *Women's Own magazine*, 21 June 1993, quoted in Donald Macintyre, *Mandelson: the Biography*, HarperCollins, London 1999, p. 241.
3 Hugo Young, *The Hugo Young Papers: Thirty Years of British Politics – Off the Record*, Allen Lane, London, 2008, p. 418.
4 Ibid. p. 289 and p. 390.
5 Gould, *Unfinished Revolution*, p. 191.
6 Ibid. p. 190.
7 A point made forcefully to the author by Murray Elder in 1993 and repeated in 2005.
8 John Sopel, *Tony Blair the Moderniser*, Michael Joseph, London, 1995, p. 150.

 9 Ibid.
10 John Rentoul, *Tony Blair: Prime Minister*, Little Brown, London, 2001, p. 208.
11 Gould, *Unfinished Revolution*, p. 187.
12 Ibid.
13 Ibid.
14 *Independent*, 12 June 1992.
15 Anthony Heath, Roger Jowell and John Curtice, with Brigit Taylor, *Labour's Last Chance?: The 1992 Election and Beyond*, Dartmouth Publishing, Dartmouth, 1994.
16 David Butler and Dennis Kavanagh, *The British General Election of 1992*, Palgrave Macmillan, London, 1992, p. 296.
17 Martin Westlake, *Kinnock, The Biography*, Little, Brown, London, 2001, p. 519.
18 Mark Stuart, *John Smith: a Life*, Politico's, London, 2005, pp. 217–22.
19 MORI/*Sunday Times* panel survey, March/April, 1992, cited in Lees-Marshment, *Political Marketing*, p. 171.
20 Gould, *Unfinished Revolution,* pp. 24–9.
21 Ibid. p. 24.
22 Report of the trade union review group, 1993, p. 6.
23 Letter from Tom Sawyer, Deputy General Secretary of NUPE, NEC Minutes, 27 May 1992.
24 Tony Blair, Walden, LWT, 26 September 1993.
25 Tony Blair, GMB Conference, 7 June 1995.
26 The Organisation sub-committee had agreed the motion by 11 votes to 2, NEC Organisation sub-committee minutes, 18 May 1992.
27 NEC Minutes, 24 June 1992.
28 Lewis Minkin, RG14, 'A Framework of Working Principles, Themes and Values, submission to the NEC trade union review group', 5 September 1992.
29 Interim Report, Labour Party-Trade Union Links Review Group, 1992, p. 16.
30 *Guardian,* 30 November 1992.
31 Gould, *Unfinished Revolution*, p. 191.
32 BBC Transcript of *On the Record*, 17 January 1993.
33 Macintyre, *Mandelson*, p. 240.
34 Ibid.
35 Ibid.
36 Selection of Parliamentary Candidates: Report of the NEC consultation, 1990, p. 4.
37 Final Report, Labour Party Trade Union Review Group, 1993, p. 34.
38 Notes of the author.
39 *Guardian*, 2 June 1992.
40 *Sunday Mirror*, 7 June 1992.
41 Interview with Tom Sawyer, Deputy General Secretary of NUPE, 5 June 1993.
42 Interview with John Smith, Labour Party Leader, 19 January 1994.
43 Ibid.
44 Card vote 59.617 per cent to 9.817 per cent, LPCR 1993, p. 177.
45 Meg Russell, '*Building New Labour*', p. 113.
46 Interviews with Murray Elder and Sally Morgan at various stages during 1994 and 1995.

47 Colin Brown, *Fighting Talk: the biography of John Prescott*, Simon & Schuster, London, 1997, p. 222.
48 LPCR 1993, pp. 161–4.
49 Voting confirmed by Russell, p. 56.
50 Labour Party document, 'Democracy and Policy-making for the 1990s', 1990, p. 8.
51 For a full discussion of the developing arguments see Minkin, *Contentious Alliance*, pp. 376–7.
52 'A GPMU View', trade union review group paper, January 1993.
53 For the range of possible block vote reforms see Minkin, *Contentious Alliance*, pp. 362–94.
54 Rulebook 1993, Clause VIII (i) (a) and (b).
55 Report of the Trade Union Review Group, p. 31.
56 LPCR 1993, p. 168.
57 Rulebook 1993–4, Membership Conditions Clause III 7(b).
58 Gould, *Unfinished Revolution*, p. 191.
59 Rulebook 1993–4, Membership Conditions Clause III 7(b).
60 Sidney and Beatrice Webb, *Industrial Democracy*, Longmans Green, London, 1920, pp. 61–2.
61 Minkin, *Contentious Alliance*, p. 357.
62 *Tribune*, 8 August 2008.
63 Tony Blair, *New Statesman and Society*, 15 July 1994.
64 Stuart, *John Smith*, p. 340.
65 Interview.
66 Trade union review group, RG18, 1993.
67 Interview with John Edmonds, 19 July 2005.
68 Paul Routledge, *Gordon Brown: The Biography*, Simon & Schuster, London, 1998, p. 182.
69 In the consultation, of the 35 per cent of the CLPs who were not in favour of any of the four main options (all of which included the unions), only 10 per cent wanted just CLP OMOV – i.e., 3.5 per cent of the total.
70 For 69 per cent the issue made no difference to their voting intention. ICM/*Guardian*, 14 October 1993.
71 Ibid.
72 NOP/*The Independent*, *Newsnight*, 26 May 1994.
73 *Daily Telegraph*, 7 February 1994.
74 Robert Worcester and Roger Mortimer, *Explaining Labour's Landslide*, Politico's, London, 1999, p. 88.
75 JPC Minutes, 30 November 1992.
76 Letter from the Policy Director, Roland Wales to M. Jones (not NEC representative Maggie Jones), 1 December 1994.
77 Domestic and International Policy Committee minutes, 2 November 1992.
78 NEC minutes, 19 May 1993.
79 NEC minutes, 23 February 1994.
80 Rulebook 1993, Clause IX 2(p).
81 NEC Minutes, 28 October 1992.

PART II

Forging 'New Labour' management

4

'New Labour' and the culture of party management[1]

The new management

New management and the vanguard

On the face of it, the election of Blair and Prescott as Leader and Deputy Leader implied a balanced relationship reflecting a duality of different traditions. At leadership level the Shadow Cabinet then Cabinet was also a fusion of the 1992 modernisers with those who had been on the traditional right and the soft left. In practice, the direction, strategy and central policies of what was self-ascribed as 'New Labour'[2] (as opposed to 'old' Labour whose attitudes and policies they very successfully caricatured and castigated) were created mainly by the group of three – Blair, Brown, Mandelson – plus Alistair Campbell and Philip Gould. They shared many perspectives and touchstones in relation to the forging of 'New Labour' and also a diagnosis and prescriptions in relation to managing problems of the party.

Unique in Labour history, the 'New Labour' leadership team was a modernising vanguard both in their self-ascribed purpose and their circumstance. They had developed a strong sense of their historic distinctiveness when contrasted with Smith and even Kinnock – not just modernisers but *the* modernisers. Although they carried various uncertainties of purpose, their greatest unity was in the negative appraisal of the party including and particularly its affiliated unions and its associated collective body – the TUC (see more on this in Chapter 9). This was coupled with an aspiration to transform it in form, identity, culture and image based on different forms of representation, and different attitudes to leadership. This task was historically unprecedented in its scope and content but it was seen as fitting the imperative arising from the condition of the Labour Party. In the face of constant change in modern life and politics, the party had to undergo a more or less permanent revolution. Following this and the election would come the modernisation of Britain. The 'out of date' Smith management had to be replaced by a management which would advance and protect the wide project that Blair and his allies had in mind.

The rolling coup

The problems faced by that management ambition were considerable, as they sought also to prepare for a crucial General Election. But adding significantly to the difficulties was the fact that behind the landslide victory of Blair in the leadership election and the spin of overwhelming popularity and supremacy, those who fully shared the Blairite ambitions for the party were a small minority. They operated from that minority position in relation to, and at times against, the mainstream of the party. A Blair-sympathising journalist, Martin Kettle of the *Guardian*, reported in 1996 that one Labour MP had estimated 'perhaps a dozen of her colleagues' were Blairites. In an article headed 'Blair's Shadow Army', Kettle's view was, 'that was about right'.[3] A well-informed but anonymous piece of journalism later had a wry comment from Blair describing 'New Labour' as 'the newest political party on the scene and the smallest. It has a membership of about five people'.[4] From within 'New Labour' the take over of the party by this small minority was quietly and sometimes boastfully acknowledged to be a *coup d'état* over the party.[5]

It was a peculiar coup in the sense that the leadership was won openly through procedures which were not Blair's first preference, and in a contest which involved a choice. It is, however, much more illuminating to see the 'coup' following Blair's election and his replacement of the General Secretary (see Chapter 5, p. 155) in terms of what happened following Blair's election. He drove party officials to adopt a new managerial identity, followed by the creation of an extended managerial organisation which produced greater powers and protection for the Leader. It can also be usefully described as a rolling coup in that it involved a series of unilateral major moves over several years. Those will be uncovered as this study develops.

Leadership

The strong party leader

There was already a major element of procedural security for the Leader, noted in Chapter 3. And the wide electorate gave the new Leader the authority of formal majority support in every section of the party including the unions. With this backing, Blair found good reasons and opportunities to expand the role and status of the Leader. His view was that the modern party needed effective ways of decision-making and that that was realised best in a singular powerful Leader with room for boldness and risk-taking. He declared that his attitude was always summed up by the phrase 'if you don't like the Leader get someone else to do the job'.[6] Yet Blair knew how difficult such an eviction would be; he had been unsympathetic on the Trade Union Review Group to alleviating those difficulties.

Back in 1992, the Shadow Communications Agency focus group material presented to the NEC had indicated that people thought that the Labour Party had too much democracy and bureaucracy. This finding got lost in the focus on democracy and the battle for OMOV in 1992–3 but was remarkably fitting to the Blair ideal of a Leader who should be left to get on with the job. Though he operated (more or less) through the formalities of the Shadow Cabinet, his informal personal decision-making and small-group policy-making style twinned by that adopted by Brown fitted well also into this new leadership model. He was impatient with the procedures of Labour's internal democracy and the plurality of power centres. It contravened his sense of effective leadership which should be able to enjoy the creative flexibility of informality without immediate constraints in policy formulation coming from the NEC or the unions.

An adroit tactician with a particularly strong sense of the manipulable weaknesses of others, he and his aides operated from a 'New Labour' perspective on ambition which had been raised in importance as a worthy socio-economic aspect of character and a salient electoral motivation. That also became more useful as a focus of leadership patronage. Encouraging the desire to 'get on', unrestrained by any hang-up of old moral criticism, became part of the new order. In his relation with the various officers and representatives that came his way, he knew the seductions of a personal contact which implied inclusion. He knew also a mastery of different faces assisted by, as Rentoul said later, 'the empty insincerity of the good actor'.[7]

One face which he preferred as his own was that of the bold, 'myself-alone', Leader. He had told Philip Gould at one stage – almost in the form of a pledge – 'I will never compromise. I would rather be beaten and leave politics than bend to the party.'[8] On the other hand, the boldness appeared to be tempered by the fact that he did not enjoy personal confrontations.[9] Put more strongly by Toynbee, he was 'by nature almost pathologically averse to confrontation'.[10] That may well have been true of some of his dealings on personal failures, promotion and relegation. There was also a special sensitivity to those with major power resources in politico-economic life (see Chapter 9) and international politics with the most powerful, where major confrontations were best avoided.

But he had shown on the NEC Trade Union Review Group a bravery in being almost alone, and the assertion to Gould was revealing of an instinctive attitude towards the Party and the drive of a man who always wanted more freedom from the collective. This left him permanently frustrated by the obstacles and made open conflict – in 'taking on' the party – natural and, for the managers, predictable. It was also on occasion provoked by them to bring his hard response into play. In practice, however, no Leader with any pragmatic and calculating subtlety could fully abide by the Gould commitment and Blair was not lacking in that quality. Nevertheless, it was the strength and ease of movement in distance-pull from his own party, its traditions and ways of operation, without losing control of the party, that marked him and his party management as historically different. It was a difference he and his close supporters thought of with pride.

The Thatcher example heightened Blair's confidence that strong leadership would pay off in electoral terms. He had no doubts about his own vote-winning capabilities carefully projected by his spin doctors. In action, he was refreshingly eager, and telegenic, remarkably secure and effective in his presentational capability facing audiences large and small. The personal qualities he brought to bear were eminently suited to the image of a quasi-presidential role and as the heroic modernising leader fighting to overcome the forces of traditionalism and conservatism. His middle-England projection free of the old Labour image made an immediately expanded appeal to a broader socio-political constituency at a time of increasing party dealignment and a growing disillusionment with the Conservatives.

His image of the strong party leader fitted the policy aspirations to lead in Europe, to lead the international community and assert a strong defence through NATO and other international organisations. A theory of effective governance held with fervour was built around the ideal of one charismatic bold individual prepared to lead from well to the front. This arrangement was seen as applicable in facilitating organisational dynamism. It fitted not only the party but the Blair idea of changing British governmental forms which worked within a residue of monarchical authority.

Strong leadership together with strong and extensive party management control could also act as a means of ensuring governmental management of the unity and coordination of the United Kingdom against the pulls of the new devolved institutions. Focused on modernisation of British government and effective delivery of the 'New Labour' objectives, and alerted by the memories and myths of Labour's past experience of forming the government, these could provide an important counter to the dangers from corporatist, centrifugal, and departmental conservative forces whilst strengthening the necessary coordination and communication processes. With this perspective it was not surprising that his attitude towards central government after Labour came to office in 1997 moved much further towards Prime Ministerial Government, with the Cabinet office in effect a Prime Minister's Department and No. 10 as a driving force of policy and information. Blair told the Newspaper Society that 'we will run from the centre and govern from the centre'.[11] This would be what the constitutional analyst Peter Hennessey characterised as 'a command premiership of a highly personalised and driven kind'.[12]

The complications

In his relations with his Shadow Cabinet and then the Cabinet, Blair did not aim to be 'first among equals'. He aimed to be in charge. In the perpetual individual competition around him the increasingly cultivated quasi-presidential style was also a means of showing supremacy over rival senior figures and potential challengers for leadership. Yet to assuage suspicion and disgruntlement, at times in Opposition he had to involve the leading parliamentarians Brown, Cook and Prescott in a team meeting of 'the big four'. More significant in disturbing this lone leadership and command model was the accommodation he had arrived at in 1994 when Brown, the senior of the two, withdrew in favour of his friend and rival. Blair made an agreement that Brown, who became Shadow Chancellor then Chancellor, be given not only command over economic policy but also oversight of the whole field of social policy. This led to some productive tensions eased by the sharing of purpose but it also led to increasing conflicts and frustration for Blair in what became more of a duopoly which set the two on a different level to others in the parliamentary leadership.

Matters were further complicated because in the Brown camp his withdrawal became seen as forced on him by a manipulation engineered by Mandelson using his media-management skills whilst acting as Blair's close but hidden advisor. It produced a deep belief that their man had been cheated of his natural and proper role by the illegitimate leader. But for the moment, although mutual suspicion touched issues of party control and Brown's party activities, the two leaders of New Labour and their close aides and allies saw eye-to-eye on the main thrust of party management.

The Leader's strong party management

Controlling the party organisation

In that management, success was not to be left to the Leader's character and skills, nor to chance and, least of all, to the free flow of democratic dialogue. The party organisation had to be brought immediately under leadership control and changed to make it fit for purpose. This involved the Leader's control over the senior offices of the party and the mechanics, facilities and role of the party's organisation (see Chapter 5). It provided a major strengthening of the position of the Leader within a consolidation of the dominance of the Parliamentary leadership as a whole. It was reinforced also by some organised cultist presentational features heightening his quasi-presidential status. From this, he could take pride in his personal ascendancy over the party as a public expression of the contrast with a weakening Conservative Leader, John Major, telling the House of Commons on 25 May 1995, 'I lead my party, he follows his'.

As a party manager, over and above the authority of his leadership, Blair had many helpful attributes. Like Kinnock, he was very focused on what he wanted and, if what emerged was not as he wanted it, he would return to it through some other route. As with Kinnock, he liked to get his coat off to engage, to educate and to inspire movement. He prized talking things over as a means of creating understanding of his position. Unlike Kinnock whose past feelings often remained uncertainly attached to his feelings about his new political outlook, there was a lack of sentimentality in Blair over his new radicalism. There was also an element of a calculating Zelig who could contrive to fit naturally into what persona was required, and with a mastery of contrived ambiguity enabled people with different views to hear what they wanted to hear.[13] This 'talent for creative ambiguity'[14] where necessary, assisted creative management in dealing with blockages.

Seen through 'New Labour' eyes, the party was a permanent source of frustration. Not only were there special problems of party and union conservatism embedded in the culture, creating obstacles to the modernising dynamic, but the Smith leadership had agreed with the unions a set of arrangements now asserted to be a 'settlement' which left the unions in a potentially still influential position within the extra-parliamentary party. The NEC defended its rights and there were deeply ingrained party-union 'rules' and protocols. Some entrenched existing policy commitments and union mandates also stood in the way. In addition, there were in place officials bequeathed from previous Leaders, MPs elected long before and candidates who had already nursed the seats. The new party had to be nurtured and managed so as to drive urgently through all these obstacles and to reshape the party to make it more subject to the Leader's supremacy.

Here another encumbrance sometimes emerged. Prescott's labour-movement roots and manual social background was especially valuable to Blair's party management. As a loyal deputy he could be used as a front and symbol of the party's concern for the wider coalition, asserting 'traditional values in a modern setting' in influencing sections of the party where Blair found a difficulty. As with other figures from the soft left like Cook, Short and Dobson, Prescott developed some areas of independent policy initiative but, like them, had in the main to make a loyal accommodation to the new and dominant force and to legitimise an agenda which was not necessarily always their own. He kept to that policy loyalty; nevertheless, as will be shown, Blair's politics of 'keeping JP on board' on party issues had other restrictive implications for party management when developed by JP himself.

Vanguardists

Historically, as we have seen, the politics of party management had been influenced by a majoritarian democratic perspective on the leadership's relations with the party and the party's relations with the electorate. Management was traditionally considered to be operating on behalf of the working people and the majority of the party against the unrepresentative minority, normally the left. They were perceived as the vanguardists, or prepared to ally with vanguardists, seeking not to represent the working class as they were but as the left hoped that they would be, with their socialist consciousness raised. The past leadership which wanted to focus on immediate electoral concerns saw their task as fending off or neutralising unrealistic and unrepresentative demands.

In one major respect that perspective was consolidated under Blair. New Labour became closely associated with its methods of focus groups and polls connecting and keeping in close touch with the shifting views of the electorate. There was always some question about how far the products were what the pollster Gould wanted to hear. And if it was considered necessary to move past public opinion notably over taxation of the wealthy, privatisation and some aspects of labour law, it went the way that the vanguard felt they needed to travel. In this respect it is doubtful whether the 1997 election was really won as 'New Labour' as opposed to the emphatic rejection of the Conservative party with 'New Labour' defining what the people needed. From 'New Labour' confidence of both rectitude and political nous, as later experience was to illustrate, it was easy also to slip into the manipulative denial of electoral choice also over candidates who might have public support but did not fit into the vanguard's plans.

Blair, party and tribalism

One major difference linked Blair and the vanguard uneasily with the mainstream of the party. Kinnock had also found the party a source of frustration and difficulty but as with other Labour leaders he showed enormous pride in the long march of the Labour Movement as the vehicle of 'a thousand generations of Kinnocks'. By contrast, Blair rarely expressed a remotely similar sentiment. It was suggested later that the Blairites were 'tribal Labour' loyalists.[15] Perhaps so, more or less, but it was a most peculiar tribalism, finding so much wrong with the party that it was difficult to express its historic virtues. Blair was particularly influenced by a perspective on the party's history in which the split between Labour and the Liberals was an electoral tragedy which had fundamentally damaged 'the Progressive Alliance'.

Openness to new forms, including rebuilding that alliance, became for some but by no means all[16] of the Blairites an essential part of *the* project. There was even a flirtation by some with amalgamation, but rebuilding the alliance was perceived primarily in terms of a joint movement of ideas and party linkage initially over constitutional reform[17] possibly ensuring a place for the Liberal Democrats in a future Labour Cabinet. The anti-tribalism included a hearty welcome for ex-SDP defectors and centrist Tories. It also welcomed a creative openness to ideas not only from the progressive centre but even from the Thatcherite right without any sense of disloyalty or guilt. This fitted into the comfort zone of Blair's denial of the modern relevance of ideology.

Though they could not start from scratch, both in their separationist wistfulness towards the fundamental reshaping of the relationship with the unions, and the uncomfortable attitude of some of them to Labour Party history before Year Zero of the modernisers, Blair and some of his closest allies appeared to have that longing for a clean sheet. Lance Price noted that at the centenary celebrations, Blair could not hide a body language that hardly expressed a deep love of the party.[18] His at times ostentatious lack of normal leadership feelings seemed to bring with it a touch of the alien.

Counteracting the alien quality in easing the management was that Blair was an attractive and likeable figure, lacking side and pomposity. Perhaps most important of all, he had a special electoral appeal representing 'us' in the Labour Party to occupants of normally Tory territory. Gould, captivated by his own portrayal of the qualities of Blair's leadership, was sure that Blair had 'a sense of the destiny of the nation and of the pulse of the people'.[19] His electoral victories evoked enthusiasm, and long-lasting gratitude in large sections of the party. In that sense he was always 'ours'. Nevertheless, there remained some hesitation in the party which revolved around anxiety about where he was going, how he was going there and even, to some realistic admiring loyalists, a regret about what had been lost.[20]

The new party: positioning and the imperatives of management

Radical 'New Labour'

Electoral positioning was a major influence on the priorities of party management. The positioning developed under 'New Labour' was given shape by the report back of emissaries to the Clinton Democratic experience – victorious in the 1992 United States presidential election. That amalgam involved an extraordinarily flexible constellation of avowed values practices and tactics from which to draw successful techniques, responses and messages. The decline of old ideologies and what was considered to be the unimportance of old distinctions between left and right justified Blair's rejection of the attempt to forge a new ideology, although that did not mean the absence of values or an ideological fervour over some prohibitions and prescriptions. What emerged was a formation well suited to the pragmatic targeting of different audiences in segmented markets, but with a general appeal pulled together later as the promotion of four values of a just society – equal worth, opportunity for all, responsibility and community.[21] It was an appeal which in itself also did not cause affront to the party.

Positioning to win the election involved adapting the party's appeal to the changing composition and attitudes of the electorate in building a winning social coalition. 'New Labour' leaders built radically on an old diagnosis that the working class was in fundamental decline and the middle class now the numerical majority. Whilst Blair thought in terms of expanding the constituency of support without sacrificing the existing base, the primary target was in practice an attempt to win over white-collar, middle-income voters by a party appeal which did not cap individual aspirations and could not to be identified with 'holding people back'. The potential unity of appeal built on the American definition of middle class which included what in the UK would be the working class who, in the

'New Labour' view, identified strongly with middle-class aspirations. An unremitting focus on 'hard-working people' had a wide social appeal but implicitly drew a distinction between them and the undeserving.

The positioning was managed to calibrate around the attitudes and preferences of the swing voter, especially wavering Conservatives, in the marginal seats. In focusing on this task, the party would abandon off-putting old political baggage and 'move forward from where Thatcher left off'.[22] From increasing conviction, 'New Labour' leading figures had accepted the neo-liberal economic framework of Thatcherism and the value of the financial activities of the City of London. They accepted also a significant injection of the Thatcherite policy legacy. On economic policy the priority remained stable, low-inflation conditions for long-term growth and competitiveness. There would be no substantial state intervention in the economy but a renewed emphasis on private-public partnerships.

Fusing with opinion in the party was that some of the most offensive aspects of Thatcherism were diluted particularly in establishing minimum standards, introducing elements of social justice and in establishing social democratic objectives in the public sector. It could be regarded as post-Thatcherite.[23] This combination of continuity and innovation was influenced by Clinton's US election tactics of triangulation. That involved a disassociation from the most unpopular and offensive features of the policies of both left and right, albeit here within a ballast of party commitments to the centre-left and what proved to be a tactical electoral pull towards floating Tory voters on the centre-right.

Management culture and business

There was another dimension to these considerations of positioning which was to be a permanent – even the primary – pressure on party management. There must be care in nursing new support within the business community. The generation of credibility in the City and more widely in the international finance markets would be vital for the economic success of a 'New Labour' Government. Integrated within this aim was an attempt to radically change the party's image by clarification of its allies and identity. Historically it had seen itself as 'the people's party', but defined in such a way as to associate 'the people' with the workers by hand or brain. Whereas in the past there had been history of defining finance capital as 'the Big Interests' and therefore 'the few', now the 'New Labour' leadership moved towards moving business to the centre of 'the many'.

The 'prawn cocktail offensive' leading up the 1992 election, aimed at the City of London, did win support for the party from the *Financial Times* but otherwise it had no electoral pay-off. In contrast, the public endorsement of the Conservatives by business representatives in a *Times* advertisement just prior to the General Election was seen by the Blair-Brown-Mandelson grouping as especially influential in consolidating Tory support from Middle England and in mobilising the wavering Tory voters in marginal constituencies. It was essential for 'New Labour' to neutralise that appeal and if possible win the public support of progressive business representatives so that it would reassure the election waverers that Labour's economic management was credibly prudent. This business support now became not only an essential goal in attesting to economic credibility but also an agency of the party's electoral strategy in ways which had a major influence over policy and the party's relations with the unions. (See particularly Chapters 6, pp. 181–2 and 9.)

Caution and priorities

Anxieties over internal argument, electoral responses and the creation of positions vulnerable to media assault led to more caution in immediate policy change than might have been expected from the rhetoric. It was a feature noted by Anderson and Mann.[24] But there had to be early adjustments of policy in areas where there was a clear electoral vulnerability or the need for an immediate public signal of 'New Labour' intentions within a constant reassurance that the party had changed. Rentoul emphasised a series of changes pronounced before the 1995 Special Conference involving moving policies closer to the Conservatives on taxation, inflation, exam league tables, opt-out schools, Northern Ireland, regional government and the House of Lords.[25] Of these the most important involved countering the accusation that Labour was addicted to 'tax and spend'. Policy development had to be managed to avoid uncosted promises and refrain from any public expenditure that implied major taxation commitments.

Amongst the Leader's early management priorities was also the restatement of aims and values in Clause IV of the party's constitution – a heavily symbolic gesture which differentiated the party from its past (Chapter 6, p. 176). This was followed by an attempt to reform other fundamental elements of the party's constitution (Chapter 6, pp. 187–97). Under new arrangements for Party into Power (Chapter 7) the party's relations with the future 'New Labour' government must be reorganised and managed so as to avoid past problems. In the PLP also a new emphasis was placed on building a better relationship with the government (Chapter 13, pp. 416–17). In all this, union-related issues must be defused and, most distinctive of all under new Labour, a changed policy relationship forged immediately with business (see Chapter 9, pp. 266–7). Intensified party management was essential to facilitate the best outcomes.

Trust, electorate and party management

Policy change in the party and the constant message of 'more on the way' were related to the problem of electoral trust identified by 'New Labour' strategists in 1994. Blair's election coincided with growing awareness of the 'sceptical electorate's' decline in political trust.[26] Curtice and Jowell diagnosed that with the decline of deference and a diminution of party commitment there was increased cynicism about the integrity of politicians, their honesty and ethical standards.[27] From Blair there was a recognition that it was 'crucial for the Labour Party to build up trust and then retain it'.[28]

This encountered the difficulty that potential causes of distrust were various and, though often obvious, sometimes not so easy to distinguish. Distrust could be focused on one particular feature or on a combination. Relationships could involve both trust-undermining and trust-enhancing features. Thus, with all this complexity, dialogue about trust sometimes consisted of people talking past each other. Although context could make for clarity, polling questions focused on trust did not normally clarify meanings and could be received differently by those who answered them.

Within these complexities for Blair and the 'New Labour' strategists, some major sources of distrust were apparent in 1994. One was the long-held public suspicion that politicians were self-interested in seeking their own or their party interests rather than that of the public – with an inclination to corruption.[29] An increasingly unpopular Conservative Government became the target of 'New Labour' attacks focused on what was held to be 'a more widespread culture of sleaze which the modern brand of Conservatism has nurtured'.[30] The attack combined financial self-serving scandals and sexual misconduct in ways which were made to embrace the whole Tory leadership. This repeated expression of repugnance over sleaze also became the 'New Labour' assertion of moral superiority and a reinforcement of the claim to new trust.

In more positive mode, trust for 'New Labour' was to be won by a focus on confidence in the government's competence, particularly its economic competence and delivery of what had been promised. This had been historically Labour's Achilles heel and was now regarded as a potential source of policy distrust that damaged both business confidence and Labour's electoral standing. Economic competence was to be shown now by emphasising stability rather than 'boom and bust', and avoiding profligacy in public expenditure that might necessitate unpopular tax increases.

A sense of reliability in living up to promises was to be achieved by focusing only on what was deliverable. It was the guiding rule not to promise what could not be delivered. Considerable management went into ensuring that policies regarded as undeliverable did not emerge from the party, and great care was taken in making only five limited but explicit pledges – one of which focused on tough economic rules; the others were cutting class sizes, fast-track punishment for young offenders, getting 250,000 under-25s into work and cutting NHS waiting lists. Keeping these particular promises would be 'a new contract between Government and citizen'.[31] Nevertheless, such was the force of the critique of Conservative government policies on the public services, especially the NHS, that the expectation of extra financing to save the NHS came over as virtually also a pledge. That expectation was shared within the party.

Much more controversial in the party was the belief and marketing that the major source of distrust was 'Old Labour' – a broad brush and caricatured repository of what was regarded as the misapplication of values, outdated and extreme attitudes and policies, off-putting images and antiquated organisational forms. Only by being seen to be creating 'New Labour' could trust be won to a sense of shared purpose and the fulfilment of the aspirations of the majority of people. In pursuit of that objective the leadership sought to shed or neutralise any negative associations and to convince the distrustful electorate that Labour had changed markedly and preferably totally. That became a primary objective and also a consistent source of party management problems.

The most fundamental claim in all this came from Blair: 'Not just that our vision for Britain is different, but also our means of achieving it'. It would involve 'a new politics' of 'courage, honesty and trust'[32] . . . 'because those most in need of hope deserve the truth'.[33] As the Queen's speech said in 1997: 'My Government will seek to restore confidence in the integrity of the nation's political system by upholding the highest standards of honesty and propriety in public life.' In this, Blair attempted 'to try to address the deep seated and damaging disaffection with politics which has grown up in recent years'.[34] It was a focus and commitment which had strong party as well as public appeal.

Behind these considerations was also a belief that 'New Labour' would be judged to be trustworthy because the 'New Labour' way was the rational way to moral purposes, untainted by the flaws of either left or right, and rooted in a realism about what needed to be done. From that realism, however, they also made some discreet but vital qualifications about the nature of politics, especially Labour politics and its tactical means and techniques. These qualifications, to which detailed attention will be paid later in this chapter, sanctioned ways of behaving which were to be a major influence on the party management, generating a problematic flank of distrust in relations with the party and eventually also in relations with the electorate.

The new party: transformative aims

Accompanying immediate policy objectives was an ambitious project of party transformation. In bolstering the possibility of changing the party's electoral appeal and taking steps towards its transformation, a managerial priority was to expand the membership of the party making it representative of the whole community. This included joining up many more union members as individual party members. It would be a member's party rather than one dominated by activists, thus undermining what managers referred to as a 'dogmatic activist-driven culture'. The more members there were, the less likely it was that the local parties were to be taken over by the unrepresentative left, and the more effective it would be in reconnecting with voters.

Alongside this development and encouraging it, Blair and the moder-nisers sought new provision for plebiscitary policy-making linking the Leader and the members. There would be ballots on the programme as Blair had sought on the Trade Union Review Group, ballots on major policy issues[35] and increasing adoption of direct elections to all significant posts by OMOV ballots.[36] OMOV, said Brown, would be the basis on which 'every member feels they can contribute to policy-making'.[37] This would replace, according to Matthew Taylor later, 'What masqueraded for democracy' which was in fact, he said, 'the capture of the party by key interests (principally trade union hierarchies) and an unrepresentative cadre of hard left activists'.[38]

The reinvigorated party would include those on low incomes who could be attracted by a low membership fee – paying what you could afford – and those drawn from the affiliated organisations encouraged by the levy-plus arrangement to become individual members of the party. It would draw in an increasing membership rooted in, and in close communion with, local communities and neighbourhoods. Indeed, Phil Wilson, a leading Blairite organiser, interpreted the origins of Blairism as the expression of working-class communities and their interests.[39] The Leader's own con-stituency of Sedgefield provided a very impressive model of what could be done with a huge rise in membership. For Brown also, mass membership was 'a way of ensuring that our political power comes from its proper source; the men and women in the neighbourhoods in which we live'.[40]

Overall, it was expected that the new members would be less bowed down by the traditions of the past – drawn into participation by the new Labour leadership with its modern and relevant appeal. They would be easier to educate into the realities of the hard choices of political life. The expectation was also that the results of such elections would produce allies much more congenial to the leadership. They would circumvent concentra-tions of Conservative Party activists and would bring forward more people open to the dialogue with the Blair leadership.

Modernisation of the party would include modernisation of the relation-ship between members and the local party organisation. This would involve a complete breaking down of off-putting barriers, antiquated practices and old institutional forms. Campaigning and the involvement of party members working in communal activities were emphasised more than obligations to attend boring bureaucratised meetings. This was tolerant of the different ways in which people wanted to be involved, but also compatible with the view that people did not want to participate and that it was not necessary anyway. It could be left to the modernising elite.

For some time after 1994 a view continued around Blair that the union collective affiliation was but a temporary arrangement. They still looked to continuing shifts in the distribution of votes at the party conference making it easier to phase out collective affiliation of the unions and finally end the electoral and power problems of union affiliation. This would also make the party more attractive to other social forces to an extent that would allow 'the people's party' to be receptive to a new and much closer relationship with business. As the individual membership of the party rose, so there would be continuing shifts in the distribution of votes at the party conference towards the CLPs with their new membership. As the membership rose, so the PLP and its more recalcitrant members would be subject to greater disciplinary sanctions urged and supported from below.

In this way, and others, a framework of organisational reforms would, it was thought, interlock into a significant transformation of the party and would facilitate a range of management objectives. The new membership and the weakening of the unions would strengthen the possibility of a modernisation which would involve major reforms of the NEC, making it more effective and representative of a broader range of party identities. It would be less oppositionist and more cooperative. Through these changes the party would be publicly more attractive, changing its image and distancing from its historic negative associations.

The framework of reform would also have significant appeal within the party. Blair promised in 1994 that in the new democratic members' party there was to be the birth of 'a new politics' and a new dynamism to democratic life in the party. 'A party which values all its members earns the respect of the wider community' . . . 'We must be a tolerant party, which respects and encourages the different views of its members.'[41] Plans he said, were in hand to give members 'greater say in Conference decisions'.[42] All this, plus new commitments to devolution of government (implemented speedily after 1997) and reinvigoration of local government (never achieved and always over-controlled from the centre) created an initial optimism within the party about Blair leading democratic change accompanied by open dialogue rather than procedural control. It was not to be.

No going back

A major immediate organisational objective of Blair's reinvigorated management was to avoid replaying the breakdown of party management, repeating the damaging failings of the party in relations with the governments of 1964–70 and 1974–79 and then the divisive experience of Opposition leading to that huge defeat in 1983 and long years in the wilderness. This feared past was a deeply ingrained mind-set producing in 'New Labour' what one minister described later as 'an icy determination that it was not going to happen again'.[43]

The party conference must not be allowed to drive the party and expose multiple divisions. There must be no repeat of the experience of 1979–82 with an NEC controlled by the left or behaving as an alternative government in exile. The PLP must be brought under disciplined control. In party elections and selections, the oppositionist left must be impeded whilst the path forward of those sympathetic to the aims of 'New Labour' should be assisted and eased.

For all its preoccupations with the future, 'New Labour' was obsessed with the battles against the ghosts of yesterday. The greatest obsession was with the image of the 'Bennite' War in the 1980s when the party 'lurched into extremism'.[44] There was little inclination to recognise either the distinctiveness of the factors which operated in the late 1970s and early 1980s, the degree to which the party had already changed under Kinnock and Smith, or the extent to which in the more distant past the leadership had itself contributed to the problems. For Blair and his allies, the party had simply not changed enough and needed the will and recipes of the 'New Labour' party revolutionaries.

Unity and accommodation

In its present state, the party was viewed as having a dangerous proclivity to public exhibitions of internal conflict. That would be very damaging in suggesting that it was a party incapable of the competence to govern, and a party internally rather than externally preoccupied. This must, therefore, be managed to maximise unity or at least to limit the public image of dissent. Tactical delay and advantageous ambiguity were helpful in not forcing too much of a differentiation of electoral and party appeal. On this, loyalist allies and loyalty could be mobilised to give the new leadership time and 'a chance' to tackle the problems and achieve the successes that the party also wanted. Woven into the presentation of managed unity on the basis of the new electoral positioning, there was also an element of controlled and limited accommodation with the party.

Whilst keeping control over a 'big tent' coalition and its party voices, 'New Labour' management would be assisted in dealing with controversial measures and disappointments, by measures and rhetoric assuaging concern for what had been lost. There was a significant continuation of elements of past policy even as 'New Labour' succeeded the 'Old'. An adjusted minimum wage and policies for union recognition loomed large in a social justice agenda. There was support for overcoming racism and poverty, moves to greater gender equality, civil partnerships, child care, family-friendly rights, advancing international economic and social development, securing human rights – nationally and internationally. A programme of constitutional change which had few costs to the Treasury gave 'New Labour' its most radical appeal. There was commitment to freedom of information, House of Lords reform, a new government for London, and Scottish and Welsh devolution (the latter depending on the outcome of referendums). These were not all of the same major public concerns but they had a significant place in party inspiration and managed party accommodation.

Shared values were often adjusted in focus and meaning; a familiar language of old values could be used in new ways. 'Our insight' said Blair in his first conference speech as Leader, is 'a belief in society, working together, solidarity, cooperation, partnership'.[45] These concepts, as with others of 'New Labour', lost some meanings and associations and gained others. There was an emphasis on fairness but 'equality of outcome' was superseded by 'equality of opportunity' and by 'equal worth'. Against the Thatcher analysis there was counterposed a new socialism, a concern for a strong active interdependent society in which individuals would have communal obligations and expanded opportunities, including the right and duty to work.

That opportunity would be provided by a fundamental reform of the welfare state with a special focus on the young and long-term unemployed receiving a hand up rather than just a hand-out. Social cohesion and the diminution of exclusion of the marginalised would take on a new priority in diminishing inequality. From these changes and later the four values of a just society, whilst disclaiming an ideology, 'New Labour' developed a flexible basis for moving away from traditional Labour policies yet differentiating the new political identity from the Conservatives and achieving a degree of unity behind the election manifesto.

Despite those and other ingredients of unity there remained in the party various uncertain and critical responses under the early Blair. There were new suspicions about purpose in the face of 'New Labour' avoidance of 'old' solutions to policy problems and there was always the problem of building into internal acceptance some of the limitations deemed essential for the display of public 'change' to the electoral waverers. The heavy focus on the advancement of business cooperation and efficiency was a deep-rooted problem in relation to justice at work considerations. For these and other reasons, appeals made to the party over policy and organisational reform through argument alone was considered not enough for a successful party management which had such ambitious goals. Other methods were needed.

Motivation and the exigencies of management

Moral ends and moral means

Anthony Howard confessed later what he and others noted about Blair at the time of his election as Leader – that he seemed capable of bringing an entirely new ethical dimension to politics.[46] Others, even some critics, would have agreed that Blair, a deeply religious man, had 'strong moral convictions'.[47] For him, it was said that 'political activity was an extension of morality'.[48] According to biographer Philip Stephens, he acted with more than normal confidence of the innate goodness of his own character and the unerring conviction that his decisions were the right things to do.[49] Perhaps so, but given the disciplined acting of a man always aware and on a stage, many professions of convictions, particularly 'the right thing to do', were at times the advocacy script. That may well have been true of Blair's affirmation that a strong sense of moral purpose to life was why he joined the Labour Party.[50] But he was not immune from some changes in confidence. There were noticeable waves of uncertainty late in 1999 and in 2000, but he recovered and in the second term the 'I'm always right' tone came so strongly and irreversibly to the fore that it was remarked upon by Campbell.[51]

Initially the appearance in British politics of a moral and unusually trustworthy politician was taken at face value by many of the public and in the party, although IpsosMORI noted a tendency still, to see all politicians as bad as each other.[52] However, his 1995 emphasis on moral purpose was well received in the media. It was much later, after the second-term Iraq War, that there began to be a more vigorous media reappraisal of Blair and the problematic morality of means rather than just ends. By 2006 his very acute and sympathetic biographer John Rentoul had come to suspect that he was 'a man who takes a macho pride in his man of the world realism' and was then 'caught bang to rights' over loans for peerages.[53] Geoffrey Wheatcroft put it more harshly. He believes 'that his inner virtue justified any means he chooses to employ. As a result, his government and party have acted more corruptly than for generations'.[54] Yet long before this change in the diagnosis of Blair's approach to politics, there was much to learn that was significant about the real character of Blair and 'New Labour' from a study of the practices of party management.

Re-forming and reforming management

Two worlds of management

The party officials who were party managers operated within what can be described as two behavioural worlds. In the first world, there was a primary concern, shared with all party employees, for doing the allotted task as well as possible in building and preserving a first-class electoral machine. A growing emphasis on professionalism and the 'the need for flexibility, competence, commitment and adaptability'[55] was also heavily encouraged. There were consensual goals, sharing the search for a healthy party rooted in the community, a stronger active membership, and seeking a broader representation with new categories of identity. Much of the management of specific outcomes involved a neutrality of supervision with open and specified procedures and with roles played by officials in harmony with wider party-behavioural values. These involved a circumspect and non-partisan concern for application of the party's rules, the reasonable settlement of internal conflict and the building and conservation of trust. In terms of the volume of day-to-day operations of management, this mode of behaviour was a dominant feature. That said, there was a second behavioural world fusing at times with the first but generally not as open, nor as neutral as the first nor as acceptable within the party. It could be said to be dominant in another sense, that it was operational in important areas and venues and over what were regarded as major issues and decisions.

Motivation and justification

An analysis of how this behaviour grew in importance has to begin with the 'New Labour' view of itself and of the condition of the Labour Party. The core leaders of 'New Labour' were (mainly) men with a range of impressive talents which gave them the elan of being special people. As culture-carriers of the party revolution which would become the basis for a historic modernising revolution in Britain, they considered themselves having the right not to be thwarted by inconveniences and obstacles emanating from within the party. This party was also special but in a derogatory sense; it was in a condition that to them provided multiple justifications for the hard lines of their political outlook. The party was theirs, and especially Blair's agency, yet it was considered unready in its fitness and dangerously capable of reviving past off-putting associations, thus providing ammunition for the party's enemies. That now demanded a greater freedom of behaviour by those who would change it.

There was another prime motivation and justification for relaxing inhibitions in this second behavioural world under Blair. It was the special urgency arising from the need to differentiate present behaviour from what was seen as the failings of the party's past managerial and organisational defects. 'We let people down by a lack of direction and leadership and by a failure of organisation', as one party official explained. 'We could do nothing for them', was another lament. Millions of people depended on the party. They were as Blair described them, 'young people huddled in doorways, families made wretched by unemployment, the poor unable to make ends meet'. 'They do not need our anger ... get into government and do something for them'.[56] The task must be met by a Leader-manager who was always in a hurry with only three years to prepare the party before the next General Election. The scale of the problem was seen as huge and pressing; the obstacles to change were seen as deeply rooted. There was little time to waste on philosophical introspection about management. Questioning the behavioural niceties of the way that the party was handled could delay or compromise the chances of winning.

The priority task was to secure an effective modernised professional party with a new organisational culture. This party had to be modernised comprehensively and fast in order to play its part in the continuous political war which was the new electoral politics. This would embody and pursue the urgent changes needed to be made for it to become the government and then to sustain it in office whilst the new culture-carriers operated on the British political system. In the electoral war and with these priorities there was little respect for the consideration that long-established traditions, conventions and institutions of the party might embody some accumulated wisdom of past experience and a past creative adjustment of trial and error. Traditional processes and culture were part of a decadent order – a view carried through media allies as 'a troublesome anachronism'.[57] Their feeling was that it had no right to stand in the way.

Modernisation – generally understood as the adaptation of the party to the new exigencies and opportunities of the social, economic, technological and political environment – became an integral component of the 'New Labour' identity and its dynamism. The consistent drive in every area had to be towards newness and the modern. This was inherently legitimate. Moving in tune with the modern was fusing with historic progress. And you were either moving forward or you would fall back. You had to sustain momentum in a permanent revolution. It was also fundamental to the outlook of 'New Labour' that the modern party should not be tied to any particular historical means in the way that it achieved its purposes. It must be free to move away from old shibboleths. This perspective also made easier the rejection of old procedural values and constraining rules.

In facing this party condition, Blair did prefer to see himself as an educator and persuader of change and he liked to see himself winning the arguments. But winning was the priority, not necessarily winning members over. Mandelson and Liddle told that 'getting your way can require a degree of intrigue and manoeuvring' that Blair 'would prefer was unnecessary'.[58] Perhaps so, but from the first steps in the managerial coup, facing the major tasks and the obstacles to change, intrigue and manoeuvring with multiple impositional and manipulative ways of behaving had become regarded as a necessary feature of the armoury of influence.

Precedents and new conditions

A knowledgeable sophisticate might take the view that, as an element in Labour's organisational political life historically, control and a degree of manipulation linked with the pursuit of what was considered the greater good had been the normality. Mandelson's grandfather Herbert Morrison noted in 1951 'a good deal of undesirable manipulation' at the party conference[59] – although saying it then with a note of considerable regret. In the Gaitskell-Wilson modernising period there can be found some major examples of past ruthlessness and manipulation in agenda politics.[60] More recently, although the Smith leadership was not seen as a manipulative regime, in 'the victory over OMOV' in 1993 not all of the behaviour was according to a political Marquis of Queensberry rulebook. In internal politics, when the pressure was really on, the tendency was for somebody to try to move that extra yard across the line looking for a means to win; sometimes it succeeded, sometimes not. Blair's party management involved not only a continuation and replication of this kind of activity but it was now part of a broader, deeper and more systematic change in the role and behaviour of Leader and management.

For Blair, the historical experience of past management controls and conduct offered useful examples, but it was regarded as problematic and inadequate. It had involved the central and active role of the unions as managerial auxiliaries, and they had expectations about how the relationship should be conducted. Blair's search for supremacy involved accepting no such limitations, which were regarded as especially damaging to the public image and the party's search for new identity. Past management had involved what was regarded as inadequate personal powers for the Leader. He had to operate within shared institutional powers with an element of constraint from countervailing forces in the PLP on the NEC and at the party conference.

There had been an element of traditional rule-book fastidiousness and inhibition about going beyond what was considered to be a proper civil-service role of the party officials. There were also practical limitations on the central communication facilities in relation to the party. Historically, there were sometimes differences within the leadership and between different party forums over leadership and managerial measures, with the ever-present difficulty that they could precipitate public rows. All that also had to be overcome in a modernised party with an image of unity. Media management required a more central integrated role, yet under Smith's leadership there had been a new concern to move away from the party influence and methods of those managers.

New opportunities and new justifications

What became different about the second world of managerial behaviour in this period of Blair's leadership, shown in the chapters that follow, were the changes in all these features. Central to the change was that the attempt to tackle all the problems and make the party fit for purpose evolved into what was intended to be a comprehensive interlocking managerial machine operating under the guidance of the Leader's Office and headquarters. There were many new opportunities (and facilities) for management activities as one modernisation of procedure and process followed another. The countervailing forces were weakened. There was an unprecedented build-up of the role of Leader, not least in its dismantling of checks and balances which limited his role; there was a lack of reverence for party traditions and rules of different kinds, and there were new objectives and behaviour which would have been regarded as out of bounds to the older generation, especially the rolling coup. Less publicly observable, the major change around the Leader was the change in management organisation and culture with new conditions of managerial operation. Within that, there were new leadership-encouraged justifications for a militancy in pursuit of management goals, influencing the perspective on the relationship between means and ends and reducing inhibitions on the behaviour of the managers.

Code of conduct

From managerial behaviour and what they said in private about it, under Blair they were influenced by a covert code of conduct which included three pivotal elements. There was a rejection of 'processology' in adherence to the delivery ethic. A new meaning and application of 'what works' was applied to procedural values. And there was a view of 'serious politics' which justified a ruthlessness of behaviour.

Processology and the delivery ethic

In all spheres, adherence to routines can produce a rigidity of mind which reduces the possibility of an imaginative response to problems. Blair was determined to free the 'can – do' personality from the constraints of 'bureaucracy' and obsessive attention to procedures, regardless of the problems this might cause for internal democracy and accountability. An over-strict attitude towards the propriety of process in facing problems became disdainfully considered as obsessive 'processology'. Under Blair's management, barrack-room lawyers and procedural philosophers were held to stand in the way of progress. In judging managerial actions, what was done was not to be regarded as a test of integrity but of effectiveness in creating arrangements which produced 'a good result' for the strong Leader, his purposes and his managerial capacity. In contrast, there was an under-developed concern for the potential collateral and consequential damage to party life, its traditions and institutions, established procedures, and unwritten rules, which might arise from this behaviour. Rentoul put it benevolently in 2004 that the Blairite core were 'so loyal to the Labour Party that they were prepared to do almost anything to help it win'.[61] That attitude to process was to be the ethic of delivery.

'What works' and procedural values

In a Labour Party in a state of perpetual internal conflict it had always been difficult to be consistent in applying procedural values. Left and right, party groups and individuals on occasions trimmed the adoption of procedural values in the attempt to secure favourable outcomes. Blairite party management produced some specially abrupt and significant shifts in values and practices. The 'New Labour' focus on 'what works' was offered publicly to refer simply to the avoidance of 'outdated ideology' in policy-making.[62] Less understood yet crucial to the internal politics of Blairism was that workability also had a power-oriented meaning which guided behaviour in process and procedure in relation to organisational change. The test was not simply was it practicable?, but did it deliver for 'Tony', or 'for us' – the management. There was an illuminating converse to this, operative where other organisational options were being pushed that the Leader did not like. As one Blair managerial ally put it, 'If that is what Tony doesn't want, it doesn't work'.

'Serious politics' and virtuous ruthlessness

In winning in the party, a complete moral purity of means would have been a daunting standard for anybody, let alone a hugely ambitious practitioner of politics with minority support. But what we have here is not an occasional and exceptional case of breaking lines, in contrast with the purity of unremitting fastidiousness. Party management was regarded as a special activity operating in a specially degenerate realm and under pressure from specially ruthless enemies. Politics was not to be treated as an 'academic exercise', as an irritated Blair pointed out privately in 1997.[63] Although ideally it was helpful to win by persuasion and consensus, 'serious politics' involved an acceptance that an at times brazen ruthlessness in pushing the boundaries of managerial conduct and seeking 'what we can get away with' was integral to the capability of being effective in playing to win. That view of seriousness was its own expression of tough determined virtue and in that sense as one central organising figure put it, challenging the criticism of manipulative unfairness, 'Labour was not a serious party till Tony'.

Manipulation and trust

Operating within this code of behaviour had a major distorting effect on the avowed pursuit of 'a new politics'. Skilful politics was regarded, by its history and nature, as involving guile, contrivance and deception often aimed at affecting behaviour without the recipient being fully aware of what was happening, or being able to prevent it. Under the pressure of 'New Labour' management exigencies, and in accordance with its code, this behaviour was accepted as having a prominent and regular place within the core management culture. It became accepted, even encouraged, that managers should not be inhibited in pursuing the necessary sophisticated activities of the ethic of delivery, 'what works for us' and at times 'serious politics'. For some it went further. The skills not only heightened self-regard, they gained respect amongst like-minded colleagues in the achievement of what were judged to be virtuous objectives.

However, that constellation produced a wider potential problem of the acceptability of manipulation. Although it was possible to label any tactical manoeuvring behaviour as 'manipulative', cultures differ in this appraisal. Normally that description was rationed in British political discourse to especially unfair contrivance or deviation from the straight and honest which was deemed unreasonable or excessive. The boundaries of acceptable behaviour for managers within the 'New Labour' culture on the other hand were wide in terms of political conduct, and what went on within the culture was at times of such a character, scope and repetition as to go beyond the lines of acceptability amongst sections of the party, This slowly became an ingredient of the rising internal distrust of 'New Labour' management, sometimes even affecting managers' reactions to each other.

This activity under Blair took place within a situation where there was already an element of mutual distrust. It involved a particularly strong 'New Labour' belief that the activist culture in the CLPs made them susceptible to ill-informed, impractical, emotional and rigid attitudes towards the party's values, objectives and priorities. Their shared purpose with 'New Labour' could not be trusted. The unions were considered always likely to distort the 'New Labour' message, become involved in self-interested conflict with Labour government purposes, and subject to influence by leftward 'out of date' ideology. From the party and union view, especially on the left, there was suspicion that parliamentary leaders would be seduced by various influences and interests hostile to, or a diversion from, the party's objectives and interests. But to all this distrust was now added a new important and more deep-rooted element of distrust, given the assumptions, attitude and practices of 'New Labour' party management.

If challenged, some managers would accept that extensive and repeated manipulation might lose the trust of the party, and they would in principle have preferred straight behaviour and honest persuasion. But, faced with various enemies and problems, within the managerial culture it was assumed to be a price worth paying if the behaviour secured the immediate objectives. If there were objections to the methods then they could live with that. 'Tough!' as they sometimes responded dismissively to the objections in 'serious politics' mode. As for relations with the electorate, the main focus of gaining electoral trust had become differentiation from the 'Old Labour' past and the showing of shared purpose, plus the exhibition of competence and of delivery. There was a much more limited appreciation of the dangers of slipping from acceptable to unacceptable in the honesty of public communication or, later, in party procedural controls that affected the public.

John Reid noted in 1997 that trust can be lost in ten minutes but 'it can take years to win it back'.[64] It is also sometimes said, more subtly, that trust 'once lost' is 'often questioned'.[65] However, there were, as noted, various potential sources of trust which could be in play at the same time with the trust-enhancing factors mitigating reactions to those that undermined trust. Even if the reaction to manipulation was dominant, there were still opportunities which presented themselves for the skilful manipulator. It was possible to cover manipulative activities with misleading titles. Support could be sustained through emphasis on other traits of character and a variety of possible achievements. Aspects of the devious could be reluctantly tolerated when the perpetrator was otherwise impressive in competence and delivery of consensual objectives. The reasonable belief amongst managerial manipulators was also that memory was short and if you had got away with it before, you were likely to get away with it again. All this gave confident room for manoeuvre but it was not unlimited, as Blair and his managers were to find out.

Awareness of manipulation had broader as well as deeply serious effects. It was a behaviour which often aroused a value-laden indignation, which could deeply imprint itself on the critical memory. Cynicism with regard to trust could produce distrust of evidence presented to substantiate other potential sources of trust including the evidence of shared purpose, competence and delivery. All that could contribute to a decline in satisfaction with performance and could be crucial in limiting the success of the attempt to secure internal party and public change. Memory is a mixed storehouse with fluctuating recall. A bad experience could be revived in memory and clarified in the face of experience of repetitive behaviour and in that recognition it could become extremely difficult to shift the reputation and its effect on willingness to believe and to cooperate.

The political enemy as model

Heavily reinforcing the manipulative disposition was what was judged to be the character of the enemies that the party faced. 'The Trots', only recently pushed to the far edges of the party's life, had thrived through the institutionalised deceits of the entryist tactic and its secret organisational form. They were a reminder of the war of politics as it was played under Trotsky's guidance in *Their morals and ours*. On the other side, the Conservative Party had always been seen in the Labour Party as involved historically in defending an unfair expression of unequal wealth and power, using their political linkage to the press with an absence of discomfort. Three election victories attained by ruthless efficiency were assisted by new US political marketing techniques which moved British politics towards increasing stage management; they also highlighted the politicising Whitehall role of the No. 10 spin doctor, Bernard Ingham. In the operation of unrestrained election politics as all-the-year-round campaigning salesmanship, privatisation was advertised at huge public expense. The crisis over Westlands, as a temperate commentator, Hugo Young, saw it, 'put on display' a governing mode of 'manipulation, vicious division, hole in the corner dealing'.[66]

In 1985–6, Conservative reforming zeal went into the extra imposition of political-fund ballots on the unions which, if lost, would have changed the Labour Party's form and crippled it financially. Nothing was said about a similar requirement to be placed on companies. Those in the Conservative Party who thought that financially undermining the Opposition might be damaging to the spirit of parliamentary democracy were brushed aside. There was corruption, gerrymandering and financial mismanagement of the Conservative flagship Westminster council from 1986 to 1989 under a policy finally judged illegal by the district auditor in 1996. The late calling to account of that council barely dented the resentful Labour view that the Conservative Party was specially ruthless and 'always got away with it'.

Under Major, frustration with Tories 'getting away with it' became particularly focused on the Arms-to-Iraq Affair which concerned the uncovering of the government-endorsed sale of arms by British companies to Saddam Hussein and the abuse of public-interest immunity certificates to prevent disclosure of information. In 1992, detailed costings for Labour's moderate proposals for government were undermined by the misleading Tory 'Tax Bombshell' campaign which with press allies successfully generated electoral fear. This added to the Labour Party managerial folklore that truth was unimportant to the Conservative Party. Only effectiveness of the message mattered.

The self-serving corruption of Conservative behaviour was also thought to be getting worse. Two proven Conservative liar-politicians, Jonathan Aitken and Geoffrey Archer, finished up in prison, and another MP, Neil Hamilton, was removed from his parliamentary seat in 1997 by Martin Bell, a 'clean-up-politics' campaigner in a white suit. What was seen by the Conservative journalist Peter Oborne, in a very insightful study, as signalling the discarding of old codes of conduct in the Conservative Party[67] was seen in the Labour Party as further confirmation of their suspicions of a degenerate ethical tendency in Conservative culture. That sense of something new and reprehensible, exploited by aggressive 'New Labour' media managers, led to the Nolan Inquiry into standards in public life set up by the Major Government, but it was seen in the Labour Party as a tardy defensive move.

Blair famously proclaimed on Day 1 in Government the need 'to be extremely careful that we are purer than pure'. It reflected an awareness that they had to be seen to live up to the 'New Labour' moral criticism of the Major government, but also a fear of the predatory dangers from a historic alliance of Conservative headquarters and the right-wing press. The enemy was seen as ever looking to use and misrepresent anything that was happening in the Labour Party, presenting democratic division as 'a split' and acting at times as the malicious reputational assassins of Labour and union leaders.

Media sensitivity, media management and the proficiency that went with them became a major preoccupation of 'New Labour' leaders, with considerable and varying effects on party management (see Chapter 5, pp. 167–8 and references in subsequent chapters). It had a cultural impact in dealing with attempts to at least neutralise the role of the party's media enemies, including the traditionally hostile *Daily Mail*. And there was a permanent special concern with the opinions of Rupert Murdoch, owner of News International Corporation, which through the *Sun* newspaper was held to have made a major contribution to the 1992 election victory. It had involved a trip across the world in July 1995, putting the case of a supplicant to the powerful that Labour was virtually a new party. Blair continued to be 'very concerned to keep Murdoch on board'.[68] Various constraints were involved in what was privately described as 'riding a tiger' whilst keeping a wary eye open for the next problem and opportunity.

That difficult ride, interwoven with acrimonious daily hostilities with devious elements of the media, reinforced what was understood to be the nature of serious hand-to-hand politics in the 'real world'. 'The game', as Ivor Gabor described it, 'was played with an unprecedented degree of bitterness and brutality'.[69] It was a war for which Labour had to train media and management warriors. They worked in a state of permanent preparedness, anxiety and aggression. Victory could never be assumed, however far ahead Labour was in the polls and however long the lead had been held. Ever aware of the enemies, managers were often filled with the neurotic concern that something would go wrong which would be seized on bringing the whole project into danger. It reinforced the controlling and manipulative outlook. You could take risks with behaviour towards the party, but in relation to the media strategy you had to make sure of what the party was doing – a major managerial precept. Hidden away around Blair and the party managers was a perception of the enemies which some-times bobbed into discreet justification in defending heavily manipulative management practices. It took the general form of 'how can we afford to be over-scrupulous? They are not. This is serious politics'.

Anxiety, confidence and zealotry

All political movements have their elements of neurosis, a potential to develop a pathology of dysfunctional behaviour, and a tendency to blind-ness about themselves. The politics of party management illuminates the origins of what became 'New Labour' pathologies as well as its successes. For the managers in 1997 what they did had 'worked' and the landslide victory was hugely confidence-building for the special people of 'New Labour'. What had been achieved was qualitatively different from previous Labour victories in the scope of its socio-political support and the 418 seats won, making it the party's most ever and its largest ever parliament-ary majority of 179. The scale of reversal for a discredited and desperately weakened Conservative version of Britain's natural party of government would take nearly ten years for that party to recover from. 'New Labour' was the master now.

A strong case could be made that Smith would have won this election albeit with a smaller majority, and without the extraordinary penetration of so many traditional centres of Conservative strength. But the suggestion that the victory was more a rejection of the deeply unpopular Conservative Party rather than enthusiasm for the special character of Blairism was brushed aside in discussions with ministers of the new government. They 'had won as "New Labour" and would govern as "New Labour"'. This would be ' "New Labour" undiluted'.[70] Governing as 'New Labour' was not only a statement of purpose and policy, it was also a statement of intent in relation to power and process. Rawnsley held the view later that what manifested itself as arrogance in government was sourced in 'New Labour' chronic insecurity about itself.[71] But it was a very important element of the 'New Labour' psyche by 1997 that as a party leadership it had mas-tered arts of management control. This allied with the self-ascribed status of culture-carriers of the future was a heady combination. They were in this sense confident people who were sure that they knew how management was done and why.

Important internal party failures and frustrations there were, as we shall see, but these and other problems were mainly hidden in presentation and easily out of mind in the overview. Watching them closely in 1997 the party observer could be reminded at times of *Dizzy with Success*, the title of Stalin's famous reproof to the 1928 cadres on the excesses of the collectivisation of agriculture which he himself had initiated, except that no public reproof ever came from Blair. Then again, the long honeymoon of Blair with the British electorate, the economic success in office and the systematic implementation of the 1997 manifesto seemed complete vindication of the management and no reason for change. In the chapters that follow will be shown how this worked out in practice and, in Chapter 15 especially, why this passionate confidence became challenged and, for the moment, undermined.

Notes

1 Sections of this and subsequent chapters on managerial politics and behaviour are heavily influenced by information, observation, interpretation of behaviour and discussions as adviser on the Party into Power process, 1996–7, and also by interviews with major party managers from 1994 to 2006.
2 'New Labour' emergence as a concept was presented at the 1994 party conference. The phrase was claimed by Mandelson, Campbell and Gould; see Derek Draper, *Blair's 100 days*, Faber & Faber, London, 1997, p. 177. Some academics in seeing the continuities with Kinnock, defined 'New Labour' as what emerged after 1983. Meg Russell, *Building New Labour*, Palgrave Macmillan, London, 2005, has this perspective, but the view taken here is that it is interesting but unhelpful in portraying the important distinctiveness of the Blair experience.
3 *The Guardian*, 28 September 1996.
4 'Profile: New Labour', *Independent on Sunday*, 26 September 1999.
5 Discussions with party officials and MPs. Also Dennis Kavanagh and Anthony Seldon, *The Powers Behind the Prime Minister: the Hidden Influence of Number Ten*, HarperCollins, London, 2000, p. 245.
6 Michael Foley, *John Major, Tony Blair and a Conflict of Leadership: Collision Course*, Manchester University Press, Manchester, 2002, p. 116.
7 John Rentoul, *Independent*, 15 April 2007.
8 Philip Gould, *The Unfinished Revolution: How the Modernisers Saved the Labour Party*, Little Brown, London, 1998, p. 216.
9 Peter Mandelson and Roger Liddle, *The Blair Revolution: Can New Labour Deliver?* Faber & Faber, London, 1996, p. 57.
10 Polly Toynbee, *The Guardian*, 30 May 2001.
11 Peter Hennessy, *The Prime Minister, The Office and its Holders since 1945*, Penguin, London, 2000, p. 478.
12 Ibid.
13 Cabinet Minister Jack Straw, 'Blair: the Inside Story', *BBC2*, 20 February 2007.

14 Andrew Rawnsley, 'The Blair Years 1997–2007', *The Observer*, supplement 1997, p. 23 referring to success in Northern Ireland.

15 John Rentoul, *Independent on Sunday*, 2 May 2004.

16 A significant section of Labour leaders including Gordon Brown, David Blunkett, Frank Dobson, Mo Mowlem, John Reid, Clare Short and Jack Straw had various reservations about an alliance with the Liberals.

17 In October 1996 a joint consultative committee on constitutional affairs was set up between the Labour Party and the Liberal Democrats. It was wound up in September 2001.

18 Lance Price, *The Spin Doctor's Diary: Inside No. 10 with New Labour*, Hodder & Stoughton, London, 2005, p. 198.

19 Gould, *Unfinished Revolution*, p. 193.

20 John Golding, *Hammer of the Left*, Politico's, London, 2003, pp. 371–2.

21 Tony Blair, *'The Third Way: New Politics of the New Society'*, Fabian Society, London, 1998.

22 Mandelson and Liddle, *Blair Revolution*, p. 1.

23 Stephen Driver and Luke Martell, *New Labour*, Polity, Cambridge, 2005, p. 28.

24 Paul Anderson and Nyta Mann, *Safety First: the Making of New Labour*, Granta, London, 1997, pp. 45–7.

25 John Rentoul, *Tony Blair: Prime Minister*, Little Brown, London, 2001, p. 264.

26 John Curtice and Roger Jowell, 'The Sceptical Electorate', in Roger Jowell et al. (eds), *British Social Attitudes, the Twelfth Report*, Dartmouth Publishing, London, 1995, pp. 141–72.

27 Ibid. p. 141.

28 Tony Blair, 'My vision for Britain', *What Needs to Change: New Visions for Britain*, HarperCollins, London, 1996, p. 15.

29 Paul Webb, David Farrell, and Ian Holliday, *Political Parties in Advanced Industrial Democracies*, Oxford University Press, Oxford, 2002, p. 455.

30 Mandelson and Liddle, *Blair Revolution*, p. 186.

31 Ibid. p. 39.

32 Tony Blair, LPCR, 1994, p. 104.

33 Ibid. p. 104.

34 Tony Blair, Speech to Charter 88, 14 May 1996.

35 Mandelson and Liddle, *Blair Revolution*, pp. 228–9.

36 Ibid.

37 Gordon Brown, annual Tribune lecture, July 1992, quoted in Paul Routledge, *Gordon Brown: The Biography*, Simon & Schuster, London, 1998, p. 166.

38 Matthew Taylor, *Changing Political Culture*, 'First Thought' Pamphlet, LGA Publications, 2000, p. 10.

39 Interview with Phil Wilson in 1998 on the origins of New Labour.

40 Gordon Brown, *Making Mass Membership Work*, 1994, p. 2.

41 Tony Blair, *Change and National Renewal*, 1994, Blair's personal manifesto for the leadership of the Labour Party, p. 19.

42 Tony Blair, speech to Fabian Society, 5 July 1995.

43 Helen Liddell, *The Politics Show*, BBC1, 30 January 2005.

44 *Sunday Times*, 13 July 1997.

45 LPCR 1994, p. 100.

46 Anthony Howard, *The Times*, 8 July 2003.

47 Christopher Foster, *British Government in Crisis*, Hart, Oxford, 2005, p. 175.
48 A.J. Davies, *To Build a New Jerusalem: The British Labour Party from Keir Hardie to Tony Blair*, Abacus, London, 1996, p. 438.
49 Philip Stephens, *Tony Blair: The Price of Leadership*, Politico's, London, 2004, p. 108.
50 LPCR 1995, p. 96.
51 Alastair Campbell and Richard Stott (eds), *Extracts from the Alastair Campbell Diaries: The Blair Years*, Hutchinson, London, 2007, entry for July 17, 2001, p. 557.
52 IpsosMORI, Political Report, 2007, p. 35.
53 John Rentoul, *Independent on Sunday*, 23 March 2006.
54 Geoffrey Wheatcroft, 'Inside the Blair psyche', *Mail Online*, 2 February 2007.
55 Paul Webb and Justin Fisher, 'Professionalism and the Millbank Tendency: the Political Sociology of New Labour Employees', *Politics* 23(1), February 2003, p. 18.
56 Tony Blair, LPCR 1995, p. 97.
57 *Financial Times*, 28 April 1996.
58 Mandelson and Liddle, *Blair Revolution*, p. 57.
59 NEC Minutes, 12 December 1951. I am grateful to David Howell for bringing this to my attention.
60 See Minkin, *Labour Party Conference*, pp. 67–83, pp. 210–13 and particularly pp. 324–6 covering revisionism and public ownership.
61 John Rentoul, *Independent on Sunday*, 2 May 2004.
62 'New Labour because Britain deserves better', p. 4.
63 Handwritten personal message to me, circa February 1998.
64 LPCR 1997, p. 151.
65 Stanley B. Greenberg, *Dispatches from the War Room: In the Trenches with Five Extraordinary Leaders*, Thomas Dunne, New York, 2009, p. 231.
66 Hugo Young, *One of Us: a Biography of Margaret Thatcher*, Macmillan, London, 1989, p. 455.
67 Peter Oborne, *The Triumph of the Political Class*, Simon & Schuster, London, 2007, p. 64.
68 Price, *Spin Doctor's Diary*, entry 10 April 1999, p. 95.
69 Ivor Gabor, 'Lies, Damn Lies . . . and Political Spin', in Andrew Chadwick and Richard Heffernan (eds), *The New Labour Reader*, Polity, Cambridge, 2003, p. 302.
70 *Sunday Times*, 13 July 1997.
71 Andrew Rawnsley, *Servants of the People: The Inside Story of 'New Labour'*, Hamish Hamilton, London, 2000, p. 24.

5

The Leader, the machine and party management

The general secretary and the Leader

Party managers generally operated under the strong influence of the culture explored in the previous chapter. But who were the managers? What was their relationship with the Leader? What attitudes and behaviour did they carry into their activities in practice? These questions provide the main focus in this chapter. The General Secretary was formally responsible for the party organisation and had historically been the senior person in party management. In 1994–5 Blair's attempt to transform authority and control over party management and establish a new culture was prefigured by the first significant internal party action and the initial step in the Blairite managerial coup. It was the replacement of the General Secretary.

According to the rulebook, a General Secretary was recommended by the NEC, and elected by the party conference.[1] They remained in office 'so long as his/her work' gave 'satisfaction to the National Executive Committee and party conference'.[2] Occupants of this post in past generations had lasted for many years and their length of service depended mainly on themselves and their support on the NEC. It was not the normality for a new Leader to immediately replace a General Secretary, but in August 1994, just a month after Blair's election, there was sudden pressure from the Leader on Larry Whitty to resign as General Secretary whilst the NEC was on holiday.

There was a case for new blood under a new Leader, yet there might have been benefits in keeping Whitty in post for a while. Over intra-party democracy he was a thoughtful managerialist, and also a party and union moderniser. His far-sighted financial arrangements included the building up of high-value donors with union agreement. In addition, the Leader might have gained from having a figure that had retained the trust of both left and right in the difficult years since 1985. But Whitty was considered too committed to the traditional union-party link, and perhaps also too committed to restraint in intervention by officials in party activity. An immediate change in the most senior party official would make the first public statement about the Leader's determination to change the party. It would also be the first step to ensure a new scale of domination, although some of the mechanisms for it were initially opportunities that were found rather than planned for.

The moving of the General Secretary went ahead, even in the face of an NEC meeting at which no member of the front bench could be found to openly support the Leader's action and virtually the whole of the trade union section expressed its deep reservations. The involvement of Prescott did secure a new role for Whitty in the post of European Coordinator and later, as a life peer, Whitty became a respected government minister in two Blair governments. But, with his departure, it became established that, under Blair, General Secretaries would last in office only as long as the Leader thought it right. Whitty had been there for nine years. In the years that Blair was Leader, from 1994 to 2006, there were to be five departures and new appointments.

General secretary and the managerial network

Some of what is described here of the managerial politics from 1994 to 2000 does not accord with what might be expected of the surface hierarchies, alignments and territorial claims around the core culture. It involved some personality influences with individual divergences, and a variety of twists and turns in fortune that had important political consequences. Tom Sawyer, who was Blair's candidate to succeed Whitty, was unsurprising. He was considered to be a more politically flexible moderniser – 'more malleable', as Anderson and Mann put it.[3] On the NEC trade union group, there was a concern about what Blair's choice might indicate about intentions towards the party, the unions and the NEC. The group produced their own right-wing loyalist candidate, another NEC member, Richard Rosser. However, he was persuaded by the Leader not to stand. That became a common practice under Blair.

One result of these manoeuvres was that Sawyer, when he was elected by the NEC, had the strong authority of the new Leader behind him but had no committed majority base of personal support on the committee. He continued to face some suspicious critics. However, he was a resourceful political operator, effortlessly relaxed in handling new developments and different political relationships. He supervised a major shift in the location of party headquarters to a central property at Millbank, and working outwards from a narrow base he gradually won particularly committed support from a group of capable loyalist union representatives on the NEC. Maggie Jones from UNISON was one such figure, and Margaret Wall of MSF (later Amicus), Chair of the Policy Committee, emerged as integral to the management of changes in process and in defence of the Leader. Margaret Prosser, TGWU, the party's Treasurer and convenor of the trade union group from 1997, also became a pivotal and very forceful figure in this supportive role although acting with more consensual discretion.

Sawyer kept alert control over what was happening in headquarters, but he was also committed to a degree of administrative delegation. This was welcomed in the regions, although it did leave them more open to a variety of pressures from different national sources. It was welcomed also by many in the party headquarters as leaving them room for manoeuvre. One such figure was the head of his office, Jon Cruddas, a graduate from a working-class background with a PhD and a worker-like manner. He developed into a creative sharp-end party manager and became a key figure in union delivery at the party conference, both as an official of party headquarters and later as Deputy Political Secretary in Downing Street. He had worked closely with Blair as a member of the policy staff when Blair was Shadow Secretary of State for Employment, although, as it emerged later, they held some divergent philosophical views on trade unionism, and Cruddas always saw the party in more pluralistic terms.

The increasing role of the Leader and his office in party management activities was reflected in the freedom of Peter Mandelson in that area. The very sharp, innovative but distrusted politician had to be covered by the code 'Bobby' so that his role during Blair's campaign to become Leader could be kept from Blair's allies, let alone the party. Quickly, he became discreetly but very actively involved in influencing the culture and some of the mechanics of the new party management. His party influence was also enhanced by interventions through selected journalists, as well as allies in the party machine. Both in opposition and in government he remained a close and all-purpose personal advisor to Blair,[4] covering party issues, sometimes with the knowledge of Sawyer, sometimes without it. As a Minister without Portfolio after 1997, and then as a Secretary of State in the government, through two controversial resignations in 1998 and 2001, he retained a permanent back- and front-door channel to and from the Leader.

Building Blair's staff

After the 1994 conference, Blair quickly strengthened the staffing of his own office and to improve party management brought in Sally Morgan, the party's Director of Campaigns and Elections, as his aide. Morgan had been a party organiser in the National Organisation of Labour Students. As a Labour official she was often categorised as a soft-left Kinnockite, and had doubts about Blair before, in January 1995, she was appointed to liaise between the Leader's office and the party. She then became a close loyalist and developed into a highly influential figure, a cunning adviser and experienced political operator with a wider management remit.

After 1997, as the Prime Minister's Political Secretary she tended to move away from the coal-face of fixing, but still preserved a managerial steering role more party-sensitive than many in the 'New Labour' core. Despite her low-key, sympathetic 'I agree with you' style, when necessary she was confrontational with a very sharp edge. She was also a subtle and fierce infighter in periodic turf-war battles with two other powerful women,

Angie Hunter in the Leader's office and Margaret McDonagh in head-quarters (sometimes both at once) but always keeping close to the Leader and in the end outlasting both rivals. Her value, not always appreciated in No. 10, was that at times she was a frank and stable restraint on the bold Blair's limited grasp on consequences.

Unusually, Blair retained from the office of John Smith one of his advisers, Pat McFadden, who came from the traditional social-democratic right and became valued for his tough-minded pragmatism and common sense. He worked easily and closely with Cruddas in conference-management activities. Both Cruddas and McFadden went into No. 10 after 1997, with McFadden as a member of the policy unit then the Deputy Chief of Staff. Faz Hakim who had come into party headquarters to work on ethnic minorities in 1994 also became part of the managerial organising team. Quiet-spoken but very effective, she was involved in various activities in managing the CLPs including the choice of conference speakers, and later NEC links. In government a deeply loyal supporter of Blair, she could also be a strong inside voice on some Home Office issues articulating the delegates' concerns.

Phil Wilson was a close friend of Blair and had been centrally involved in his selection and election, and then in the building of Blair's local party at Sedgefield. He was unusual in seeing Blairism in term of the latter's sensitivity to 'real' working-class attitudes and he tied this in with a vision-ary sense of a mass party linked to the communities of 'New Labour'. A born political campaigner, he was brought into the Leader's office playing various roles, including expanding the membership, but always with special managerial responsibility for organising linkage to CLP loyalists at national and regional level. With Labour in government in 1997, he moved into Millbank headquarters till 1999.

A major change in senior managerial personnel ensured a shift towards Blairite policy loyalism. Roland Wales stayed as a left-of-centre Director of Policy, nursing the democratic development of the National Policy Forum, until the end of 1995 when, feeling out of place in the Blair culture, he resigned and was replaced by Matthew Taylor, a dedicated Blairite from the policy staff, with a student-activist background. The new Director was a creative thinker and talker who combined an impressive theoretical per-spective on reform and policy innovation with a strong enjoyment of the tactics and manoeuvres of hard-line party management. After a period as Assistant General Secretary under McDonagh from October to December 1998, he moved to the Institute for Public Policy Research, but always remained close to No. 10, and he reappeared later in a Downing Street policy role.

Peter Coleman in 1996 moved from the post of Director of Organisation to become Secretary of the European Parliamentary Labour Party. A cap-able circumspect old-school party organiser, he retained that mixture of rule-governed propriety and the realpolitik of assisting party management which had traditionally characterised the role. He was followed as Director of Organisation, and then Assistant General Secretary, by David Gardner, a sharp and precise Blairite, more comfortable than Coleman with the new order, but also carrying with him elements of an older perspective on procedural consistency and restraint.

Other figures around the new Leader moved on the influential periphery of party management. Angie Hunter, Blair's long-term confidante, became Diary Secretary, and brought with her a sensitivity to business and middle-class concerns about the Labour Party and radical views on its reform. Murray Elder, Smith's head of staff, was kept on temporarily but departed in 1995 when Jonathan Powell became the Chief of Staff of the Leader's office and then of No. 10. He had moved from the foreign service at Blair's request and his civil service expertise was highly regarded. Although he brought no depth of understanding of the Labour Party, he was not inhibited in occasional heavy involvement in discussion about party management and reform.

Much more central to regular party management was Geoffrey Norris, an ex-Labour councillor, who moved into the Leader's office as a policy specialist, and then into the No. 10 Policy Unit with responsibility for liaison with business. In that role he developed a huge expertise and a politically delicate touch. With it came managerial influence over anything in the party which affected relations with business and its organisations. Ian McCartney, MP was the son of a political family from a working-class background and, in a sense, a son of the Labour Party as an active trade unionist and an ex-party organiser. He was unusual in the Blair circle in that class, union and party pedigree. Because of his class style and wicked humour his considerable intellectual abilities were sometimes underestimated. After 1997 he became a central and innovative player who worked the sensitive interface between government, party and trade unions from different posts.

Sawyer, McDonagh and the general secretaryship

Sawyer as General Secretary had a weekly meeting with the Leader and a day-by-day dialogue with the Leader's office and later the Downing Street Political Office. He also had regular contact with Mandelson. Yet by the summer of 1995 he had become more of an outsider figure following his failure to deliver his ex-union NUPE (now UNISON) to vote for the change in Clause IV of the party's constitution in 1994 and 1995. According to Campbell, Sawyer had been relaxed about delivery of that union's support.[5] Problems also emerged over the weak management of Blair's attempt to push his agenda on abolition of union sponsorship. In the aftermath, Sawyer began to reconsolidate some of his links to the soft left with whom he shared a genuine perspective that relations between the party and the Leader ought to be more of a two-way process.

The new ascendancy of the Party Leader and his office over the party organisation, and Blair's carelessness over protocol and territory, sometimes had the effect of adding to the internal administrative problems of the General Secretary. New figures could simply 'emerge' in various roles in party headquarters sent by or in the name of the Leader initially because of work they were doing on his behalf or recommendation. Sawyer's position appeared to be challenged in 1995 by a young Labour Party assistant organiser placed in headquarters at Blair's insistence to mobilise support for the change in Clause IV. Following that campaign Margaret McDonagh emerged as a hero of delivery and was almost immediately touted by some around the Leader as 'the next General Secretary'.

But she and Sawyer forged a close understanding. He gave her room to operate, indeed passed a lot of initiative to her, and then backed her to be the next General Secretary when the time came. They had very different personal styles, particularly in terms of consultation and delegation, and they always differed over the party's role in the new policy-making institutions where he was supportive and she was uninterested. But with his backing, and under her own great steam as general election campaign coordinator, McDonagh became a weighty presence in relation to the development of party organisation and party management long before she became General Secretary. Sawyer was neither by philosophy nor by instinct a knee-jerk authoritarian and, at times, he and Morgan attempted to guide Blair towards a more accommodative stance towards the party. But there was increasing pressure to deliver in pre-election preparation, and by the end of 1996 over the project called Partnership in Power he and Morgan had moved well in tune with the 'control and drive it through' agenda, as did most other managers (see Chapter 7).

Election victory and new management posts

The election victory, organised with impressive energy and professionalism, cast all of them in a good light and, following approval for the introduction of what became Partnership in Power covering party-government relations, Sawyer initiated a major change in senior management. It involved the creation of a new post of Deputy General Secretary with upgraded Assistant General Secretaries covering organisation, policy, campaigns and communication. On 25 June 1997 this was accepted by the NEC with some reluctance over top-heavy appointments. McDonagh was made Deputy General Secretary, a position which she had in practice already been occupying since late 1995. Sawyer aimed to concentrate on a roving political role encouraging Partnership in Power.

In the Downing Street Political Office, there was scepticism about the value of these new managerial arrangements. Much of the political role, including much of the party management and relations with the unions, was now being played in the Political Office. From 1997 it was run by three highly skilled political managers, Morgan, Cruddas and Hakim, all of whom were long-time critics of McDonagh and Sawyer. Sawyer's role was now very unclear to No. 10, especially as McDonagh was, with a great deal of independence, acting as an assertive and interventionist Deputy General Secretary. There were some periods of particularly unstable relations between her and Morgan. They were politically not far apart, but were old rivals, and temperamentally and in style and their intra-party allies very different. McDonagh was particularly close to Hunter, Morgan's rival in some No. 10 power struggles.

Relations between the two managerial offices deteriorated, particularly over the tactics for NEC elections (see Chapter 8, p. 239). In May 1998, Sawyer saw that he was losing Blair's confidence and resigned as General Secretary after the party conference. He was given a peerage. Despite opposition from the Political Office and a wide range of others, Blair, supported strongly by Angie Hunter, stuck to his own judgement and the advice from Sawyer that McDonagh should be the next General Secretary. She was the first woman and youngest-ever person in that post. The post of Deputy General Secretary was immediately abandoned.

To Blair, McDonagh's prime appeal was that she was someone who progress-chased and delivered anything the Leader and the party required her to do, or that she herself thought necessary in the party's interest. She had been in charge of what was seen as the successful target seats strategy in the General Election of 1997 and, with Blair focused on winning a second term, it was vitally important that her talents remained at the centre. If you anticipated, as Blair did, that the Labour Government might have problems with the party and particularly the NEC, then again there were attractions in having an iron controller as General Secretary, schooled in the electricians' union, famous for its no-holds-barred infighting.

McDonagh was unusual in the devotion of her commitments. As General Secretary she continued grass-roots work for the party to a degree probably not seen in a senior official since the days before the First World War. Her prime purpose was that the Labour Party won and retained power. That it was necessary to rigorously manage those who might prejudice the purpose followed with absolute logic. In full heavy-footed-delivery mode on behalf of the Leadership – 'the control freak's control freak' – she could be a ruthless and feared figure, bold in dealing with anybody and any situation, 'in your face' about who she was and what she wanted.

As a result, the number of critics within other sections of the party organisation, including those who had been passed over and those who had been treated with less than gentleness, grew steadily during her period in office. Nevertheless, she retained a hard core of admirers and allies in the organisation who, whatever their disagreements, appreciated her drive and election skills; to an important extent, later they carried on her legacy through different Leaders. She also had her own shrewd political appeal, based on gaining a protective circle of support amongst a small group of powerful women trade unionists on the NEC all also called Margaret – Maggie Jones, Margaret Wall and, later, Margaret Prosser. A fifth Margaret, Whelan from UNISON, Chair of the Conference Arrangements Committee, was also part of the group. But to the No. 10 Political Office, McDonagh became the source of deepening aggravation and not infrequent cold-war relations. After a while they regarded her as 'out of control', a remarkable comment in these heavy management times.

In the aftermath of the crisis over the election for the London Mayor (Chapter 12, pp. 394–6) McDonagh took to herself (and was given) much of the odium which began to attach to 'control freakery' and became a symbolic negative reference point as the tactics of party management were re-evaluated. Her close association with 'command and control', and with what was labelled by critics 'The Millbank Tendency', began by 2000 to look out of tune with the changing public mood and the party's needs. For Blair and the party she delivered again in terms of an election victory in 2001. She had planned to leave the job sometime after managing another Labour election victory but in any case, following the general election of 2001, the new post of Party Chair (long discussed around the Leader) was now at the point of introduction (Chapter 15, pp. 485–6). McDonagh's resignation followed and three years later, somewhat reluctantly, she accepted a peerage whilst keeping an active unofficial involvement in party management.

The expansion of management

Meanwhile, following the organisation of management after the 1994 conference which was not the success it was spun to be (see Chapter 6, p. 177), there had begun a major intensification of management to avoid failure happening again. That had developed its own momentum as the 1995 Clause IV battle developed and the building of party management for the next annual conference became a greater priority. As Cruddas and Harris described it years later, there emerged 'An informal cross-departmental task force within the party's head office . . . charged with party management and the delivery of votes within party structures, especially the annual conference'. The unit's work became 'formally built into the core duties of head office, and in particular the role of the general secretary'.[6] From there came also a party managerial linkage to designated officials in the regional offices.

In the next two years, there was a spread of managerial concerns to ensure that the party's officials at all levels were geared up for the next general election and the necessary intra-party changes that lay ahead. In that process more officials were brought into party management roles. There was a greater integration of the policy directorate, organisation

directorate and communications directorate in managerial activities covering every facet of the party's activities, and a greater integration of the
regions in early mobilisation on policy and selection issues. In that sense
national and regionally, although they were often over-stretched, there
were more 'managers' than ever before. Webb tells us that there was a
substantial increase in central-office resources after 1994,[7] and in the twelve
months following the post-election cutbacks of 1998 the number of staff
employed in regional offices increased from 75 to 142.[8] Although it is
difficult for an outsider to discern the lines which differentiated the party
political-managerial activity from other aspects of the work of party staff,
that increase, the changing ratio of central party staff to members[9] and the
diagnosis of ex-party officials indicated a strengthening of the managerial
as well as electoral capacity of the machine.

Adding to the significant management strength after 1997 was the big
increase in Downing Street and Whitehall political staffing under the new
Labour government. The senior posts were held by Special Advisers including Chief Press Secretary, Chief of Staff and Chief Economic Advisor to
the Treasury. As Dennis Kavanagh notes, there was a particular increase
in the size and importance of the Downing Street Political Office and
Policy Unit.[10] Brought into government, in the first few days, were over
20 people who had worked with Blair in Opposition.[11] This had significance
for their links to party management as much as the operation of government. The Political Office, particularly, was closely involved in party
management. Blair had thought in terms of running the party via No. 10
with Margaret McDonagh focusing on elections. But this was not seen as
practicable by his staff, and McDonagh was strongly opposed. Things were
left as they were, but there was a regular territorial tension, even a repetitive tug of war, over some functions.

Developing central control

Under Larry Whitty there had been some assertion of regional financial
autonomy, but under Sawyer there was little in the way of formal organisational change in the relations between headquarters and the regions.
However, there was a slow attrition of regional conferences and, in 1995,
a new NEC power to ballot the members directly (Chapter 6, p. 187).
Sometimes through the direct influence of the General Secretary, but also
at times bypassing the party hierarchy, came a drive for control over the
whole party. From Blair's office and then No. 10 Downing Street were sent
the messages of 'what Tony wants'. Through the reinvigorated operation
of the party machine at and after the 1995 party conference came new
managerial priorities. The considerable influence of Margaret McDonagh
in various roles and campaigns emphasised delivery of what the centre
called for. Meetings with the regional officials followed the 'New Labour'
pattern. There were always 'trusties' put up to speak, proposing what the
centre wanted.

Repoliticisation, redefinition and the Leader's vanguard

Blair may not have been too clear in 1994 about the future mechanics of management but he knew exactly what he did not want from the Labour Party and what kind of attitudes he wanted from the officials. The radicalism and minority vanguardism of 'New Labour' made it essential for Blair to create a political machine of officials in his own image to drive through success. Before 1994, loyalty was heavily emphasised by and in the machine, but it was an abstract multilayered loyalty to the party, 'the movement' and the Leader. Now, the changes in the culture of party management (analysed in Chapter 4) were accompanied by what amounted to a major coup, making the party machine of officials into a repoliticised instrument of the Leader, responsive to his purposes, driving through his priorities and protecting him.

The most important change on the inside but not much noticed by the world outside was a covert shift imposed on the functional responsibilities and role-definition of party officials. There were clear signals to the party officials that the party organisation must be fully focused on delivery of all Blair's party agenda. Whatever was said in public, the officials had to cast off the old neutrality of 'civil servants' of the party and redefine themselves as 'political organisers' working behind the objectives of the new Leader. In the 1995 campaign to change Clause IV of the party constitution, not only was the party organisation totally involved in the mobilisation, staff were encouraged to get more active within their own parties for the same purpose.

The contrast with the past was so important it is worth emphasising. In the days of the traditional model of party management, as noted previously virtually all officials thought of themselves as party civil servants. Reg Underhill, a senior national official of the party from 1945 to 1972, author of the Underhill Report and an official not averse to occasional discreet political intervention in the party's interest, always saw himself and other officials as 'civil servants of the Party'.[12] Jim Cattermole, a superveteran regional organiser, often seen in the past as political in his activity as a party official, said in 2003 that he had been very pleased with that civil service description.[13]

In practice, they had always been political organisers in the sense that their priority work was in development and assisting the organisation so that the party could win elections, and there was often some mix of this neutral civil service role with the occasional political steering of internal decisions. But the crucial feature was that it was the 'civil service' role that they affirmed as the legitimate role. Now under Blair the change in legitimacy was sharp and clear. 'We are not civil servants' was said to an observer in a challenging tone. Its full implications were not generally talked about but widely understood. There was a positive responsibility to intervene to manage and redirect the party with diminished inhibition and less concern for not crossing boundaries. In 1994 during Blair's election as Leader, Whitty had sought to restrict the political activities of militant Blair supporters in the machine. For a period after Blair's election there was some tension between the old and the new. But generally for the national and regional machine it settled down to the acceptance of the new role definition.

A study of Labour Party employees found that 88 per cent of the party staff were members before they took up paid positions, and two-thirds of these claimed to be very active.[14] It was said by the party managers in defence of their new role that the staff had joined the party as politicals and therefore naturally remained political. The redefinition and repoliticisation of the Blairite managers was defended by senior party officials as a right as individual citizens of the party. All of this should have precipitated an especially sharp delineation of roles which ensured that activity as a party official within a democratic hierarchy was clearly circumscribed. It did not happen because, although they may have acted at times in pursuit of their own values and purposes, that was not the dominant pattern. They were in practice the core of the Leader's faction, organised in a national system of management run subject to the influence of the Leader's office but arranged from the office of the General Secretary, through a senior official, prompting organising and coordination activity down to regional level.

This political role of the party staff was all the more important because under Blair, in terms of their political opinions party employees were to the right of Labour MPs, members and voters,[15] a location resembling that of Blair himself. The new role-definition and political alignment of the party officials had created the Leader's vanguard organisation, and it stayed that way. It was an example of the virtue of boldness and what might be achieved if operations of the party were altered outside formal constitutional authority. This 'coup' process and its repetitions will be explored further in Chapters 7, 10, 11, and 15 and 16. All of this strengthened the powers and broadened the opportunities and choices available to Blair's enterprising party management.

The potential dangers slowly became apparent to critics. MPs Fatchett and Hain complained that 'the skills and expertise of the Party's professional staff should be devoted to the functions of organisation. It is not their job to usurp the internal democratic process'.[16] The dangers were even greater when developments came near to challenging the old unwritten rule that the party bureaucracy was excluded from formal representation within party policy-making processes. That possibility hovered over the proposals for representation of party stakeholders during Partnership in Power discussions in 1996 before eventual retreat, and reappeared again with more confidence in 2003. It remained a crucial feature of the success of the rolling coup that the reality was never subject to a formal party authorisation. In great measure it was covered by secrecy and lack of accountability.

Power, constitution and the mutability of rules

Managers, professionalism and two worlds of management

Reverence and rulebook

This secrecy and lack of accountability was characteristic of the whole of the second world of management (described in Chapter 4) covering important facets of the party's internal life. The character of that second world was heavily influenced by the attitudes valued by the Leader including his urgent focus on delivery and his perspective on the constitution and rules of the party. In encouraging a new flexibility, Blair sought escape from all facets of what he regarded as the 'Old Labour' prison. He had little respect for 'antiquated' practices and was determined to avoid anything which implied constraint on the development of 'New Labour'. That became reflected in the status of the rulebook. Historically, in its constitutional aspects, that had not changed very frequently. It had long been a symbol of the party's history and identity, an expression of what was regarded as 'this great movement of ours'. It was also the familiar and faithful instrument of a multitude of barrack-room lawyers at the grass roots. Some keen and well-off CLPs, up to the late 1980s, even gave all new members a copy. It could be quoted alongside 'Citrine', the guide to the conduct of meetings, in argument over proper procedure.

A change from the moderate constitutional conservatism noted in 1978[17] had begun with the pressures from the Campaign for Labour Party Democracy and was, with new management purposes, continued under Kinnock. Now after 1994, in an atmosphere where there was a ready Blairite rejection of much of Labour past, the rulebook lost its reverential respect as a symbol of history and identity. Instead, undergoing regular change, year by year, with more expected in the future, it became a set of transitional arrangements, no longer so closely tied to what had been thought of as a 'magnificent journey'.[18] In Blair's eyes, Labour history had no such magnificence.

Availability and accessibility

It also became less easily available and less understandable by ordinary members. A big change took place in the 1995 rulebook. This change was to separate the 'constitutional' element of the rules from the 'procedural' aspects which over time, it was said, 'had got mixed in'. It was in that respect a rational tidying process. But with a multitude of new procedures, some of which were guidelines which allowed regional and central officials to initiate precise rules taken out into separate books, it was less immediately available as a collection, other than for party officials. The multiplicity of rules meant that even the most conscientious CLP Secretary had to ration their concern and expertise. By the second term, even an NEC member with years of union and party experience admitted privately to not being able to understand the rulebook. That impoverishment of knowledge did not trouble a management deeply suspicious of an activist's democracy. It had the advantage of undermining the possibility of the rulebook being used by what was described by one manager as 'pedants, barrack-room lawyers and troublemakers', to impede the purposes of 'New Labour' and its Leader.

The Blair managerial era was heavily concerned with establishing rule-making supremacy. New power relations between the Leader and the party machine, between the NEC and the Leader and between the NEC and the senior officials ensured that generally, with a few important exceptions (noted below relating to the traditional right and loyalism), proposed rule changes from outside the leadership met obstacles and vigorous opposition whilst Blairite rule changes became, in effect, unimpeded declarations. And down from Blair came signals which implied that officials should use rules in the light of Blairite purposes; they were to be regarded as means to the practical ends of delivery, not ends with a rigid reverence that could get in the way.

A well-hidden conflict on the eve of Blair's first party conference as Leader, in 1994, revealed Blair's attitude towards a rule that got in the way of what needed to be done. It revolved around the application of the constitutional provision prescribing equal women's representation as delegates. Blair worried that if male delegates were excluded by vigorous application of the rules, it could leave Labour vulnerable to attack on grounds of 'political correctness' as well as causing some internal rows. A fierce and significant argument was waged over this between Blair's office media aides on the one side and the Director of Organisation Peter Coleman, the Constitutional Officer Mike Penn and also the Conference Arrangements Committee on the other. The bullying behaviour of Blair's aggressive young media enforcers on this issue was described by one moderate official as 'behaving like little Hitlers'. As the Leader was later privately informed, older party officials developed a feeling that the Leader and the newer younger members of his office had 'insufficient respect for abiding by the party's constitution and rules.'[19]

At this stage, none of the party officials and representatives would give way. They regarded defence of the agreed rules as protection of the stability and cohesion of the party. Blair's response to them was to regard the actions of those defending the rules as 'ludicrous', and lost his temper. As it happened, after 1995, the rule about women's representation – having been found to be a managerial godsend in bringing into the conference substantial numbers of more easily influenced novice delegates carrying what was now to be 50 per cent of the vote – it was then strictly adhered to.

Under the new role definition and repoliticisation of officials, the organisation moved more fully into line with the Leader on managing such tricky delivery issues. The experience over women's representation joined other signals about what Blair found acceptable and what he did not. It was made clear that the can-do Leader expected the party to be run as a can-do organisation operating with a resourcefulness which took it for granted that any problem could be 'fixed' one way or another. There continued to be spasmodic in-house tensions between the incumbent Constitutional Officer and those around the General Secretary who gave more robust priority to risk and unrestrained delivery. But that private constitutional argument revolved around a protection against legal comeback rather than a defensive protection of the spirit of the rules within party values. In that sense delivery became the spirit of the rules. This delivery was now assisted also by a much greater degree of managerial flexibility in creating and amending rules driven by an attempt to make it more fit for purpose. The NEC had the final right to decide in the case of any dispute as to the meaning, interpretation or general application of the constitution. But the content of the developing Blairite rulebook of 1995 introduced and strengthened a high degree of delegation of the powers of the NEC to its elected officers, committees, subcommittees, the General Secretary, other national and regional party officials, and designated representatives.[20] This delegation could be legitimised retrospectively by the NEC, as advised by the national officials who had an important tactical power of interpreting the rulebook. Acting for the NEC could involve using the constitutional power to adjudicate on disputes with decisions which were 'final and conclusive'.[21] In the name of flexibility some rules under Smith had been left deliberately and consensually unclear in avoiding rigidity in development, especially in relation to the new experimental arrangements of National Policy Forum policy-making. That carried over into Blair's period in seeking to extensively develop organisational change and new unwritten rules outside the formal rules and sometimes without formal announcement. It also secured opportunities to avoid votes where recommendations on rule changes were likely to have been rejected.

In an accentuation of past managerial behaviour but now within the expanded and flexible rulebook, the code of the 'political organisers' involved seeking an advantageous choice of what rule to emphasise. There was also a developing political precept that creative managerial skills were reflected in testing how far individual rules could be taken in their interpretation and application to see what could be achieved without undue internal reaction. That was eased by the fact that the NEC was precluded from supervision of the covert operation of the managers, indeed not given any formal acknowledgement that it existed. From this came a confident expansion of the powers of the central officials. At times, this managerial skill also involved a dextrous contrivance of communicational as well as organisational resources in order to handle a difficult constitutional situation and to generate a satisfactory outcome.

The latter was an example of what Blairite managers referred to when they talked of 'managing' a problem. It was here also where 'serious politics' could at times venture 'beyond the line' of general party acceptability, depending on the importance of the issue, the pressures from above and, to some extent, the personal proclivity of the manager. The new scope and intensity of this beyond-the-line activity aroused the ire of some past managers. Ex-Kinnockite and Smith managers, and more veteran officials, including a famous past manager, Jim Cattermole, commented critically on the changed standards of conduct of central party officials.[22] They developed the disapproving view that the key managerial feature which distinguished their era from that of the Blair ascendancy was the change in attitude to the party's rules, written and unwritten.

Rules and conventions

In spite of this movement towards new unwritten rules, an important contrary change in attitudes took place towards past unwritten rules. This became clear, although unannounced, within weeks of Blair becoming Leader. In examining Labour's ethos from the vantage point of the 1970s, Henry Drucker had emphasised the party dependence on formal written rules in specifying how the party should be governed.[23] But there was another dimension of regulation that he and others missed. As we have seen, feeding into the party's rule consciousness and respect had been the framework of mainly unwritten 'rules' and protocols of the union-Labour Party relationship derived from traditional party and union values.[24] Labour management had always been run with the aid of a mixture of the written and the consensually conventional. Now, in a crucial development, the old 'rules' and protocols of the union-party relationship were unilaterally rejected by Blair and his managers without announcement. As a method of political change, the unilateralism was a sign of things to come.

The Blairite machine and the Blairite movement

The traditional right and loyalism

The historic sense of coalition of the leadership, the machine and the faction known as the traditional right had been an integral feature of management activity, especially in the loyalist behaviour of union NEC representatives. For his part, although Blair always wanted some distance from this old right, seeing them as a part of Labour's sunk-in-the-past problem, being a realist in party management he continued to connect with them as an important loyal party support. However, there remained something very unusual about their early relationship with Blair. His unwillingness to abide by old conventional rules and protocols of the relationship marked a new type of leadership behaviour. His flirtation with the ending of collective affiliation was also a worrying development. On the NEC, there were some surges of distrust over his direction, his treatment of the committee and his plebiscitary ambitions for the party, coming from members who were proud to have fought to 'save the party' in the past. Some of his total-modernisation advisers, Philip Gould in particular, were regarded with disdain as having little sense of practical politics. At one point the attitude of the modernising ultras was likened by the MP John Spellar to 'rightwing Trotskyism'.[25]

All this created a disorientation which left room for some unusual responses which for the moment complicated the process of 'turning the working machinery of the Labour party into a decorative ornament'.[26] At an early stage under Blair, the NEC trade union group produced some significant discreet critics from the traditional right. Gordon Colling of SOGAT, Chair of the Organisation sub-committee and convenor of the trade union group, was the most notable. In the 1994 leadership campaign there had been a substantial imbalance in the resources available to the three candidates. The extent of it was never clear, as supplying information was voluntary, but Whitty's view was that Blair's resources were five times that of his main opponent Prescott.[27] There was also a sudden rise in expenditure by some politicians for elections to the NEC and complaints about glossy brochures sent out to CLPs. A procedure committee, chaired by Colling, recommended strict new rules in party elections, limiting candidate expenditure and individual donations as well as prohibiting the soliciting of funds. The NEC on 30 November decided to ban all expenditure on NEC elections, with only the statement by the candidates, issued officially by the party, allowed to be circulated.

These controls over expenditure were never fully adhered to but at the time they reflected both unease at unfairness and suspicion of wealthy donors seeking influence through and around Blair. Over this and other organisational issues, the idea of solidarity with the party took on at times a change of emphasis which differentiated it from support for what the Leader wanted. Some of it was very important, particularly over Clause IV (see Chapter 6, pp. 180, 182–3). Partnership in Power and the NEC role (Chapter 7, p. 222) and over the acceptance of the new organisation TULO (Chapter 9, p. 271). But the traditional supportive role by union representatives on policies and on most major organisational reforms continued.

The system of management and the primacy of Blairism

Alongside the national system of management operating through the party machine, with its links to the traditional right including the AEEU union and to the organisation Labour First, there might have been built a distinctively Blairite movement. The journal *Renewal*, set up in 1993 by a grouping from the Labour Coordinating Committee, proved to be too free-thinking and critical for any such purpose and, by the end of the first term in government, ultimately went more or less into internal opposition. In 1995 a new Blairite journal and organisation, *Progress*, was set up with cooperation from within party headquarters, and with the approval of Blair providing that it centred itself around the Leader.[28] Its function was to be a modernising educational medium, and it gained a nod from Prescott on the reassurance that it was not to be a faction. The organisation was not noticeably successful in gaining grassroots adherents, and after 1997 the

LCC – which had in great measure become a vehicle of Blairite objectives – was wound up. That left what appeared to be a political gap in Blair's operations.

Amongst Blair's aides the evangelical organiser Phil Wilson privately urged after 1997 a turning of the NEC's Healthy Party project in that direction, linked to the expansion of the party through community involvement. But it met other functional perspectives on the party and was not publicly pushed. In 1998 proposals in No. 10 for a broader-based managerial organisation were shelved and the Blairite operation remained heavily reliant on and dominated by the repoliticised party machine. It was an arrangement that generally worked to Blair's satisfaction before and after Labour came into government. The party officials were also very happy with it. They were proud of what they did to benefit the party. It raised their status and interest in the work, and in any case they saw Wilson and others around Blair as ultimately depending on them. The officials also operated generally with deep discretion and without grandstanding. They operated in a well-oiled hierarchical structure and a system of management which was not beset by internal conflicts that compromised Blair's overall control by developing its own political objectives. An alternative arrangement might have opened up another flank to the party factional influence of Gordon Brown, a worry that grew stronger towards the end of the first term in government (see below).

Blair and the encouragement of delivery

As Leaders exemplify attitudes and tactics, so others are influenced to follow – particularly the young and subordinates who need to win approval in order to keep status or gain preference in climbing the greasy pole. Leaders educate and socialise their political followers by what they do as much as what they say, and by what they don't say as much as what they do say, what they want to know and what they don't. In 1995 a discreet 'thank you' reception was instituted by the Leader's office for the political organisers' covert operation, away from prying eyes following the end of the conference where the platform won on every issue. Blair expressed his pleasure about the outcome to managers who were eager to share with him the ways and means of their multiple successes. But he indicated his reluctance to know how they did it. Similar indications were given at subsequent private 'thank you' receptions.

This fitted the persona of a man not madly interested in detail, and not so at ease on questions of management – indeed, as some of his loyal aides would say privately and affectionately, 'lousy at it'. He was, they agreed, 'an outcomes not a processes man'. His avoidance of the details of what the manager may have been doing could also have been the natural reaction of someone who liked to see his own persuasive role as the crucial feature. Because of this it is possible to see Blair's early attitude, as one senior party manager described it to me in 1995, with a laugh, as, 'He thinks that it's him'. But given his many later references to party management in reported private conversations, it is difficult to believe that Blair kept his pristine ignorance, or that he failed to understand the impact of the signals he was emitting. Rather, he was keeping a defensible 'do what you have to do' distance from the dark side of Blairite politics. 'Bobbying' again it might be said.

Some defenders of Blair's management argued that what some in the machine thought was the Blair message and what he was really saying were two different things. Tony's position, it was said, was distorted by others with different values, in Millbank or in the party machine 'where they are all 21 years old', full of the sense of their own accomplishment in 'going beyond the line'. They possessed an eager interest in the thrill of 'NUS style politics', as it was occasionally described. Yet hawkishly militant young organisers sharing a 'tomorrow belongs to me' enthusiasm were not absolutely deviants. They responded to a culture which was a mix of the permissible and the encouraging to activities on behalf of the culture-carriers of the future. Managers learned that there would be no problem in being boldly and militantly controlling in search of 'what delivers' and 'what works'. Nor was there reproof for those who in their management moved beyond the publicly defensible line in appreciation of the 'serious politics' of a situation. The consistent pattern of evidence from party officials was best summed up as seen through the eyes of one national official, prominent in the first term of government. Privately, striving for accuracy, he described Blair as a man 'not too obsessed with the niceties'.

To most of the managers, following the private managerial codes was what made you good in both a professional and a moral sense. In the new order, successful political manipulation was simply politics and something that you could be proud of. It could also provide some of the psychic highs and satisfactions of political life, a sense of superior power and of risk taking worthiness, earning respect among colleagues by skilful achievement. Until shaken by public reactions near the end of their first term in government (explored in Chapter 15, pp. 465, 471) with the possible exception of managerial reactions to the Road to the Manifesto ballot in 1996 (Chapter 6, p. 196) the managerial culture established by the 'New Labour' core had little place for a sense of regret. Where that did exist it had to be hidden.

That was the way to get on, and getting on was another thing that 'New Labour' applauded. Pressed political organisers were not expected to spend time thinking, let alone arguing, about process, especially the integrity of the process they had been told to implement. That non-questioning approach was part of a routine of showing loyalty and zeal in conditions where urgency was being driven down the hierarchy often in a highly bossy and pressurising style. There could be an element of fear if not enough energy was shown in delivery. Whistleblowing about managerial practice was out of the question.

Generation, differentiation, and variation

In the period from 1994 to 2001 so much of the organisation and culture of Blair's party management took root that all had in some way to respond to it. Yet, the broad circle of those directly involved did have some significant differences in attitudes towards the managerial imperatives with varying conceptions of 'taking the party with you', 'partnership', 'the activist culture' and 'the healthy party'. This could add a complicating feature to the operation of the management culture under Blair, unrecognised in the world outside. As explored in detail later, the staff of the PLP Office, under Alan Howarth, had their own autonomy and traditions reflecting both the distinctiveness of the Parliamentary arena and an older view of rules and the role of party officials. Jon Cruddas, first in party headquarters and then later in No. 10, worked very successfully managing links to the unions as one of the two major front-line managers. He brought to this role a pluralism which at times moved and pushed past the understood Blairite positions on organisational reform.

Cultures are not changed overnight and are usually always changing in some imperceptible way. In 1994, within the machine, in the PLP and on the NEC there was still a heritage of past values, attitudes and practices as well as some leading-edge forerunners of new outlooks. As the culture and messages were passed down the hierarchy within and from headquarters, the Leader's office, and then No. 10 and across to the PLP, the strong centre and the disciplined expansionist managerial culture did sometimes come into conflict with other influences and beliefs. In spite of the attempt at command and control there remained elements of traditions within the party which influenced commitment to different amalgams of management and pluralism. The union presence in particular, however much curbed by 'New Labour', was always in some interaction with the managers varying in each forum.

As for what lines of propriety were kept and what were crossed, beneath some general behaviour patterns knowledgeable ex-managers locate some significant individual variations, even eccentricities in behaviour. It is worth noting also that the biggest manipulative control freak could be the most righteous in handling money or expecting perks. One experienced ex-manager drew more general categories, said to be in use distinguishing between a zealous group of managers developing under Blair who were labelled by him and others as the 'new fanatics', for whom 'anything goes', and contrasting them with those concerned only with limited 'fit-for-purpose' activity.

New party managers

Background and appointments

In the past, party officials were from a working-class background. They had generally not been to university but were committed to the party from their youth. They started from the bottom often as constituency party agents and worked upwards on long-term contracts, normally staying in post as the regional organiser till retirement. The NEC was then loath to fire anybody[29] and the Leader himself could not sack long-serving employees.[30] The national officials were then drawn from those working in the field after long experience of the Labour Party – and a deep education into its history and culture.

The members of the Blair machine were markedly different from the past generations. Where the organisers appointed during Smith's leadership were in the age group 30–40 and generally with experience of other occupations, those appointed under Blair were 20–30, and virtually all university-educated with limited other experience. Some of the new intake would stay in the machine but most, although highly motivated in the party employment, were people who came to see this job as a stepping stone which might take them to other fields and occupations.[31] They would stay working for the party with average length of service of only around five years.[32] Many of these party officials were on short-term contracts and there could be rapid movement not only from post to post in the machine but also through termination of employment or resignation. At the top, with each change in the General Secretary and sometimes more frequently, came a similar short tenancy affecting the occupancy of other senior party offices. Appointment of staff became much more informal and mainly in the hands of the General Secretary with a gradual exclusion of NEC members from appointing committees.

This potentially freed up the new officials to play a more flexible, creative and less hidebound role. It meant that they were keen, energetic and eager to make a quick mark. But it also meant that in their insecurity they were easier to socialise into the new norms of party behaviour. And it meant that they had limited knowledge of past problems, less life experience to draw on, less integration into the local community and shared less of a collective political memory. Because they were younger and less secure they were less independent and had less authority in relations to the centre and to leading politicians.

Insecurity, in-house trade unions and the curtailment of intra-machine pluralism

Insecurity was not only produced by the terms of contracts, it was also brought about by the changes in union representation. Over the years, headquarters and the regions had developed strong union branches. The National Union of Labour Organisers had its own traditions and its own journal, *Labour Organiser*. It had been a force to be reckoned with by the central management. Although there was a reduction in the militancy of all the in-house unions under Kinnock, NULO could still present discreet collective resistance and was also (with other union branches) the sources of various organisational reform initiatives. All that changed under Blair.

With new contractual arrangements, a new membership, a powerful head-office management and an emphasis on delivery, the culture of the party was much less conducive to active trade unionism. NULO amalgamated with the GMB and their journal on party matters was wound up. As the General Secretary – particularly McDonagh – asserted a widely defined operational freedom from the NEC in conjunction with its loyalist allies, there was no effective policing of the managerial process by party representatives. All this helped create a sense of managerial invulnerability providing that they were not clashing with the Leader's objectives.

That and the relentless drive from the centre created a sense of powerlessness amongst many working at lower levels of the party organisation. It also meant a decline in the political role of the internal trade union branches both as alternative generators of a different form of repoliticisation and at times as campaigners for internal party reform. Ironically the internal union branches were brought into significant vociferous involvement later defending the managerial officials and supporting their political rights when they were under criticism for their covert interventions. It was another addition to the commanding character of management developments under Blair.

Managerial components

Two kinds of manager in unity

Panebianco, in his highly influential study of political parties[33] drew attention to the confusion about different bureaucracies in the government of parties but does not relate his clarifications to the function of party management and does not explore the possible tensions between two kinds of managers – managerial officials and managerial representatives. In the first category were the Leader's aides and those of his colleagues, later acting as special advisers to members of the government, together with party officials at headquarters and in the regional offices. They had the main tasks of party management. They interacted with the second category of managers. These were the elected representatives on key committees of different forums which for some purposes had managerial functions, particularly the Parliamentary Committee, the National Executive Committee and the Conference Arrangements Committee. Most prominent in this were figures with leading roles which linked with activities of the managerial officials.

It might have been expected that this distinction would be the basis of a divergence between the two types of manager with pressure from the representatives' constituencies constraining the role of managerial officials. In practice, however, normally – although not exclusively – the interaction between the two kinds of managers was, as described above, an influential linkage from managerial officials to managerial representatives rather than the reverse, and a unity rather than a divergence. Under cross-pressures, the role of representational managers could at times, to various degrees, take on the character of honourable double agent seeking to reconcile managerial representational responsibilities. However, as will be shown, it was possible for the divided management to become a significant problem for the Leader later, as pressures increased from below (see Chapter 18, pp. 615–16).

The managerial use of communications

Media management and party management

The hour-by-hour operation of Labour's spin-doctor media managers grew to be judged the epitome of sophisticated and effective political action in dealing with a proliferation of 24-hour media outlets. Political marketing was noted by political specialists,[34] and a wide range of political commentators, as a new factor contributing strongly to changes in internal power relations especially during Blair's leadership. The status of media management and its role within the party was enhanced after 1994 by Alastair Campbell as Blair's press officer, with Mandelson still playing an element of his old role.

In 1997 Campbell became central controller of No. 10 communications and Whitehall information officers. His means of influence grew as the number of Special Advisers grew from 34, under the Conservatives in 1994, to 78 by 1999–2000; half the increase was in No. 10.[35] He regularly attended Cabinet meetings and was given, with Jonathan Powell, Blair's chief of staff, authority to issue instructions to civil servants. In the biography of Campbell by Oborne and Walters he is described as 'Blair's vizier or grand chamberlain'.[36] Scammell described Campbell as securing a personal relationship with the Leader which was nearing equality with his master.[37] Yet there was no doubt that in setting the direction for taking the party and its policy, Blair was the master.

For this study it is important to note that Campbell and less-senior media managers were a differentiated entity in the organisation and yet, as agreed with Blair, heavily integrated into the party managerial arrangements for policy and decision-making to a degree which had no precedent in Labour's history. They shared a common diagnosis of the problems from the major enemies, the behaviour appropriate for dealing with them and the necessary coordination within the party. Campbell was not only regarded as the maestro of his vitally important media trade. His closeness to Blair, his unparalleled new governmental powers as press secretary, his control over ministerial public statements and his strong personality made him an authoritative source streaming tactical and strategic influence down into the party management process across the whole field of policy-making at its earliest stages.

Internally the spin doctors carried special managerial prestige. 'The folk hero in this building', said one senior headquarters policy adviser looking backwards from the second term, 'was the person who shouted down the phone at the press and got a headline changed.' That abrasive quality of combative complaining added to the muscular impact on the party where media managers were influential in limiting and deflecting attention from any development considered to be not in accord with their strategy, and in creating and projecting the dominant media messages of the policy framework. A positive agenda was carried in speeches by Blair, Brown and other leading figures which were extensively prefigured and emphasised, making sure that the case was defended against attack, emphasising and highlighting the causes which Labour took forward in unity and counter-ing those features of the party and its relations with the unions which were most easily distorted by the media or otherwise considered damaging.

In spite of the rhetorical commitment of the Leader's office and head-quarters to a members' democracy and, later, to partnership, the party had always to be shown in the media as subordinate. The Leader had always to be shown to be winning and always to have the best messages even if that meant at times taking them from his colleagues. Although there was a big and successful initial push for increased party membership, the research which showed the importance of active grassroots party membership in determining constituency election outcomes[38] met a very muted welcome for fear of the problematic implications of an active and assertive member-ship for internal party relations and the media strategy. The rhetoric of 'a members' party' was always combined with close supervision of the potential problems raised for the media managers adding to the forces driving a controlling centralisation of power. In carrying the message of Blair's supremacy and neutralising anything which might darken the Leader's image, the spinners were constant drivers, reinforcing a favourable public perception of Blair which deepened and extended his political honeymoon.

Media managers regularly interfered directly in party management. Campbell regarded himself and was regarded by other managers as 'a Labour Party person', but he and his managerial colleagues judged it naive to think that facing the media enemies the Labour Party could afford to be involved in an uncontrolled democratic process with abstract ideals at a detriment to the exigencies of realism and media power. A measure of intimidation was regarded as necessary to inhibit the internal obstacles as well as to limit opportunities for the party's enemies. There was an uninhibited enhancement of the routine management practice, begun under Kinnock, of focusing publicly on what was going to happen to sources of opposition – groups to be weakened, institutions to be curbed, etc. An exaggeration of the political blood spilt on the floor in any significant vic-tory (said to be the Mandelson doctrine) was used to heighten the impres-sion of supremacy.

Spinners anonymous and party management

The question of who was doing what in this media management and on behalf of whom was sometimes very uncertain. The prized techniques of spinning became integral to a common view of managerial professionalism that could spread easily into competitive personal advancement by any ambitious politician, aide or managing official who could use them to illustrate and to advance status. Establishing full managerial discipline over this was not easy. Campbell had to contend with a multiplicity of sources of spin, including the continuing individual operation of Mandelson. Millbank was an important conduit of media-management messages but also had its own communications staff who appeared to operate with some autonomy even under a 'New Labour' government.

There was a particular irritating problem even for party managers trying to locate the authenticity of what was said to have come on behalf of the Leader. The media messages created at times a disjunction between the voice of Blair operating in formal party or party-union relations and the voice of the spin-masters who worked the wider media strategy. This phenomenon, sometimes labelled sarcastically amongst internal critics as the 'two voices of Blair', was reflected also in a steady stream of stories, said to be telling what the real attitude of the Leader was, or announcing proposals coming from the Leader within and against the party, even if the move had not been supported by party bodies and did not fit the priorities of party managers. A similar process specially affected relations with the TUC (see Chapter 9, p. 280). It was a recipe for regular aggravation and for the longer-term deepening of distrust.

Managing internal communication

Building on changes introduced during the Kinnock era, the party's internal communications had developed various new technical capabilities which added to the capacity for control. The central party-membership lists were now built into the managerial process. Using the pager to keep people abreast of the latest message enhanced the capacity for public unity and also acted as a reminder of the party line and positioning. The pager and the headphone intercom enabled managers to keep close contact with each other at party venues. Telephone conferences facilitated coordination from the centre and more influence over the regions.

Non-communication, it might be said, also expanded. 'New Labour' management, from the first, had few qualms about manipulative secrecy – not making some key information available – usually justified in terms of costs or not letting the press get hold of it. Until the second term, it was hard for National Policy Forum members to get lists of the addresses and telephone numbers of other representatives to the NPF. It was also hard for NEC members to get figures on the size of constituency representation at the party conference and difficult to get accurate membership figures. The verbatim annual conference report became less available.

At its away day in October 1998 one of the themes which emerged from the NEC discussions was that 'there needs to be more communication with an involvement of party members'.[39] Polling of members was then agreed as part of the new communications but it became colonised by the official responsible for intelligence relating to the party. Members of the NEC were not kept informed of the poll results and the party member in the field was never given any details. Private suggestions to senior officers that the results should be shared were met with a bold grin. Amongst the ideas which also emerged from that away-day discussion was 'a member's magazine' replacing the free *Labour Party News*. The new magazine, entitled *Inside Labour*, went into production in 1998 but it was an uninspiring affair, issued at uncertain intervals two or three times a year and drawn up mainly in accordance with the old top-down specifications. It did not appear to have an eager readership awaiting it.

In the years of opposition, the party's persuasion into 'New Labour' cultural and policy change had been encouraged through three large-scale campaigns which were also aimed at influencing public opinion. There was a Clause IV campaign in 1994–5, a Rolling Rose programme in 1995 and the Road to the Manifesto campaign of 1996. In addition there were large-scale political-education conferences putting forward the 'New Labour' world view from 1995, at a venue and time which paralleled the National Policy Forum. In 1996, at its peak, over 5,000 attended national and regional political-education conferences based on small study circles. It remains surprising, given the lessons drawn from the developing weakness of the 1974–9 Labour Government in relations with the party, that there was virtually an abandonment of the political-education programme in government, affected in part by a package of financial measures which also affected plans for local organisers for the Partnership in Power project. Political education was brought back only in very limited electioneering form in 2000.

It had been expected that the new technical facilities and the membership list would produce better and greater volume of vertical internal political communication between leaders and members, and would replace horizontal political communication within areas, regions and constituencies, thus weakening active grassroots dialogue.[40] In practice, although horizontal communication did decline, vertical communication from the leadership to the membership was found to be costly and was very limited in political content. In practice also, as it became clearer that a targeted communication within a reconfiguration of communicational advantages was working effectively at the party conference and that at the NPF other restrictive controls were in place, the pragmatic need for direct heavy top-down party-political communication declined.

The fact that internal communication to the members was weak and spasmodic compared to the role of the mass media meant that influencing the media so as to manage the party was also a regular activity. More productive in connecting with the party, when necessary, was the influence, through radio and television news and key friendly journalists on the *Guardian*, the *Independent*, and the *Observer*, papers read by the party members, Labour supporters and supporters of targeted progressive causes. But whether focused on the party or not, in the early years, raising Blair's profile and applauding his skills, together with the exciting and bold colours of the 'New Labour' portrait that the media managers painted, affected many in the party who, whatever their other sentiments, were vicariously sharing the sense of the Leader's special mission, special charisma, special supremacy and special success.

The Leader's machine and competitive control

There were, however, important complications working against the full realisation of the Leader's supremacy, especially from tensions and wrangling amongst the major 'New Labour' politicians. Although there was a high degree of unity between Blair, Brown and Mandelson over the problems which faced them from the party and the unions, and over the need for these to be closely managed to reinforce discipline, the lack of media discipline between leading figures and between their aides at times proved very difficult. Spinners and counter-spinners became integral to the repertoire of power shared to some extent by most of the parliamentary leadership, exacerbating rivalries at the highest level.

The most serious was an antipathy dating back to Blair's candidature for the post of Leader, and the tensions over Brown's broad central-economic and social-policy role. Persistent conflict between Mandelson and Charlie Whelan, as spin doctors, apparently on behalf of Blair and Brown, regularly created alarm and at times frustrated anguish amongst party managers. To Campbell in No. 10, Whelan was seen as a regular source of mischief in the unattributable-briefing game and as the source of growing distrust of Brown amongst his colleagues.[41] Brown supporters saw Mandelson as the inventor and compulsive exponent of the interpersonal attacking and defending game. Neither Campbell nor Blair could put a complete stop to the media-oriented factional battle, partly because both were seen as complicit in the battles; no sooner had one truce been arranged or promised, than off it went again, publicly indicating and accentuating disunity.

Added to this, it was also held by Brownites that there had then been an understanding between the two men that Blair would at, some stage, concede the position of Leader to Brown. Denying this, close-in Blairites, from an early date, regularly suspected him of preparing the ground for a takeover and working towards that, seeking to control the party. Because this was being fashioned into a remarkable instrument of the Leader's power, it was understandable that in the Leader's office there was a worry that somebody else might seek to control it. Mandelson, in his biography, details Blair's opposition to a Brown proposal in September 1994 that Michael Wills be installed as Labour's Deputy General Secretary.[42] Mandelson dated his own refusal to support Brown on this and refusing to work together in giving advice to Blair, as the point where Brown began to view him as an enemy.[43] Not mentioned in his account is the specific allegation, to be found in Peston, that Brown propositioned him about working together to control the party.[44] Whatever the truth of it, around the Leader, it was later given some nervous credence.

In 1996 the Blair–Brown conflict surfaced to public view and thereafter spasmodically emerged and re-emerged. Brown was viewed around Blair as a driven man who never slept in pursuing his ambitions, working 'incredibly hard in building up his support'.[45] In the first stages of the 1997 election campaign, Brown's team were seen in headquarters as operating as a separate grouping and, by Mandelson, as running a parallel campaign until Blair brought the campaign together.[46] Brown did take a welcoming interest in new MPs and a consoling interest in those who lost ministerial jobs. In the PLP after 1997 there developed a recognisable grouping of 'Brown's friends'. Nevertheless, as Routledge pointed out in his biography of Brown, 'evidence for a prototype machine for a potential leadership bid' was 'slim'[47] Certainly, an examination of the political complexion of the Parliamentary Committee, PLP officials, NEC or senior party staff suggests that this characterisation of a Brown organisation was much exaggerated.

The Routledge biography appeared to be a Brown-sanctioned attempt to give publicity to its tale of the wronged prince who should have been king. But in 1998 the removal of the Chief Whip, Nick Brown, and his deputy George Mudie was more about the practicalities of the job and who was top dog between Blair and Brown, than a full frontal countermove over party control. For the moment Brown kept his allies Geoffrey Robinson and Charlie Whelan in office whilst Mandelson was promoted to Secretary of State at the DTI. At the end of 1998, Mandelson had to be sacked following a newspaper story that Blair later described as a political assassination likely to have come from Brown's associate Whelan.[48] After the second forced resignation of Mandelson in 2001 and the enforced departure also of Robinson and Whelan, the internal government battle and the spin that accompanied it still continued.

The evidence of conflict amongst the leaders, captured in fine detail in Rawnsley,[49] heightened suspicion and tensions over relations within the party headquarters. In the pre-2001 election period. Brown had two senior figures in Headquarters. Douglas Alexander, brought in as head of election planning, and Nick Peccorreli as Policy Director who moved to campaigns. These caused some extra agitation in No. 10 and amongst headquarters Blairites. Campbell's Deputy Lance Price in his diary noted 'worrying signs that Gordon's people at Millbank are becoming difficult'.[50] In contrast, McDonagh, who was watching these things closely and acutely and was not above being suspicious herself, was derisive about the fears of Brown's attempted takeover of the machine.

Worries in the Political Office in No. 10 were not confined to what Brown was up to, although that raised the most palpitations. They at times had some aggravation over the role of the much misunderstood elected Deputy Leader, John Prescott. Without drawing obvious public lines of difference with Blair, he had used Blair's acceptance of the need to 'keep JP on board' on party issues to establish some restrictive implications for the conduct of party management. In semi-private contributions, he involved himself in speaking for the party's members, defending the rights of MPs and attempting to exercise some check on 'New Labour' bouncing and authoritarianism. This meant discreetly moving at times against the Leader's preferred options and particularly those of his aides and ultra-loyalist enthusiasts.

That may have added to the problem of Ian McCartney, who was a close ally of Prescott. Working from the Cabinet Office, at one stage in 1999 he appeared to have had Blair's general support to move in and sort out the headquarters. But true to Blair's form he was never given a specific commitment[51] or any clear terms of reference.[52] It seemed he was to become the new party chair and was reported in the *Times* as having set up a team at headquarters to 'kick-start the party into action'.[53] Yet lacking clear authority and an advance understanding with party officials as to what he was doing, McCartney had a very circumscribed role fighting a General Secretary determined to defend her territory.

Blair's aides advised action in June 2000 to protect Blair's primacy against what were described as 'the politicians'. A senior Blair aide, Pat McFadden, was inserted into party headquarters. Again, as was the Blair managerial style, he was not given the clearest of briefs. 'Go into Millbank and represent us' seems to have been the injunction. 'Looking after the politics' was how it was also described in No. 10. Though very diplomatic, McFadden found great difficulty when faced with a very formidable General Secretary who had not been consulted. Lance Price was also moved into headquarters from his No. 10 spin-doctor role to gain control over Millbank communications management as director and to assist in getting Millbank up to speed in its attacking role. There was, however, another function – watching with McFadden what 'the politicians', especially 'Gordon's people', were doing in order to ensure no loss of political control. Blair's view of that problem was pointed and a sign of what Blair had in mind for after the 2001 General Election. It was, he said, 'essential Millbank was properly locked up'.[54]

Notes

1 Rulebook, 1993–4, rule 7.
2 Ibid.
3 Paul Anderson and Nyta Mann, *Safety First: the Making of New Labour*, Granta, London, 1997, p. 51.
4 Peter Mandelson, *The Third Man: Life at the Heart of New Labour*, Harper, London, 2010, p. 194.

5 Alastair Campbell and Richard Stott (eds), *Extracts from the Alastair Campbell Diaries: The Blair Years*, Hutchinson, London, 2007, entry 2 October 1994, p. 18.
6 Jon Cruddas and John Harris, *Fit for Purpose: a Programme for Labour Party Renewal*, Compass, London 2007, p. 12.
7 Paul Webb, *The Modern British Party System*, Sage, London, 2000, p. 242.
8 Ibid. p. 244.
9 Paul Webb and Justin Fisher, 'Professionalism and the Millbank Tendency: the Political Sociology of New Labour Employees', *Politics*, 23:1, February 2003, p. 10.
10 *The Times*, 28 September 1999.
11 Ibid.
12 Interviews with Reg Underhill, circa 1968–70.
13 Accompanied interview with veteran organiser Jim Cattermole, 24 November 2003.
14 Justin Fisher and Paul Webb, 'Political Participation: the Motivational Vocation of Labour Party Employees', *British Journal of Politics and International Relations*, 5(2), May 2003, p. 168.
15 Ibid. pp. 180–1.
16 Derek Fatchett MP and Peter Hain MP, 'A Stakeholder Party', *Tribune* pamphlet, 1996, pp. 8 and 19.
17 Minkin, *Labour Party Conference*, p. 335.
18 Francis Williams, *Magnificent Journey: the Rise of the Trade Unions*, Odhams Press, London, 1954.
19 Letter from Lewis Minkin to Tony Blair via Murray Elder, then head of Blair's Office, 10 October 1994.
20 Rulebook, 1995, Chapter 1, clause VIII 5.
21 Rulebook, 1995, Chapter 1, clause X 5.
22 Interview with Jim Cattermole, 24 November 2003.
23 Henry Drucker, *Doctrine and Ethos in the Labour Party*, Allen and Unwin, London, 1979.
24 Minkin, *Contentious Alliance*, Chapter 2, pp. 26–53.
25 *Tribune*, 8 December 1995.
26 Francis Beckett and David Hencke, *The Blairs and their Court*, Aurum Press, London, 2004.
27 Larry Whitty, speech to Labour History Group, 6 March 2007.
28 Tom Watson, *Labour Uncut*, 16 March 2011.
29 Richard Rose, *Influencing Voters: A Study in Campaign Rationality*, Faber & Faber, London, 1967, p. 68.
30 Ibid.
31 Fisher and Webb, 'Political Participation', pp. 177–9.
32 Webb and Fisher, 'Professionalism and the Millbank Tendency', p. 15.
33 Angelo Panebianco, *Political Parties: Organisation and Power*, Cambridge University Press, Cambridge, 1988, pp. 224–6.
34 Bob Franklin, *Packaging Politics*, Arnold, London 1994; Jennifer Lees-Marchment, *Political Marketing and British Political Parties: The Party's Just Begun*, Manchester University Press, Manchester, 2001; Margaret Scammell, 'The Media and Media Management', in Anthony Seldon (ed.), *The Blair Effect: The Blair Government 1997–2001*, Brown, London, 2001, pp. 509–34; Dominic

Wring, 'From Mass Propaganda to Political Marketing: the Transformation of Labour Party Election Campaigning', *British Elections and Parties Yearbook*, 5:1, 1995.

35 Peter Riddell in Anthony Seldon (ed.), *The Blair Effect: The Blair Government 1997–2001*, Little, Brown and Company, London, 2001, p. 27.

36 Peter Oborne and Simon Walters, *Alastair Campbell*, Aurum, London, 2004, p. 359.

37 Scammell, 'Media and Media Management', pp. 519–20.

38 Patrick Seyd and Paul Whiteley, *Labour's Grassroots: The Politics of Party Membership*, Clarendon, Oxford, 1992, pp. 186–7; David Denver and Gordon Hands 'Measuring the Intensity and Effectiveness of Constituency Campaigning in the 1992 General Election', in D. Denver, P. Norris, D. Broughton and C. Rallings (eds), *British Elections and Parties Yearbook*, Harvester Wheatsheaf, Hemel Hempstead, 1993; Ron Johnston and Charles Pattie, 'The Impact of Spending on Party Constituency Campaigns at Recent British General Elections', *Party Politics* 1, 1995, pp. 261–73.

39 Notes on NEC Away Day – 27th October 1998, General Secretary, 2 November 1998.

40 Patrick Seyd, 'New Parties New Politics? A Case Study of the British Labour Party', *Party Politics* 5, 1999, p. 401.

41 Interview with Campbell in Hugo Young, *The Hugo Young Papers: Thirty Years of British Politics – Off the Record*, ed. Ion Trewin, Allen Lane, London, 2008, entry dated 19 January 1998, p. 542.

42 Mandelson, *Third Man*, pp. 181–2.

43 Ibid.

44 Robert Peston, *Brown's Britain*, Short Books, London, 2005, p. 51.

45 Lance Price, *The Spin Doctor's Diary: Inside No. 10 with New Labour*, Hodder & Stoughton, London, 2006, entry 19 September 1999, p. 142.

46 Mandelson, *Third Man*, p. 212.

47 Paul Routledge, *Gordon Brown: The Biography*, Simon & Schuster, London, 1998, p. 337.

48 Tony Blair, *A Journey*, Hutchinson, London, 2010, p. 220.

49 Andrew Rawnsley, *Servants of the People: The Inside Story of 'New Labour'*, Hamish Hamilton, London, 2000.

50 Price, *Spin Doctor's Diary*, entry 15 5eptember 2000, p. 251.

51 Ibid. p. 112.

52 Ibid. p. 130.

53 *The Times*, 1 October 1999.

54 Price, *Spin Doctor's Diary*, entry 23 May 2000, p. 223.

6

Transforming fundamentals and laying new foundations

Changing clause IV

Breaking from the past

After constructing the first elements of systematic party management in 1995 there was an immediate engagement with the primary agenda of transforming fundamentals and laying foundations for a reconstruction and re-presentation of the party. This process brought into play a style of leadership, a view of politics and a range of managerial methods which would come to epitomise Blair's party management. It would have some highly publicised and striking successes but it also involved some unacknowledged major limitations and failures. And it would consolidate a philosophy of bold and unrestrained governing, recognisable years hence.

It began with the battle to change the party's old ideological objectives as set out in Clause IV (4) of the rulebook. The clause committed the party to 'secure for the workers by hand or by brain the full fruits of their industry and the most equitable distribution thereof that may be possible upon the basis of the common ownership of the means of production, distribution, and exchange, and the best obtainable system of popular administration and control of each industry and service'. It was no surprise that the 'New Labour' leaders should have no sympathy for this clause but it was not expected that Blair would regard changing it as a priority. John Smith had rejected bothering with it, seeing reformulation as a divisive distraction, irrelevant to the priorities. Blair's view expressed during his leadership campaign was a deliberate obfuscation, planned at the time with Jack Straw, who was the leading public advocate of taking it on.[1]

Once elected, after much hesitation and consideration, his inclination was to press ahead with it in his major speech as new Leader to the 1994 conference. For the party it would be, as Blair told Gould, 'electric shock treatment'[2] in making a symbolic break with Labour's past. That would also reassure potential new allies and electoral supporters that the party had changed, making a major contribution to the struggle to win their trust. Much of the consultations within a small group at the Blairite core was taken up with 'should I or shouldn't I?' and 'if I do, how do I tackle the speech and handle the media?' questions. It was judged that John

Prescott needed to be persuaded about the change, and he became part of the consultations.

Blair's tour de force speech on the Tuesday afternoon was very effective; its 'no more ditching, no more dumping' emphasis seemed to be pointing in another direction for the delighted audience and it ended in highly skilled ambiguity about his intentions with no specific mention of the old clause. The last three pages of his speech were held back for fear that the news would leak and those hostile to the change might organise an adverse reaction, although interruption to the first speech of a new Leader had no precedent and was extremely unlikely, given that he had been backed by a huge and impressive victory across the party. They had to 'make sure'. At the end of the speech, the spin doctors moved in to explain to journalists what it meant. This was portrayed as a brilliant manoeuvre by Blair's media and party aides. That judgement was followed by others, including some potential critics, sharing the view that 'The lightning raid had paid off'.[3]

This was overgenerous. In Chapter 5 there was a description of considerable pressure put on party officials and the CAC, over the agenda, by the aggressive young communication staff in the Leader's office. It was backed up by the edict that 'Nothing gets through the conference unless Tony agrees it'. But Campbell, who had the key role managing tactics and presentation,[4] was focused on the latter. Tom Sawyer the future General Secretary was 'in the loop' over the proposal,[5] but Jon Cruddas from headquarters and Pat McFadden from the Leader's office, the two key conference managers then and in the years that followed, were not informed of the decision to 'go for it' until it was too late. So the CAC (also not previously informed of this move) simply applied the rules to the resolutions which had been submitted and accepted them. The costs of this extraordinary lack of foresight only became apparent when it was realised that the conference had before it a composite resolution No. 57 (of three resolutions and an amendment) supporting the old Clause IV. There was no alternative position, not even in the form of a stalling operation. In terms of conference management it was inept and not simply an 'accident of timing'.[6]

Despite heavy pressure to remit, the mover refused and on Thursday morning the Leader was defeated on this issue by 50.9 per cent to 49.1 per cent. Robin Cook was blamed by supporters of the Leader for his choice of speakers which produced five speakers for the composite but only three against. In future all this would be brought under concerted management control but it would not be the last time that media management complicated, even undermined, party management.

Looking to the future: unions as a base of support

In Blair's memoirs he described this support for the resolution as being passed 'at the insistence of the unions'.[7] 'Insistence' is misleading. Certainly there was some reaction in the unions against what was seen as 'a bounce' without consultation, and the natural response of delegations was to follow their mandates in favour of the clause. They were just going through the old democratic routines. Why was that unexpected? The whole exercise over Clause IV was later to be described as Blair's 'bold challenge to the unions'.[8] Again, in reality things were rather different. In the conference defeat of 1994, whereas the affiliated organisations had voted against the no-change resolution by 36.6 per cent to 33.3 per cent, the CLPs had voted in favour of it by 17.4 per cent to 12.5 per cent. Looking to the future and a re-run of the vote, the party activists in the CLPs seemed the basic source of opposition. Seeking overwhelming union support for a new clause, particularly the support of union leaders, seemed the route to future victory – a very old managerial story.

A large block of unions and their senior officials associated with the traditional right constituted a loyalist core at the conference. USDAW, led by Garfield Davies, could be reliably expected to help the leadership on all issues. Under Gavin Laird and Bill Jordan, then Ken Jackson, the AEEU was a loyalist-led union, closely linked to loyalist Labour First network. Alan Johnson of UCW had been the only union leader to speak out immediately in favour of changing Clause IV. The GMB led by John Edmonds had also come out in support. MSF under Roger Lyons was also likely to be very helpful. The managers' rule-of-thumb assessment looking to the 1995 party conference also included the GPMU, ISTC, RMT and TSSA as positives about the change.

The worry was that experience had shown that a momentum of decisions could be built up through the mandates of union conferences which would tie the union leaders into opposition at the party conference. In 1959, Gaitskell's proposal for a change in Clause IV had been halted in this way. How was that to be avoided now? The first managerial answer to the problem was to hold a special conference in the spring, prior to the conferences of the unions. Sympathetic union leaders signalled privately that this could be helpful in giving them more flexibility in how they responded to any draft. This has to be borne in mind when we come later to the huge row about union leaders not consulting their members.

NEC consultations and timetables

There had now to be a campaign in favour of the change. What form would it take? This also had not been a significant part of the pre-conference discussion. An important initiative from the linkage of Cruddas and McFadden backed by the new General Secretary Tom Sawyer proposed that there would be an extensive consultation of the party together with a programme of meetings. Blair accepted it although at one stage in headquarters the word was that he was hesitating. He had a more immediate problem in getting the change through an NEC where the overwhelming majority were not immediately enthused by the focus on Clause IV and there was also suspicion of Blair's tendency to 'bounce'. His proposed timetable provoked concern that the period of consultations would be followed by a very limited time for the party and the NEC itself to discuss the substance of the new clause. The partisan and anodyne questions in the draft consultation document were also an irritation. Because of all this, although support for the document advocating the change was overwhelming, at its November meeting the NEC refused to agree to the timetable and the consultation questions.

By December, with the backing of union leaders, the NEC agreed that the special conference would be moved back from 8 April 1995 to 29 April – still leaving only a month for discussion of the new clause. The questions had been improved, although not to everybody's satisfaction; the party was not to be asked whether it wanted to retain Clause IV. Most important, there was insistence at the NEC that they should have a special meeting on the new clause on 13 March, before another meeting two days later at which they would vote on it. With those changes, the NEC overwhelmingly agreed the document. Clare Short with Dianne Abbot and Dennis Skinner still favoured it going to the annual conference and giving more time for debate and decision within the party, but this was defeated by 20 votes to 3. The crucial feature remained, however, that when the wider party saw the new clause there would be no opportunity for it to be amended.

Targeting

The initial signs from the CLPs were not good. A significant number were already bound by mandates to preserve the old Clause IV, and the momentum seemed to be in that direction. The campaign to take the fight into the party was organised through Margaret McDonagh and the party machine but also through a leadership-instigated but formally independent 'New Clause IV Campaign' in south London. The campaign involved all avenues of communication, with Blair himself campaigning energetically and impressively at meetings of invited party members. What those meetings indicated was a confirmation of the findings of a Seyd-Whiteley survey that the blanket commitment to common ownership indicated by Clause IV no longer represented grassroots opinion.[9] As the consultation exercise was later to illustrate, there was a party consensus on the mixed economy.

With these indications, and conscious of 100,000 new members since 1994, Blair wanted the NEC to oblige CLPs to ballot all their members, but the NEC did not have the constitutional power to do so. What he could do was to get the NEC at the January meeting to agree to a recommendation that, 'to encourage the maximum involvement of party members, membership ballots should be held in every constituency'.[10] The consultation involved extensive political debate with Blair and Prescott, whose formulation of 'traditional values in a modern setting' was often quoted, addressing meetings all over the country. It was declared, justifiably, 'a huge success'.[11] The press agitation for ballots and the CLP receptivity to the principle led to overwhelming support for the procedural change, even in some of the CLPs where the General Committee had already taken a decision on Clause IV.

The new clause

As for management of the formulation of the draft of the new clause, it had a complicated gestation around the Leader's office with friendly sources encouraged to add to the pool of ideas but a small group of policy people involved in the first draft. The consultation of wider party opinion had no direct impact on the drafts, in part because its answers were predictable and guided by the questions. The formulation was never simply the pure expression of the party's aims and values. The drafts of the new clause were written and rewritten with a wary eye on the appeal to the target electoral audiences who were not (as yet) committed to, or reassured by, the 'New Labour' party. Blair's advisors differed in the degree to which this electoral objective should submerge other considerations, and it seems to have been from around this time that the notion emerged amongst some of them that there were, around the Leader, 'Labour Party people' and 'the others'. Producing the new clause became a delicate and protracted operation. Quite late on in the process, Blair decided that the draft which was emerging from his policy staff was not what was needed, and there appears to have been some loss of confidence in that operation. The task of drafting was then given to Derry Irvine, a long-time friend of the Leader. Blair himself then took over the draft which went to a meeting of the party officers group and then the NEC on 13 March.

It became one of the managing tactics of the next decade to undermine, and in the spin publicly downplay, the significance of the NEC under Blair. The important but hidden reality of its role in the policy battle over Clause IV was that as a result of meetings involving NEC representatives, which continued throughout the drafting period, not only were various small amendments made to the draft but so were some which were of great significance. Amongst the criticisms voiced in the NEC trade union group, when they saw the Blair draft marked 'DI' on 8 March, was a strong reaction against a weakening of the commitment to collective activity. A similar complaint was raised later at a meeting of Blair with Tom Sawyer the General Secretary and the Party officers Gordon Colling the Chair, Tom Burlison the Treasurer, and Diana Jeuda the Vice Chair, plus Richard Rosser, all of whom were members of the trade union group and all elected on the right-wing slate, held on the morning before the final NEC meeting. Rosser was its convenor. At this meeting it was argued strongly again, particularly by Jeuda and Rosser, that this was a defining principle of the party.

Though initially resistant (saying it had been in but had since been 'dropped'), Blair agreed to take it back for further discussion. With the assistance of Sally Morgan, who was responsible for the linkage to the NEC, when the final version came before the NEC it now contained the statement that the Labour Party 'believes that by the strength of our common endeavour we achieve more than we achieve alone'. This was eventually highlighted on every Labour Party membership card and was for years proudly displayed, as the central theme of New Labour's clause, in the foyer of the new party headquarters in Old Queen Street (later sold).

Blair was using it publicly within 24 hours of the NEC meeting, on BBC *Newsnight* on 13 March. Further, even more striking, 'achieving together what we cannot achieve alone' was given to the October 1995 Conference as one of Blair's prime reasons for him joining the Labour Party.[12] By 2003 he described this section of Clause IV as 'a fundamental restatement of ideology'.[13] Yet the fact remains that 'collective endeavour', the central message of the party, had been left out and then pushed back in under pressure from the NEC trade union group.

The night before the final NEC meeting authorised the draft, support for 'a dynamic economy serving the public interest in which the enterprise of the market and the rigour of competition are joined with the forces of partnership and co-operation' was more clearly differentiated from 'A dynamic market economy' which was proposed in the Leader's draft but judged by the NEC to carry more right-wing implications. By this, as Plant pointed out later, the market was placed in a moral framework.[14] However, the phrase 'the dynamic market economy' could easily fall into a short-hand managerial usage which lost that framework as it did in the 1997 business manifesto and the 1997 party manifesto.

Clause IV 2 and the party of business

Building a much better relationship with business was, as Brown explained later, one of the reasons why 'we rewrote our constitution'.[15] There was no question of portraying the power of the transnational corporations as a problem for democracy. This was raised in an input to discussions of the new draft but ignored even to the point of failing to seek a way to register that corporate interests were not necessarily the same as the public interest. Working with the corporations was working with the future. Working to control them might be regarded as Old Labour and unfriendly.

After the 1994 conference, Blair had been reminded that Clause IV involved not just a statement of values but a statement of sundry other 'objects' including a commitment to cooperate with the TUC or other 'kindred organisations'. Rewriting this was potentially of huge significance in terms of changing perceptions of the party's main allies and, in that way, helping to redefine its identity. Years later Blair announced that 'support for business' was 'a founding principle of New Labour'.[16] It might be thought, therefore, that the change in Clause IV was the opportunity to argue the case and validate the new relationship. Mandelson apparently thought so. Macintyre's study reported him making and failing in an attempt to prevent the singling out of 'the trade unions' as allies, preferring instead 'to co-operate with others, at home and abroad, who share our values'.[17] Blair aides later privately acknowledged that there was an attempt at this time also to push in a reference to working with the CBI. But over these there was an important step away by Blair.[18] With continuing anxiety over a possible defeat at the conference, and some uncertainties over what exactly was to be the new relationship with business, it was decided that it was better to secure a series of feasible tactical victories in the right direction. That was tactically wise, but much of the later problems of party management, and the sense of grievance and distrust about relations with business, followed from this lack of debate and authorisation of a development which was to be of central importance influencing party management.

Clause IV 2 and trade unions

Amongst NEC members, the 'DI' draft of this section was also considered inadequate in its reference to the trade unions and was still considered inadequate when it went to the final meeting of the NEC. Jack Straw, who had some extra prestige here as a pioneer of Clause IV reform, together with Clare Short pushed for a rewording, otherwise it was 'going to provoke trouble'. After a talk between Straw and Blair, the 'trade unions and co-operative societies' were now given first place over 'voluntary organisations, consumer groups and other representative bodies', and the former were now described as 'affiliated organisations', making the union link explicit.[19] The final version read, 'Labour will work in pursuit of these aims with trade unions, cooperative societies and other affiliated organisations, and also with voluntary organisations, consumer groups and other representative bodies.' This could not have been very welcome to the Mandelsonian school and it ran counter to general demotion of a special relationship with the unions. But the Straw-Short amendment was the version announced publicly and prominently displayed in the March/April edition of *Labour Party News*.

However, without any further meeting of the NEC, by the time the new clause was placed before the special conference on 29 April, the formulation had mysteriously changed both from the original version proposed to the NEC and the version agreed by the NEC. Although the unions retained primacy in the list of allies, the words 'and other affiliated organisations' had disappeared from the draft.[20] That now read, 'Labour will work in pursuit of these aims with trade unions, and cooperative societies and also with voluntary organisations, consumer groups and other representative bodies.' With all eyes on the main substance of Clause IV, nobody who knew of the background politics of the NEC seemed to have noticed the wording of the list of allies.[21] Given the understanding that, as the media indicated, it had all been 'settled', few would be looking for that kind of additional detail. That is how Clause IV was voted on, went through and remains in the rulebook to this day.[22]

In a further twist much later, the Straw-Short version reappeared in the NEC Report to the 1995 October Conference, even though the other version went into the rulebook. Perhaps it was simply a multiplicity of cock-ups, or even a cock-up within a conspiracy. Who knows? The suspicious observer, discovering it after years of studying the methods of party management under Blair, ponders whether this was an early important example of 'serious politics' and 'what works', and also further confirmation of the developing new attitude towards decisions of 'the party's ruling body'.

Contents and continuity

In the new clause the first statement of new aims and values was that Labour was a democratic socialist party. This had not been specified in the original clause but had long been widely regarded as its essence. Now it was more of an unserious genuflection. Acceptance of the document was, however, carried along by a range of consensual objectives not there in the previous version. They included 'a spirit of solidarity tolerance and respect': 'a just society which judges its strength by the condition of the weak as much as the strong': 'delivers people from the tyranny of poverty, prejudice and the abuse of power' with 'security against fear'. What later became characterised as a quintessential 'New Labour' emphasis on individual aspirations and ambitions was nowhere explicit although there was a consensual commitment to creating for each of us the means to realise our true potential.

There would be 'an open democracy' with 'fundamental human rights' and a new concern for 'a healthy environment'. The focus on 'a community where the rights we enjoy reflect the duties we owe' was integral to the new party appeal, but also consistent with Labour traditions of fraternity and mutuality. There were other important continuities with Labour's traditions. 'The party', it declared, aims to achieve 'a community in which power, wealth and opportunity are in the hands of the many and not the few'. This emphasis on Labour serving the many was implicit in the populistic elements of the programme of 1918, and of Clause IV (5) of the old constitution. It was in line with a long tradition of claiming Labour as 'the people's party'. Altogether, there was much here on offer to appeal to a party anxious to win an election and move forward to a better society.

Innovation

The great advance secured by Blair was that the continuities were now clearly divorced from the anti-capitalist prescriptions which traditional socialists had held to be central, and were instead linked with a market economy and a thriving private sector. The previous common-ownership commitment, traditionally interpreted as implying comprehensive public ownership, was replaced by a formulation that undertakings 'essential to the common good are either owned by the public or accountable to them', which was compatible with various institutional arrangements. In addition, the old labourist commitment to ensure that workers secured 'the full fruits of their industry' has been replaced by the objective of 'justice at work', and 'the opportunity for all to work and prosper'. These were much more flexible commitments. Also 'equitable distribution' had been replaced by 'equality of opportunity'.

Managing the special conference

The unions and ballots

In spite of the huge backing that NEC gave to the document – a vote of 21 to 3 with 5 abstentions, with all the trade union group voting in favour – astute party managers were all too aware that adding the opponents to the abstainers represented organisations with 40 per cent of the vote of the special conference. Major efforts were now made to get the unions to ballot their individual members. Here we come to a persistent problem for Blair and his managers. In a federal party in which the unions were auto-nomous, the party leadership had no right to formally prescribe a ballot for them, although the NEC's trade union review group had given the nod to expansion of party rights at the interface. In any case, this was very late in the day from a leadership which had, after the 1994 conference, made its first tactical focus the attempt to give union leaders freedom to make the decision without union commitment. It was not surprising that the Union of Communication Workers (UCW), led by Alan Johnson, the most prominent advocate of changing Clause IV, responded to the new appeal. Others retained their normal method of representative and delegate decision-making, in some cases supplemented by consultations.

In unions which voted for the victorious outcome it was often a judge-ment of priorities. As John Edmonds told the Party conference, 'It's no secret that the GMB would have written this clause differently but' (to Arthur Scargill who attempted unsuccessfully to move reference back) 'we are not prepared to make a self-indulgent gesture'.[23] It was helpful in secur-ing support that the consultation document replies made clear that there was a broad consensus in the party and the unions that there should be 'public ownership of essential services'.[24] This confirmed another Seyd and Whiteley finding, that the members' belief that a limited number of public utilities should be entirely within the public sector was still a touchstone issue.[25] Blair himself in his speech to the 1995 special conference emphasised 'why we fought off the privatisation of the Post Office' and 'why we will fight to keep our railways as a proper public service, publicly owned, publicly accountable to the people'.[26] This was what members thought that they were getting, and running sores were produced for years as 'New Labour' policy developed in other directions.

Just to make sure of the outcome, in the final voting there was no means by which any alternative to the new clause could be expressed. The ballot paper supplied by Head Office to constituencies who were balloting their members asked only about support for the NEC statement, which had come with an NEC explanation of why it was necessary to rewrite the clause. Faced only with the choice of accepting the new clause or rejecting it, there were good reasons to do so for a party – desperate to get rid of the Tories and impressed by what they saw of Blair – to give it a hopeful interpretation.

The outcome

The overall vote on the new clause was 65.23 per cent for with 34.77 against, with the CLPs overwhelmingly in favour, by 90 per cent to 10 per cent. In the end 441 out of 630 CLPs had balloted their members. All the ballots resulted in substantial support for the new clause. It is worthy of note that Millbank did not issue total figures of turnout but unchallenged information given to the *Tribune* political correspondent Hugh Macpherson was that only around 85,000 out of 320,000 members – less than a quarter of Labour members – participated,[27] perhaps reflecting the lack of choice.

At the special conference a majority of the union vote went in favour but the five major unions voted different ways. The AEEU, USDAW and the GMB voted in support of the new clause. Morris, not for the first time, had trouble with the TGWU Executive Council and failed in his attempt to persuade it to go with the change. Bickerstaffe, not himself a supporter of the change, also had the problem of UNISON being a newly amalgamated union and thought it should be left to the union which way it decided. An internal vote of union representatives went against Executive Committee opinion and against the new clause.[28] So two large unions, the TGWU and UNISON voted against.

A poll, which had 85 per cent support for the change amongst all union members,[29] was contrasted with the way that these two unions voted, and the fact that the UCW balloted and the new clause had been supported by a 9 to 1 majority was hurled at the two large dissentients. The spin crudely and robustly against 'the unions', was that 'Blair's rewrite had "seen off" the unions',[30] in spite of the majority vote of affiliated organisations (less than 1 per cent of which were not unions) going 54.6 per cent to 45.4 per cent in favour of the change.[31] For some this passed into history (or rather represented as) 'pulling the rug from under the trade unions',[32] and much later, in 2005, at a time of new pressure from No. 10 for reform of the union vote, an influential study of the unions said that they had opposed Clause IV reform.[33]

Aftermath: mismanaging the union problem

The battle to change the party

Having won overwhelming constituency party support over the new clause on an individual basis, the individual members were now seen in increasingly benevolent light. After giving one impressive performance after another to the responsive members, the Leader was reported as saying 'The Labour

Party is much nicer than it looks . . . full of basically rather decent and honest people'.[34] It was a comment which from any previous Leader of this party would have been regarded as astoundingly patronising. That aside, it was of course only human to feel good about people who agreed with you. The exercise had, as Blair claimed, been an opportunity for greater mutual understanding.[35] Out of the unity forged with the union majority in the battle over Clause IV there might have been created a new internal accommodation with new conventions and protocols assisting a more trusting relationship.

Yet on a wave of victorious euphoria, for the Leader and his allies there was a particular appeal in aggressively pushing union reform with an anti-union tone. All union activities, within or outside the party, industrially as well as politically, through the TUC or through other affiliated union organisations, were still seen in Blairite eyes as potentially damaging to the party's electoral chances as well as to the success of a 'New Labour' government. The public had to be assured of their subordination and 'an arm's length relationship'.[36] Spin doctors and outriders began aggressively and unrestrainedly driving forward the momentum for further change and new measures with the message that the Leader was stepping up 'war with the unions'.[37]

Stepping up the war

These attacks caused deep exasperation, especially from the unions who had voted with the Leader. On the left, from Livingstone this again aroused the reaction that they were 'trying to break from being a trade union-linked party'.[38] This regular reprise had some basis in reality; the Blair-linked Labour Coordinating Committee had produced a proposal that year for a non-federal party of individual members.[39]

At the height of the media onslaught, it suddenly became apparent in the Leader's office that the impact of this historic majority party decision over Clause IV, which had both union and CLP majority support, was now being lost. Out of the great victory the spin-manager had managed to create an image of a divided party with a 'union problem'. Campbell warned privately that they 'had to be careful that division and disarray did not become our main backdrop'.[40] He wanted Mandelson to stop doing his own thing.[41] There was a screeching halt of political brakes in the Leader's office.[42] What had happened, as the *Evening Standard* on 3 May 1995 described it with reference to Mandelson's role, was 'an inept piece of freelance spinning that went disastrously wrong'.[43]

Yet, as we now know, it was not simply Mandelson acting alone. According to Campbell, Blair was still defending 'Peter's line' on the grounds that it 'was forcing the unions to sue for peace'.[44] But it did nothing of the kind and was never likely to do so. This was not Blair at his most perceptive. The attack simply heightened union defensiveness and, from some, created further distrust. In that it added to the longer-term problems of the relationship, as it happened it also managed to create a further sense of grievance in the Brown camp over the way that the attack on the unions diminished the impact of Brown's launch, at that time, of his economic-policy statement.

Other features of this declaration of war raised questions about the management focus and priorities. The 'New Labour' leadership continued to regard these waves of hostility towards the unions as likely to contribute to popularity. Yet each year in Opposition under Blair, on the question of which party had the best policies on the trade unions, those naming Labour actually dropped – from 54 per cent in 1994 to 39 per cent in April 1997.[45] Meanwhile, around the time of the argument over Clause IV, the proportion of those in the working class who identified with Labour fell and continued to fall as the image of the party changed.[46] That may have had other contributing factors but the 'New Labour' mind was content with the changing electoral support and continued to prioritise its reassurance to business and its appeal to the middle class.

The new reform agenda

Party referendums

After the vote on Clause 1V, the first reform item to be dealt with was a strong one for Blair, the national power to call for a party referendum. In the rulebook in 1995, a new constitutional provision was enacted at the party conference giving the NEC 'the power to require constituency parties to hold ballots on such matters as they deem to be appropriate'. The ballot papers, timetable and procedures would also be as decided by the NEC.[47] From the NEC the conference was assured that the rule only involved consultative ballots and such ballots 'would have no right at all to amend the constitution or to overrule Conference and this is quite clearly not the intention'.[48] However, that was not what the rule said, and the intention was by no means so clear-cut.

Reforming NEC composition

Blair's intentions remained all-encompassing. It was to 'rebuild this party from its foundations'.[49] In the face of this aspiration the unions neither sued for peace nor waged outright opposition. Proposals for constitutional and organisational change were accepted as Blair's right and function as the Leader, though met with overall defensive unity against a fundamental attack but otherwise with a degree of flexibility and restraint. The restraint was reinforced by the old traditions of party solidarity and the old 'rules', including avoidance of sanctions, but it was also a restraint forced by the exigencies of their own political vulnerability and their desperate priority to see the election of a Labour Government. In practice on the details of reform, much as in 1992–3, there was a mix of positions, with different alignments depending on the issue.

On reform of the NEC, the sensible view of the trade union group was regarded as seeing it in broader terms. It should be considered in the round in the context of an examination of representation on the NEC. Party officials joined in an attempt by the Leaders' office to move forward this part of their agenda. At the 1995 conference, delegates had before them a composite resolution 63 calling for reform. But the party office recommendation to 'remit' was changed to 'oppose' by the NEC, and in the conference the resolution was overwhelmingly defeated with the unanimous vote of the unions.

Block vote: redistribution and abolition

The next part of the reform agenda was the huge and symbolic issue of the conference block vote. The 70:30 reapportionment of votes, proposed by the trade union review group and instituted for the 1993 Conference, was agreed to be the starting point for a phased series of changes to be reviewed when the CLP membership reached 300,000 and changes made until they reached 50:50 between CLPs and affiliated organisations.[50] This would leave the unions at fractionally below 50 per cent of the vote. The long-term decline in union membership and affiliation continued, but individual membership had risen substantially from 266,276 at the end of 1993 to 305,189 at the end of 1994, affected by publicity around the funeral of Smith, then the leadership campaign and the attractions of Blair as Leader. It was 400,465 by the end of 1996, and 405,235 by the end of 1997.

The membership increase encouraged those around the leadership, who were always anxious to keep the momentum going, to move fast to an immediate increase in the CLP vote to 50 per cent. But there was no unity of approach. Cruddas, the manager most involved with union liaison, continued to advocate privately only an incremental change. Various NEC representatives and senior politicians took the same view, focusing on the union role in ensuring stability. There was, therefore, an element of boldness to Blair's decision to push ahead, giving another huge hike in the vote of the CLPs. The victory in the CLPs over Clause IV, plus the new potentially plebiscitarian procedure now agreed by the NEC, reinforced a vision of how the Blair-led party might operate.

The unions for their part were, as indicated, prepared to forgo their preponderant position, but opinion was divided over when this should happen. Most had thought in term of gradual change, but almost all (the exception until 1997 being the AEEU) thought also in terms of absolutely no further move below 50 per cent for affiliated organisations. Eventually agreement was reached that there should be an immediate reduction in the affiliated organisations' vote to 50 per cent, which would become operative at the 1996 Conference. The new voting arrangements would, as agreed, have consequential changes at regional conference level and also have the effect of diminishing the trade unions' votes in relation to six places on the NEC – the women's section and the Treasurer. But there was still a disagreement over whether this was to be confirmed as 'a settlement' on the basis of partnership and power-sharing between the affiliated and individual membership (the review group position and now the overwhelming majority union view), or was to be regarded as a stage in a continuing evolution in which the union collective vote could be reduced much further.

What Blair wanted most at this point was an announcement that there was an agreement that the unions' vote could move further down at some future date. There was no such agreement. The union consensus was for 50:50 now and then leaving it for the foreseeable future. They would quietly live with what he said publicly but should there be any attempts to move the affiliated organisation vote to under 50 per cent they would oppose it. At the 1995 party conference the unions accepted the managerial sidelining of other options, but, speaking for the NEC, Dan Duffy (TGWU) described the equal weighting as 'just and right . . . to settle matters once and for all'.[51] The victoriously gung-ho Blair might have disturbed this by pushing for a further reduction of the union vote to 30 per cent the following year, but caution was urged successfully by Sally Morgan.[52]

This reform was heralded as 'the abolition' of the block vote. It could be taken to mean the end of union delegates all voting together according to their union mandates. Provision for individual voting in the union delegations had been provided in the constitutional changes in 1993. The new formulation of Clause 3 moved the emphasis on to hand voting rather than card voting. And for card votes after 1993 each delegate of an affiliated organisation cast an equal percentage of the organisation's vote. CLP votes were similarly divided if there were more than one delegate. In practice the unions generally (although in hand votes not exclusively) still cast their votes as collective units in accordance with their delegation meetings and union policy mandates. These arrangements had long been a source of concern to reformers of various kinds both within and outside of the unions.[53] But in an atmosphere of high distrust, on this it was felt on both sides that reform had gone as far as practicable and it had to be left to the unions to cast their votes as their traditions dictated. It was, however, accompanied by spin from the Leader's office via party candidates that there would be further reform of union representation.[54]

Sponsorship

Sponsoring of Labour candidates by trade unions predated the birth of the party and has always had its controversial aspects. A major political vulnerability was that sponsorship was often misunderstood and easily misrepresented as unions paying money into the pockets of MPs who could therefore be subject to improper pressure. But not for many years had unions been involved in this kind of payment. Indeed, in a period when observers were noting that it had become easier for MPs to accept payments from other organisations, the unions were phasing out the last remnants of financial arrangements.[55]

The sponsorship that remained was focused entirely on the organisational and election expenses of constituency parties. Within the Labour Party, these were regulated by the Hastings Agreement of 1933, which specified maximum amounts of such payments and was accompanied by a prohibition on the mention of finance in candidate selections. Unions were generally very circumspect in avoiding anything which suggested a contravention of parliamentary privilege in their relations with MPs, and aware of the need for some insulation between finance and policy-making. Although sponsored MPs were not the 'kept men' of legend,[56] the accusation of financial pressure remained easy to make. A second problem of sponsorship was that by its nature it tended to produce a maldistribution of union-party resources focused primarily on safe seats. Various ad hoc arrangements had been found by the party and the unions to ameliorate this maldistribution but a wider reform which might produce a general sponsorship fund which the party would administer was held back by the problem of dealing with union autonomy, insecurity and protection of their individual interests. The trade union review group had proposed various reforms to these arrangements, mainly to assist the party financially.[57]

The impending report of the Nolan committee, which had been set up by the Major government in a climate of growing public concern at MPs being involved in financial 'sleaze', led to union concern that it might take reform out of the hands of the party. Discussions between the party and union leaders led initially to a high-level agreement on an immediate change in procedure. An irony here was that, for various reasons, the union leaders were themselves not anxious to hold on to the idea of sponsorship. Not only did they want to end misrepresentation of their financial leverage over MPs, but some of the leaders, particularly in the GMB the TGWU and UNISON, agreed that the present arrangements were often a waste of money. This pointed to changing procedures quietly and consensually so that the finance went clearly and directly to the constituency party together with some agreed new redistributive mechanisms for allocating money in ways which better assisted the party.

Unfortunately, once the negotiations were under way they became bedevilled by the union-hostile and party-insensitive weekend spin that had been experienced from the Leader's office time after time before. For the wavering Tory voters and business it was again couched in aggressive terms that Blair was on the 'attack'[58] and 'set to axe trade union sponsorship'.[59] In both the GMB and the TGWU these further examples of being publicly 'pushed about' were made worse by what appeared to be the Leader apparently telling them through the press how they should spend the union members' money. The proposals also became once again mixed up with the issue of potential divorce. At an important meeting between Blair and the PLP trade union group on 11 July 1995, a few frank but not unreasonable comments by Blair changed the atmosphere. Labour was a party of government and had to relate to the social partners, but 'you can't have a partnership if the bias is to one of the partners'. Unfortunately again, this was backed up by the only MP present who supported separation, and it confirmed the worst fears that getting rid of sponsorship was part of another agenda of ending union affiliation to the Labour Party. It became another example of the regular reappearance of the distrust created by Blair and his allies in 1992.

Over this, there was not the adequate reassurance given to the NEC trade union group that there might once have been from the Leader or the General Secretary. Eventually, in line with the initial discussions and on an initiative from the unions, new arrangements for development plans, in which sponsorship would be ended and the money would go directly to designated constituency parties, gave the unions an arrangement they were perfectly happy with, but did not give the party the new pooling arrangements for marginal seats that it wanted. Later, in practice, the unions did provide more finance at regional level for organisation in the marginal seats, but this was at the unions' own discretion. After 1995 the TGWU became much more circumspect in its attitude towards paying money into the party (see Chapter 8, pp. 260–1). As for the effect on the union role in the party in the House of Commons, other forces at work changed the organisation of that relationship in such a way as to strengthen it (see Chapter 12, pp. 380–1, Chapter 14, pp. 443–5).

The Road to the Manifesto

The Road to the Manifesto ballot of 1996, for those close enough to observe the inner politics, was a bright illumination of Blair's leadership style and the problems of his management. Blair had always been attracted to the idea of a pre-election composite of policies which would be subject to a 'yes or no' response. Now there was to be a national ballot on a document which would be an early version of the manifesto. Discussions about this proposal had been going on privately around Blair since the previous December, but it says much about Blair's leadership that the General Secretary and senior party officials were not involved in these prior discussions and, by the time they found out in April 1996, the decision to go for a national ballot of party members on the document had been taken.

The aim was that the document would clearly show to the electorate that the party was a new political force united behind its leadership. It would generate a new relationship of trust with the electorate. Backed by the party, this would also add authority over potential dissidents. However, to those receiving the news of the proposal it suggested something else – the possibility of a new party policy-making structure, one based on direct quasi-presidential, plebiscitarian rule, circumventing the party activists and the authority of the party conference, producing not a party decision based on policy choices but simply an endorsement of what the Leader had already decided.

It also emerged that there was potentially another agenda. Blair's initial proposal of a ballot of *individual* members excluded the unions and the affiliated membership from participation. The union leaders could see immediately that this exercise could be, in some respects, a positive exercise but it could also start a hare running in the party about the inauguration of a new form of decision-making which would set off an angry reaction and a constitutional row. In any case it might well look bogus, and might result in a low turnout which would be damaging and, in any case, would be hugely expensive. As for their own role it might well herald an attempt to permanently reshape the party's institutions and procedures in ways which put them permanently outside the policy-making process. A precedent for the delegitimation of the trade union role in policy decisions, once established, might be used to ease the path towards full separation.

A new unity amongst the unions now got in the way of Blair's plans. The decline in sharpness of old Cold War political divisions between right and left in the unions and the suspicions surrounding the separationist spin led to an unusual new cross-factional current. A pan-union network had begun to operate across the political officers on issues of deep concern to the unions. Between 1995 when in the AEEU Ken Jackson became General Secretary and 1997, he and GPMU Leader Tony Dubbins began to mend fences broken during the Wapping industrial dispute. Jon Cruddas, performing the managerial role, managed to build a trusting entry into this network with his own independent voice which also became a voice for the unions around the Leader. This assisted in organising defence against attacks on the union position within the party, and the unified network later had a significant influence over developments in the PLP.

On the Road to the Manifesto it encouraged a mix of union cooperation and resistance, subtle but absolutely firm; they behaved as if it was taken for granted that they too would of course ballot all their own 3 million affiliated members. Told by Blair about the ballot, the GMB leader Edmonds said yes, certainly, he was in favour of balloting the union's members but overall 'it will cost about 1.5 million of our political fund resources which would otherwise be available to the party'. Margaret Prosser of the TGWU, shortly to become the convenor of the trade union group of the NEC, said something similar. Many other unions responded cooperatively in the same vein. Around the Leader this was not at all welcome, as the question then emerged: how could this be a symbol of unity if the unions were excluded against their will? No satisfactory answer was forthcoming. It appears not to have even been considered in the months of gestation of the 'good idea' before party officials were informed.

After some resistance and hesitation, the issue was left to further discussion with the Deputy Leader, John Prescott, to examine the practicalities of involving the affiliates. Meanwhile, the argument now turned to the procedure itself. Diana Jeuda had already proposed to the Leader that the concept of a ballot be replaced by that of a pledge. It was much more compatible with the idea of seeking 'endorsement' rather than making a choice. It was much more honest and would deflect criticism that it was a manipulative exercise. This suggestion was taken to the trade union group of the NEC at its meeting on 27 March 1996, and received enthusiastic agreement.

In anticipation of this proposal the NEC meeting which followed was faced with a motion phrased, ambiguously, in terms of 'a full ballot . . . to provide a firm pledge'. The proposal to shift entirely to a pledge appeared to be supported overwhelmingly by contributions or indications made at the NEC, including – as far as can be ascertained – all the senior politicians either speaking in favour or nodding their assent. Blair gave his own consistent nods of acknowledgement and this was taken to be his agreement. The motion was then carried by 22–2 with only Diane Abbott and Dennis Skinner opposing. Yet what followed was a classic 'New Labour' manoeuvre. The emphasis of the press release was on a ballot not a pledge. The next morning much of the media carried versions of the spin that the ballot would go over the heads of the activists, outflank the dissidents, and downgrade the trade union role.

The unions were first astounded then fierce, and in the next month there were a series of bilateral and joint meetings, privately reported in detail to those involved in the Party into Power steering group meetings (see Chapter 7, pp. 202–3). The reports described a politics confrontational to a remarkable degree even by the standards of the poor relationships at this time. At one point in the robust exchanges, Blair is said to have acknowledged, 'you don't trust me and I don't trust you'. This was in an exercise designed to show the electorate that it could trust the new party and to show just what a united party 'New Labour' was. Blair, highly skilled at deflection, also at one point counter-attacked vigorously over the inadequacies of the unions' own policy-making procedures. Officials there report him as saying 'I want you to stay but I want you to reform'. Much later, in one private meeting with a senior member of the NEC, Blair admitted that he did bounce the NEC but said frankly 'I did not know any other way'. All this was the source of near despair amongst members of the NEC and in the union leadership. How could you deal with him? How do we build trust?

The extent of the alienation in the unions, and the increasing ferocity of the antagonism, threatened to spread into protracted public conflict overshadowing the launch of the document. Slowly, with assistance from Prescott, the reconciling voices around Blair began to hold a greater sway. Accommodations began to be made through a new linkage of Cruddas, Morgan and Joe Irvine, John Prescott's Special Adviser. The story from Blair's office began to be that it had been an error; he had failed to tell them not to spin it. At a meeting with the trade union group before the April NEC meeting, Blair let it be known that he had found out who had done the spinning and had a word with them. Later, on 2 July 1996, Blair agreed that the spinners' description of the NEC meeting in March had been inaccurate.[60] It was the first time that he had admitted that the spinners had got it wrong, but there remained some deep disbelief over his explanation of an 'error'. 'Been there before and got the T-shirt', as one senior NEC member commented later.

It was now agreed that the unions would ballot their political-levy payers. The Road to the Manifesto would emerge on the basis of four major policy documents drawn up by the Leader's office and by key members of the Shadow Cabinet. At the April meeting of the NEC a statement from the General Secretary confirmed that the unions and the whole party would participate in extensive debate and consultation in a policy-making process which would include the national policy forum. A draft Road to the Manifesto would then, it was promised, come to a final meeting of the NEC, thus further integrating it with normal party procedures, and be taken for authorisation by the party conference.

Following this process the draft document was discussed by a special national policy forum but was unamendable. It then went through a heavily controlled policy process (covered in Chapter 9, see pp. 276–8). On 2 July, at the NEC meeting, suggestions but not amendments were acceptable. An attempt by CWU Leader Alan Johnson to change the qualifying period for unfair dismissal failed to gain insertion. On 4 September the document was launched as *New Labour, New Life for Britain*. At the October party conference, the process around the document was agreed. No amendments were accepted and, without announcement, the document itself was not taken to a vote. This might have been used as a precedent for procedural change, but the following year, Partnership in Power arrangements further integrated the role of the conference in policy-making. Immediately following the party conference, members received a short summary of the document, with a letter from Tony Blair urging a 'Yes' vote, and a yes/no response paper. Although the summary of the document was free, the full document itself had to be purchased. It is understood that not many people did. Necessarily the summary was not just a shortened but a selective version.

Getting out the vote

The unhappy and problematic gestation was not the end of the difficulties. There was an immediate problem of how to ensure a turnout which was at least respectable. The anticipation was that the return of ballot papers would be highest in the first and last phases. But the initial turnout figures (which were made available to the organisers) were very disappointing. There was a fear that the final result would not top 50 per cent. It seemed to be difficult to get enthusiastic about an exercise with no alternatives and no sense of any conflict. One regional party official said later without irony that 'What we really needed was a good row'. Such are the difficulties of heavily controlled plebiscites. Gould, a leading proponent in initiating the

Road to the Manifesto, noted later that 'without conflict . . . people are simply not convinced'.[61]

There was a problem also for the hard-pressed but eager party organisation. The machine had been geared up to multiple priorities agreed by the General Secretary and the NEC at the beginning of the year. Nobody around the Leader appears to have thought over what might be involved for the party organisation in abruptly adjusting activities and the priorities to a task of this scale in getting out the vote. There was from the beginning some irritated scepticism about the whole Road to the Manifesto enterprise and a reluctance to sacrifice too much time. With Margaret McDonagh in national charge, the exercise was enthusiastically driven and as far as possible dovetailed into the key seats strategy in getting those constituencies to raise the turnout.

Responsibility for the field work was given not to a team around the General Secretary or the Director of Organisation Peter Coleman, but to a team around the Membership Development Officer Phil Wilson. To Wilson it was an opportunity to further develop a new grassroots 'New Labour' organisation in each constituency, thus rooting the Blairite agenda much more firmly in the party where all constituency parties and branches had been asked to appoint Road to the Manifesto coordinators. In a process which had much in common with the normal election work there was canvassing, marking cards and 'knocking up' and then marking the cards again. Greater pressure was also put on the politicians, including the most senior, to get involved in the work of encouraging the CLPs to get out the vote in favour.

Facing the immediate evidence of low turnout there were some panicky responses. In addition to regular membership mailings, there was an expanded role for telephone canvassing by a private company and also by the party in the regions and occasionally headquarters.[62] Videos were produced. Sponsorship was encouraged. Freephone facilities were offered to the members with a message from John Prescott (paid for by the *New Statesman*) urging recipients to vote. In the end, 'We threw money at it', was the majority description amongst the key managers. All of this depleted resources which might have been spent elsewhere The total cost including to the unions was estimated to be probably over two and a quarter million pounds. Ten of the unions did eventually drop out of the exercise because of shortage of finance or because, as the ISTC put it, 'spending 45p per member on a public relations exercise was . . . a waste of resources and a diversion from the campaign'.[63] Still, the problem of turnout seemed to remain.

The result, 5 November 1996

And yet, in terms of the final turnout, the ballot result was a considerable success – a very surprising, even puzzling outcome, measured against the estimates and fears of the managers. The CLP turnout was said to be

61 per cent, amazingly, much higher than in the Clause IV vote. Less surprising given the absence of choice was that 95 per cent of those voting voted 'yes'. The turnout in the much larger ballot of affiliated organisations was as expected much smaller. In the affiliated organisations including the 15 unions, there was a 92.2 per cent yes vote on a 24.2 per cent turnout, which was near to what was expected.

Significance

A pragmatic organisational view about the significance of this exercise was that the document had clarified the details and contours of policy and through the media reinforced some important messages on problematic issues. But the attempt to sideline the unions had failed; the impact on Labour's policy-making procedures was marginal and left the constitutional position intact. The 95 per cent vote of individual members and the 92.2 per cent vote of affiliated members did provide a useful symbolic expression of party unity behind the manifesto which, it was thought, could be used as a means of reinforcing discipline – but as far as can be judged, did not.

The process, as said by Blair, would 'breathe new life and new hope into our politics'.[64] Yet across the media the exercise met another reaction – that it resembled a very old and dangerous form of political life. 'Is it a joke?' asked the interviewer Andrew Rawnsley, 'Vote either yes or yes?', reminding viewers of the disreputable historic figures who were keen on referenda.[65] John Pilger likened it to 'the sort of black joke that juntas play on nations'.[66] As for the new political life breathed into the party, in September it was agreed by the NEC on a steer from the Leader's office that all deliberation of new policies and resolution submission should cease in the party.[67] This was in anticipation of an election the following summer. Yet new policies continued to emerge from around the Leader.

Perhaps the most significant reaction actually came privately from the central managers themselves. They had been proud of their role in the change to Clause IV. But this one was an embarrassing episode for many of them – something they were always a little bit uncomfortable about, passed off with a mutter and a shrug or a weak smile. What came over from most of them afterwards was a sense that it was too much of a manipulative fix and lacking in public legitimacy. It was described variously as 'just a PR exercise', 'not an exercise in democracy', 'a fake', and even (pause for thought here from a leading figure) 'a bit iffy'.

Although after 1997 in the New Labour government there was a regular discussion about direct communication with the citizen,[68] and the government authorised public referenda for a variety of constitutional purposes, effectively by the end of 1996 such a referendum was never again used within the Labour Party itself. It was not recommended in the Partnership in Power document for the 2001 election. Blair was later reported by a close aide as admitting that it was 'just a gimmick'. One thing was made clear privately but emphatically. Most of the managers who had to do the work did not want to do it again – ever. It also brought home to the managers and to the future ministers that they had additional enormous potential practical problems on their hands in holding ballots on major policy issues in government, as Mandelson and Liddle had advocated.[69] How much time would it take up? When would the ministers govern? Would many people want to take part? How would the party look united?

There was something else to be derived from sudden acute awareness of these questions. That few of the potential downsides to this whole Road to the Manifesto venture appeared to have been evaluated and confronted in the months of management planning suggested something significant about the change-focused Bolshevik culture of 'New Labour', also showing in other aspects of changing fundamentals and laying new foundations. There was a tendency to focus on the immediate benefit, especially the impact of bold announcements and initiatives, and to underestimate or even not consider the accompanying costs and problematical consequences. It was an insight into the insensitivity of Blair and many, but not all, of his advisers, to collateral and consequential damage produced by their way of conducting politics.

Notes

1 Interview with Jack Straw.
2 Philip Gould, *The Unfinished Revolution: How the Modernisers saved the Labour Party*, Little Brown, London, 1998, p. 218.
3 Paul Routledge, *Gordon Brown: The Biography*, Simon & Schuster, London, 1998, p. 218.
4 Peter Mandelson, *The Third Man: Life at the Heart of New Labour*, Harper, London, 2010, p. 184.
5 Alastair Campbell and Richard Stott (eds), *The Blair Years: Extracts from the Alastair Campbell Diaries*, Hutchinson, London, 2007, entry 3 October 1994, p. 18.
6 Peter Riddell, *The Unfulfilled Prime Minister: Tony Blair's quest for a legacy*, Politico's, London, 2005, p. 27.
7 Tony Blair, *A Journey*, Hutchinson, London, 2010, p. 85.
8 Stanley B. Greenberg, *Dispatches from the War Room: In the Trenches with Five Extraordinary Leaders*, Thomas Dunne, New York, 2009, p. 186.
9 Patrick Seyd and Paul Whiteley, 'Red in Tooth and Clause', *New Statesman and Society*, 9 December 1994.
10 NEC Minutes, 25 January 1995, 49(ii), p. 6.
11 About 8,500 responses came in: 6,500 from individual members, over 1,400 from party branches, over 200 from CLPs, and over 20 from affiliated organisations, LPCR 1995, p. 287.
12 LPCR 1995, p. 96.
13 LPCR 2003, p. 98.
14 Raymond Plant, *Guardian*, 20 March 1995, cited in Steven Fielding, *The Labour Party: Continuity and Change in the Making of 'New Labour'*, Palgrave Macmillan, Basingstoke, 2003, p. 78.

15 Introduction, Labour's Business Manifesto, *Equipping Britain for the Future*, April 1997.
16 *Daily Telegraph*, 16 November 2001.
17 Donald Macintyre, *Mandelson: the Biography*, HarperCollins, London 1999, p. 277.
18 Mandelson, *Third Man*, p. 185.
19 NEC Minutes 13 March 1995, amended version of draft statement of aims and values (GS: 19/3/95), p. 3, and telephone interview with Clare Short, March 1995.
20 Conference Arrangements Committee Report, Labour Party Special Conference, 1995.
21 I knew about the amendment at the NEC, yet for years I misread the wording of the clause that was submitted to the Special Conference. When I did notice this about 2002, I asked discreet questions of different people who might know, but got various versions of 'Really? Ha! No idea . . .' or blank stares. Both Short and Straw said that they had genuinely forgotten all of it by this stage.
22 Labour Party Rulebook, 2005, Clause IV – Aims and Values 4.
23 LPCR 1995, p. 292.
24 Labour's Aims and Values: the consultation report, 1995, p. 1.
25 *New Statesman and Society*, 9 December 1994.
26 LPCR, Special Conference 1995, p. 290.
27 *Tribune*, 12 May 1995.
28 John McIlroy, 'The Enduring Alliance? Trade Unions and the Making of New Labour, 1994–1997', *British Journal of Industrial Relations*, 36(4), 1998, p. 552.
29 Leo Panitch and Colin Leys, *The End of Parliamentary Socialism: From New Left to New Labour*, Verso, London, 1997, citing MORI, fn 42, pp. 322–3.
30 *Guardian*, 10 June 1995.
31 Derived from figures presented in the Labour Party special conference report 1995, p. 307 and confirmed by a senior manager.
32 David Mitchie, *The Invisible Persuaders*, Bantam Press, London, 1998, p. 292.
33 David Coates, pamphlet *Raising Lazarus*, Fabian Society, 2005, p. 29.
34 John Rentoul, *Tony Blair: Prime Minister*, Little Brown, London, 2001, p. 262, quoting from the *Guardian*, 1 May 1995.
35 Tony Blair, speaking on BBC *Newsnight*, 13 March 1995.
36 Peter Mandelson and Roger Liddle, *The Blair Revolution: Can New Labour Deliver?*, Faber & Faber, London, 1996, p. 227.
37 *London Evening Standard*, 1 May 1995.
38 Ibid.
39 Labour Coordinating Committee pamphlet 'New Labour: a Stakeholder's Party', 1995.
40 Alastair Campbell and Bill Hagerty (eds) *Alastair Campbell Diaries*, Vol 1, *Prelude to Power*, Hutchinson, London, 2010, entry 1 May 1995, p. 191.
41 Ibid., 2 May, p. 192.
42 Interview with Clare Short who had been in discussions with Blair at the time.
43 *Evening Standard*, 3 May 1995.
44 Campbell and Hagerty, *Campbell Diaries, Prelude to Power*, entry 2 May 1995, p. 192.
45 MORI, Poll archives, August 1995.

46 John Curtice and Stephen Fisher, 'The power to persuade; a tale of two Prime Ministers', in Alison Park et al., *British Social Attitudes 2003–2004: Continuity and Change over Two Decades – The 20th Report*. Sage Publications, 2004, p. 241.

47 Rulebook 1995, Chapter 1, Clause VIII 3(j).

48 David Ward (NEC), LPCR 1995, p. 64.

49 *Guardian*, 6 July 1995.

50 Final Report of the Trade Union Review Group, 1993, p. 26.

51 My notes.

52 Campbell and Hagerty, *Campbell Diaries, Prelude to Power*, entry 4 March 1996, p. 390.

53 Minkin, *Contentious Alliance*, 1991, pp. 364–86.

54 *Independent*, 30 September 1995.

55 Minkin, *Contentious Alliance*, p. 242.

56 Ibid.

57 Final Report of the Trade Union Review Group, 1993, p. 19.

58 *Observer*, 11 June 1995.

59 *The Sunday Times*, 11 June 1995.

60 This is derived from various sources including party officials and members of the NEC and intensive discussions on the steering group of the Party into Power project. In Campbell and Hagerty, *Campbell Diaries, Prelude to Power*, March 28, p. 406, Campbell wrote that 'we hadn't pushed it in that direction'. What the 'it' was, and who the 'we' were, made for a very interesting disassociation, but was not clarified.

61 Gould, *Unfinished Revolution*, p. 263.

62 Seyd, '*New Parties, New Politics?*', Note 7, p. 402.

63 General Secretary's Report, NEC Minutes, 31 July 1996.

64 Press release, 29 March 1996.

65 *A Week in Politics*, ITV, 30 March 1996.

66 *New Statesman and Society*, 25 October 1996.

67 NEC Minutes, 1 September 1996 and 30 October 1996.

68 Bob Franklin, 'The Hand of History: New Labour, News Management and Governance', in Andrew Chadwick and Richard Heffernan (eds), *New Labour Reader*, Polity, Cambridge, 2003, pp. 307–8.

69 Mandelson and Liddle, *Blair Revolution*, p. 229.

7

Creating 'the Party into Power' project

Problems and potentiality

From 1994 to 1997, although the attention of Blair, his colleagues, advisers and party officials was heavily focused on winning the election, there was also a continuous private management dialogue on the kind of problems a 'New Labour' government could be expected to face. This was inevitably mixed with reflection on previous experiences of Labour in government. Their determination not to 'go back there' focused on unrealistic expectations and oppositional instincts in the CLPs, and the possibility of a shift to the left and a new militancy in the unions, all becoming enmeshed in the assertiveness of an NEC led by PLP dissidents. Blair worried also over the potential gap which might emerge between the party and the government, reflected in critical resolutions at the party conference and possibly open confrontation. All this would be a gift for a hostile media and the party's opponents.

The move towards a new more cooperative arrangement between party and government, which had already been supported in principle by the 1990 conference, gained much of its support in acknowledgement of the inadequacy of the existing party policy-making process. The development of the new National Policy Forum had, in experimental form, offered a practical example of another kind of process and politics, whilst not precluding constituency parties and affiliated organisations from putting down resolutions to the party conference as in the past. So the momentum was already under way for a change in the way that the party operated which might blend into major new arrangements for government.

Cranfield and a new approach to change

Urged forward by Blair, the decision was taken to move into detailed discussions of future relations and arrangements. After consultations with John Monks who had been carrying through a cultural and structural re-launch of the TUC, Sawyer made the first adroit move at the NEC in July 1995. The perspective was that, 'Changes in culture require us to examine critically our ways of working, our relationships, institutions and communication and then to modify them effectively as required'.[1] Under the supervision of a specialist in organisational culture, Gerry Johnson from the Cranfield School of Management, a methodology was introduced which contrasted the operation of the existing party with that of the organisation which NEC members would prefer to see; discussions explored how the possible ways of working, relating and behaving together might be different after effective change. Out of this came a recommendation that the NEC set up a project which would be called 'Labour into Power'.

The focus on the party and how it might be changed was natural, but in this context was one-dimensional. The questions not being directly addressed were of how the leadership could learn from past experience at that level and how it might change its present behaviour to accommodate a new relationship. At this stage the plebiscitarian model of the strong Leader had some very enthusiastic Blairite radical adherents, reflected in the Road to the Manifesto plans. The day that the discussions began at Cranfield, there had appeared in the *Guardian* an article by Michael White headed 'Blair shuns MPs and party chiefs in policy group' which announced that Tony Blair had set up 'a secret committee of trusted moderates led by Peter Mandelson' to examine policy changes before the next election.[2] It was said to exclude Brown, Cook, Prescott and the then Policy Director Roland Wales.

Two days later, in a letter published in the *Guardian*, the article was rejected by the Leader's office as 'absurd',[3] but it had done nothing to assist the General Secretary in building trust for the objective of 'strengthening of new relationships'. There were even suspicions that the announcement of a secret committee was an attempt at sabotage. Was this another example of the two voices of Tony? If the Mandelson committee was active, what was the point of the Cranfield meeting? At Cranfield also there was a clumsy late-night attack on trade union membership of the NEC from Jonathan Powell, the new and, on this, hawkish chief of staff of the Leader's office. That fed another flank of suspicions already re-aroused over the Road to the Manifesto that this review might turn out to be yet another thin end of a wedge of planned union–party separation.

The process

The project and the Task Forces

The discussion and thinking behind the Party into Power project were reported to the NEC on 31 January 1996 and authorised there with only one person, Dennis Skinner, voting against. Four Task Forces of NEC members had been agreed at Cranfield on a proposal by the General Secretary and these also were authorised to begin work: Task Force 1 The NEC at Work, led by Maggie Jones from UNISON, Task Force 2 Relationships in Power, led by front-bench MP Mo Mowlem, Task Force 3 Strengthening Democracy, led by Margaret Wall from MSF, and Task Force

4 Building a Healthy Party, which would be carried out by an existing regeneration task force led by Diana Jeuda.

Together, the task forces involved only 16 members of the NEC, and attendance by members of the NEC at Party into Power project meetings was low, as were NEC attendances and morale generally in this period following two years of Blair's policy ascendancy. Apart from Mo Mowlem, there was no direct regular input from the senior front bench. Formally, to coordinate the general process there was to be a quarterly meeting of a committee of chairs of the NEC, receiving a report of task-force activities. With so many general election preparations under way, no promises could be made of much staff involvement, but two facilitators/advisers were appointed, Bob Fryer who was the head of Northern College – a specialist on trade unionism and organisation management – and Lewis Minkin.*

The steering group

In practice, much of the initial drive and detailed work came through an informal steering group of five people called together by the General Secretary. The political composition of the group was predominantly soft left with no Mandelsonian influence. That was surprising at this stage of Blair's ascendancy and was in part a reflection of old alliances and personal friendships. Diana Jeuda, who was the Chair of the NEC and Party Chair that year, chaired these meetings. Jon Cruddas, Head of the General Secretary's office (and after the General Election, Deputy Political Secretary in the 10 Downing Street Political Unit) became General Project Coordinator. Fryer and Minkin were also members of the group. Sawyer was comfortable with this composition as by late 1995 he was more 'on the outside' in relation to Downing Street decision-making and attempting to rebuild his own links with the soft left. It also reflected his attitude towards policy-making at that time. All taking part, including Sawyer, could be described at this stage as inclined towards a cooperative, pluralist, inclusive relationship through a process marked by dialogue and mutual education.

At the first steering group meeting, held in a room at the TUC on 19 March 1996, the General Secretary's suggestion was that 'occasionally' the five in the steering group would later be expanded to eight, adding three of the chairs of the task forces Maggie Jones, Mo Mowlem and

---

* These were initially reported to the NEC as 'facilitators' although this was never conveyed to me or the Convenors' Group where we became 'advisors'. In practice, we played different self-allotted roles and, as divisions opened up in the group, followed different political alignments. Bob Fryer defined his role mainly as 'technical' adviser involving some administration and organisational advice and document drafting. I defined my role as a political advisor, proposing and commenting consistent with the original approach of the steering group and my papers on partnership in July 1996.

Margaret Wall. That change with implications for the political composition did later take place, to what became called the convenors' group. Others, including Sally Morgan from the Leader's office and Joe Irvine, adviser to John Prescott, also attended the most important meetings. Although a degree of creative discretion was left to those working on the project, the Leader's priorities were conveyed from his office through the party officials and some of the task-force chairs. Bob Fryer, a skilled writer, was given the job of drafting a document. That responded to Sawyer's direction and drew from and fed back into the views of the task forces and the steering/convenors' group.

Problems and purposes

The atmosphere on the steering group, as this exercise commenced, was cooperative and positive, particularly as the focus on the regeneration of the party was one to which those involved gave a high priority. The General Secretary secured general agreement on 'the necessity for the Cabinet/Shadow Cabinet to take the NEC and the Party seriously and develop proper mutual relationships'.[4] It was agreed that there should be a cultural change, particularly in ways of working, relating and behaving together.[5] That ambition received a troubling rebuff in March of 1996 when the plebiscitarian proposals for the Road to the Manifesto analysed in Chapter 6 (see pp. 00–00) suddenly emerged without consultation with the General Secretary or anybody else closely involved in the Party into Power discussions, and that was seen as working to a different model of politics and power.

Partnership and sharing

However, by the early summer of 1996, there was a broad agreement that although the prime responsibility of a Labour government was to the people and parliament, it also had responsibilities to the party. Representation through both party democracy and parliamentary democracy must be safeguarded whilst recognising the different functions of party and government. The form of the National Policy Forum strengthened the case for building a new politics of dialogue and mutual education, and engendered some enthusiasm about the party responding to the creative possibilities of sharing in the process of policy formulation. The mood in the party already expressed a desire for cooperation with a successful Labour government after so many years in Opposition. Out of this discussion in the steering group and the task forces came a move towards the idea of a 'partnership' – a concept which had been part of the proposals in 1990.

Minkin's view, put forward in papers to the steering group, was that there was a new basis for a cooperative relationship in support of the much-desired Labour government, but it should be a two-way relationship.

This involved the need for the party 'to strengthen the breadth of the discourse around Ministers', and warned that 'a Labour Government cannot afford to show persistent disrespect for (party) support without adverse consequences'. It criticised the gap between the rhetoric of democracy and the present realities of centralisation of power.[6] The analysis was welcomed by Mowlem, but drew her pessimistic initial response that 'If you talk to Tony about a partnership he will tell you to fuck off. He will say what can you do for me?'[7]

The cautious development of the draft document was influenced by Mowlem's alert, and tended to become dominated by a homogenous view of the party's oppositional culture as the source of major problems. This, in turn, was contested by those who saw the Bennite period as unrepresentative of either the loyalist history of the NEC or its current attitudes and as failing to consider the special circumstances of the late 1970s. New arrangements, it was agreed, would emphasise the different responsibilities of the government and party and that the NEC should not aim to operate as a shadow or watchdog of Labour in power. As was pointed out, the Labour culture has always had strong loyalist traditions with elements of realism, governmentalism and partnership encouraged through the experience of trade union leadership and local government.[8] In present circumstances of the overwhelming desire for a new Labour government, much could be built in terms of partnership, without one partner substituting itself for the other.[9]

However, those involved could never fully explore in the formal processes of the steering group the question of what kind of leadership culture, as opposed to what kind of party culture, was needed to make a new relationship work. It would seem to be opening up the old critical confrontation. As the General Secretary warned, the project had to aim at the best that could be done which avoided the Leader going his own way. With that objective, the Party into Power discussion was not just about establishing new attitudes, procedures and process but also about keeping an eye on whether Tony would 'buy into it'. Jones from UNISON, an influential loyalist, put the sophisticated case that Blair would find acceptable the argument that this would relieve him of some of the (managerial) burden so that he could do other things.

Given the new awareness of the problems of the plebiscitarian option (and its discrediting amongst the managers noted in Chapter 6) and the persuasiveness of the case made to Blair for avoiding past problems, the key managers moved closer together in support of partnership. Morgan, Mowlem, Sawyer and also Blair's agent John Burton began to influence the Leader in these terms. The Leader's confidence never wavered that he was the best person to take decisions but the idea of 'a partnership' had some very appealing features to a politician who was attracted to the self-image of persuasive leadership, providing there were adequate mechanisms of management control. That proviso was always part of the private reassurance given to him, although not openly shared at the time with all the Party into Power participants. His role and how it was protected became a pathology in deep tension with a spirit of a partnership which might generate sustained enthusiasm and trust.

The cross-pressures and the process

Partnership and consensus

Even though some different views on the practicalities opened up on the steering group, there appeared at this stage to be a unifying openness about the conduct of the process and general agreement on its new partnership purposes which came out in several ways. There was overwhelming support for the general process of a rolling programme which would be reviewed annually over a three-year period. Each major policy statement on a different policy area would take two years in preparation and deliberation. The first year would be consultative; the second would be decisional.

The most attractive new policy-making feature for the party in the evolution of the draft policy-making document, eventually titled *Labour into Power: a Framework for Partnership*, was its openness to the party's input within a shared process. It was envisaged that there would be a first-year process which was sensitive to a broad range of opinion. The documents from the policy commissions 'would include options, alternatives, minority positions and so on, as necessary',[10] and the NPF would then also be free to add 'comments, ideas, proposals, options, etc'.[11] The NEC would publish the final document 'including all options, alternatives, and minority proposals as a consultation paper' and it would then be discussed and voted on at the conference.[12] In the second year, when the final decisions were made at the conference, these documents would also include 'any necessary options, alternatives or minority reports'[13] which would be voted on. There were technical issues raised here about the organisation of the process but at this stage no challenge was made to it.

Within the model some conflicts were inevitable, but it was thought it should be possible with the appropriate cultural changes to deal with them in ways which were a major improvement on the past. This would be 'based on acceptance of the clear and different functions of Government and Party, whilst seeking the highest possible level of cooperation between them'.[14] In integrating the various inputs, the Joint Policy Committee would discuss, adjust and harmonise, and where necessary would add 'comments or proposals of its own'.[15] In the policy commissions there would be a regular dialogue between the party and the government not only on the rolling programme but on issues as they arose.[16] It was also agreed that there had to be a strategy to minimise or avoid conflict by prior confidential advance consultations and communications. Easing the harmony within a culture of partnership would involve a new close coordination between party officials and political advisors to government ministers.[17]

Partnership turns to subordination

This mood of apparent consensus on purpose in the steering-group discussions was reinforced by awareness of leadership approval of a similar cooperative sharing in proposals for the future PLP-government relations (see Chapter 13, pp. 416–17). The consensus appeared to be consolidated on 11 July 1996 at an enthusiastic away-day. But the following day, a shock was caused by an interview with Tom Sawyer in the *New Statesman* which began by saying that, 'The former Trade Unionist and Bennite plans to create a new party structure under a Labour government which makes loyalty to the leadership paramount and discourages dissent'. In the whole article there was only one mention of partnership. There was, reported interviewer Steve Richards, 'no attempt to disguise the purpose behind the reforms'.[18]

This was accepted by some loyalists close to Sawyer as a necessary part of the 'reassuring Tony' agenda but it caused consternation amongst others. At the NEC meeting there were contradictory signals. Responding to Blair's emphasis on listening to the party, optimists did feel that he was 'buying in to it'. But Blair also complimented Sawyer on his article and said that it did reflect his own views. It was not surprising that the atmosphere around the NEC chairs meeting from this point was described by one of Blair's aides as 'grudging and negative', nor that the cooperative unity within the Party into Power discussions should give way to a developing split. These tensions have to be seen in terms of key issues which dominated the steering group discussions for the next five months.

Key issues

Partnership and its obligations

The general agreement about partnership on the steering group was that it involved the benefits of mutual obligations. The draft document and subsequent versions said that 'Successful partnership will be based on mutual support and effective two way communications, providing opportunities for consultation and discussion and constituting a valuable means of mobilising wider support for Labour amongst the electorate at large'.[19] That mutual support included alleviating the pressures on government ministers who had a range of practical difficulties in working with the party and enough trouble fighting with the Opposition. A remarkably frank and effective intervention by Mo Mowlem at this time appealed for a supportive party behind new ministers 'who will be feeling fear and panic'.[20]

The document declared the obligation of the leadership to be 'to take the NEC and the Party seriously and to develop proper mutual relationships based on trust'.[21] There was a warning that a partnership should be based on 'acceptance of the clear and different functions of Government and Party'.[22] Yet there was always another view which saw the dominance of the government as both inevitable and desirable, and that later became reflected in the document in a way which proved more important than appeared to be the case. Following a statement of joint responsibility, it was asserted that 'Once in power, a Labour Prime Minister should take a leading role' in defining 'the main parameters of the partnership and agree its principal forms and practical manifestations'.[23] The view that his leading role would be the dominant role was an operative assumption of the key party managers and it was a fair representation of much of what was to happen in practice.

Partnership and Institutions: NEC and JPC

It was agreed that when Labour was in government it was 'essential that the NEC worked closely with the Cabinet in Party policy formulation'. A new Joint Policy Committee of party and government would be established which would be drawn equally from the government and the NEC and would be chaired by the Prime Minister.[24] The evolving document, in places, and the steering/convenors' group discussions at times, appeared to confirm that the NEC would still have the opportunity for a collective policy expression – albeit one which was to be carried out with restraint, and NEC representatives on the Joint Policy Committee would report back to the full NEC.

In the section on the NPF, which constitutionally had been a consultative body of the NEC, the NEC kept its central policy-making authority. The document said that the NPF would be connected more fully with 'the wider membership, with the Party Conference and NEC'.[25] The NEC, it said, had a strategic role in relation to the principal goals of the party,[26] and in line with the existing constitution it should be consulted about priorities for the Queen's speech.[27] However, some indications in the draft document hinted at a different view. It was said that the current split between the Joint Policy Committee and the Domestic Policy Committee (of the NEC) had 'proved problematic'.[28] At one point it even said that the JPC would be the 'executive' body overseeing the party policy-development process and reformed NEC working arrangements.[29] That indicated a major extension of the JPC role. These inconsistencies in the document were not clarified. There was too much else to discuss and only later did it become clear how important this was as a managerial project.

The conference and the problem for the managers

Party officials and Sally Morgan were very anxious for the steering group to move the agenda onto the reform of the conference. Indeed, ex-Regional Director Jon Egan argued later that in a sense Partnership in Power had served its managerial purpose by 'providing the alibi for reforms of conference'.[30] A public exhibition of 'a divided party' was an electoral nightmare to the leadership, the managers and the spin doctors, exemplified in the memory of a Labour Chancellor of the Exchequer Dennis Healey speaking from the floor of the conference in 1976 and being booed. Yet by contrast they could see the huge opportunities of a conference operating within the glare of media attention acting as a shop window for a Labour Government in registering its record and presenting its appeal to the party and the people. They also needed to keep control over the rule-making powers of the conference, a source of much trouble for them in the past.

Under Blair, these problems appeared at first sight to have already been substantially overcome. Controls had become very tight and comprehensively organised (see Chapter 11, pp. 333–5). Privately, however, in 1996 the managers were saying something subtly different. That year virtually all the resolutions actually tabled for debate came from instigated sources. For all the talk of 'a new party' and 'a Blairite consensus' there was considerable unease amongst the managers about whether the party was 'safe'. There was also no guarantee that a consensus won 'to get rid of the Tories' would be sustained in two terms of Labour Government. The managers also knew that part of their own inventiveness in finding different promises to hold off adverse votes were not necessarily fully deliverable, and such tactics were likely to be much less effective when the party was in government. Thus, the appearance of the Blair supremacy and the Blairite juggernaut hid some significant vulnerabilities. The private view of one 'coal-face' manager was that the conference victories would not be sustained far into the Labour Government. Another put it simply, 'by the second year we will be in the shit'.

Difference opened up over the speed of the change and its completeness. There was a particular problem that the practical operation of the conference under a new policy-making system was very uncertain. Convincing the party and gaining acceptance of the new arrangements would be difficult because rights and powers would be taken away from the existing conference before the members could be reassured about what would be gained through the NPF process. The greatest fear expressed was that concern for the defence of the government and the public relations possibilities might make of the conference a political graveyard, demoralising party members and lacking authenticity for the public.

Initially, few seemed to be thinking of a complete break with the present conference process. One indication was that there was even some discussion of earlier compositing before the conference rather than no compositing at all. But suddenly into this discussion there was a very powerful push for immediate total change from the General Secretary responding to Blair's demand for urgent 'modernisation'. Phased change was said to be 'too conservative'. The party conference was pronounced by No. 10 'ready for complete reform'.

NEC stakeholders and reform

It had been accepted by the NEC that reform of the structure and representative character of the NEC could best arise in the context of discussions of its capacity to deliver various objectives.[31] In particular, there was general agreement that other party entities ought now to be represented alongside the older sectionalisation of trade unions, constituency organisations, a women's section, youth section and other affiliated organisations. Reform was also now located within a framework now described as that of a 'stakeholder party'. This could be used to prescribe a variety of different stakeholders, rights and processes and had been taken up in the context of party reform by the MPs Derek Fatchett and Peter Hain[32] from the soft left, and by the Labour Coordinating Committee close to Blair.[33]

Task Force 1 chaired by Maggie Jones began by specifying the stakeholders with new rights of membership of the NEC to be Labour councillors, Labour MPs, the MEPs and the EPLP, and the Cabinet. There was no agreement on this composition or the numbers involved at this stage. Blair's main worry was over the composition of the CLP section of the NEC. Here there had always been a dominance of leading MPs for whom the CLP membership chose to vote. In the past this had meant that members of the Shadow Cabinet and Cabinet were strongly represented, a feature which had on occasion produced tension with the primacy of government collective responsibility, especially in the time of Tony Benn as Chair of Home Policy. It also presented a public position from which rivals for the leadership could strengthen their visibility and exercise a degree of additional influence through the party. For all these reasons, Blair was looking for a basic minimum position of prohibiting Cabinet Ministers from membership of the NEC.

But the argument amongst his aides went further. It was now suggested that because ordinary members were not represented on the CLP section it would be better reserved completely for 'rank-and-file members'. All Labour MPs would be prohibited, and have to stand in the PLP section. This pleased Blair but raised some uncertainties and drew some reservations. Who would know who the rank-and-file candidates were? Alternatively, if the CLP section elected big media names, these could downgrade the seriousness of the process. Clare Short pointed out that participation might diminish. From the traditional right there was the worry that left-wing rank-and-file ultras might break in. CLPD on the other hand saw some of the dangers acting as an undemocratic bar to the CLP members voting for whom they wanted to support, especially as it would remove some important left-wing MPs. In the Party into Power discussions no agreement was reached at this stage.

NEC and trade union representation

From the General Secretary and from around the Leader one powerful argument was that with a composition expanded to accommodate new stakeholders there had to be a reduction in the trade union section of the NEC. After Powell's intervention at Cranfield and in the face of a regular press spin that they were a target, the NEC trade union group sought clarification. The General Secretary attempted a special reassurance in a letter to the TGWU General Secretary in January 1996.[34] Blair himself also did it, at a meeting of the Trade Union Liaison Committee on 20 September 1996, stressing that he understood their role and that his concern was with the Shadow Cabinet members on the NEC, not with union representation. There the matter rested, uneasily.

Non-executive directors and business representation

It took on an acutely controversial new aspect when it began to be argued that the NEC could only have a limited size and therefore trade union representation might have to be reduced. At the same time, supported by the General Secretary, Task Force 1 came up with a recommendation for 'non-executive' directors on the NEC. These it was argued would bring an independent perspective and expertise to the NEC's role. Immediately obvious critical questions were raised on the steering group. How would these directors emerge? Would they be in practice nominees agreed by the Leader as a means of producing a Leader's block vote? Weighed down by its lack of democratic legitimacy and the inconsistency over reducing the size of the NEC and trade union representation, the proposal was lethally damaged but not abandoned.

Behind the reaction was another concern at proposals that if the party stakeholders included the unions why not business representation on the NEC now that close relations with them was becoming a priority? It would of course be a step miles too far for the party conference to accept. But it became clear later that Sawyer saw this as a means of bringing in a new representational linkage between the party and the business community sympathetic to the Blairite agenda, a position to which he saw himself as well suited. Around this time the *Daily Express* owner Clive Hollick, an enthusiastic supporter of Blair and a task-force participant, made an important contribution to the discussions, minuted to the steering group. He tried to focus on the problem for a members' democracy of dealing with powerful socio-political forces outside the party. But this was outside the frame of reference of the party managers and not developed.

Consultation, contemporary resolutions and the drive for delivery

In January 1997 there were three important political developments which brought tensions in the steering group to a head. The deadline for delivery of the document titled *Labour into Power: a Framework for Partnership* was now approaching. A previous deadline had already been passed. The Leader, always a man in a hurry but, with reasonable concern here, wanted to ensure that the whole thing was ready to be put in place by the time Labour became the government. The pressure was felt particularly by Sawyer. Work on a range of complicated and contentious issues had fallen behind schedule. As the arguments progressed, and the attempt was made to encompass the different positions and points raised, so the document had become long, very long – over fifty pages.

Another version of the document was completed on Friday 17 January 1997 for an important Task Force 3 meeting to take place on the following Monday afternoon, 20 January. At that meeting, three union representatives from the NEC – Margaret Prosser of TGWU, Mary Turner of the GMB, and John Mitchell of the GPMU – made strong criticism of the construction of the document and urged that there should be a shorter document with more emphasis on the principles underpinning it. They were emphatic that it must go out to consultation by the party and the unions before the proposals were accepted, 'allowing people to produce their own ideas' as Prosser put it, but also giving people some ownership of it. No vote was taken on this at the task-force meeting but it was not opposed and it appeared that consultation had been agreed.

At that same meeting, after consensual discussions on the main agenda items, there was a long and tense discussion on a memo from Minkin. Following concerns first expressed at the Northern College discussions in 1990 (see Chapter 2, p. 74) and recent discussions with Cruddas, the memo focused on giving the CLPs and affiliated organisations the right to submit to the conference motions on 'contemporary issues' alongside both the continuous programmatic process and the emergency resolutions – which covered only a very tight category. In support of this, Minkin argued that there had to be some means of discussing such issues as they arose, if only as a safety valve to an untried system, and, more controversially, 'it was not clear where Blair was taking the party'.

That comment aroused some robust indignation. The proposal was opposed by Sawyer, Morgan and others on the group, particularly Margaret Wall, defending the totality of the new process and protecting a future Labour Government against 'being undermined'. All resolutions, it was said, must be sent direct to the policy commissions for consideration and be part of the continuous dialogue. That would be the strength of the new process compared to the old. All this was discussed without reference to the possibility that if the exclusion of resolutions was complete it could also mean that there could be no constitutional change initiated from below and no formal way at all of removing a Leader, a process made covertly more difficult by the managers later. The memo was not put to a vote but there was again an important intervention from Margaret Prosser of the TGWU. She noted that the argument had changed the atmosphere and would have to be taken on board. Jon Cruddas, who saw it as a further means of building cooperative managerial links with the unions, also saw virtue in the proposal and gave welcoming signals. Prosser's messages appeared to have gone home.

That evening at 8 pm there was another meeting of the Party into Power steering group to examine the final document. As normal, it did not include the GMB, GPMU or TGWU representatives. It did, again as normal, include Jeuda, Jones and Wall. It also included Mowlem, Morgan, Cruddas and Joe Irvine, Prescott's special advisor, as well as the General Secretary together with Fryer and Minkin. There were discussions on improving and shortening the document, during which it became clear (though not announced) that the amended document was to be taken to the NEC without going out to consultation. There was then a denial that an agreement on a consultation had in fact been reached in the afternoon. But in the next few days as word leaked out, strong representations were made by union leaders, particularly Bickerstaffe and Edmonds, and also NEC representatives including those who had proposed the consultation. Prosser again argued that it would be very unwise to push on in this way; in her union it could undermine support for the whole thing. Eventually it was agreed that this document would now be consultative and seen as interim.

Once the consultation had been agreed, although it left behind some grievances on the part of the General Secretary and his allies, there was a more relaxed atmosphere at the next steering group meeting on 23 January. Commitment to partnership, which was surprisingly weak in this draft (just one reference) was strengthened, as was the role of the party in policy-making, although within the limitation that it would be the government which would define the main parameters in what was said to be a partnership. After an intervention by Joe Irvine speaking for Prescott, the proposal for non-executive directors was removed and it never reappeared. Support for the facility to consider and make decisions on matters of current importance was now described as 'necessary and to be the subject of further discussion'.[35] Also, in this atmosphere it was possible to bring forth a compromise on CLP representation on the NEC. This involved accepting the idea of a quota of rank-and-file representatives but also their right to choose others for some seats. A quota of four rank-and-file members out of seven was mentioned.[36] The document moved to another rewrite by Fryer and other agreed verbal changes before submission to the NEC.

NEC meeting 28 January 1997

At the trade union group meeting prior to the NEC and on the NEC itself, there were reservations expressed over the prognosis in the draft document that it was the government alone which would define the main parameters in what was said to be a partnership – but no alternative wording was offered. There were also calls for strengthening further the idea of partnership and the need to emphasise that this was the beginning of a genuine consultation. At the NEC, Skinner was the most highly critical. Otherwise, what reservations there were focused on details and areas of uncertainty in the document.

The most significant conflict came over the NEC women's section. Since 1996 under the new quota system there had been 15 women on the committee out of 29 members, including five in the women's section, but by

1996, pressure grew to abolish the women's section and move totally to quotas. The fact that the women's-section elections were dominated by the votes of the unions added another dimension to reduction of their representation. Task Force 2 had moved towards abolition, but on the NEC trade union group there was strong opposition to proposals which would reduce union influence. Finally the phrase in the document 'sympathetic to the argument' for quotas was weakened to 'worthy of further consideration'.

Spinning Blair's supremacy

The leaders of GMB and UNISON and TGWU had already let it be known that they were not prepared to accept the document without seeing the detailed application following consultation. On a formulation proposed by Robin Cook and Margaret Prosser it was 'agreed as a basis for consultation'. The vote on this was 22–1 in favour, with Skinner against and David Blunkett one of the abstentions after expressing deep reservation about the loss of conference powers over resolutions.

Although the NEC had approved the draft only as a consultative document, in the media it was hard to find any mention of the consultation. The emphasis there was again on Blair's supremacy; he had imposed himself over the left, the NEC and the conference, which would have a more presentational role. BBC Ceefax summed it up on 29 January as, 'Blair acts to curb activists' power'. In retrospect, in view of what was to follow, much of this was accurate enough as a forecast, but it went strongly against what the majority of the NEC and many of those involved at this stage thought that they were doing. Once again it caused a gnashing of teeth. One again there were the 'yes isn't it awful. It's not him' denials from Blair's office.

At the next NEC meeting on 26 February there was a robust critical post-mortem on the spin. Eventually, in response, Blair suggested that in future Margaret Beckett and Robin Cook make statements to the press after the NEC made decisions of this kind. This was welcomed as a step forward but of course within three months both of them would have collective cabinet responsibility and, if Blair's proposals for reform of the NEC went through, they would come off the NEC as well.

Consultation and drafting

The consultation was hampered by the fact that the document, though shorter than it had been, had never been intended as a consultation document and remained very substantial. It was also unsatisfactory that the consultation period was to be very short. Because of the widespread call for more time, at the NEC's May meeting the deadline was extended from 20 June to 4 July, but this still left a strong body of CLP opinion dissatisfied. In May, a shorter consultation paper drafted by Tony Grayling of the policy directorate was put out in more natural consultative mode, together with a question-and-answer briefing. In early July, partly for contingent reasons (Fryer was going on holiday), Taylor (closer to Morgan than to Sawyer), now took over the drafting of the main document with Grayling. Shortly afterwards it was agreed that the document be renamed as *Partnership in Power*.

Shifting alignment

Changing the steering

In terms of the content of the interim document, as was pointed out by John Blevin in *Tribune*, it could be said that there was 'little to back up claims of a leadership stitch-up'.[37] But the struggle that had taken place in January indicated more to come. The General Secretary now prepared to change the balance of forces. There was an attempt to 'shadow' the original steering group (now generally referred to as the convenors' group) by a new convenors' group which would operate discreetly and not include Jeuda and Minkin.[38] As it happened, some of those invited to the shadow meeting doubted the wisdom of the tactic and most did not attend. This meant that the first group continued to function and to deal with the main business.

But now the existing convenors' group was to have an increased membership, justified by the exigencies of strengthening the nuts and bolts on tricky procedural issues, which became a heavy emphasis of the discussions from February to the May general election. Party officials Matthew Taylor, his deputy Tony Grayling, David Gardner and Phil Wilson became much more involved alongside Cruddas. There emerged still a pluralism of views with some significant differences over OMOV, the trade union role, handling contemporary resolutions and reform of the NEC, but the group was now dominated by party officials and in the end they would have to subordinate their views to those of the Leader and the General Secretary working to him.

Supremacy and enhancement of control

The election victory on 1 May aroused enormous party and public enthusiasm. Blair's role in the victory raised his authority even further. Later some managers would privately assert that the controls since 1994 were about getting this Labour Government, and were not intended to be a permanent set of arrangements. That may well have been in the minds of some of the managers, but analysis of the managerial behaviour in the phase immediately following the completion of Party into Power discussions (see Chapter 8, pp. 230–2) and how Partnership in Power was operated (see Chapter 10, pp. 305–8) points in another direction. What can be said is that what followed was a remarkably creative exercise not only in getting the technicalities right but also in ensuring the maximum of future control.

On some key issues dealt with in the period following the 1997 victory, it also became more clearly a power struggle. It still involved an interplay of persuasion and receptivity, but it now also had a stronger sub-current involving imposition and manipulation. Within this there were the usual personal complexities of competitiveness, ambition and the pull of leadership preferences and patronage. In an insecure politics under a dominating Leader who had achieved an unprecedented victory, it was natural for some officials and representatives to make their own appeal to the Leader by showing how skilful they were at achieving the fusion of their own interests, those of the party and 'what Tony wants'.

'What the big man wants', 'what works' and managing OMOV

The power meaning of the code of 'what works' was made starkly clear in continuing steering group discussions about the method of electing NPF representatives from the constituencies. Before 1997 CLP representatives to the NPF were elected two by regional conferences and four to six (depending on constituency size) by meetings of regional delegates after hustings. *Labour into Power* had noted that a proposal that Constituency Labour Party representatives on the NEC be elected by CLP delegates at the party conference was under consideration.[39] In the extensive discussions in and around the steering group, it had been suggested to those with doubts about it (of whom Diana Jeuda and David Gardner were the most forceful advocates of OMOV) that elections held at the conference could reinforce its sovereignty and give activists an independent democratic role. This was potentially true, if it had been allowed to operate that way. But given what had happened in management thinking and later in management moves to 'make sure' over OMOV voting, it proved to be an illusion.

A majority of the managerial officials had moved against an OMOV ballot because since 1993 they had become even more aware that OMOV in CLP selections made political management more difficult. Revealingly, at this time, 'the big man' was said in the convenors' group meeting to be 'relaxed' about the form of voting for the NPF, depending upon whether 'we can get a reasonable result': a clear signal to his managers. The procedural argument then became dominated by considerations of 'more manageable' versus 'less manageable' arrangements in judging 'what works'. NPF manageability was regarded as so important that there was even a protracted discussion of experimentation with different procedures to see 'what worked'. This whole case study became an important illumination of the Blairite subordination of procedural values to management.

The group received updates on what the consultation was producing. When the full replies to the consultation came in, in the open form of response only 4 per cent believed that NPF elections should take place at the party conference. The strongest support (43 per cent) was for regional elections by OMOV.[40] But this led to no alteration to the favoured managerial form. In spite of the evangelical role of the modernising LCC closely linked to Blair, who had advocated in their 1995 reform pamphlet *New Labour: a Stakeholder's Party* that OMOV be widely extended, that organisation went quiet over what was now being proposed.

The dialogue with the members

It had been recognised for some time that the confidentiality of the NPF process was both an asset, in encouraging dialogue free of media interference and a problem in that, unlike at the party conference, members in the constituencies did not have information provided by the media. It was therefore essential that Forum members kept close contact with their constituent groups and reported back to them. Discussions on the process were thin on suggestions for how this might better be achieved. Much emphasis was placed on the encouragement of local and regional policy forums and there was great enthusiasm for their growth and style. But the link to the national level was never established, other than in terms of generalities that continuous dialogue was essential and that if the local forums were to be submitting their ideas on a regular basis it needed a robust organisation of response at headquarters.

On this it was said, with great emphasis by party officials in Party into Power meetings, that though expensive and time-consuming it must be done thoroughly. In the final version of the Partnership in Power document, the policy commissions and the National Policy Forum were 'charged with ensuring a continuous dialogue with local branches and constituencies'.[41] It was agreed that there would be a report from the commissions to the NPF 'on submissions and motions received and action taken or recommended',[42] also that to keep the flow of information to the party there would be a comprehensive annual report to the party conference from the National Policy Forum.[43]

In the Party into Power discussions, formal and informal, it became increasingly accepted that the main thrust of the party's role would be its part in developing future policy leading to the production of the manifesto.[44] The special focus of the process and the test of its integrity was accepted to be the content of the party's manifesto for the second term. Little attention was paid to how this might operate in term of the manifesto-making process itself and there was no inclination to open the Clause V arrangements for producing the manifesto. As part of a discussion at a convenors' group meeting on 16 July of how the party might deal with necessary changes in policy after authorisation by the NPF, there was a proposal from one manager for a party plebiscite as in 1996. But it was clear that the other managers at the meeting were not anxious to return to the Road to the Manifesto experience, and even the proposer said that it should be, 'a genuine programmatic manifesto ballot – not the previous democratic farce'. The proposal received no support.

The focus on the Party's role in sharing the generation of future policy through the partnership process meant that the emphasis was taken away from contemporary policy. However, though it was never properly thrashed out, it was suggested that the close new two-way process between government ministers and their aides and the NEC and party officials would cover issues as they arose as well as the rolling programme. In the final document, it was also said that the policy commissions would provide an opportunity for on-going dialogue between the party on the ground and the government throughout the year.[45] These features were assumed by some of those involved in the discussions to involve a sensitivity to the party on contemporary issues as they arose. Some of those party officials linked closely to No. 10 had other views, it turned out (see Chapter 8, pp. 230–1).

Minority positions, cross pressures and alternatives

By this time in the Party into Power discussions there was also a growing managerial concern with getting the document through the party conference, especially as alternative positions would be restricted to the end of the second year, with the first-year report simply setting the agenda for the second year, 'identifying key issues and priorities and reflecting on currents of opinion inside and outside the party'.[46] There would be no first-year conference votes. The emphasis was on the facilities for the second year. Not only would the NPF, if it was 'unable to reach a consensus view', have the responsibility of including 'alternative proposals representing different constituencies of opinion within the Forum and the Party as a whole',[47] but, the conference would 'for the first time be able to have separate votes on key sections and proposals in the policy statement'.[48] Here then was (apparently) a major improvement in the capacity of the party conference to influence policy.

Unions and representation

The future position of the unions was still a background argument. Around the Leader, it was contended that regional officials in the unions were generally more representative, more accommodating and easier to have a dialogue with than the General Secretaries. Proposals for regional rather than national union representation were regularly flirted with as part of the policy process, but the senior union officials saw themselves as the unions' elected representatives and those proposals as divisive. This could not be resolved by imposition from the political wing, and even the proposal of a split representation, regional and national to the NPF, caused problems. At the Task Force 3 meeting on 5 June 1997, it was finally accepted that it might not be possible for the group to resolve the intrinsic difficulties.

Eventually, it was agreed that there would be national representation of the CLPs and trade unions plus a regional representation to be dealt with by consultation within the party at regional level. It led eventually to three representatives per region, and by custom one of them was generally from the unions. There was much disagreement within the unions about the distribution of the twenty national union representatives. This was left to discussions within TULO and, late in 1997, the issue was settled with representation roughly proportionate to membership. But there was no obligation to review these arrangements, nor any party say on how the representatives were chosen.

A healthy party

The task force on building a healthy party was a continuation of regeneration discussions which had been going on since 1992. It was poorly attended even by the low standards of NEC involvement in the Party into Power. Much of what emerged in the draft and then final document was primarily a fusion of the work of the Millbank official Nick Smith, who was involved in codifying imaginative good practice, and Diana Jeuda. Their contributions reflected a consensus on building party membership, stimulating active and outward-looking campaigning parties rooted in the local community. They would be fully representative, raising standards and innovating through new local structures and methods of organisation.

But Jeuda had a major disagreement with the more centralist party officials over the ownership of change. Her view was that this belonged properly to the party in the country rather than to party professionals. She accepted that leadership needed to be underpinned by a degree of management but had major reservations about the methods and scope of the Blair version. Her warning at one stage was that if you do not address the party's doubts you can't get them to cooperate with change. The NEC should facilitate a step-by-step approach to addressing their concerns, rather than instructing.[49] There should be more room in the rules for local experimentation. This devolutionary facilitating perspective lived uneasily with a central drive for delivery, a tension which never came into the document but emerged later as a push from above for the abolition of the local General Committees and their change to all member meetings (see Chapter 8, pp. 254–5). There was also another tension not registered in the document between Jeuda's liberal pluralism and Wilson's ideal of building a community-based Blairite party. The healthy-party task force was abandoned in 1997 but then re-established as the party-development task force under a new chairman, Ian McCartney.

The finale: Bishop's Stortford, 24 July 1997

The Composition

The composition of the final convenors' group meeting held at Bishop's Stortford was radically different to that of the original steering group. There were four senior Party officials (Sawyer, Gardner, Taylor, and Grayling), three NEC Task Force convenors (Wall, Jones and Jeuda) and two advisors (Fryer and Minkin). For a key but potent period of the meeting three members of the Downing Street Political Office staff (Morgan, Cruddas and Hakim) attended as the Leader's representatives and Morgan announced the Leader's position on key issues.

The draft of the document, and the rule changes, had been sent over to Downing Street, but were not available to the convenors' group until the morning of the meeting. It became clear at that point that much advance liaison work had ensured a maximum movement behind the Leader's position. Although Sawyer and Morgan had moved in and out of alliances during the Party into Power process, and divisions had opened up between the managers, at this stage they became absolutely united on the agenda that the Leader wanted and Morgan announced. In response to the Leader's message, Minkin – who had no official party employment – as before played an independent role in line with the original discussions of the steering committee. He drew attention to adverse comments made on Blair's attitude to parliament and the cabinet as well as the party, and argued that over-control which affected the people's choices could lead eventually to a hostile public reaction.

Composition of the CLP section

Probably the most important aspect of the Leader's message concerned the CLP section of the NEC. After long discussions Task Force 1 had agreed on 2 July a proposal to make the CLP Section eight members with a maximum of two MPs and four reserved women's places.[50] It was, it seemed, a victory for the members, a negotiated compromise and choice. The proposal caused some concern on the traditional loyalist right of the NEC, anxiously questioning whether rank-and-file representation could lower turnout and the section be captured by 'small groups'. At that stage major disagreement had broken out amongst the managers and the idea of elected regional representation of CLPs (which had been rejected at Task Force 2 meetings) suddenly re-emerged. Cruddas, Wilson and McCartney (involved in Task Force 1) now favoured just taking the reform decision in principle, leaving the NEC unreformed for the moment. The committee was considered to be working well and radical reform should follow the development of Partnership in Power and the NPF.

According to the final analysis of replies to the consultation, the largest body of explicit opinion, 22 per cent, said that the grassroots of the party would be better represented on the NEC by ensuring more representation from CLPs if necessary by having a 'non MPs quota'.[51] In a crucial development, in the weeks that followed Blair hardened his position, possibly in response to media stories about the unions putting on pressure and especially an article reporting that that he was being forced to do a deal with the unions.[52] In No. 10 this spin was blamed on Edmonds, but, as he pointed out later, it was very advantageous to hawks around the Leader.[53] What is certain is that 'the Big Man's view', as it was described by one official, meant that the draft before the final Bishop's Stortford meeting on 24 July was different to that agreed in Task Force 1 meetings. It now supported all MPs being taken off the CLP section.

Also, where the old CLP section had been seven and the 2 July proposal had been eight, this would now have only six members. The No. 10 representatives moved united behind it at the final meeting, as did all the party officials and NEC representatives. That unity spread to the PLP where Fatchett and Hain, who had earlier developed a thoughtful critique of the managers, and of what they called the LCC 'centralised elite model' version of the stakeholder party, now also moved behind what was emerging in Partnership in Power. A resulting split developed on the left, out of which emerged a new coalition organisation joining the Campaign for Labour Party Democracy with Labour Reform, calling itself the Centre Left Grassroots Alliance (Grassroots Alliance and GRA for short). They became the main critical grouping.

Contemporary resolutions

As already indicated, there was a strong body of managerial and some NEC loyalist opinion, which was, like Blair, not happy with the procedure of contemporary resolutions at all. 'Tony hated it', it was said from his office, because it 'allowed people to go to the rostrum and slag off the government'. Jon Cruddas took a different view and accepted the safety-valve argument. He, and later Phil Wilson, continued to argue that these resolutions and the compositing process that they would reintroduce could be an addition to an armoury of interactive party management. The signs were also that submission of resolutions was supported in the party at large. As Fryer reported in his final analysis of the party's response to the consultation, there was 'substantial concern that branches and affiliates should continue to be able to submit motions directly to the Conference' and that 'real debate' should still take place.[54] Support for contemporary resolutions built up in the various meetings after the consultation. Here was one area where Blair could not get his way even in the later phase.

There had been particularly strong managerial resistance to any resolutions on party organisation and administrative issues as well as policy. It was argued initially that if there was a continued right of submissions, on these issues the local parties might flood a conference having lost the right to general submission on policy items. Eventually, at the suggestion of the General Secretary, contemporary resolutions would include also organisational issues, but only one could be submitted, whatever it covered. Now, with audacious managerial brio, that became another selling point of the proposed new document.

Remarkable creativity was elicited from the managing officials in a long battle with Jeuda and Short to produce definitions and procedures which would, on one interpretation, protect the Partnership in Power process by the limits placed on resolutions, or on a more critical interpretation, in the search for control through eventual suppression of resolutions, be as off-putting as possible to those who thought of submitting. That, some thought, would also help the procedure to fade out.

The rule that emerged involved a heavily restrictive formulation of contemporary issues, not differentiating organisation/admin issues from policy (and making no reference to constitutional issues which had to be fitted in later as organisational issues). The wording became 'a topic which is either not substantively addressed in the reports to Conference of either the NPF or the NEC or which has arisen since the publication of those reports'.[55]

Understandably, not all such resolutions could trigger a debate given the time available, therefore an attractive element of democracy was suggested. There would be a priorities ballot to decide which contemporary issues should be debated. But, very obsessive in 'reassuring Tony', some of the managers became very nervous at the idea of publishing for the delegates a list and details of the resolutions which had been submitted. They visualised this dominating the media agenda and becoming the source of many stories of party splits. The agreement that emerged now, after a lengthy informal argument, was Kafkaesque in form. There would be a list but just of the topics. Delegates would vote on the priorities for contemporary resolutions but would not be allowed to know in detail what was in those resolutions. Eventually it was agreed that there would be a list of subjects nominated for debate, a list of those submitting resolutions on these subjects and a comprehensive summary of their content but not the content itself. This detailed process was not disclosed to the 1997 conference and therefore not open to a challenging vote there.

The union leaders and support for partnership

Most union leaders had generally kept some distance from the detailed politics of the Party into Power discussions as internal party business. Some ultra-loyalist NEC trade union representatives discouraged information going to their senior officers who might have reacted against it. The consequences of this interplay can be gathered from one very significant meeting which was held on 22 July where the six major union leaders from AEEU, GMB, GPMU, MSF, RMT and UNISON were told by Cruddas of the final outline of the drafting, including the ending of regular resolutions, and they learned that this was a fait accompli. That left them, in descriptions from both sides, as 'stunned', 'gobsmacked' and feeling 'railroaded'.

Cruddas was able to give them some reassurance and, in effect, a managerial agreement that four contemporary resolutions would be acceptable and that this would involve the four largest unions. It did not fully assuage their discontent. Potentially important, but not at this point a pressing concern, was that if they focused on the spread of policy priorities in their contemporary resolutions (as they did), unions could not submit organisational or constitutional resolutions, and though not an immediate priority, they might one day need to do that.

On the day after this meeting, the *Independent* reported that the unions were determined to confront Blair.[56] It was another story the origins and motivation of which were argued over but the fact was that whatever their misgivings, the union leaders had accepted the wisdom of trying to balance the needs of government with the traditions of the party; partnership with intra-party democracy. They had come too far since 1990 in terms of commitment to the general principles of a more joint, diagnostic and deliberative process of policy-making. It was in their view simply a better way of making policy. Less obvious was that they and the managers stood to gain also in the sense that the private process and the new deliberative culture gave the union leaders themselves more room for manoeuvre in relation to their own mandates.

It could also be convincingly argued, as it was by Roger Lyons, that this was 'emphatically not the link-breaking project'.[57] There was an agreed reduction of trade union voting weight at the NPF compared to what it had been before, and also a reduction in the weight of their influence in the composition of the NEC. But the NEC trade union section itself had not been touched, and union representation at the NPF cohering with regional representation proved to be more influential than it appeared. Minority positions would go to a party conference, once again declared sovereign, where the affiliated organisations still held 50 per cent of the vote. That now became all the more crucial. Driving the point home, at this stage the AEEU publicly drew a line in the sand, voting for the changes but with Jackson making clear that they would fight any future move to cut the voting strength of the unions at the conference.[58]

The NEC final decisions, 30 July 1997

At the trade union group meeting, held the night before the NEC, it was clear that they were going to support the document. The normal pull towards loyal support there was accentuated in the light of the great election victory. There was particularly resolute support from those directly involved, Maggie Jones, Margaret Wall and the new TGWU representative Margaret Prosser, who was in the process of becoming the party Treasurer and chair of the trade union group. Nevertheless, in the background dialogue of that group they had indicated strongly that it wanted the NEC to retain its formal constitutional powers of submitting to the party conference its own resolutions and declarations affecting the programme, principles and policies of the party. Following an argument in the convenors' group, the NEC also retained its conventional power of declaring its attitude towards conference resolutions. These could not be touched.

On the NEC, the debate on abolition of the Women's Section in favour of quotas showed the different positions of Clare Short (ex-Chair of the NEC Women's Committee) with doubts on the healthy effect of this change on the women's organisation, and Hilary Armstrong (the present chair and a forceful advocate of change as well as a further reform of the women's organisation). The debate was not conclusive. But the consultation of the party had indicated 'on balance' support for strengthening of quotas (15 per cent) over a separate women's section (8 per cent) with 5 per cent opposed to any positive action.[59] In practice, the decision to move forward on the basis of the report went ahead in the rule changes accepted by the 1997 Party Conference.

Most attention here and in various advance meetings again focused on contemporary resolutions. The 'secret' wording of contemporary resolutions stimulated some difference of perspectives over what the media might say and how delegates might react. Short, supported by Blunkett, attempted to loosen the criteria for contemporary resolutions as Jeuda had done without success in the trade union group, particularly in the way they affected constitutional and organisational issues.

The new partnership policy process which it was said justified the constraints on single policy resolutions could not be applied to these constitutional and organisational topics, as there was no process on these matters through the National Policy Forum. Though the NEC endorsed the document 19–1, with Skinner dissenting, the argument continued. In the end Matthew Taylor suggested an adroit compromise that the NEC Report each year would contain alternative positions on organisational reform which could be voted on. It was unclear how this could work but support was given in principle and went to the conference with the formula although, as it turned out, with little commitment. Still, though this issue was never raised in the open discussions, the preservation of contemporary resolutions on organisational questions left open the unwanted (by No. 10) possibility of resolutions from the party to choose a new Leader. That was dealt with by the party secretariat later, outside the knowledge of the party, and established a procedure which in effect protected the existing Leader (see Chapter 13, p. 431).

Delivering the votes

On the surface, in delivering the vote for Partnership in Power, there was little cause for managerial anxiety. The Leader was on an unprecedented roll of popularity. His standing with the electorate had surged post-election and, following his handling of the death of Princess Diana, reaching a height unprecedented for a party in office. Nine in ten Labour supporters said they were satisfied with him.[60] There was enormous pressure in the party to follow the chorus of admiration and approval.

Of the total of 570 motions, almost one in five was on the Labour into Power project, with 44 calling for delay for one year, 27 objecting to the ending of the right to submit resolutions and a further 29 making a variety of different complaints. But the consultation disclosed a large measure of support for the key principles of partnership, stakeholding and a healthy party. And only 7 per cent of the responses indicated opposition to, or general dissatisfaction with, the key proposals.[61]

In their replies to the consultation, the majority of the unions had also indicated their support for the general thrust of the document, with UNISON and the AEEU the most enthusiastic, although with virtually all expressing some detailed reservations. It is worth noting also that in terms of union priorities and what a Labour Government might deliver, winning union support was eased by some re-commitments on rights at work contained in composite 12. This had been formulated by Cruddas in conjunction with the union officers and accepted by the NEC. It was not over-specific, and not a direct quid pro quo. But as one of the managers described it, it became 'a help in consolidating support in the final weeks', and it was said on the left to have had particular influence in the GPMU and TGWU.[62]

The unions were satisfied that the new process overall appeared to bind Labour ministers into a dialogue with the party involving the sharing of future policy-formulation. There would also (without qualification) be alternative positions offered for the first time in the policy documents as well as on the organisation issues contained in NEC Report. The opportunities to have votes on key sections and proposals in the policy statements were especially appealing. Even the restricted right to submit contemporary resolutions was now presented to the party as giving them more rights.

The fact that the document said that the reports 'would be circulated in time for conference delegates to consult with their constituencies and seek guidance on issues to be determined by Conference'[63] seemed to indicate approval for the CLPs retaining their conventional mandating role. This was in line with historical practice and the 1993 trade union review group report[64] that voting at Conference 'did not preclude mandating of delegates in line with their organisation's rules and policy decisions'. But there was another emphasis in the private briefing by managing officials at the party conference. In regional liaison meetings in the years that followed, it was made clear (correctly) by the officials that mandating was not part of the constitution, but it was then discouraged as though it were prohibited.

The rule relating to new representation on the NEC by rank-and-file members had a misleading aspect. Rule 3C4.3 read that 'Commons members of the PLP and EPLP shall be ineligible'. A note in explanation of the changes said that the change was to provide for 'genuine grass roots representation from CLPs'. Officials later argued that peers voted as ordinary members for the Leader of the party, and therefore they should be allowed to be represented in this genuine grassroots section. But the fact was that on the convenors' group no discussion had taken place about representation from the House of Lords and there was no reference to it in Partnership In Power.

The voting

Conference procedures gave little scope for specific amendments: only three opposition resolutions were taken to this entire complex set of proposals. This was an initiative from the headquarters organisation department, accepted by the Conference Arrangements Committee by only 4 votes to 3. On the NEC CLP section argument, the compromise position on composition was not put, just a composite 50, favouring the traditional right of CLPs to nominate and support whom they wanted for the section. The result was overwhelming conference opposition, 62.85 per cent to 37.15 per cent. Only 15.78 per cent of the CLP section voted in favour of the traditional position whilst 21.38 per cent of the affiliated organisations vote went in support, a total vote for of 37.15 per cent. Support in the unions might have been greater had not a group of unions including the GMB, AEEU and GPMU agreed to abstain on the grounds that they ought not to determine CLP representation.

Composite 51 on the right to submit resolutions and amendments to documents direct to party conference without going through the Partnership in Power process was supported by 20.98 per cent of the CLP vote, but only 11.54 per cent of the vote of the affiliated organisations went in support, another indication of cooperation with the partnership arrangement agreed by the unions in spite of the gut reaction of some of the union leaders. It was still overwhelming victory for the platform – 67.48 per cent to 32.52 per cent.

In the end, the only danger for the leadership was over delay. The consultation analysis had shown that 32 per cent believed that insufficient time had been allowed. A further 15 per cent believed that the decisions should be left to the 1998 conference.[65] At the conference, on composite 53 although a substantial minority – 20.98 per cent – of the CLP went for a resolution in favour of postponement, only 11.54 per cent of the affiliated organisations did so. That was a mixture of union realism and the union position on partnership since 1990. The overall vote was 67.48 per cent to go ahead without delay. The vote on the changes to constitution rules was 82.54 per cent in favour, only 17.46 per cent against.

Significance

Party acceptance became a matter of hope and willingness to participate in the apparent spirit of the enterprise. Edmonds told the Conference, 'this debate is not just about policy-making, it is about trust'.[66] The managerial response was to bring in especially trusted individuals to front the distrusted change. Ex-General Secretary Whitty was asked to address the conference in support of the new document. Mo Mowlem was asked to wind up the debate for the NEC and asked to promise that 'the annual report' covering organisational change 'will give us alternative statements to vote on'.[67] It was applauded but the document had a looser phraseology referring to 'where appropriate' and did not mention a vote.[68] In practice, it never happened.

The final version of Partnership in Power did have a strong idealistic appeal in anticipating politics as open dialogue, in the emphasis on participation by all the members, and in the idea of a partnership. It had its negotiative elements, including the (reluctant) consultation and the (resisted) acceptance of contemporary resolutions. It had some heel-digging over retention of some formal powers of the NEC. The process sometimes involved a tense pluralism which embraced union representatives and more surprisingly a few of the managerial officials. But it had its impositional elements as well, particularly about the CLP section of the NEC and the large-scale obliteration of direct resolution submission which became for union leaders a fait accompli.

It also had its important manipulative features – particularly in the realpolitik of the discussion over elections for the NPF, the special arrangements for organisational issues which failed to happen and, as revealed later, the covert change in nominating procedures for the election of the Leader. It involved a changing relationship between the officials and the NEC, and also, in the crucial final stages, some media interventions which stimulated the hawk in Blair and encouraged hard management. In addition, as will be shown in Chapters 8 and 10, there were a range of developments which in different stages later undermined what had been sold to the conference and the party. No clarifying amendments which changed the partnership towards what was thought to have been agreed in 1997 were allowed through the contemporary resolutions procedure at future party conferences. The reassurances being given to Blair indicated the opposite of partnership and drove a management which made it more 'fit for purpose'. There was more of this management to come.

Notes

1 NEC document. GS:31/7/96.
2 *Guardian*, 15 July 1995.
3 *Guardian*, 17 July 1995.
4 NEC document GS: 13/1/96.
5 Ibid.
6 Lewis Minkin, 'The Party into Government: The Case for a new Partnership between the Party and a Labour Government', July 1996.
7 Notes of the author, published with Mowlem's permission.

8 Lewis Minkin, 'Labour in Power: Partnership for Effectiveness', 18 July 1996, *Partnership in Power* file, Manchester Labour History Museum Library.

9 Labour Party document, *Labour into Power: a Framework for Partnership*, January 1997, p. 9 of final version.

10 Ibid. p. 16.

11 Ibid.

12 Ibid. p. 14.

13 Ibid. p. 15.

14 *Labour into Power*, p. 9.

15 Ibid. p. 16.

16 *Partnership in Power*, Executive Summary, p. 3.

17 Minutes of Task Force 2, 1 July 1996, and discussions following it.

18 'Interview: Tom Sawyer', *New Statesman*, 12 July 1996.

19 *Labour into Power*: section 2.2.2, p. 5 of final version.

20 My notes, published with Mowlem's permission.

21 *Labour into Power*, p. 2.

22 Ibid. p. 9.

23 Ibid. p. 10.

24 Ibid. p. 23.

25 Ibid. p. 13.

26 Ibid. p. 21.

27 Ibid.

28 Ibid.

29 Ibid. p. 10.

30 *Tribune*, 15 October 1999.

31 NEC document GS 13/1/96.

32 Derek Fatchett and Peter Hain, *A Stakeholder Party*, 1996.

33 LCC, New Labour: a Stakeholder's Party, 1996.

34 Letter from Tom Sawyer to Bill Morris, General Secretary of the TGWU, 1 February 1996.

35 *Labour into Power*, p. 16.

36 This was formulated at the time by Minkin but may have been derived from an article by Peter Hain in *Tribune*, 1 September 1995, which argued for a quota-ised NEC in terms of activists, councillors and backbench MPs as well as women.

37 *Tribune*, 12 February 1997.

38 A letter from the General Secretary dated 17 February confirmed, for those invited, plans 'to review Party into Power every Thursday evening until the end of March'. The core of this grouping became Sawyer, Jones, Wall and Fryer. Invited also were Jon Cruddas, Margaret Prosser, Mo Mowlem, Phil Wilson, Sally Morgan and Joe Irvine, but they, it appears, did not attend.

39 *Labour into Power*, p. 14.

40 *Partnership in Power*, Appendix, p. 18.

41 *Partnership in Power*, p. 11.

42 Ibid., Executive Summary, p. 3.

43 *Partnership in Power*, p. 15.

44 Ibid. p. 9.

45 Ibid. p. 14.

46 Ibid.

47 Ibid. p. 18.
48 Ibid. p. 20.
49 Ibid. p. 30.
50 Project Report of Task Force 1, The NEC at Work, 2 July 1997, p. 2.
51 *Partnership in Power*, Appendix p. 19.
52 *The Times*, 9 July 1997.
53 My interview with Edmonds.
54 Results of the Consultation Exercise, 23 July 1997.
55 Rulebook 1998, Rule 3C2.3.
56 *Independent*, 23 July 1997.
57 *Tribune*, 13 June 1997.
58 *Morning Star*, 29 September, 1997.
59 *Partnership in Power*, Appendix, p. 19.
60 MORI/*Times*, 2 October 1997.
61 *Partnership in Power*, Appendix, p. 19.
62 Party Conference Socialist Campaign Group Newsletter, Monday 29 September 1997.
63 *Partnership in Power*, p. 16.
64 Final Report of the Trade Union Review Group, p. 28.
65 *Partnership in Power*, Appendix, p. 18.
66 LPCR 1977, p. 19.
67 LPCR 1997, p. 28.
68 *Partnership in Power*, p. 10.

8

Managing the changing NEC: partnership and shifting power

The policy process and the NEC in Opposition

When Blair was elected Leader in 1994 the National Executive Committee, still an important institution, was often reasonably described as 'the party's ruling body'. It had general supervision of the party administration and it had a crucial position in terms of the formulation and filtering of constitutional and organisational changes. Blair was bequeathed from Smith the new Joint Policy Committee and the new National Policy Forum. Although the JPC (a body not noted in the party's constitution) had taken over much of the NEC's work, it was still through the NEC that party policy documents emerged and it was the NEC which made recommendations to the party conference on the acceptability or otherwise of resolutions under discussion.

In general the union group on the NEC continued to play their traditional supportive role over policy and despite some reservations from individual unions over arms expenditure in 1995 and particularly over an existing party commitment over rail ownership in 1997 (see Chapter 11, p. 343). Blair was never opposed on policy by a united union group. Nevertheless, Blair retained an ambivalent attitude towards the group. On principle he thought that the group should not be there, but they became acceptable when they assisted him – as they did most of the time. The NEC's power remained a complication for his version of strong leadership and was viewed as potential trouble when Labour moved into government. From the first, Blair's intention was to move all policy authorisation away from the NEC and make the party's policy officials focus more on campaign assistance. Sawyer as the new General Secretary began an early reappraisal of the NEC role with that understanding. Around the NEC there developed a more flexible policy process with much less respect for formality and protocol and much more attuned to the needs and convenience of the Leader. Even at the Joint Policy Committee, 'It was found difficult to find a time to meet and papers were not always circulated in advance',[1] most items were simply rubber-stamped as products of the new leadership.

Yet Sawyer was unable to stop the NEC policy process from defending its existence alongside that of the JPC. In October 1994 there had been a move to merge the Domestic, International and Joint Policy Committees on the grounds that there was too much duplication. That attempt was fought off. In December, replying to a query, the Policy Director still noted that the JPC reported to the NEC which 'apart from the Conference is the primary policymaking body of the Party'.[2] Policy statements had to be cleared by the JPC and the NEC.[3] And when in July 1995 the regional policy consultative document was launched without going through the NEC, this was accepted only on the basis that it was an exceptional procedure because the shadow minister would be abroad at the time of the NEC and this should not be used as a precedent.[4]

Partnership in Power and the NEC

From 1998 Partnership in Power was presented as the party and government working together in a joint and mutually supportive operation which would acknowledge the distinct responsibilities of the party and the government. The interim document specifically warned against subordination of the one by the other. But what happened in practice after 1997 in the third phase of development of the plans could be judged a manipulative master-stroke even in this, the era of such actions. The key development for which there was no authorisation either in Partnership in Power or a decision by the NEC was the closing down of the NEC Policy Committee and in practice the end of the party's collective policy voice.

The policy role of the NEC

Although there had been a sign in an LCC pamphlet of 1995 that the NEC was to have no policy role,[5] it's doubtful whether there was any understanding amongst those consulted in the party in 1997 that this would happen. Little in the union submissions indicated any support for it. The shorter Question and Answer briefing with the Grayling consultative document did not enlighten them. In section 5, 'establishing a credible political programme' was still specified as one of the NEC's two strategic political functions. In section 3 it said that the policy-making process would go through the JPC *but would end with the NEC*. In Section 8, it said that alternative policy positions would emerge from the secretariat working with the National Policy Forum and the NEC. The NEC's constitutional position in relation to its resolutions and declarations affecting the programme, principles and policies of the party was the same as it was before the PIP meetings began.

Although at a convenors' group meeting on 17 July 1997 it had been reported verbally that Blair was adamant that the JPC must be the final authority on policy, and the emphasis placed on the government consulting with the NEC on the Queen's Speech, which had been in the Interim Report, had disappeared in the final version of Partnership in Power, agreed by the party conference, it still specified that the NPF would report to the JPC, the NEC and the conference.[6] The new rulebook established in 1997 specified that it was part of the duties and powers of the NEC 'to establish and oversee . . . a Joint Policy Committee'.[7] What happened in practice without announcement was the most audacious feature of the rolling coup. The composition of the NEC Policy Committee was formally established but meetings were simply not called by its secretary Matthew Taylor, the Policy Director who, in May 1998, announced to the NPF that the NEC had 'devolved its authority to the JPC'.[8]

Even the devotedly loyal chair of that committee, Margaret Wall, who had not been very protective of the committee's agenda, was not told that the committee would be wound up. As had other unions, Wall's own union, MSF, had made clear in its submission to the consultation on Partnership in Power that the NEC must remain 'the supreme policy-making body between Conferences.'[9] She privately protested to Taylor and the General Secretary Sawyer, but they were deeply resistant to re-establishing the committee's role, and her loyalty ensured that there would not be wider repercussions. As for the NEC itself, it was some time before it was realised that there was no Policy Committee in operation. Operating within a self-denying ordinance not to act as alternative government in policy-making, it was difficult for NEC members to kick up an immediate fuss about something that might be represented as an attempt to assert policy against the government. These developments also left party officials with no authoritative party voice to draw upon as a counterweight to the instructions from No. 10, although they were not looking for it.

This fitted Blair's need for reassurance of control, although it left open various odd policy areas which could be described as either policy or organisation, particularly local government. More problematic for the managers in the end were the important formal policy rights under the constitution which had had to be left untouched by the covert treatment of the NEC. The constitutional right to submit to the conference 'resolutions and declarations affecting the programme, principles and policies of the party',[10] and the conventional right to declare a view of conference resolutions before a vote, implied a continuing NEC right to discuss policy although in this period they were never used in ways contrary to the wishes of the Leader.

Whilst most of the managers hankered after closing off the loopholes, there remained a body of opinion on the NEC which never accepted the imposed change. In an unusual move initiated by Prescott, just prior to the 1998 Conference, an uncontentious draft NEC Statement on transport was initiated and had drafting amendments by the Deputy Leader and Diana Holland.[11] In contrast, on 27 November 1999 a paper on Labour in local government was produced with a controversial title 'problem or opportunity?' without NEC local government representatives being consulted.[12] In the second term, the conflict over rights of policy-making would come strongly to the fore as a contested area over some key issues, including Iraq.

Another serious loophole had been left by the failure of the attempt to ban all organisational resolutions. The original position of Sawyer and Morgan, both speaking for Blair, on abandoning resolutions would have prevented the conference passing any resolution calling for a leadership election. Now that loophole was closed by an undeclared inactivity, in which the headquarters simply failed to send out the nomination forms at the time of year that they were due. No challenge was expected at this stage of Blair's ascendancy and it took some time for this failure to be noticed. Here was another addition to the managerial coup.

History as management device

Other new managerial controls over the Partnership in Power policy process will be explored in Chapter 10. Here it is important to note that the reaction of the NEC over this unauthorised change in its policy role reinforced and reflected a broader effect on the workings of the committee after 1997. The committee's restraint was reinforced by the clever cultural blitz engineered by Sawyer, which had accompanied the Party into Power preparations and discussions. The NEC's history had been portrayed as wholly negative in relation to the past Labour Government and the source of one of its major problems. Its recent accommodating policy role was glossed over. That version of history and defence of loyalty against 'oppositionism' were used repeatedly as a management device to reinforce inhibition in not challenging the leadership.

The NEC was also influenced by the shrewdly drawn 'critical success factors' defined at Cranfield, concerning the committee's responsibility when Labour was in government. These were carefully worded to indicate a very non-assertive and non-critical role. There was a responsibility on the NEC to support a Labour Government and ensure that its work was understood and promoted: it had to produce an active and representative party on the ground. It was to act as a sounding board for ideas and reaction to a Labour Party in power, providing encouragement and constructive feedback. It was to act as a conduit between the party in power and the party on the ground. And it was the responsibility of the NEC to manage these relationships as a duty to the party as a whole.[13] In addition, 'The NEC would have a close harmonious and supportive relationship with the Leader'.[14]

There was a genuine eagerness amongst NEC members to make partnership work if the government would let them. They wanted to be part of the solution not the problem – an important expression of changing attitudes which had been building up on the NEC during the years of being out of government. Even some of those who held a different view of the history and politics found themselves very inhibited by the need to avoid disunity and not to put consistent 'oppositionist' pressure on the Prime Minister. In avoiding their past, real and attributed, they were at times psychologically ill-adjusted to defend some aspects of their own legitimate role against the managing officials. That role became defined now by the alliance of managers and NEC loyalists working to 'what Tony wants' and sometimes simply to their view of 'what Tony needs' or what the managers wanted. Years later it was possible to see the continuing impact of this restraint over the NEC's diminished role.

The new role of the managers

That was in contrast with the bold behaviour of the senior party management. What was presented to the party as a partnership was taken by senior headquarters staff as a signal that power was passing permanently into the hands of 10 and 11 Downing Street. Almost all of the officials behaved as though this was inevitable and right. The Cranfield Report had included a recommendation for a clarification of the relationship between the NEC and the General Secretary and staff. Without formal note, that clarification had now come about. The officials, working closely with the special advisors and the Political Office in No. 10, were an important contributor and beneficiary. Officials could now sail forth much more boldly confident in representing the Leader. It was no coincidence that Brown resigned from the NEC after 1996, aware that it was likely to become a shadow of its former self and probably not worth his time and his subordination if he was there only as a Blair nominee.

Changes in the NEC's operation

Partnership in Power Task Force 1, chaired by Jones, continued to produce various proposals for reform of the NEC operations following the NEC's acceptance of the Partnership in Power final report. Most of the NEC had not been involved in the detailed formulation of the section dealing with NEC arrangements. Their focus on other issues in a huge series of changes put before them left them much to argue about later, and it became clear then that many on the NEC had major reservations about what the officials were putting in front of them.

In the week before the party conference 24 September 1997, Task Force 1 produced its plans for the organisation and style of working of the NEC.[15] This drew attention to the increasing problem of poor attendance at the NEC and its subcommittees in recent times. It argued that Partnership in Power could place additional burdens on the committee members, undermining the need for more targeted involvement. The NEC was therefore not to meet monthly as it had done since the party's inception 'but at least six times a year'. As the NEC did not meet in August or December anyway, this would be a reduction from ten meetings to six. This change also fitted into the practicalities of relieving the burdens on the new Prime Minister.

The appeal of the new arrangements was in the portrayal of a modernisation of procedure in which the NEC would concentrate on strategic and bigger-picture issues, devolving more responsibility to the subcommittees and senior officers without the subcommittee debates being repeated at the NEC. In particular, there would be a new beefed-up Organisation Committee, 'representative of all the stakeholders', which would have full delegated powers but with detailed matters requiring thorough deliberation and scrutiny on the NEC which would be on the basis of reports from this Organisation Committee.

The NEC was heavily divided over these proposals, with the majority expressing misgivings of various kinds. It was argued that the decline in NEC attendance was in part the product of the loss of its influence and that these proposals would make attendances worse. There was fear of a two-tier NEC with an inner elite based on the favoured members of the Organisation Committee put there by the General Secretary. The proposals on the internal arrangements of the NEC were referred back to a subsequent meeting on 30 September then again a week later, and accepted only after a third meeting. Under pressure to move on in unity, a compromise was reached to make it eight meetings per year and, in order to move on, the Organisation Committee delegated powers were (for some reluctantly) accepted. As Russell pointed out, the changes resulted in a cycle of meetings which were not widely known and made lobbying from the party more difficult.[16]

An NEC meeting on 29 October 1997 reinforced for some members a sense of collective institutions being under threat. The General Secretary proposed that the party conference – always hitherto a five-day event – would be reduced to four days. The case for this emphasised the financial savings involved and also revealingly noted that 'the media have for some time been unhappy with the length of coverage the Party receives'. Although Jones, Prosser (now the Treasurer) and Wall spoke in favour, it was met by a wide range of critics including Prescott. The Secretarial paper on this was withdrawn although it was returned to later in 1999. Proposed changes in the timetable for the conference were also deferred.

Reform of the women's organisation, which had faced strong critics as well as supporters at various levels, nevertheless went through the NEC on 29 October 1997. The National Women's Conference, often a radical critic of the leadership but also an instrument of Labour women's advance within the party, was reformed so as to bring it in line with Partnership in Power policy-making, That would end its resolution-based nature and integrate with the national training event for women. Later, in 1999, the Women's Sections of CLPs were abolished in favour of Women's Forums.

A review of regional reorganisation was instituted after a paper from the General Secretary noted that 'the regional political structures ... do not fit easily with the new partnership principles'. But the regions proved wary of any organisation which appeared to be outside their long-established structures. There were worries also that the forum process would be difficult to enmesh with procedures of accountability and they required a different spirit – that of scrutiny. An example of a new process was set by the North and Yorkshire Region which replaced the regional conferences with two policy forums, both with steering groups and a joint Executive. But with little support in other regions, the rest of the restructuring never took place.

Under new arrangements after 1997, the Campaigns and Elections Committee, hitherto an NEC committee chaired by the Deputy Leader, became a joint committee. Facing considerable scepticism, to reassure and involve the NEC, Matthew Taylor proposed that the NEC as a whole should engage with the major strategic issues around campaigns and elections with a report to the committee from each meeting of the joint committee. That did periodically take place, with on one major occasion on 27 July 1999 an acrimonious discussion concerning results of the European elections. For the senior party officials and reforming loyalists on the NEC, all this resistance was a conservative and at times obstructionist response. In an unusual private ad hoc meeting of party officers and officials on 8 June 1998 to reconsider the future of the committee, the present NEC was described as 'unreformable', but the coming changes in the NEC composition after the new elections would be 'a window of opportunity'.[17]

Modernisation and its effects

The 'modernising' changes which were introduced and adjusted were, it was said, 'to ensure it is more strategic, responsive and effective dovetailing with the new role of the Party in partnership with government', and also in its relations with the party in Europe and in local government.[18] NEC meetings were to be focused on coordinating the party with the government, determining and reviewing party strategy and objectives and monitoring the operation of the party.[19] The push for a more effective NEC did encourage attempts at objective-driven activity with monitoring of implementation and later NEC action notes after decisions. There was a new concern to use NEC time effectively rather than having some items repeated whilst squeezing out many others. The new delegated role of the Organisation Committee did give opportunities for more strategic discussions for those involved. But increasingly some on the NEC grew unhappy that the changes had consolidated the ability of officials and their allies to drive through the NEC decisions about which it was not always fully aware, given the abbreviated nature of Organisation Committee minutes and the failure to supply papers from the committee. Ann Black later noted that 'currently too much power is delegated to subcommittees, party officers and the General Secretary'. There needed to be 'a rebalancing'.[20] But though this overall dissatisfaction, as will be shown, fed into a series of revolts, the overall pattern of power after the Sawyer reforms remained the same.

The new NEC and the Leader's block vote

The compositional changes produced an NEC of 32 more broadly representative of different sections of the party, but it was also one in which both the trade union and constituency party components were proportionately reduced. Blair on the other hand was strengthened by three new Cabinet representatives – Mo Mowlem, Ian McCartney and Hilary Armstrong – chosen by him, and this in effect much of the time created alongside the Deputy Leader a small but significant leadership block vote. The three new PLP representatives also looked likely to be a managed addition to this leadership block, although in 1999 a revolt in the PLP freed them up (see Chapter 13, pp. 423–4). Just as significant, the changes had strengthened the Leader by driving off the NEC MPs elected by the CLPs who might have built up as the Leader's rivals. They also, as it happened, drove off some who had a record on the NEC of supporting independent initiatives relating to party and government. These included Blunkett over elements of Partnership in Power, Straw over trade union representation in the party and especially Clare Short over the same issues and many more.

Managing elections

Much of the NEC representation was still outside the immediate influence of the managers. The trade union section elections were covered by various unwritten trade union rules, particularly representation by size, and the party managers continued to have little direct influence on the choice of union representatives. The elected section from local government section was independent, although if the latter had produced 'oppositionists' there might have developed more managerial intervention. The Treasurer continued to be a leading trade unionist, agreed privately between the unions with some consultation with the leadership, although then elected by the whole conference. The election for the affiliated socialist societies' seat since the counter-Bennite revolt of 1981 and 1982 was an uncontested representative of the loyalist right, in this period Dianne Hayter.

The major battles and management politics took place over elections for the CLP sections, but there was often at this time also a fierce controversy over the Youth Section seat. The outcome of these first elections held under Partnership in Power rules in 1998 were thought of as an opportunity to register a public symbol of the changing party and in practical terms to move the NEC into an accommodating frame of mind.

Youth section

The youth section was untypical in its history and organisational form, but its internal politics and elections were nevertheless an illuminating expression of Labour management values and practices. The youth organisation was always prone to fall into the hands of one grouping or another of the left, and that target ideally fitted the anti-oppositionist drive by Blairite party managers – some of whom had come through the anti-Trotskyist battle inside Labour Students. The youth organisation had a looser constitutional structure than other affiliated organisations, easier for participants to cheat and harder for the organisation to keep to timetables and rules. Hence there were invariably multiple technical infringements. The politics was complicated also by the fact that the loyalist faction worked with the assistance of the research staff of the AEEU and the right-wing organisation Labour First, helped also by their rule book which stipulated that Labour students' officers must accept the line management of national party officials. On the other side in this period, the left worked with the research staff of another union, MSF, who like their AEEU colleagues were often ex-participants in student politics.

The crucial managerial focus was in controlling the Labour youth conference, which met every two years and elected the youth representative on Labour's NEC. Party headquarters at Millbank routinely gave advice to its favoured candidates and was adept at ruling out other candidates on the grounds of technical infringement. It was a practice which could at times severely embarrass the modernising youth loyalists who did not want to see abuse of rules, and thought it too heavy-handed and undermining to their reputation for integrity. In a bold letter of complaint sent to the General Secretary on 21 March 2001, Clare McCarthy and Phil Pinder, supported by others from a wide spectrum of views and sections of the youth organisation, made known their objections to managerial behaviour, but it had little effect on the interventions. This was 'serious politics'.

CLP representation and management

The procedural background and management

As already noted, NEC results in Opposition through OMOV ballots never quite lived up to expectations of a resultant political shift. In 1994, Cook, Blunkett, Brown and Harman were elected and Straw replaced Kinnock, but the leftist Skinner came back. Under quota rules which guaranteed two women's places, Diane Abbott came on and not Mowlem.

For 1995, in response to complaints, new guidelines were issued which stopped the circulation of campaigning material by candidates to CLPs in order to create a level playing field. Candidates were allowed to circulate collectively, at party expense, only a short statement. But in practice, in the years that followed, there were no limits on expenditure, and it seems little attempt by the party officials to monitor it.

After a surge of new members and with new rules of women's representation giving them at least three out of the seven seats, there were high hopes from around the Leader's office that a big shift would take place away from the left in the CLP elections. Yet the 1995 results were fairly similar to those of the previous year. Harman held her position and increased her vote. Mowlem, one of Blair's election managers, replaced Straw who had been another manager, via the women's quota. But, from the left, Abbot and Skinner were still on, and that result contrasted with and spoiled the image of a clean sweep of leadership victories in policy votes declared at the conference. The following year, whilst Blair preserved the managerial grip on the conference policies, his second year of total policy victories, the NEC CLP section remained unchanged.

In 1997, following Brown's resignation, the NEC contest that followed was a symbolic test of support for 'New Labour', with Peter Mandelson fighting for a position against Ken Livingstone – a left bête noire of the 'New Labour' leadership. Mandelson's defeat, with Livingstone's vote up by 43 per cent over the previous year's, together with a continuing rise in Skinner's vote, were huge blows to the vision of OMOV as a mechanism for undermining the left and strengthening the leadership. The Socialist Campaign Group in Parliament diagnosed the emergence of a new left with OMOV votes more left-wing than the votes in Conference.[21] Consequently, the section began to be seen by the managers as a dangerous entry point for a resurgent oppositional left. All this added again to the sense of justification for what the managers had to do to deliver 'a good result'.

The CLP Section after 1997

In one aspect, the leadership's worst fears were successfully precluded by the new rules that allowed only 'rank-and-file' candidates to stand in the CLP section of six seats, of whom three must be women. It did become a means of avoiding a public display of CLP support for PLP dissidents and a means of impeding a move to prominence of any alternative political leadership. For their part, the left outside Parliament was now reorganised into a potentially broader base of the Grassroots Alliance between Labour Reform, a cross-factional grouping for party democracy and the Campaign For Labour Party Democracy which had a left-wing as well as an organisational reform agenda. It was essentially a procedural alliance focusing on party democracy and accountability and heavily critical of the 'New Labour' style of management. The prefix 'Centre Left' became more firmly added to the title in an attempt to show breadth and also to neutralise the attack on 'extremists', but the whole thing was a mouthful and the Grassroots Alliance (GRA) was how it had been and generally still was known inside and outside the organisation.

The main driving force behind the GRA came from the left but it was not confined to that section. The GRA slate of six, first in the field in the election battle of 1998, was Liz Davies, Christine Shawcross, Pete Willsman, Mark Seddon, and Cathy Jameson, all from the left, and Andy Howell from the right. One result of the growing reaction to management 'control freakery' was that in the summer of 1998 GRA candidates were receiving support not only from the *Morning Star*, the *Tribune* and the

New Statesman but also from the *Guardian*. Its editorial on 28 May 1998 described a party 'In the grip of Millbank' practising 'a degree of control freakishness that borders on the obsessive', and an editorial on 10 August 1998 gave the opposition support in praise of 'Labour diversity'.

This was the big party battle that the leadership and the managers had been waiting for. The GRA had to be defeated. Mandelson's candidature in this section in 1997 had been encouraged from No. 10 Downing Street. In the aftermath of his defeat there were severe internal disagreements between the General Secretary and Deputy General Secretary on the one side and the No. 10 Political Office on the other, over the political management of the elections. Following one of these rows when Blair took a different view to that of Sawyer, he decided to resign as General Secretary after the party conference of 1998.

Initially the issue was over the degree of inclusivity of the pro-leadership slate in NEC elections. Here party-headquarters managers had been the first into action. McDonagh's decision, supported by the General Secretary, to work with the traditional right – the Labour First Organisation (in a grouping here called 'Members First') – was for her a practical organisational arrangement to counter the organised left, as well as a useful link to old allies. She mixed this with bringing in some candidates with high name recognition. The six on her slate were Michael Cashman, Diana Jeuda, Jack McConnell, Margaret Payne, Rita Stringfellow and Terry Thomas. But the Political Office in Downing Street approved of neither the slate nor the way it was produced. This became a battle over political judgement but also for territory and control over the links to those who would be elected. In this melee, the traditional-right Labour First organisation put up its own separate slate of only five candidates, Adrian Bailey, Maggie Cosen, Val Price, Mary Southcott and Sylvia Tudhope, with no overlap with the other slate. The election campaign on behalf of the pro-leadership slate was thus weakened by the arm-wrestling and by too many candidates. But that was not its only problem.

Campaigning and managerial partisans

In an extraordinary election campaign fought with broad-ranging managerial assistance, the central party organisation was clearly and openly partisan on behalf of the 'Members First' loyalist slate. The General Secretary Tom Sawyer, and the ex-Leader Neil Kinnock, attacked GRA candidates, particularly Liz Davies, in the press whilst the election was going on. No NEC election campaign in history had been fought by party officials showing so little pretence of impartiality. This was 'serious politics'.

A 'clandestine spin operation' was run from No. 10 as well as from Millbank.[22] The GRA was portrayed as a cover for hard-left 'oppositionists'. The main driving force behind the GRA did come from the left but it was a varying left and also had a few significant pro-democracy recruits from the traditional right. But the counter-attack from the confident managers portrayed them as a cover for hard-left 'oppositionists'. The most left-wing Liz Davies was consistently but incorrectly described as a Trotskyist. Some journalists close to No. 10 went further. In her book Davies points particularly to the article by David Aaronovitch in the *Independent* warning that in these elections 'the Trots are back with a vengeance'.[23]

Across the party, all the party managers were encouraged to get active. The whips' office discreetly encouraged loyalist MPs to assist in getting the right outcome.[24] In some constituencies identical letters were sent on behalf of local Labour MPs, advocating support for the Members First slate.[25] The spirit of the financial controls proposed in 1994–5 over NEC and Leadership elections appears to have been forgotten in the urgency of the delivery in 1998. Party communicational facilities were used to organise and press the managerial case – a use which appeared to be the normality under succeeding General Secretaries under 'New Labour'. This was justified by some of the HQ managers as a legitimate counter to the liberal-left press which was said in headquarters to be 'ganging up' against 'the government'. At this time the behaviour of Millbank was described in a *Guardian* editorial as acting with 'a degree of control freakishness that borders on the obsessive'.[26] The AEEU gave substantial financial support to help with various forms of loyalist communication. On behalf of the loyalist slate, large advertisements appeared in the *Observer*, *Guardian* and *New Statesman*. Pete Willsman, chair of the GRA, estimated that the GRA campaign cost £3,000 whilst the Members First organisation spent £150,000.[27] We have been 'massively outspent', they complained to the media.[28]

There developed an aura of desperation around some of this managerial activity. It was clear to one candid NEC loyalist in the middle of an election that the managers had advance information of the way things were going – and they were not going well. A similar point was made later to me by an ex-senior party official: 'We knew more than we should have done.' As was becoming the norm, rules were treated with a flexibility that advantaged the loyalist candidates. To secure maximum turnout, telephone voting was allowed without the NEC being directly consulted;[29] it was said that the NEC had already approved the principle of telephone voting. The loyalist managers' slate also appeared to have access to the party's membership lists.[30]

All this failed to have the expected party response. The result, announced at the conference, was a considerable blow to the management; four GRA supporters, Davies, Jameson, Seddon and Willsman, were elected. Overall, the managerial tactics had badly rebounded. Lance Price, a No. 10 spin doctor, confessed later that they had 'successfully branded the so-called Grassroots Alliance as hard Left' but had not had much success in raising the profile of their own candidates.[31] They had also shown little anticipation that worried party members might be tempted to register a protest vote against managerial manipulation and it took a long time for 'control freakery' to fully register in No. 10 as an albatross nurtured by the managerial methods. It had been very rare for anybody from the leadership to imply criticism of the party management activities of the officials, but at the meeting of the NEC on November 17 Deputy Leader Prescott expressed unhappiness with some of the things that had happened in the NEC elections, and sought a fresh start. There were calls at that meeting for a ceiling on expenditure (which had been agreed in 1995) to be applied, and for party staff to act with impartiality. The lack of 'a level playing field' continued to be raised on and off the NEC for years to come.

The results, the backlash and the emergence of a new left-wing think tank, Catalyst, led the No. 10 Political Office to a deeper reappraisal of what might be happening. There was, from Cruddas, a focus on the dangers of contests being typecast as 'control freaks' versus 'pluralists'. A new suggestion was of the creation of a broader-based umbrella alliance as a Blairite movement. But for reasons already explained in Chapter 5, it never came about. Instead other lessons were drawn. The election of ex-TV star Michael Cashman on the Members First Slate confirmed to Millbank the value of name recognition in a vote where turnout had declined markedly from that under the old arrangements. After a long and acrimonious post-mortem between the Political Office at No. 10 and the old and new General Secretaries, the overlap of pro-leadership slates was made much greater, and managerial tactics changed.

For nearly a hundred years, there had been a fixed timetable for NEC elections based around the party conference in October and then, in 1998, in the period leading up to it. From 1999 this became a changeable date in May/June thus breaking constituency routines and ensuring that, whatever happened, it received less attention and would not affect the presentation of the conference as a triumph for the leadership. As Clare Short had warned and CLPD lamented, it also affected participation. By 1999 participation had dropped by 45 per cent on 1997, the last year of the old composition and of stable timing.

In increasing the number of extra high-profile candidates, thus heightening name recognition, the ex-General Secretary Lord Sawyer, hitherto an evangelist for rank-and-file representation, was now in the Lords and standing in the 'rank-and-file' CLP section (a possibility allowed but unnoticed under the rules drafted whilst he himself was General Secretary). Another surprise was that Michael Cashman was still allowed to take his seat on the NEC although by that time he was an MEP. The GRA lost Willsman, a result attributed by them to the two strong personal votes. But there was something else that was significant happening here. Although the Grassroots Alliance vote at 47.7 per cent was greater than that of the slate supported by headquarters, at 43.8 per cent, it had not gained in strength quite as it expected. The signs were that the organised left-wing base was shrinking, with some of its former supporters leaving the party, as CLPD acknowledged.[32] To that extent, party management was being made easier.

The following year the election was brought even further forward to April/May, coinciding now with local elections which again drew attention away from the party contest. For financial reasons, it was said, the ballot paper and documents envelope was tucked inside the rather boring party newsletter *Inside Labour*, instead of being sent separately. You might notice it, you might not. There was certainly some likelihood that it would be thrown away as junk mail. It may have helped the finances but it did not help the participation of members and it heightened the already strong suspicion of 'Millbank tricks'.

One target of the pro-leadership slate was achieved. Seddon came fifth, but as a result of the rules on the quota of women was off the NEC. Cathy Jamison of the GRA had stood down, but on to the NEC now came two very different political animals from the GRA. Ann Black has started on the centre-right and voted for Blair to be Leader. She was now an independent centrist in policy terms. But she gave huge attention and brought encyclopaedic knowledge to the defence of constitutional propriety and the spirit of Partnership in Power. Christine Shawcross, on the other hand, was a classic militant traditional socialist. With Davies from the left still on, the GRA again had three representatives. Top of the poll came Tony Robinson, another famous TV actor and party activist. He was a loyalist but increasingly critical of control freakery and the manipulations of the managers. He would have stood regardless of the slates but Margaret McDonagh saw him as an impediment to the GRA and someone who would generally support the Leader in crunch votes and he was put on the official slate. Successful also on that slate was a high-profile and articulate loyalist Shahid Malik, the first Asian ever on the NEC. Sawyer, because of his high profile it is assumed, was re-elected despite the advance indications and a poor record of attendance and activity on the NEC.

In spite of the reaction against control freakery and a new if uncertain adjustment from No. 10 Downing Street, the Millbank managers kept doing their business over organising elections for the NEC. Advance financial restrictions were still not applied to NEC elections. In 2001 Sawyer stood down from his position to give more time to his business responsibilities. Liz Davies also stood down, highly critical of Labour's business connections and government policy. In April 2001 she resigned from the party. Attempts were made to replace Sawyer by another peer, Joyce Gould, the ex-Director of Party Organisation after nomination by her CLP, Brighton Kemptown. But it turned out that they had nominated Willie Sullivan.[33] Later it was privately confirmed by a senior party official that support for Sullivan had been switched to Gould after informal consultation initiated not from Gould but from the General Secretary's Office. An NEC resolution proposed by Ann Black referred to a report from several members that Millbank party staff had initiated the switch and that this had not been denied.[34] The General Committee of the local party, which met again three days after the closing date, could not reverse the decision. The procedure was publicly reported by CLPD as 'Millbank manipulation rejected'[35] and Gould, who had not known of the circumstances surrounding Sullivan's loss of nomination,[36] failed to get elected. It showed a changing anti-control freakery mood in the party but also an extraordinary invulnerability in managerial behaviour.

Mark Seddon returned to the NEC bringing the GRA back up to three. It was indicative of the growing party resentment at control freakery that in 2001 Shahid Malik, Tony Robinson and Ruth Turner, who had all been on the Millbank slate in 2000, this year more clearly designated themselves as 'independents' and with two others stood on their own slate. Although they also again received support via the Millbank organisation, they developed a new emphasis on more members' participation and more transparency. Robinson again topped the poll, with Black in second place and two others from the GLA, Shawcross and Seddon, elected. Ruth Turner was also elected. Party-headquarters managers had some reason to be pleased that in the era of increasing challenge to control freakery, the left had been held back. But the new arrangements had contributed to a decline in participation. Using 1997 as a base, the turnout had declined each year and by 2001 it had declined by 71 per cent,[37] a blow to the health and legitimacy of the process, but that took second place to the priorities of management.

Trade union group and new loyalism

The NEC trade union group, comprising the representatives on the trade union section of the committee plus the Treasurer and union representatives in the women's section, continued to be a key element in the politics of the NEC. It met on the evening before every NEC meeting to consider its attitude to what was on the agenda. The historic tradition of group members to work in solidarity with the party and a Labour government continued under Blair albeit, as has been shown, with some difficulties in the early days. Their sense of responsibility and of political and organisational realities and their consciousness of their historic role made them a routine managerial asset. Regular representation of major unions on the committee facilitated through customary inter-union arrangements facilitated the passing on of their traditions and practices. Normally nothing of their internal disagreements was publicly revealed.

Their long service, availability and freedom to do party work meant that they were placed on all the important subcommittees and, for the ultra-loyalists particularly, the newly strengthened Organisation Committee and the Joint Policy Committee. The most senior generally took the chairs of committees and became members of an inner group called the Officers Group. As longer-serving members of the NEC they annually became in turn vice-Chairman then Chairman of the NEC and therefore also of the party. All these were also personal status gains.

As a result of these positions, after 1997 they met ministers frequently and moved closer to sharing their burdens as a part of the government political scene. That gave a new sense of personal importance and of a wider responsibility than their union representation. Through patronage from No. 10, that could also assist advancement after their occupational retirement. With the managers looking for committed and experienced loyalists who would be assiduous House of Lords attendees, a significant number of the post-1994 loyalists of the NEC trade union group eventually became peers: Tom Burlison, Gordon Colling, Maggie Jones, Margaret Prosser, Richard Rosser, Tom Sawyer and Margaret Wall.

Because members of the General Council were prohibited from sitting on the NEC the trade union section representatives were normally second-rank leaders of varying ability and personal authority. In general, there was from them more of a tendency to awe and deference than from the senior union officials, who were themselves not immune from it. The unusual distinction that had been made in the early days of Blair's leadership between solidarity with the party and support for what the Leader wanted on non-policy issues became much diminished as the election approached and then the party moved into government. Most union representatives in this period after some initial hesitation also became more personally impressed by Blair and more appreciative of his leadership qualities. The gains for working people after 1997 added to their sense of joining in an achievement. Accepting partnership with No. 10 they tended to be more influenced by governmental views about the weaknesses and failings of the unions, and suffered some disorientation about who constituted 'us' and 'our' obligations. All this helps explain a tendency over time for some union representatives to 'go native', especially if they held an official party post.

As for the policy issues after 1997, in the knowledge that the NEC had lost its policy committee, rarely did the group discuss policy at all, although on some specific issues which were a preoccupation of individual unions their concern could find an expression. Unusually, between October and December 1998, at a time of considerable anxiety over the developing employment relations legislation following newspaper reports that Fairness at Work might be diluted, that subject was raised on the Leader's report. The most significant, though low-key, contribution at that time was that of Margaret Prosser, convenor of the group, with arguments couched not as demands but in terms of justice and the ability of the party to motivate its core voters. The matter was taken no further by the union group and they made no attempt to use the NEC's initiating and responding role over policy at the conference as a means of pressure on the government.

The general secretary and 'the four Margarets'

The background relationships of the group with the party's General Secretary and the No. 10 Political Office were important. If the group-meeting discussions found a significant problem, it was expected that it would be dealt with discreetly so as not to give ammunition to the media or to left 'oppositionists'. Leading group members could be involved in phone or face-to-face discussions with the General Secretary or the No. 10 Political Office representatives prior to the NEC. Prosser, as the convenor, regularly met with the General Secretary in the afternoon before the NEC and expressed the thrust of the union-group concerns, receiving extra information about the details of the agendas and the reasons behind proposals so that they could be fed to the group. There was no attempt to bind its group members to a line, although that often spontaneously arose in taking along a sense of majority opinion.

'The Four Margarets': modernisation and management politics
The role of Jones and Wall at the core of the small loyalist group supporting Sawyer in pushing Party into Power also affected the drive for its various follow-up consequences for the operation of the NEC. Prosser had been influential in securing some accommodations against the wishes of the Leader and/or General Secretary in the Party into Power project, but as Treasurer of the party she began to wear a harder new 'party' hat. These three kept close links with Sally Morgan and also became close supportive allies of Margaret McDonagh, whose accession to the post of General Secretary in November 1998 coincided with the NEC's strengthened pro-leadership component.

Although there were misgivings on the NEC over McDonagh's appointment and some of her managerial decisions and style, the fact that she was the Leader's appointment, a young woman doing a difficult job at a time when the GRA had made its entry, served to extend loyalty to her. Loyalist union representatives from AEEU and USDAW regularly gave their support, as did even representatives of unions thought of as critical – Steve Pickering of GMB and Mike Griffiths of GPMU. But more crucial became the networking of 'the Four Margarets' and, at times, a fifth Margaret, Margaret Wheeler, who was the chair of the Conference Arrangements Committee. She received important protection. Her surprise public push for a change in the law covering all-women short lists may have been the result of their influence. In other aspects there remained a peculiarity here that, at a time when women in the PLP were advocating 'a new politics' and constraining macho management there, loyalist hard-line management by women should be in the driving seat at party headquarters and No. 10, activating at times a very old and heavy politics.

NEC members and union obligations
With two exceptions in this period, Derek Hodgson of the UCW and Richard Rosser of the TSSA, both of whom were union General Secretaries, the union representatives were subordinate within their own union organisation. It was a common misconception that because of this the twelve

trade union section representatives 'all do their general secretary's bidding'.[38] That appeared to be the general picture but it was never quite like that. The role as union representatives had to be reconciled with the responsibilities involved in party representation at its most senior level, but what this entailed for the character of the relationship with the most senior union officer had a different complexion and a variable balance depending on the personal attitude of the individuals and the position they held on the NEC.

The most common view of legitimacy around the NEC was that they must have some autonomy of action, and most of them defended their area of discretion over NEC affairs. In reciprocation, most senior union officers did give them some room for manoeuvre and they avoided close regular oversight. Under the Blair drive sometimes, and from some NEC representatives, the politics involved not keeping the senior official fully informed. This was particularly the case in the way the union leaders were bounced over the loss of the right to resolutions to the party conference. Most union General Secretaries had opposed the curtailment of the independent NEC policy role after 1997, yet once it had happened they did not attempt to intervene to change it.

Margaret Wall of MSF was highly unusual in her avowal that her first obligation was to the party (meaning here its leadership). 'I could not do anything else' was her heartfelt sentiment. It was a radical loyalist view shared in those terms by nobody else in the trade union group. Though the union's General Secretary Roger Lyons was not averse to striking out publicly and critically over some industrial policies, he was not always closely involved in what was happening politically on the NEC. Some relationships did involve the ease of closely shared political alignment. This was particularly true of representatives of the AEEU, regularly loyal and associated with the traditional right. Brenda Etchels, John Allen and, later, John Gribbon coupled this with a discreet background voice over issues which troubled the union.

In the TGWU, although Bill Morris expected to be kept informed and favoured clearer lines between the party and the government, the two TGWU members of the NEC Diana Holland and Margaret Prosser, Treasurer and union-group convenor after 1996, sometimes took different approaches on party issues or where the union position was unclear. In 1999, following the NEC internal reforms and what was seen as the general tendency of union representatives on the NEC to become sunk in party obligation, Morris complained to Prosser about the subordination of the NEC.

Relationships in UNISON were the most unusual and important. Rodney Bickerstaffe was a General Secretary well to the left of the unions' representatives on the NEC and disdainful of 'New Labour'. Yet generally he accepted the inevitabilities of the great shift after Blair's big election victory. Seeking to continue an influential insider strategy that had developed under Smith, normally he left room for the NEC roles of UNISON representatives, notably the party managerial figures Maggie Jones and Anne Picking. He also recognised that the Jones role could have gains for his union's members, whatever his personal political views.

For her part Jones was also adroit in gaining more room for herself, as she had done over the Party into Power discussions. The perspective she had articulated over Partnership in Power was carried into the loyalist reformist role on the NEC. It involved an implicit message to the Leader: 'Leave it to us. You are too busy to be involved in all this. We will deal with it for you.' Her view was that working people were gaining from a well-supported Labour Government and that UNISON representatives in different forums acting as management loyalists were listened to, especially over the issue of the two-tier workforce. (See Chapters 10, 16 and 17.)

In the first term of government, a discreet loyalism also affected GPMU representative Mike Griffiths, who kept close but not always forthcoming relations with his General Secretary Tony Dubbins, a critic of the Government and a tactician of union involvement in the PLP. Griffiths at this stage played a low-key supportive role on the NEC as vice chair of the Organisation Committee. USDAW was different again. Its votes were usually robustly loyal except on issues where there was a powerful movement within the union. Even then an opposition vote was avoided by John Hannett. What made USDAW especially different was Diana Jeuda, a women's-section representative. She played a singular and high-profile role traced already over Partnership in Power and found a self-directed role over party government and organisational issues. She could occasionally move strongly to a verbally dissentient policy position but also avoided an opposition vote.

The very few union general secretaries on the committee did not behave in the same way. Alan Johnson, a member of the committee from 1993 to 1997 representing the CWU, was an ardent Blair supporter and behaved accordingly. On becoming an MP, he was replaced by another general secretary, Derek Hodgson, a traditional Labour-right loyalist who kept close links to Jon Cruddas and John Prescott but was not a regular at the trade union group meetings, a pattern that kept him free of that influence. His distinctiveness lay in his adroit use of union and public support in defence of his own union policy, especially over a publicly owned Post Office where he was prepared to cross lines of assertiveness in party forums that others shied away from. In contrast and more typical of trade union group behaviour, the TSSA representative Richard Rosser, convenor of the trade union group from 1996 to 1997, behaved in accord with the group and right-wing loyalist tradition.

After 1997, the pressures from loyalist management were such that union representatives who stopped 'playing ball' could find their operation on the NEC more difficult. A disillusioned RMT representative, Vernon Hince, very much a pillar of the traditional Labour right in his union and desperately trying to keep up with the sharply changing political landscape, complained at the NEC about the ministerial treatment of the railways dispute. He was thereafter increasingly described as 'off-side' and was even partially side-lined when acting as Chair of the NEC. Edmonds from the GMB became increasingly frustrated with the NEC's limitations and management tactics and more anxious to keep tighter links with the union's NEC representatives, Steve Pickering and Mary Turner. In 1999, the GMB broke ranks and their duo of representatives voted with the GRA on policies to assist the manufacturing sector and also against the outsourcing of party membership, over which GMB members held administrative posts. But the alignment was temporary and continued to be highly unusual, although Turner often spoke out.

The GRA and managing the NEC

This behaviour of the NEC union representatives baffled and affronted the GRA members who came on in 1998. Their organisation had been born out of dissatisfaction with the performance of leading figures on the parliamentary left and they were always anticipating unprincipled deviance and career-oriented moves. They rarely appreciated the clash of responsibilities and the difficult reconciliation that had to take place. What they thought they saw was union representatives unwilling to stand up for union policies and they thought that somebody had to do it. GRA members were prone to produce for the NEC, without even prior informal discussion with the trade union representatives, resolutions which they saw as principled and often in line with union mandates. They would later complain: 'Why did they not support their union policy as they should do?'

Within the trade union group this aroused long-held disdain for 'impractical idealists' and 'posturers' aiming not to solve problems but to appeal to an outside audience. They were seen as causing unnecessary difficulties by placing before the committee statements worded simply to embarrass the Labour government. Even where the union representatives privately supported the criticism and proposals coming from the GRA, there was generally a determination not to give them any open boost. Tactically, it was a regular feature that whoever was the NEC Chair called them first to provide the target and to stir up loyal support. The preferred chosen method of dealing with the issue was then to find some procedural mechanism for avoiding a direct vote on the substantive issue. Side-lining their initiatives for procedural reasons, even on issues which aroused substantial concern on the NEC, became routine. All this was accompanied by a renewed secretiveness. Even to members of the NEC, information including details of internal elections results and membership could be very sluggish in appearing.

Davies, Seddon and Willsman tried to play a barrack-room-lawyer role at different times in defence of party procedures, but they were hampered by their ideological definition, and their unremitting opposition role. Later, when she came on the NEC, Ann Black's one-woman counter-management operation did add a new dimension to the GRA activities. She slowly carved out a unique position as a party commentator and constitutionalist, producing a massive output of information and judgement. Her reports were couched in tones of restrained objectivity and occasional regret rather than anger. Over time she became a significant player on the NEC although, in this period, gaining very little, a point that others registered in justification for their more open and abrasive attacks. Perhaps nothing would have significantly changed the managerial operation and its methods.

Undermining the NEC

Partnership in Power had emphasised a strengthened role for the NEC.[39] Sawyer had argued during Party into Power meetings that reform of the NEC would raise its status. The final document had proposed that 'to raise the profile of the NEC in the Party[40] there would be an annual development plan . . . widely distributed . . . for discussion at annual conference'.[41] There would also be 'a much fuller debate' on the NEC Report.[42] In practice there was no such annual plan and no systematic attempt was made to have regular fuller debate on the NEC report. That report became the 'Party report' and then in 2000 the 'annual report' with the reference to the NEC dropped. As for the options and alternatives in organisational change 'where appropriate'[43] it was never found to be appropriate and so there was never a vote on them.

Media attention on the NEC meetings was generally discouraged by the media managers' indications that it was of little significance. Elections held away from the conference also reduced media and party attention. NEC meetings which had once been closed to other than committee members, unless by invitation or advance agreement, were now filled with any number of staff and government representatives who just wandered in and out. The NEC liaison role with the Conference Arrangements Committee and as appeal court against the committee's provisional decisions was abandoned without advance information or reference within the Party into Power discussions. The Joint Policy Committee acting as arrangements committee for the NPF was chosen by the General Secretary and there was no right of appeal through the NEC against JPC decisions in that role. The NEC received no papers from the JPC. It is difficult not to see all this as the systematic subversion of the role and profile of the NEC.

Discipline and disputes

The NEC had long had the duty and powers 'to uphold and enforce the constitution, rules and standing orders of the party and to take any actions it deems necessary for such purpose'.[44] Over the years, this had involved the committee in discussion and adjudication over many internal disputes and individual disciplinary cases. But this part of the NEC's work also declined after 1994. The Disputes Committee of the NEC had been one of its most active committees, dealing with high-level cases. But in 1997 it became a subcommittee of the NEC Organisation Committee dealing mainly with low-level local cases over issues of membership, suspensions and selections. Such matters rarely surfaced on the NEC.

Much of the NEC's past disciplinary role had been taken over by the National Constitutional Committee, and after 1997 there was a big decline in the number of cases dealt with. At first sight this appeared to indicate a new tolerance at odds with the prevailing managerial mood. But what became clear later was that the image of the iron grip and the disappointments of Partnership in Power reinforcing decline in party membership led increasing numbers of left-wing dissidents simply to become inactive or to depart. Seeing this the party managers, worried over the costs in time of NCC cases, were generally prepared to play a longer game of waiting for them to move into passivity or go.

They also had other procedures which could be discreetly used. In 1999 a new local government reselection interview panel system was brought in to help improve the quality of Labour councillors. They needed improvement, but there were occasions when existing councillors who were simply politically troublesome were forced out through this re-examination. That could rebound. One well-known example was Christine Shawcross, who after twelve years was prevented from standing again as a councillor in Tower Hamlets by a selection panel in 1998. She became a cause célèbre on the left[45] and as a much publicised dissident, like Davies, was elected to the NEC in 1998 and then re-elected for years after. Experiences like that reinforced the indignation of GRA representatives.

Elections to the National Constitutional Committee became heavily factionalised, with party loyalists always mindful of the need to protect the party and the left influenced by its concern for the protection of dissenters. Pete Willsman, elected to the committee in 1996, was said by his ally to have 'tried his best to prevent expulsions and disciplinary action against left-wingers'.[46] To the loyalists this was not a recommendation. As in relation to the NEC, OMOV balloting became seen as problematic by the managers, particularly as so many of the candidates were political unknowns. On the NEC, 27 July 1999, it was agreed that elections to the NCC should change from OMOV balloting to election by Conference delegates which was a process working so well for the managers over NPF elections. (See Chapter 10, p. 313.)

Control, dissent and the growth of the new centre

Old dissenters and new alignments

In the ways indicated, the NEC became a more managed and diminished body by 1998. Significant decisions, expected to be those of the NEC, could be taken 'somewhere' without consultation with the committee. Or the attempt was made to slip them through without much observation.

When the Secretariat was constrained by the NEC decisions or reactions, the officials could later return to the agenda with different tactics and a chosen timing. Party headquarters at Millbank developed a reputation which became synonymous with control.

Because of the NEC's weakness, it was tempting for observers to follow the spin and see the NEC as a completely passive committee of little importance. Yet that tendency was accompanied by another. Behind what appeared and was often presented as unanimity of support was a rumbling reaction again the threat or practice of managerial control. That grew stronger after 1998. The developing reaction to the commanding style of McDonagh on the NEC, in the context of a wider party and public unease about managerial control of 'New Labour' over candidate selections and elections, gradually gave more room for the growth of a new centre on the NEC.

Hayter from the socialist societies and Jeuda from the women's section were part of it. In the trade union section Diana Holland (TGWU) and Muriel Turner (GMB) in different ways forcefully articulated critical positions. Helen Jackson and Dennis Skinner, representatives from the PLP, did the same. The loyalist local government representatives Jeremy Beecham and Sally Powell had an increasingly critical stance over local government, and also pressed for more open respect for rules in the management of the party. They had all also become increasingly resentful at the lack of adequate consultation of those not in the inner circle, although they had no intention of directly confronting the activities of the machine or publicly criticising the General Secretary, and they remained inhibited by the past reputation of the NEC, by their own loyalty and by a reluctance to join with the 'oppositionist' GRA in critical attacks. But behind the scenes, in networking responses with others or putting down markers in judicious contributions to the NEC, they began to exercise a greater resistance and counterbalance to the Secretariat.

Tension also built up between the management in headquarters and in No. 10. Other than in terms of the dangers of the committee sending damaging messages to the electorate, the No. 10 Political Office by 1998 became relatively unconcerned with internal NEC affairs; McDonagh was left in control or uncontrollable. Fractious personal relations between McDonagh and Morgan contributed to this distancing. Morgan's attitude towards occasional loyalist critics such as Hayter and Jeuda was that, as they were solid when the chips were down they had earned the right to put their own lines on some issues and to pursue a different course over party government. McDonagh took a heavier line against dissent.

The management of reform

The propensity to revolt that had been there under Sawyer over the reform proposals took a sharper edge on 1 November 1998, which was the first meeting of the expanded NEC with McDonagh as General Secretary. The committee had before them an NEC code of conduct requiring NEC members to inform the party's press office 'before discussing NEC business with the media'. It came also with some general guidelines on the communicational conduct of members of the NEC. The proposal had arisen out of the NEC's own away-day discussions and concerned genuine issues of confidentiality and avoiding 'helping the Tories'. It explicitly stated that nothing in the code would be used in an attempt to suppress or silence debate on the NEC or to restrict the right of NEC members to express publicly their views. But the media managers repetitive public spin about Blair's control, the partisan conduct of the NEC elections, rows over the Euro-selections, and McDonagh's iron lady reputation, all undermined the acceptability of the code. 'Control freakery is the buzz word of our times in the Labour Party' said a BBC *Today* programme announcer on 16 November 1998. Tight control, always seen by the leadership and managers as an asset in winning public support, became publicly identified as a significant problem.

The NEC accepted the paper on the code of conduct with some division of focus between those who emphasised support for collective responsibility and others with reservations and a range of criticisms. There were important suggested amendments which would narrow the range of issues to finance, membership staffing, party strategy and other confidential issues. Significantly, in a discussion held after Blair had left the meeting, Prescott moved that the code be regarded as simply a guidance note. In the end, although three from the GRA abstained and only Liz Davies voted against, the guidance note was not controversially operated. According to Davies, she had never seen a hint of the much-vaunted division between Blair and Prescott.[47] The answer to that was that in part she was never meant to see it, so mindful was Prescott of the presentation of unity with Blair and so distrustful was he of what some in the GRA would feed out to the world. But here as in other places the Deputy Leader was a significant force on important procedural issues.

NEC July 1999: Chief Whip's report

Perhaps the most important disciplinary function retained by the NEC was that under the rules it retained the right to refuse or withdraw endorsement of a candidate if they failed to accept or act in harmony with the standing orders of the PLP.[48] From the General Election of 1997 there was a strong and repetitive spin that action would be taken against repeated dissent by MPs when the time came for them to be reselected. *The Times* report 'Blair to purge left wing' was a typical early headline.[49]

The new procedural document agreed by the NEC and the 1998 conference stated that the Chief Whip 'shall present a report to the NEC detailing unauthorised absences and abstentions with votes against the Whip' and 'may recommend to the NEC that they interview MPs with exceptionally poor records prior to endorsement'.[50] In a consultation there had been over 90 per cent support from CLPs that 'the whips' factual information on attendances and voting be made available to constituency parties'.[51] Defensively the document also stated that 'it is not intended that this process be part of the PLP's disciplinary procedures'.[52] Yet that appeared to be opened up in a 1999 NEC document which said that an 'exceptionally poor record' was also to include 'honouring their undertakings to follow the Whip'.[53]

The report had been awaited with some trepidation by dissenting MPs and by *Tribune* which reported that the deselection haunted left Labour MPs. The threat of action was also fought over privately amongst PLP managers. (See Chapter 12, pp. 421–4.) That battle, plus the new awareness of the adverse opinion growing in the media and the party over 'control freakery', explains why plans to act on it in the NEC could not be straightforward, and particularly not be attached to Blair. There was no majority in the NEC trade union group in favour of NEC action, and when the report was introduced to the NEC by the Chief Whip, on 27 July 1999, she made no recommendation. The trade union group convenor Margaret Prosser, in a politically ambiguous contribution to the NEC, proposed a meeting between the officers and the Chief Whip with a view to deferring reselection of serial offenders. Some, including the PLP officials present, interpreted this as a hard-line attempt to assist the Chief Whip, the General Secretary and No. 10 Political Office by giving legitimacy to future NEC action. It met their strong opposition.

Soley, the PLP Chairman, said it was a matter between the CLP and the MP. Prescott was in favour of taking action against some absentee MPs but asserted that this was a matter for the PLP and the CLPs not the NEC; he urged that the NEC should not interfere until constituency parties had responded. That was taken by the NEC generally as that the report simply be noted, a frustration for the forces seeking sanctions. Nevertheless, in September 1999 the minutes of the July NEC meeting recorded that the committee had agreed to give further consideration to the issue of the voting records of MPs,[54] but this version of events was contested at the next NEC and the challenge was not disputed. The committee did not return to the issue and no action was ever taken on the whip's report. It grew to be the view thereafter that Prosser's intervention was a long grass signal that 'the trade union group did not favour action on MPs'. At some point also, No. 10 decided in the light of public condemnation of the managerial handling of Livingstone's candidature for London mayor (see Chapter 12, pp. 387–96) that any deselections would be divisive and would again draw more attention to what was being labelled 'control freakery'. That also became the message down the machine. Control freakery which had impeded action in the PLP had now generated an incapacity of the NEC to manage PLP sanctions.

Local party reform

The growing mood of anti-control freakery and distrust of the centre also had its effect on the reception for proposals for local party reform. A strong body of opinion amongst the Kinnockites, then the Blairites, had focused for some time on the off-putting culture and language, the priorities, the bureaucratic arrangements and the structures of local party government. On 22 June 1999, the front pages of the *Guardian* and the *Independent* carried reports of an internal report from the Director of the North West Region, David Evans, who in 1999 was made Assistant General Secretary. It had an attractive emphasis on making party members active participants in the political process, not passive bystanders. It also advocated replacing the General Committees of elected delegates by all-member meetings which would annually elect a small executive committee.[55] This specific local reform was understood to have the backing of Blair and Mandelson as a means of strengthening modernising forces and weakening 'Old Labour' elements.

McDonagh herself was not very happy with some of the proposals. She favoured more branch rather than GC activity and did not initially push the agenda. However, by 1999, after the adverse June European results in which Labour's seats were reduced from 62 to 29, there was strong party criticism of the process of selection and of the national organisation of the campaign. At the NEC meeting of 27 July 1999 it was argued that the NEC had been 'bullied' into accepting the fait accompli of a process whereby members campaigned for candidates they had not selected. It was in that context that the Millbank report on the election results refocused the criticism by precipitating a questioning of the local party structure as unsuitable for current campaigning needs. Ian McCartney, Chairman of the NEC's party development task force, emphasised the need for reform, as did McDonagh. It would be carried in a 20th Century Party document.

But given the recent history of the NEC elections, the cavalier treatment of OMOV in Wales and over the European elections, and the extensive controls over the mayoral selection in London, the party headquarters had declining credibility over issues of democratic reform, even amongst some loyal supporters and modernisers. Now to add to this problem came a Mandelson media intervention with an unfortunate title including the words 'say hello to virtual labour'.[56] Distrustful conservatism coupled with a lack of consultation with the unions also meant that this was seen as a pre-liminary to an attack on the local unions. Ken Jackson, General Secretary of AEEU, and the loyalist organisation Labour First were adamant that they would not support any weakening of the union input at local-party level. The union loyalist traditional right also saw the reform as a possible means by which the left at some point could advance.

A more basic problem was that one proposal for the form of reform had been seized on by its proponents and made into a totem with not too much evidence to support it. The case for all-member meetings was found, in practice, to produce mixed results in terms of attendance, local activity and electoral success, and to produce its own problems.[57] Enfield Southgate CLP was initially presented as an ideal model by advocates of reform, but later the CLP partially reversed its changes, as it became increasingly clear that all-member meetings were not necessarily effective in fulfilling all the different functions of the local party nor of enhancing a sense of effective participation.

The final replies to the 20th-Century Party consultation document showed that the arguments from the centre had failed to convince. Only 8.7 per cent of members favoured radical change/to get rid of the GC.[58] For the moment, the abolitionist case was dropped and replaced by a policy of encouraging a pluralist and voluntarist reform policy in local parties in which a lot of change was already happening. It also became accepted that it was rational that different types of constituency needed different models. What now became envisaged was local bodies reviewing their activities, seeking best practice with a range of pilot projects to assist them and inviting all members to the GC. The now renamed 21st Century Party document would again be a consultative document and not a commanding arrangement.

NEC and its own agenda November 1999

The Leader's weekly report to the NEC had traditionally taken the form of a speech followed by questions. It invited a regular, if bitty, policy discussion where important signals could be given of NEC opinion. After various pointed interventions by GRA members in 1999 there was increasing irritation by ultra-loyalists that this might become the scene of a series of critical interventions about government policy. It reminded them too much of what they had been told of Callaghan's experience of attacks in the 1976–9 period. Consequently Task Force 1, still led by Maggie Jones, produced a report on 'Making the NEC work better' . . . 'continuing the process of renewal and improvement'[59] and attempted to lay down some guidelines about the behaviour of the NEC following the Leader's report. They included a proposal that items raised following the Leader's report 'should be restricted to the key issues facing the Government and the party'. There was to be 'no automatic speaking right'.

As it happened, the Jones initiative coincided with other union representatives, particularly the GMB's Mary Turner, making a forceful intervention over the proposed closure of Remploy. Jones saw this as an improper use of the Prime Minister's time and of NEC procedures, but there was strong reaction to her position from various sources at the NEC including, significantly, Prescott. Vernon Hince, from the Chair, said that the paper should be noted and comments sent to Jones after which there would be further discussion in January. At the next meeting on 25 January 2000, in a new paper 'Making the NEC work better – an update', Jones's most controversial recommendations were removed. The final paper said simply that the NEC 'might want to give further consideration' to achieving 'a proper dialogue'. The NEC 'noted the paper'. In No. 10 it was said, probably honestly, that the proposals were not a great concern for Blair, and indicated that the ultra-loyalists had moved past him. He was after all supremely deft in dealing with virtually any intervention from anybody at the committee.

Management and counter control

Nevertheless No. 10 continued to support heavy and comprehensive management where it was regarded as necessary even if that did not contribute to protecting the best standards in public life. The NEC was not encouraged to get involved in supervising any of these management operational matters. That prohibition was seen as a corrective to the situation in the 1980s when the NEC was a permanent court of appeal over grievances. In 1998 there had been a leak to Andrew Grice, the *Independent* political correspondent, of the 'fixing' activities of the London liaison team.[60] Later, it was reported that the officer concerned had been removed from the team, and it was said by the party's Chief Media spokesperson Mike Craven to be 'a one-off incident'. But as indicated in Chapter 11 (see pp. 347–8) it was the normality of management practice and nothing came of the incident.

However, by early 1999 a range of issues brought the conduct of party selections and elections – and the conduct of officials – into sharp public as well as party focus. In a compelling article, Trevor Fisher pointed out the NEC elections had been 'dogged by allegations of manipulation and malpractice', and gave the causes for immediate concern being raised by the Stafford and Bermondsey CLPs.[61] There was also criticism of the scrutineer for the Wales election – the Unity Security Balloting Limited. On the NEC, as often was the case, the open complaints came from the Grass Roots Alliance. Privately, there was much more variation in attitudes amongst the loyalists but publicly there was usually a solid phalanx ready to face down these complainants. A report to the NEC on the conduct of national ballots now judged that 'It is clear that a view has developed that there is a legitimate political tactic to be employed by casting doubt on the balloting process'.[62] That may well have been true, but was compatible with the notion that there was something to complain about.

A new code of conduct was introduced, in which it was now laid down that neither candidates nor those acting on their behalf could make public or reported statements designed to bring the 'independent scrutineer' into disrepute or to question the integrity of the conduct of the ballot or the complaints procedure.[63] Legitimate concerns could still be raised privately directly with the scrutineer or appropriate party officials but no publicity should be sought. There were private anxieties expressed by some traditional loyalists about this response[64] and on the NEC by Jeremy Beecham. A proposal came from Seddon that the scrutineer's role be put out to tender. Although only the GRA group of four voted for it, there were notable abstentions by Hilary Armstrong, Jeremy Beecham and Sally Powell.[65]

The business party and sponsorship

The contribution of high-value donations and sponsorship and the huge attendance of business organisations around the party conference had the effect of making it look more like 'Labour Party plc'.[66] At the grass roots, there was growing concern over the commercialisation of the party, especially after headquarters offered a proposal that members could gain discounts on bills and in purchases.[67] There was also continuing irritation over the lack of control over finance in internal party elections and selections. A review of policy on donations, sponsorship, advertising and exhibiting at the party conference and similar activities, and the establishment of criteria for the acceptance of sponsorships, was pressed on the NEC by Davies and Jameson at the January 1999 NEC meeting.[68] But after some delay an alternative review under Professor Keith Ewing was established in March by the Finance Committee. He was asked to report on providing a level playing field for aspiring candidates in selections and equal access to information, including the feasibility of requiring candidates and their supporting organisation to declare their expenses.[69] But no decisions on limits on spending were to be taken before Ewing reported, so any question of limiting sponsorship was on hold. The draft code of practice produced by Ewing was impeccable but, as it happened, the Ewing investigation was never completed. He was asked to do other priority work for the party and eventually, beset by leaks and lack of support on the committee, Ewing moved to other things and the committee never published its work.

Nevertheless, Margaret McDonagh was reported as having accepted at the March NEC in 1999 that all employees should be impartial.[70] A New Procedural Code of Conduct for Candidates and Officers in Elections to National Committees was amended to include the statement that 'All policy staff shall act impartially in the conduct of the elections', and 'No party resources shall be deployed in support of any one candidate or group of candidates'.[71] This did not of not course provide a constraint on the behaviour of party officials who worked to another code of conduct, but that it was there at all says something about the strength of feeling around the issue.

In November 1999 GRA members Mark Seddon and Pete Willsman complained about the conduct of the conference election of the NPF including the partiality by officials.[72] This was a very sore point under Partnership in Power. The General Secretary countered by focusing on complaints received about GRA members' behaviour including, it was said, 'aggressively lobbying and intimidating delegates at the ballot box'.[73] It had become clear that there were no guidelines for elections held at the conference, and it was recommended by the General Secretary that there be a code of conduct for that.[74] The final amended version of that code stated that 'Labour Party staff employed by the National Executive Committee shall not canvas or distribute literature on behalf of any National Policy Forum candidate'.[75] To get some perspective on the operational effect of the new codes it is important to note that when, a few years later, a senior official from this period was asked privately about the application of the code of conduct, the smiling answer was, 'What code of conduct?'

Meanwhile, in the middle of the bitter battle over Livingstone and selection for the mayor's post in London (see Chapter 12, p. 393), No. 10 aides and leading figures on the NEC were now becoming more defensive in the face of a wave of now public as well as party dissatisfaction, some of it linked to the semi-public rows around the NEC. Vernon Hince, as chair of the NEC, took a step of visiting members of each section and drawing out their complaints. On 8 May 2000 he took the further unusual step of called together an ad hoc NEC meeting to discuss their role on the NEC with the General Secretary. The meeting was cleverly handled by McDonagh, who drew on their appreciation of practicalities and illustrated the difficulties of management. But it fed into the general new propensity for some members of the NEC to quietly dig in their heels.

On 25 July 2000 McDonagh attempted to push through reform of annual NEC elections making them biennial on cost-cutting grounds and because, in her view, the NEC would be better served by the change. That faced concerted opposition from a range of sources. The decision was postponed. One factor was undoubtedly worry over the party's reaction in the light of the recent controlling record. It now went out to consultation where the proposal was rejected. It was, in effect, the first clear defeat for McDonagh as General Secretary, although the battle over this was joined again immediately following the election.

What was becoming clear was that, although headquarters managers still attempted heavy control, this faced significant reservations and limitations as reaction to what happened in headquarters fused into the growing party opposition over the management of the Livingstone saga. There was now also growing electoral embarrassment, and concern in No. 10 over the public's response to accusations of 'control freakery', and much thought about how it might be dealt with. (For the further developments on this see later chapters, particularly Chapters 15 and 16.) In background discussions between the NEC trade union group, the General Secretary and No. 10, it was agreed now that the process of selections would also be part of the 21st Century Party consultative process.

Management, the trade unions and finance

Financial managers

The financial provision for the party by the unions was a controversial and often misunderstood and misrepresented feature. The unions retained a close interest in the party's financial affairs, believing that they had the right to advance consultation over all proposals for change in the financial relationship.[76] By convention, they generally took the Chair of the Finance Committee and, in a separate arrangement, the party's General Election Fund Trustees drawn from the affiliated unions. Since the late 1960s they had also taken the elected Treasurer's post, usually with advance consultation with the Leader. These posts might be thought to be positions of political power, with leverage over the policy outcomes or important organisational issues providing a counter to party management control. Yet the evidence over many years, continuing under Blair, pointed to union restraint and a Chinese wall around the union financial and political roles.[77] If anything, the roles played by these union representatives on the NEC produced a party management influence on the unions rather than the reverse.

This was particularly revealing over election funding. The introduction of four senior union leaders as trustees from 1987 to 1997 provided no policy leverage but a security for avoiding waste. The unions themselves provided a new rulebook procedure to avoid the politicians getting involved in a begging-bowl operation; election finance was provided in the form of a portion of the affiliation fee put into a special fund. This guaranteed a pressure-free fund and, from the union leaders, an assistance to management in controlling expenditure.

'New Labour' and new relations

After 1994 there was a changed situation in which the 'New Labour' leadership proved increasingly attractive to various wealthy donors. On the political side, that financial relationship was seen as a symbol of the breadth of the new party and an asset thought to be easily and regularly replenished. It also appeared to be without the electoral costs of the myths surrounding the input from the unions. Consequently, even before the 1997 election, an attitude had grown around the Leader that with these donations and an enlarged membership they did not need state funding, which in any case was electorally unpopular and could not be agreed with the Conservatives. Most significantly, it was thought, they could now do without much financial input from the unions. After the election victory, the election fund from the unions was not pursued. As for the regular union-affiliation money, by 1998 this was privately met by what was, at times, a disdainful dismissal. It was even described privately (and half-jokingly) by a senior Downing Street manager as 'take the money and run'.[78]

Union insecurity about where Blair was taking the party, the shedding of traditional 'rules' and protocols of the relationship, the grievances against the perpetual spin hostile to the unions, the sense of being outsiders in their own party, and now the new value attached to money from the rich individuals all added to distrust and a sense of alienation. From this point, some major break in the traditional restrained behaviour of the unions in respect of financial sanctions might have been expected. It is difficult even for the well-informed observer to know what went on in private conversations, and the observer of reported conversations sometimes has problems of interpretation. During the long argument over employment-relations legislation in 1998–9 there was a union unwillingness to discuss extra finance till the legislation was finalised. This could be read both ways. It could be interpreted as a warning signal of suspended judgement about whether future requests for finance would be met favourably, or it was a respect for propriety.

Another problem for the observer was that it was in the interests of No. 10 critics and media forces hostile to the unions to allege the making of private financial threats. It painted an adverse picture of the unions, put them on the defensive and was a way of encouraging extra funding without strings. There were, however, three cases where political considerations might reasonably be said to be a factor in reduction of financial provision in this period. In 1997 the AEEU held back a quarter of a million pounds in potential election-campaign contributions to signal their unhappiness over candidate selection procedure at Swindon. But it must be noted that this was not a threat in advance of a decision, and the form was more within the tradition of lament rather than demand. It did not affect affiliation payments and what was held back was put in the pot later.

In the TGWU, there had been some lingering resentment from over what was seen as managerial cheating on the OMOV decision. Morris saw most of the Blairite leaders and managers as people who treated him, the party and the unions with an element of contempt. In 1995 the Pearson Group had become the first public company to make a cash donation to Labour. Morris was very critical. 'The acceptance of such donations can only reinforce the drift of the Labour Party away from organised Labour.'[79] But the union itself now contributed to the sense of drift. Just as the Blairites drew lessons from the Clinton experience, so some in the unions, particularly within the TGWU, did the same after examining relations between US unions and the Democrats They had a freedom to use their finance to spread around and campaign independently whilst retaining support for the Democrats.

So, whilst retaining a firm hold on their links to the Labour Party, the TGWU looked to use the money for broader union objectives which did not involve giving more money to the central party. A relatively unnoticed, and unanticipated, consequence of the 1993 party-union reforms had affected the levels of affiliation. With now a fixed proportion of votes at the party conference, the unions collectively had no need to keep up affiliation levels to sustain their vote. Traditionally unions affiliated on a level close to the levy-paying membership and in some cases since the 1980s had, when asked, over-affiliated to help the Party. The TGWU had begun under Smith to reduce their national affiliation as their membership fell. Now the TGWU also became particularly reluctant to agree to a regular uprating in affiliation fees to the party. This continued even after 1997, in spite of Margaret Prosser being the party's Treasurer and Bill Morris moving closer to the Chancellor, Gordon Brown.

Alongside this, although attempts were made to build up the party's local community involvement in areas of TGWU development, the union continued to show its traditional face of political restraint. It was careful to fend off attempts by some regions to support only those who followed the TGWU line – a move thought at one stage to threaten Harriet Harman. Nevertheless, the new national parsimony of the TGWU fed into the general union mood about affiliation and it edged some other unions in the same direction. More significant in the longer term, resistance from below was now a real factor in union financial provisions at a time when there were new worries over declining membership and the financial future. The commitment involved in levy paying began to be undermined by a targeted threat from organised anti-Labour left groups, seeking to gain financial and political support out of the disappointments.

In this context at one point Derek Hodgson, General Secretary of the CWU, warned publicly that 'his members could back calls to reduce or freeze affiliation fees' because of threat of privatisation in the forthcoming Postal Services Bill. 'Our affiliation is based on the party keeping its promises'[80] was a loyalist warning about his members' reaction to any untrustworthy behaviour by 'New Labour' leaders. That had long-term significance on this issue, but it could also be read – and perhaps was intended to be received – as financial leverage. Nevertheless, overall what is striking here still was the absence of clear straight policy-finance pressure. Not until 2001 did this emerge. It came though the GMB and even then with a peculiar outcome which turned it into its opposite (see Chapter 16, p. 533, and Chapter 17, p. 569).

High-value donors and sponsorship

In spite of the confidence of the new modernising regime in No. 10 and party headquarters that high-value donors, rather than union affiliations and donations, were the unproblematic future, there were unanticipated consequences of the assiduous confident pursuit of the wealthy. A £1 million donation came from Formula One owner Bernie Ecclestone in January 1997 – while Labour was still in opposition. The 'New Labour' government announced a ban on all sports sponsorship by tobacco companies but in November it proposed that Formula One be exempted. That followed a meeting between Blair, Ecclestone and others at which no formal minutes were kept.[81] Blair denied any link from policy to finance but the full story, including the scale of the donation, emerged rather than being declared. The Committee of Standards in Public Life (now the Neill Committee), consulted by the party over the propriety, advised return of the money and that was carried out.

In the verdict of Mandelson the government had 'acted out of character',[82] but what had happened could also reasonably be construed as a confident carelessness about rule-governed propriety, linked to confidence about what could be got away with, both of which were nurtured in the practices of party management. Spin was then used in an attempt to cover it up.[83] That led to some questioning of Blair's self-characterisation as a 'straight sort of guy', although against the heavily favourable image and momentum of his honeymoon as Prime Minister it did not immediately affect his public standing.

To the apparent surprise of 'New Labour' strategists, the appearance of 'Labour Party plc' had developed a more sustained downside as it become increasingly clear that voters disapproved of millionaire donors.[84] Over time, as individual memberships went into decline, it also began to dawn on some of the media strategists, egged on by the Party's Finance Director David Pitt-Watson, that in order for the party to keep up the image of the broad coalition, as well as to guarantee regularity of income, it needed to keep up the level of union contributions with its reliable and open income drawn from the pennies of levy payers. Under the pressures of financing the forthcoming general election, the officials began to say that the party had gone far enough away from union funding.[85] In 1999 it was projected that individual members and small donors should provide 40 per cent of funding, the affiliated organisations unions would provide 30 per cent, high-value individual donors 20 per cent and commercial activity 10 per cent. The breadth of this range of funding was also seen as useful in contrast with the narrower base of Conservative Party funding.

McDonagh made an energetic attempt to revive the union source of finance, both in adding to the General Election Fund and increasing affiliation rates. But it was now a much less receptive atmosphere. All the unions would promise was an increase for the one year, 2002. Not until late on in 2000, as part of the attempt to get in union money, were the trustees appointed. But they were allowed to play only essentially a fundraising role. They had little information, including on the size of the election fund, and took few decisions. It was expected from both sides that the unions would provide £12 million, but there was resistance in the middle levels of the unions and in the end only £9 million was supplied.

In 1997, this issue of control over funding was a source of considerable puzzlement and concern to the new Party Treasurer Margaret Prosser. It seemed an encouragement to spend money and lay down no limitation on where it was raised. Blair (who had his own contacts to Michael Levy the Fund Raiser and to the High Value Donors Unit) seemed uninterested in the NEC lack of control. After 1997 the financial retrenchment which normally followed a general election was late in coming and the finance director, Paul Blagborough, resigned in 1998 after his complaint over this to Blair was rebuffed. Prosser told the NEC on 26 November 1997 that the finance committee had now agreed to exercise greater control over funding but in practice, on the grounds of fear of leaks, there was still little or no attempt from officials to assist close NEC financial scrutiny. By January 1999, the NEC was told by David Pitt-Watson, the Assistant General Secretary and formerly the Finance Director, that the party was once again solvent. But he also was unhappy with the financial controls and in 2000 he resigned.

Although it was said by one of Blair's aides that there was more concern for financial restraint by the politicians in 2001 than in 1997 and that they also found getting consistent financial information from headquarters difficult, as before, there did not seem much sign of detailed concern by No. 10 for this aspect of headquarters management. At Millbank the focus was on giving the politicians what they wanted and organising to win. This again fitted the Blairite emphasis on modernising dynamism and realism unimpeded by rigid bureaucracy. As it happened, the 2001 General Election was postponed due to foot-and-mouth disease, which added considerably to the election bills. The lack of detailed and restrictive supervision at a time when debts were again increasing was to have a series of important longer term financial and party managerial consequences.

Notes

1 'Implementing the Party's New Policymaking Processes', NEC Minutes, GS: 3 October 1997, p. 5.
2 Letter from Roland Wales to M. Jones (not Maggie Jones), 1 December 1994, JPC File. Manchester Archive.
3 JPC Minutes: 27 September 1995.
4 Minutes of the Domestic and International Committee, 23 July 1995.
5 LCC, *New Labour, A Stakeholders' Party*, 1995.
6 Ibid. p11.
7 Rulebook, 1998, clause VIII 4(i).
8 My notes, NPF meeting 17 May 1998.
9 MSF submission, 25 June 1997.
10 1999 Rulebook, clause VIII 4(h).
11 NEC Minutes: 22 September 1998.
12 Liz Davies, *Looking Glass: A Dissenter inside New Labour*, Verso, London, 2003, p. 123.
13 *Labour into Power*, section 1.3.1.
14 'Critical Success Factors', Notes on NEC Away Day, 27 October 1998, General Secretary 2 November 1998.
15 NEC Minutes: GS 24/9/97.
16 Meg Russell, *Building New Labour: the Politics of Party Organisation*, Palgrave Macmillan, Basingstoke, 2005, p. 84.
17 Meeting, 8 June 1998, to consider the working arrangements for the NEC under the new arrangements. Present: Richard Rosser, Maggie Jones, Margaret Prosser, Hilary Armstrong, Ian McCartney, Matthew Taylor, David Pitt-Watson, Tom Sawyer. Formal notes given to me.
18 NEC Committees, Task Forces and Panels: NEC Minutes, 17 November 1998.
19 Ibid.

20 Ann Black, 'Rules and Responsibilities of the NEC', NEC Away Day Paper, 9 October 2000, p. 1.

21 Socialist Campaign Group, *Campaign Briefing*, Tuesday 30 September 1997.

22 Lance Price, *The Spin Doctor's Diary: Inside No. 10 with New Labour*, Hodder and Stoughton, London, 2005, entries August 1998, p. 24, and 14 August 1998, p. 26.

23 Ibid. p. 19.

24 *Guardian*, 19 May 1998 and interviews.

25 Davies, *Looking Glass*, p. 29.

26 *Guardian*, 28 May 1998.

27 My notes, CLPD meeting, 27 September 1998.

28 *Independent*, 28 September 1998.

29 Diane Abbott MP and Mark Seddon, *Guardian* letters, 20 August 1998.

30 *Guardian*, 16 September 1998.

31 Price, *Spin Doctor's Diary*, p. 26.

32 1999 Elections, in Conference Edition, Campaign for Labour Party Democracy, No. 59, September 1999.

33 18 May 2001.

34 NEC minutes, 24 July 2001.

35 Campaign for Labour Party Democracy Newsletter, No. 52, July/August 2001.

36 Interviews with Joyce Gould, 2001 and 2003.

37 Figures supplied by Vladimir Derer, CLPD.

38 Davies, *Looking Glass*, p. 24.

39 *Partnership in Power*, p. 6.

40 Ibid. p. 9.

41 Ibid.

42 *Partnership in Power*, p. 10.

43 Ibid.

44 Rulebook 1999, clause VIII 4(a).

45 Davies, *Looking Glass*, p. 14.

46 Ibid. p. 13.

47 Ibid. p. 38.

48 Rulebook 1997, Rule 4A, 10.

49 *The Times*, 13 July 1997.

50 'Labour's Future: Keeping a Strong Voice in Parliament', NEC procedural document, 1998, p. 3.

51 Ibid.

52 Ibid.

53 Procedural document for reselection of existing Members of Parliament, NEC Minutes, 28 March 1999.

54 NEC Minutes, 27 July 1999, item 6(ii).

55 David Evans, 'Only Rules Can Cause This', *Modern Labour*, October 1999.

56 Peter Mandelson, *Independent*, 29 September 1999.

57 Russell, *Building New Labour*, pp. 229–30.

58 21st Century Party, 2000 Table 5B, p. 57.

59 Report 'Making the NEC work better', NEC minutes, 23 November 1999.

60 *Independent*, 29 September 1998.

61 *Tribune*, 25 September 1998.

62 Conduct of National Ballots DO 33B/3.99 (amended), NEC minutes, 23 March 1999.
63 Clause 2.1.b, Elections to National Committees by OMOV ballots. New Procedural Code for Candidates and Officers, NEC Minutes, 23 March 1999.
64 Dianne Hayter letter to Margaret McDonagh, 16 March 1999.
65 Davies, *Looking Glass*, p. 66.
66 David Osler, *New Labour PLC: New Labour as a Party of Business*, Mainstream Publishing, Edinburgh, 2002.
67 Deborah Mattinson, *Talking to a Brick Wall: How New Labour Stopped Listening to the Voter and Why We Need a New Politics*, Backbite, London, 2010, p. 84.
68 Davies, *Looking Glass*, pp. 47–54.
69 NEC minutes, 23 March 1999.
70 'NEC Report', *Socialist Campaign Group News*, April 1999.
71 Elections to National Committees by OMOV Ballot, New Procedural Code for Candidates and Officers. NEC Minutes, 23 March 1999.
72 GS4/11/99, NEC Minutes, 23 November 1999.
73 Ibid.
74 Ibid.
75 National Policy Forum Code of Conduct for the Constituency Section, Clause 8, NEC Minutes, 23 January 1999.
76 Minkin, *Contentious Alliance*, p. 40.
77 Ibid., Chapter 16, pp. 508–39.
78 Telephone conversation with me.
79 *Financial Times*, 17 February 1995.
80 *Tribune*, 17 March 2000.
81 Andrew Rawnsley, *Servants of the People: The Inside Story of 'New Labour'*, Hamish Hamilton, London, 2000, p. 93.
82 Ibid. p. 105.
83 Ibid. pp. 103–5.
84 George Jones and Gallop/*Daily Telegraph*, 19 January 2001.
85 'Party Finances', Annual (NEC) Report 2000, p. 14.

9

Managing policy relations with business and unions

Section 1: creating the business alliance

How was the extraordinary new relationship with business initiated within the party? One answer is that the new moves involved only limited indications to party bodies of what was involved and where the relationship might be going. Some of that was an uncertainty on the 'New Labour' side about how far it might travel. Much of it was anxiety about how much the party might react. 'Keep it moving' appeared to develop as the precept. The Institute for Public Policy was used as a useful initial agenda-setting body of the dialogue between 'New Labour' leaders and the CBI. As early as April 1995 it set up a helpful Commission on Public Policy and British Business, which included leading business figures and some trade union leaders.

Informally, its discussions covered a broad agenda of hitherto contentious issues which fed into a dialogue given especial impetus by the extraordinary public excitement generated after Blair's emergence as Leader. The possibility of a government from which 'things can only get better' elicited even more and wider optimism than had been anticipated. The business community led by the Director General of the CBI, first Howard Davies then Adair Turner, under heavy and continuous reassurance, were not anxious to be left out of the developments and increasingly they saw 'New Labour' as genuinely committed to working with them in the common endeavour of wealth creation.

Invited to address the CBI conference in November 1995, Blair gave them an impressive mix of some of Labour's basic policy commitments together with emphasising the creation of an encouraging environment for business. He and Brown had made clear in meetings with business representatives that there would be no return to flying pickets, secondary action, strikes with no ballots or the trade union law of the 1970s, but there would have to be re-regulative adjustments of the Thatcher industrial-relations inheritance. This would produce a balance between social justice and economic efficiency and a new cooperative relationship with the labour force. In this they came up against the CBI opposition to both the minimum wage and union recognition. But Blair and Brown gave and kept a promise that these changes would be constructed and consulted on in such a way as to create an industrial-relations 'settlement' which would end destructive conflict in the workplace and bury the whole industrial-relations issue as an area of major controversy. In doing so, it would also give business the stability that it needed.

Attractive as that was, the CBI had spasms of wariness about being pulled too far into the sharing of 'New Labour' identification, for fear of causing damage to its relations with the Conservatives, unsure also of its own members' willingness to accommodate with policies to which they had been opposed. But the momentum in building the new relationship enabled the political leaders to think in terms of 'getting ahead of the game' in establishing the relationship. How this complex politics was managed, and what the reactions to it were, will be dealt with below and drawn out further in subsequent chapters, particularly Chapter 14, dealing with employment relations. Here it is important to begin by exploring the developing attitudes and behaviour of the 'New Labour' leaders generated in the party management of nourishing this new relationship. What began as instrumental 'New Labour' moves now took on a new socio-psychological dimension which further nurtured relations.

The psychology of affinity and politics of party management

Asserting 'New Labour's' differentiation from 'Old Labour' involved making clear that the party was now subordinate, and that in its management the party's leaders, particularly Blair, were now dominant over the trade unions. The image of Blair's supremacy was seen as crucial in response to the continuing concerns expressed by business leaders. In a survey in 1995 just 5 per cent of business leaders would vote Labour; two of their main concerns were an increase in corporate regulation and fear of a revival of trade union power.[1] The more they expressed their fears the more receptive the 'New Labour' leaders – carrying policy commitments to re-regulation – sought to be, and the more it affected management of relations with the party and the unions.

As far as practicable all consultations with the affiliated unions and the TUC which covered issues of employment and labour law were paralleled by consultations with business and employer organisations. The document which covered labour law as part of the Road to the Manifesto exercise made clear that it was 'based on our extensive consultation with business, employer and employee organisations'.[2] To facilitate a two-way movement towards consensus starting in Opposition, those elements of the party's past commitments which were retained through conviction or pragmatism in spite of CBI opposition, were at different times adjusted to assist acceptability.

It was made clear that the minimum wage would be retained only within a process of consulting the employers. Union recognition would be covered by legislation but with restrictions on its operation after more consultations. On the windfall tax on utilities to assist the New Deal on youth employment, the CBI was assured that this form of taxation was exceptional and privately promised that the tax would not be repeated. Following strong lobbying by the CBI it was agreed that European social legislation would be treated on a case-by-case basis.[3] The processes of Partnership in Power also brought business informally into an inclusive liaison that helped move business opinion to acceptance of the amended minimum-wage policy. All this dialogue also had its effect on those involved on the 'New Labour' side, further encouraging the sharing of business perspectives, difficulties and aspirations.

Historically, through periods of conflict and crises the sense of involvement with the unions in a common movement had been a source of emotional and practical strength, enhancing the underlying mutuality of obligation and joint endeavour.[4] Now, there developed a changing sense of affinity as the 'New Labour' leadership became heavily involved in a dialogue and understandings with business which reinforced the pull towards that relationship. The psychological responses to what was experienced as the burden of Labour's history bred an acute desire to atone for Labour's past. A predisposition to almost obsessional acts of contrition which had affected ministerial attitudes towards the party after Labour's last period in office ended in 1979, now swung in an entirely different direction as this generation became anxious to reassure business that a fundamental change had now taken place.

Within the new socialisation from contacts with business, the union role in the party became seen as even more of an embarrassment. Their affiliation to the Labour Party, creating an entrenched constitutional relationship, could be dismissed as 'largely an accident of history'.[5] Business by contrast was, by its nature, an admirable innovative force of successful wealth creators. Labour must not be anti-success and keeping business close was also an expression of 'New Labour' modernisation. It also provided an opportunity to facilitate strong leadership and national self-assertion; association with the neo-liberal perspective became the basis of a new evangelism in which Britain under Blair aimed to take the lead in social democratic Europe away from old versions of the social market economy.

Although Blair declared that a New Labour government would govern for the whole nation, amongst the higher aspirants in society who must not be 'held back' were particularly those who drove innovation. This made them specially interesting people whose purposes were in tune with the public interest. It was the unions especially in the public sector who were seen as problematic vested interests. In his introduction to the 1997 manifesto Blair lumped together 'that all parts of the public sector live within their means; taking on vested interests that hold people back; standing up to unreasonable demands from any quarter'. Business, on the other hand, was never linked to vested interest, and substantial personal incentives and rewards were necessary to encourage their risk-taking and entrepreneurial spirit.[6]

Blair shared the view, associated with Mandelson, of being 'intensely relaxed about people getting filthy rich', providing that taxes (which must not be onerous) were paid. Brown was less personally wealth-admiring and discreetly preserved some redistributive instincts, but he was increasingly inspired by entrepreneurial businessmen and at times fearful of the potential reaction of the dynamic business colossus.[7] Those in the top positions in business became role models of British creativity for the 'New Labour project'.

There was also a broader set of attitudinal consequences for the Labour Party of this unprecedented relationship with business as it became closer and more cosy than had been foreseen. What were seen as the admirable qualities of management in the private sector were contrasted with the problems of inadequate management of the public sector. That made it easier later to accept the spread of privatisation and later still private involvement in the operation of the public sector, and to develop a new attraction to marketisation, indeed almost any solution that had business origins, association or support. Attraction to the business community was fused with a strong orientation towards making Labour Party management itself more 'business-like'. This also became an expression of modernisation, although as the finance manager David Pitt-Watson pointed out, there was no clear perception of what model of the party could easily be equated with being like a business. Admiration for the businesslike and the modern produced a sharp movement towards out-sourcing to private companies of the administration of Labour Party membership on terms which became problematic.

Building business into the party

These socio-psychological motivations added to the considerations diminishing respect for the virtues of a 'labour movement', keeping the unions under management control and, as noted in Chapters 6 and 8, motivating attempts to integrate the direct business relationship with the party. The honours list became a means of building into Labour's representation in the House of Lords talented Labour sympathisers with business experience, some of whom took on ministerial roles. But political ambition for change in 'getting ahead of the game' reached further, seeking to build business representation into a new stake-holding relationship *within* the party, as direct partners.

The nearest to institutionalisation of the Labour Party link to business that was achieved was in a headquarters reform. Under Smith, there had developed a movement of opinion amongst party staff, including Ann Cesik and Nick Matthews, seeking to build a better dialogue. From 1995 this intensified and, with no party consultation, in 1996 a new Business Unit was created within headquarters, coordinating and building upon the various contacts lists of shadow ministers. The unit had three interrelated tasks: locating business support, liaising with business and eliciting business endorsements for the party – particularly in general election campaigns. On 1 December 1997, a reorganised Business Liaison Unit was established which was also now to increase the level of understanding of business in the party – although it was a limited exercise, again done without party debate.

These activities sustained and intensified the attempt to secure a better representation of the interests of business within the Labour Party. There was an opportunity here, or a risk, identified later by Colin Crouch of Labour becoming 'more or less a business party'.[8] But in practice, as indicated earlier, it met resistance. Following the nervousness about party reactions exhibited over Clause IV in 1995, the attempts to bring business in had been based around some bi-functional arrangement which could be justified in other terms. As noted in Chapter 7, one such attempt had been made in 1996 in the Partnership in Power draft proposals for Non-Executive Directors on the NEC but it had been opposed and killed off. In the review of the Labour Party's regional organisations which ended in October 1997, the principal roles of the regions were recommended to include 'liaising with business and affiliated organisations', in that order.[9] The regional reforms were rejected by the regions.

However, the proposal for elected mayors in local government became potentially far more important. At first sight, a reform whose immediate focus was the search for regeneration in local government had little connection with integrating business into the party. Elected mayors were seen as a means of introducing civic pride, dynamism, an increased public interest in local government. Blair also saw the new post in terms of his philosophy of strong individual leadership. The kind of people for the job would be those 'who could run things' and 'who could get things done'. Ideally, it was said by a spokesman for a supporting organisation, 'they would be progressive businessmen, entrepreneurial and innovative and capable of shaking up old structures and relationships in local government'.[10] In line with that view, the first candidate sought by the Labour Leader to stand for London mayor in 1999 was the entrepreneur Richard Branson. Key managers also discussed the possibility that this office might also very discreetly provide a national cadre of local notables, stimulating the creation of local partnerships with business and also embedding representatives of the business community within the party within the broader pattern of new links with business envisaged at this time.

The initial problem for this mayoral election policy was that it had few supporters within a party where presidentialism and personality politics were less favoured than around Blair, and the more collective form of local government still had many supporters. The proposal had been opposed at the NPF in 1995 and responses to a later internal consultative document showed little support for it. In the party conference debate on local government that year nobody referred to it, including shadow ministers. In the 1999 policy document Renewing Democracy: Rebuilding Communities, the elected mayor or the appointed mayor with executive powers were offered as a suggestion for 'possible experiments . . . if there is a local will to that end.' The 'it will happen' spin and the later imposition of policy continued. But public support proved hard to fix or sustain.

The affiliated unions reorganised

Trade Union and Labour Party Liaison Organisation (TULO)

Whilst the focus on strengthening links with business and weakening the role of the unions within the party was taking place, a new union problem emerged for the Leader in the launch of the Trade Union and Labour Party Liaison Organisation (TULO). It operated with a regional structure and income from all of its affiliated unions, making it more united than its immediate predecessor. Blair had deep reservations about it participating in policy discussions in any form. There were tensions also with the TUC who saw its own role and specialised staff expertise being challenged. But, reinforced by the agreement with Smith, supported by Prescott and backed by the NEC trade union group, the new organisation did get under way in 1994 soon after Blair's election as Leader.

In an accord ratified by the party conference, it became formally a joint committee of the unions and the party and jointly chaired by the Party Leader Tony Blair and by the General Secretary of the TGWU Bill Morris. There would be a general committee of all unions and a smaller executive committee. To establish a closer link with the party, a Trade Union Liaison Officer was now to be based in party headquarters. The party wanted the post to be responsible to the General Secretary but the unions wanted it responsible to the TULO Chairman. Eventually the unions got their way but over the years such were the tensions that it could at times be an uncomfortable position for the different incumbents: John Mann 1994–2000, Natascha Engel 2000–2001 and, especially later, Byron Taylor (see Chapter 16, p. 507).

TULO's fundamental role, as with its predecessor organisations, was to assist the party in its campaigning and organisational work. Some of the unions continued to press for it to improve collective dialogue, including over policy. But Blair was strongly opposed to this, seeing it as a potential Trojan horse for policy influence. In the longer term, this turned out to be not far wrong, as will be shown, and it was only after the specific right to discuss policy was replaced by an inclusive formula of 'matters of common concern' that there was an agreement to proceed. Blair never cooperated with using the committee as a forum of joint policy discussion, and the union leaders, led by Bill Morris, did not for years push to make it work that way. The organisational discussions it spent time on did not attract the involvement of the front bench and mainly TULO operated as a union voice with some attendance by the General Secretary.

Leadership dominance, 'rules' and protocols

Though union leaders had generally accepted the leading role and responsibilities of the politicians to formulate the major policies of the party, they had also regarded it as within their rights as affiliates to submit their own resolutions to the conference. Such resolutions had sometimes been and continued to be instigated in cooperation with the managers, but not always. Blair did not approve of the procedure. When he told the TGWU conference in 1995 that 'persuasion is in, demands are out',[11] this was not just a message about language. It was made clear that the use of trade union votes in order to initiate and determine policy in ways which ran counter to those favoured by the Leadership was itself illegitimate. The distinguished academic and influential revisionist figure Alan Flanders had in the past held this to be the case over political issues,[12] but it had never been widely shared. Now, it had become subsumed in Blair's declaration to the unions that 'we are making the decisions'.

Blair well understood the ethics of community reciprocal obligations, so the most significant early development was that not only did Blair make clear his rejection of the old 'rules' and protocols of the union-party relationship but he refused to negotiate new ones. All would be decided by the political leadership and, where necessary, by the unilateral declaration or action of the Leader. This fitted into the perspective of a politician who had little respect for 'antiquated' practices but also was determined to avoid anything which implied constraint. In relations with both the affiliated unions and the TUC (see below) there was deep resistance from the Leader to even specifying protocols of advance warning, let alone consultation, although these had been an integral feature of past understandings operating within this relationship.[13]

Showing supremacy by occasionally insulting union leaders who appeared to stand in the way was also thought to be an essential feature. In an early incident, during the debate over Clause IV after Bill Morris the TGWU General Secretary had called, reasonably, for a clear commitment to public ownership, an unidentified party source described him as 'confused, muddled and pusillanimous'.[14] It had always been held that within the 'rules' and protocols of the movement there must be no interference by politicians in the internal affairs of a union.[15] That had never stopped discreet political influence, working with allies in the union. But around Blair there was no respect for protocol lines, especially those preventing him or his staff from carrying through change within the unions including the election of sympathetic officers. When Morris became involved in a battle over his re-election in 1995 it was reported by critics that 'the press conference launching the campaign of his opponent, Jack Dromey was organised from the office of Peter Mandelson'.[16] This was explained in the

Leader's office as Mandelson's office being used for a press release without permission. The campaign failed to get rid of Morris and he later built a very close relationship with Gordon Brown, also an enemy of Mandelson.

Victory with majority union support over Clause IV in 1995 might have been an ideal time to establish newly defined and unifying 'rules' and protocols. Union acceptance of Partnership in Power in 1997 was another such moment when the partnership might have been reinforced by an attempt to build a new settlement with the unions. But mutuality, rules and an internal settlement was not what Blair and Brown were after. It would be too great an acceptance of the union role, it would disturb the business view of 'New Labour' and it would qualify the projection of the Blair supremacy. The result was that it left an impression of impermanence to the traditional federal form and created permanent insecure suspicion.

To union leaders it was disorienting in view of the valuable historic contribution of the 'rules' and protocols for unity, a workable solidarity and cohesion in the relationship. It was now a 'why don't they play the game?' puzzle. Privately, some managers would admit that they were trying to behave as though the game, as they had known it, did not exist. As one of Blair's aides put it, the unions had to be treated as nothing special. Looked at another way, it was a bold and extraordinary attempt to manage the relationship in such a way as to make the unions outsider lobbyists in the party they had created. Publicly, in order to appeal to potentially floating Tory voters and to satisfy the new relationship with business, the treatment of the unions was domineering and disrespectful to a degree which touched deep historic nerves about class and status. This became a perpetual form of neurotic overkill with inevitable consequential damage for internal party relations.

Privately on occasions, Blair justified his behaviour and style of party management to union leaders by arguing that the unions would get more if people saw that he was not being bossed about. They should keep quiet and take the punches. He was, he said, treating the unions as fairly as the political exigencies allowed, indeed giving the unions a lot. They must not boast about what they had secured. They had always publicly to lose or at least achieve only a draw in relation to business. Most union leaders followed his behavioural edicts but they stored up long-term problems in persuading middle-rank officials and active rank-and-file trade unionists that their commitment, their organisation and their affiliation was being rewarded.

Major union leaders and their political role

Under Partnership in Power, unions had the right to be involved in the policy-making process which passed through the NPF and the party conference where, as will be shown in Chapters 10 and 11, they were expected to play their historic role of loyalist auxiliaries in party management. Some were very anxious to play this role. It was their tradition and they also regarded it as the most sensible thing to do in the circumstances. The five largest unions, AEEU, TGWU, GMB, UNISON and USDAW, continued until 2000 their restraint in relation to the policies that emerged from the political leadership. But they developed some significant differences in their political role and behaviour. Following EEPTU's incorporation into the AEEU in 1995, Ken Jackson became AEEU General Secretary. After the merger of AEEU and the Manufacturing, Science and Finance Union (MSF) to form Amicus, Jackson assumed the role of Joint General Secretary of the AEEU Section of Amicus with Roger Lyons from MSF as the other Joint General Secretary.

The union was now reorganised on the model of the EEPTU and had close links with international traditional centre right-wing trade unionism. It resourced and became closely linked to the loyalist organisation Labour First. Jackson had an affinity with the moderate 'New Labour' policy agenda strengthened by realism over partnership with employers which made new relations with business acceptable. From that he became a favourite Blair trade unionist. However, with this he coupled a strong sense of party and class patriotism which involved organising opposition to links with the Liberals, antipathy towards proportional representation and to personality-focused elected mayors. He strengthened the unions' antipathy to breaking the link with the party in response to Blair's agenda, but otherwise the union tried to go with the flow of loyal support, and even on its keynote policy issues tended to lay down markers rather than forcing a confrontation that imposed the union's view.

Carrying on from the politics of the battle over OMOV, leadership relations with Bill Morris from the TGWU and John Edmonds from the GMB were more complex, although both were very suspicious of Blair and his policy intentions. Bill Morris, working with a left-wing culture at the TGWU, was very critical of Blair's party management and the closeness of 'New Labour' to the CBI. He also resented the attempted interference in his union and the personal insults emanating from around the Leader. Nevertheless his instinctive response was not to rock the political boat. Until 2000 he refrained from using his role as Chairman of TULO to create coordinated union policy and even then saw it in limited terms, as will be shown in Chapter 10.

John Edmonds became a bête noire of 'New Labour'. He was the most likely to intellectually challenge 'New Labour' political assumptions and even to criticise Brown's economic policies, although most of this never surfaced to public attention. He was increasingly resentful and distrustful of Blair's methods of controlling policy, and scathing about subservience to CBI and business opinion. It made him unusually alive to any possibilities of creating new political leverage and he was early to suggest that the unions could attempt to coordinate policy. He and Morris were both very supportive of the revived role of the PLP Trade Union Group (see Chapters 13 and 14). Yet, as Chairman of the party's trustees he remained very supportive of the move to end the leadership's 'begging bowl' operation and never sought to use it for policy purposes. He also moved easily into a restrained and party-neutral role as annual President of the TUC in 1998.

From UNISON, Bickerstaffe as shown in relation to the union's NEC representatives had a singular mix of attitudes. He was never at home with 'New Labour' and was heavily critical of close relations with business, but he had an aversion to political battles which were unwinnable and kept most of his more pointed criticisms private but regular. After the Clause IV row until the pensions issue was forced back into the Labour Party Conference in 2000, apart from an intervention on treatment of immigrants he gradually narrowed his focus to his TUC economic role and defence of the public sector and public sector workers. His party role was paralleled by his priorities within the union itself where his priority attention was focused on ironing out problems of the newly amalgamated union. He often left the UNISON-Labour link organisation of Labour affiliated members, which determined political policy, nationally dominated by Blairite loyalist officials, with Jones as an initiating figure. Through the UNISON-Labour link activities, Labour loyalism on policy became increasingly 'New Labour' loyalism. Bickerstaffe participated in the Labour Party Conference but did not attend other internal Labour Party meetings of the NPF or TULO. (See also Chapter 8, pp. 246–7 and Chapter 10, p. 317 for his unusual relations with UNISON representatives operating in the party.)

Although there was a left wing in all the unions, there remained at this stage only a small group of unions who were consistently left-led, more committed to traditional left objectives and more confrontational. Rejecting the partnership agenda industrially and politically ASLEF, BFAWU, FBU and the NUM all remained openly hostile to New Labour. Still, the fundamental policy predicament of all the union leaders was that however aggravating was their treatment under 'New Labour' and however aggrieved they were by the new courtship of business, the priority was a Labour government as soon as possible. In the face of adverse socio-economic and technological change and hostile Conservative government legislation, the union membership had declined from a peak of 13.2 million in 1979 to 8.2 million in 1994. A fundamental battle over the party's relationship with the unions and business was likely to promulgate a huge internal row that gave tactical ammunition to the party's opponents. There remained always the background threat of new legislation proposed by the Conservative Party. In 1996, the government's green paper on industrial disputes proposed various further restraints and restrictions on strikes. Leaked papers showed that this was deliberately intended to highlight difference with the Labour Party.[17]

Unions, business and policy development in Opposition

Policy and party management

Before and immediately after Labour moved into government, the main management role at the party conference was done through Jon Cruddas, Head of the Secretariat in headquarters, working sometimes on this with Pat McFadden from the Leader's office. The two differed in that some discreet back-door management contacts on policy were kept open to the unions by Cruddas, using the pan-union political officer links that sometimes operated independently of the Leader's preferences. But the managers' primary responsibility was to deliver for Blair – which they did with great success. The managerial task was not an easy one. It had both to maintain a party control in which the unions were often key auxiliaries of management and yet also to face down the adoption of strongly held union policies that impeded the favoured electoral positioning or caused a problem for developing relations with business. In assisting this delicate operation, significant verbal commitments from the party leadership went wider than the justice-at-work issues. Blair's appeal to the TUC in 1995 on the futility of being in Opposition included the importance of the power to do something for the poor, the unemployed and the homeless.[18]

Leadership policy and keeping control

Blair told union leaders more than once: 'I know how to win', and electoral results seemed for a long time to confirm that he was right. What also became clear was that his knowledge meant to him that he had the right to decide whatever process and timing was suitable and convenient. Any traditional informal procedure could be ignored or be changed to something else. Any normal procedure could be altered at short notice. Some of this could be explained in terms of a poor managerial competence but it was also an expression of his thrusting supremacy, and the realpolitik of his attitude towards the unions. Blair was a man in a hurry to get things done. He could use loyalty and also abuse it for the greater good. Brown had a similar attitude to the unions with a close-to-the-chest style and also, as with Blair, accompanied by a spin that often rubbished the union positions.

Union leaders causing Blair a public problem brought out in him an uncompromising fighting streak. The very few union leaders, notably Edmonds and spasmodically Lyons of MSF, who appeared in the eyes of the Leaders's office as unhelpful in using the media, or worse, challenging publicly Blair's authority, were met with punishment reprisals. There were routines on this – an obvious snub, some undermining media spinning and a withdrawal of leadership cooperation in any further serious discussions.

Road to the Manifesto and policy-making

Over and above its tactical failures in changing the party, the Road to the Manifesto document was, as Michael White pointed out, 'a useful exercise in stripping down policy commitments, jettisoning those which might embarrass the leadership, getting the ditching and dumping over with'.[19] Blair himself largely wrote the final version of the Road to the Manifesto document,[20] which became titled *New Labour, New Life for Britain*. It contained a range of policy commitments and the five specific pledges. Working with Brown, Blair dominated the policy process at his most determined as well as his most cavalier, especially over the treatment of the section on labour law as it went through party processes.

In June 1996, the Joint Policy Committee was given the task of examining a section of the Road to the Manifesto document, *Building Prosperity, Flexibility, Efficiency and Fairness at Work*. The meeting to discuss the document was called at very short notice and with no advance warning, even to the party's General Secretary. Consequently there was a low attendance – particularly of trade union representatives. Although Blair was not present he still dominated the meeting. Shadow ministers made it clear that they were working to tight instructions and could only refer back to Blair any issues raised at the meeting. As one NEC member said 'We were all bounced'. David Blunkett, Shadow Secretary of State for Education and Employment, described the committee operation in this process as 'neither joint nor policy nor a committee'.[21] It was Blair's imposition by proxy.

The 'New Labour' economic policy emphasised improving the quality of the workforce making the employed more skilled and the unemployed employable. Over this, the policy of a compulsory levy on employers for training, urged by the unions, became a defining issue for them. It would be a symbol of the Labour leadership's preparedness to assert the public interest on uncooperative and often selfish employers. Yet the policy was dropped and replaced by individual learning accounts. The justification – to be heard time and again in different circumstances – was that they did not want to burden employers, even though the new policy was found to be inadequate in solving the policy problem. It was also produced in a classic 'New Labour' move. It began as a sound-bite to the media by Gordon Brown before the Shadow Minister David Blunkett was told and before the unions knew anything about it. The union expertise in this area was ignored and the work they had done in moving the employers on the issue was lost.

There were continuing arguments over taking rail back into public ownership. This had been in Blair's 1994 conference speech as a firm commitment. Now, in 1996, in spite of an opinion poll which had shown a majority of the electorate in favour of this public ownership as well as the renationalisation of water,[22] the document confirmed that 'we will create a publicly owned and publicly accountable railway system' but added 'as economic circumstances and the priorities of transport policy allow'. The message was read in the unions as 'not going to happen'. The policy was, said Blair's biographer Rentoul, 'an insincere pledge' which was 'simply dropped when the final manifesto was drawn up'.[23]

In line with what Blair had said in advance, the document accepted 'the key elements of the trade union legislation of the 1980s – on ballots, picketing and industrial action'. In its omission it also made clear that protection from unfair dismissal for all workers, including those with short service from day one of employment – the Smith commitment in 1993 – was shelved. For many in the union leadership that was regretted, as for some was the use of PFI as the best combination of public and private finance to renew infrastructure. Labour had opposed it when it was introduced by the Conservatives but now became a central policy.

A range of positive commitments did appeal to the unions. Britain would be part of the European social chapter. The staff at GCHQ would regain the right to belong to an independent trade union. There would be a legal obligation on employers to recognise a trade union. Employers would be encouraged to develop family-friendly policies. There would be procedures for information and adequate consultation and the right to present a claim for unfair dismissal where industrial action had been lawful, with the right also to be accompanied at disciplinary or grievance procedure meetings.

The trade-off

At the core of the new labour-law proposals there was an important economic-political case being argued. In *Building Flexibility Efficiency and Fairness at Work* it was asserted that there could be no unqualified claim to labour rights because rigidity in labour market regulations and the overburdening of employers with legislative restrictions which clashed with efficiency and competitiveness must be avoided. It was argued that the fairness of minimum standards would assist the cooperation of partnership in the firm, enhancing commitment, competitiveness and wealth creation. There was, it said, 'self-evidently a balance to be struck'.[24] But at times front-bench speeches were made, and documents written, declaring another view. With an eye on the right-wing listeners who might doubt entirely the compatibility of social justice with the primacy of economic efficiency, and half an eye on the wider Labour Party audience who would welcome a clear commitment to social justice, Blair said simply that 'a choice between economic efficiency and social justice . . . is false'.[25]

Yet the discussion taking place behind the scenes when Labour moved into government was to be all about areas of incompatibility between rights and efficiency, with no precise agreement on criteria for the trade-off. Nor was the case for the trade-off fully argued in the wider party and unions. Most of the people balloted over the Road to the Manifesto only saw the abbreviated version of the document. Some in the unions continued to hope that a more confident Blair and succeeding Labour Governments would ratchet the rights to the level that social justice demanded. Around the terms of this balance or trade-off were to emerge some huge and difficult arguments in government that had never widely been prepared in a hearts-and-minds persuasion.

In Blair's view an accommodation of sorts had to be made without frightening the employers or stirring up the Tory press. The document did mark a crucial differentiation from what the labour force were receiving and suffering under the Conservative Government, and in that gave the party managers important ammunition. Overall it was as one critical union leader admitted at the time, 'a lot better than it could have been', a wistful and in various degrees disappointed worldly wisdom which was to be heard many times in relation to 'New Labour'. For others focusing on what was left out and what was still not clarified, it was the shortfall in commitment which was striking.

The TUC re-launched

Party significance of the TUC

In terms of the politics of party management, there was always another territorial dimension. The TUC as the voice of organised labour, regardless of political affiliation, had long asserted its autonomy from political parties, even from the Labour Party. But most major unions were affiliated to both. Policy often arose from similar union resolutions, and in some periods there had been background liaison and a body, like the Contact Group under Kinnock, aiming to keep some discreet coordination between the two organisations. This had been important for reaching an agreement with the TUC union majority and then using it in the processes of party management.

Under its own talented new leader John Monks, the TUC was very aware that the media presentation and electoral mood which had boosted Thatcher had seen the unions as politically over-mighty in a way that damaged both them and the Labour Party. Backed by an enthusiastic staff, in 1994 Monks re-launched the TUC as a modern and moderate new force of trade unionism. He was supported by the traditional right and generally by the mainstream of the unions. A new pluralistic parliamentary strategy was led inside the TUC by John Healy. Nigel Stanley was appointed as the first TUC Parliamentary Liaison Officer, working towards a strategy of coalition lobbying issue by issue with a broad appeal not confined to representatives of the Labour Party. Encouraged by Charles Clarke's consultancy advice, the TUC even sought to win a new working relationship with the Conservative Party as well as the Liberal Democrats.

It was envisaged that there might ultimately be an all-party trade union group of MPs. One possible culmination of the new TUC strategy might also have been the adoption in Britain of the framework favoured by Monks of national social partnership on the European (Rhinish, Scandinavian or later the Irish) model in which government, unions and business would be involved in an institutionalised set of consultative and negotiating relationships. Unions would be equal national social partners, seeking consensus in working collectively and constructively with the employers and the government. This agenda had developed under Kinnock and Smith. Ideally this would operate with any government, and Monks thought that it would have a particular appeal to Blair. That expectation was reinforced by a view that in their early affable personal relationship one moderniser could talk to another.

In a receptive memo to Blair on 26 April 1996, Monks even made it clear that he envisaged a broadly based union alliance looking to widespread public support rather than expectation of the Labour Party providing a separate 'fast track to influence'. In effect, at the time he was offering an alternative to the internal pressures from affiliated unions. He even thought, initially, in terms of working quietly behind the scenes with allies from Labour's traditional right to assist Blair in encouraging the unions to play their traditional stabilising role in party management, whilst at the same time encouraging further reform in relations between the unions and the party. Years later, it was from Monks that an observer could get the most sensitive and fair-minded union understanding of the 'New Labour' project.

Responses, disappointments and managing the unions

In spite of all that, although the re-launched TUC gained a favourable press, a new image, and a wider respectability, important elements of Monks's major political ambitions were regularly thwarted. Links with the Liberal Democrats improved but the Labour Leader's office did not like the TUC consorting with the Liberal Democrats where Labour's electoral interests might be at stake. The Conservative Party response was at best tepid and at worst hostile. Hostility to the unions was strongly entrenched within the culture of that party. John Major refused to meet John Monks – unusual behaviour even for a Conservative Leader.

But the heaviest and most sustained blows came from the spun voices of 'New Labour'. In 1995 the first Congress following the re-launch was 'hijacked' by a Labour Party management controversy. A week before the TUC the *Guardian* reporter Seamus Milne leaked a confidential document written by Blair advisor Philip Gould. Though more than six months old it was sensational in its content and provocative in its leaking. It sought as 'the only ultimate future . . . a genuine one member-one vote party'.[26] But at the same time it advocated a centralised command structure under the personal control of the Leader. The memo confirmed many of the worst fears of the affiliated union leaders about the Blairite perspective on party democracy and union affiliation. It enraged the Leader at the destructive character of the leak and it dismayed Monks because it undermined the emphasis he wanted for the Congress.

This might have been a one-off event but, far from the relationship becoming consensual, the modernising, cooperative TUC was subject to the same belligerent attitudes and treatment as were the affiliated unions. For Blair's positioning and management the two entities were indistinguish-able, and a majority of both came to see him as an exceptionally difficult man to come to terms with. He had little appreciation of, or respect for, the delicate protocols involved in differentiating the two and could easily break into discussion about what he wanted at the party conference whilst meeting the TUC on economic issues. Yet at the same time he would have reacted fiercely to any attempt from the TUC to tell the party what to do.

Though Blair retained, pre-government, the use of the contact group between the party and the TUC to discuss policy issues, this was not given the same respect nor did it work in the regular efficient way as it had under the previous two party Leaders. There was rarely a paper from the party side. Joint preparation was much less thorough, agendas were more uncertain and some issues were even dealt with by a formal letter. The document *Building Flexibility Efficiency and Fairness at Work* went to a meeting of the contact group in what the TUC expected to be the first of the discussions on its content, only for them to discover that it was the last. The major difference from the Liaison Committee experience in the period before the 1974 election victory was that now there was no discussion of future relations between trade unions and the government, nor did that even take place informally.

The TUC as part of the management problem

The 'New Labour' leadership had an electoral diagnosis which not only shaped the reform agenda in connection with the place of the affiliated unions within the party but was also a severe limitation on the role envisaged for the TUC. 'New Labour' was, it was argued by Philip Gould, 'defined for most voters by Tony Blair's willingness to take on and master the unions'.[27] That did not seem convincing in the light of the poll data (see Chapter 6, p. 187) but it fitted the tactical party management project. Nearer the mark was his view that Conservative defectors and centrist floating voters were 'always nervous about Labour regarding it as potentially unsafe'. They needed 'relentless reassurance'.[28] Looking back to the previous Labour government as in effect the last war, Mandelson – who had been employed at the TUC – writing with Liddle saw relations between the unions and that government as 'too close and incestuous'.[29] In their view the TUC had been too dominant and was responsible for the major political reaction which helped undermine Labour in office. Protecting the interests of their current members was bound to make them conservative about change, a sectional interest, likely to shift to the left and challenge 'New Labour's' ability to govern.

Central to all this was again that Blair's supremacy must always be on display. The TUC leader found himself regularly 'bounced' on sensitive issues, even where a new consensual agreement might have been forged. Important new party ideological-policy developments which might affect the workforce were sometimes simply announced without advance warning, and they could be abandoned in just the same manner. On 8 January 1996 Blair publicly adopted for the first time 'the Stakeholder Economy'.

Characteristically, his speech was given without any advance warning or discussion with the TUC, although one of its implications, involving companies acting in partnerships in which all employees had a stake, was of central concern.

It was made in Singapore to a conference of businessmen, then reconstructed once it came under attack for its potentially 'corporatist solutions'[30] and after its potentially non-'New Labour' implications had been fully recognised.[31] Under pressure from Brown, who regarded this as his area and had also not initially been consulted, it virtually disappeared and was totally absent from Blair's speech to the 1996 Party Conference even though it was the heading of the economic-policy section of the agenda. He told one of his briefly questioning shadow ministerial colleagues that this was because 'it hadn't taken off' and 'didn't resonate'.

Disputes and the voice of labour

The organisation and conduct of industrial disputes had always been held to be a matter for the union or unions concerned. There was a prohibition against open political interventions by politicians; these were likely to make a situation worse. Public distancing from the unions had been the strategy developed by the Labour leadership since the miners' strike of 1984–5 but always accompanied by background liaison between the Leader's office and the TUC. This background work was highly developed between Charles Clarke (then Head of Kinnock's office) and John Monks (then Deputy General Secretary of the TUC), with a strong sense of a common project. This was not the case with Blair as Leader. Concerned to avoid 'New Labour' being portrayed by the Conservatives and the media as 'the striker's friend', he had neither empathy nor sympathy for what Monks thought he had to do as the union-movement leader.

In 1996, over the handling of industrial disputes in the Post Office (involving the CWU) and on the London underground (involving the RMT), there were interventions by Blair calling for arbitration on the Post Office and then by the Shadow Employment Secretary David Blunkett, calling for an end to the underground strike and for arbitration. These were badly received in the relevant unions and at the TUC as being a breach of established protocol, industrially unhelpful as well as, in effect, partial towards the employers. The irony was that some of the ministers involved, including Blunkett, and Prescott, shared the TUC's misgivings. Prescott was particularly worried that intervention in the RMT dispute would undermine negotiations and establish pressure on shadow ministers to give an opinion on every dispute.

Blair and his media advisors were unrepentant, indeed happy that they had safeguarded their electoral strategy in a highly sensitive area, disregarding the fact that it also became clear that both disputes had public support. The loud and repeated signals to the media were not without internal party management costs. The loyalist AEEU General Secretary Ken Jackson, writing in his union journal about Blair's intervention, said that 'New Labour simply displays its ineptitude when it interferes in industrial disputes'.[32] There was also a union reaction on the postal dispute at the party conference which very unusually, in the form of an emergency resolution, Blair's managers could not stop (see Chapter 11, p. 339).

Monks's anger

At the TUC Congress of 1996 there was to be no Blair speech, although as usual he attended the General Council dinner. In a context where Monks thought that he had an agreement that there would be no new legislation on strike balloting, Blair spoke there only of 'no immediate plans'. Blunkett spoke of possible new restrictions on strikes. Later that week, the Shadow Minister Stephen Byers, in what became a famous 'fish supper' discussion, was reported as telling journalists something to the effect that if the Labour Government had industrial trouble with the unions, the Leader would hold a ballot of individual members to break the links with the unions. How practicable this might be and how it might produce an intelligent solution to the industrial problems did not appear to be part of the dialogue. Byers, much later, in 2003 denied privately that he had ever said this, but his role at that TUC was never clarified to Monks. It may have been a media managerial attempt at a deflection from the launch of the Institute of Employment Rights campaign at this congress for improved workers' rights.

The TUC regarded this treatment of them as irresponsible and shocking. Historically, they were the originators of conventions intended to make for the smoothest possible accommodation of organisations which had different functions and responsibilities. Consensual procedural understandings enabled people to deal with their problems together with appropriate consultation whilst preserving their legitimate autonomy. On TUC territory it was expected that the protocol of autonomy would be respected. Campbell noted in his diaries that 'as ever . . . they felt bounced'.[33] This was a point where Monks, the normally amiable diplomat, openly lost his temper with Blair. It gained him little. Blair kept to his electoral and media priorities.

Spin and the union role

The exaggerated suspicion of the unions as aspirants to control the Labour leadership and the heavy overriding media-management message of 'we are in control' never adjusted for the historical examples of restraint in the behaviour of the unions. The positive case for trade unionism, the example of union leaders helping the 1974–79 Government, the degree to which Monks's own modernising agenda had won support within the TUC and the presentational importance of allowing the TUC to get its own message across, were all expendable.

In the media strategy as Monks was later to express it, the unions had been allotted the role under New Labour 'of defining what New Labour isn't'.[34] Privately the party managers responsible for links with the TUC,

Cruddas and McFadden, took a more relaxed view of policy differences than others in No. 10 and headquarters. To the TUC they simply said 'That's your policy, it is not ours'. But with grim and it seemed to union leaders blinkered inevitability the doctors spun. It was subsequently argued in No. 10 that this treatment of the TUC had succeeded in its main purpose, the neutralisation of the union problem as an electoral issue, although much of the change in public opinion had, as indicated, already taken place under Smith. Also, the more that publicised hostility to the 'Old Labour' problem of the unions came from around the Leader, the less they did to help change perceptions of the unions. Perhaps it would have happened anyway, but in the longer term, as we shall see, this way of 'dealing with Monks' strengthened the internal union critics, weakened the TUC's position and, through the rise of left-wing forces in the unions, eventually helped destabilise Blair's own party management.

Minimum wage reformulated

Whilst this was going on another way forward in policy-making was developing. Labour had fought the 1992 General Election with a minimum-wage policy based on a formula of 50 per cent of male median earnings – £3.40 per hour in that manifesto. That had caused problems in the election campaign, particularly over the danger that the policy could cost jobs. Its renewal would also face considerable employer resistance which would threaten the desired 'New Labour' closeness to business. Blair committed himself to the minimum wage in his personal election campaign in 1994. Brown also was heavily committed to assisting the low paid and alleviating poverty particularly through a tax and benefit system. The minimum wage was seen by both of them as an important element of their anti-poverty measures, but it was also for Brown a means of reducing what the state had to pay.[35] It was also very helpful to party management in the short and long term that it fitted the old Labour view expounded at this time by Brown that 'exploitation in the workplace we know is immoral'.[36]

Blair made it clear when it came to the policy discussions of 1995 that though he remained committed to the principle, he wanted a policy which would gain consensual support and defuse the electoral problem. Under Harriet Harman, the Shadow Secretary of State for Employment, these commitments and reservations developed in line with Blair's steering and specifically an idea of Geoff Norris in the No. 10 Policy Unit. There would be an independent low-pay commission of employers and union representatives, who would, after the election, establish the rate by agreement based upon economic circumstances.

UNISON, whose General Secretary Rodney Bickerstaffe had fought long and hard for the minimum wage, feared that what was in the offing could involve a major dilution of the policy. That union and several others had a policy based on mandates which could not be ignored or quickly changed and constituted a democratic obligation for them. Blair found these union policy-making processes were clumsy in relating to 'the process of change and development in the party'.[37] At one point in May 1995 the issue went to the contact group with the TUC because it was meeting at the time when the argument blew up, but there was no agreement.

Nevertheless Blair was convinced that the new policy was the right one and he went ahead. The key development here was that the Leader's position found more support at regional level in the unions than indicated by the formal commitments. Harman, encouraged also by discreet signs of acquiescence by union leaders, and assisted by some unusual managerial procedural dexterity or good fortune (see on this Chapter 11, p. 341), succeeded in gaining remittance of the crucial resolution which might have precipitated a policy crisis. Monks walked a delicate tightrope between its formal commitments, his loyalty to Bickerstaffe, his pursuit of workers' interests and his willingness to help the government.

Now Blair sought to push his agenda along by gaining CBI agreement to the principle whilst giving their representatives a say in the detailed formulation and application. As the creative nuts and bolts man, Ian McCartney, Shadow Minister for Employment Relations, became involved in discreet advance consultations involving both unions and business, including the establishment of two advisory groups aimed at the two sides. As a result, within the trade unions, support for the new process was accepted and consolidated. By 1997, most union leaders, focusing as always on the priorities, came to accept that the change of process had been the right one, although in UNISON particularly there remained scepticism about the rate that would eventually emerge. At the same time, the CBI began to shed its opposition.

Social partnership as aspiration

On the success of this first phase of consultations, more hopes were raised in the TUC that this would be the forerunner to a series of social-partnership arrangements between the future government, unions and employers. From time to time, Blair had privately indicated or appeared to indicate that the unions would get more out of a social-partnership context than through the party. But when the call for new social-partnership relationships between employers, unions and the government came publicly from Monks in December 1996 and on the same day from Edmonds, for tripartite structures to discuss jobs, training, the European social chapter and low pay, they were slapped down by Stephen Byers, the Shadow Employment Minister, with the approval of the Leader. This was said to be too much like old labour corporatism and it appeared to be 'turning the clock back'.[38]

Winning the election and keeping close to business

Taxation and social justice

An initiative from the Leader's office led to the NEC agreeing on 30 October 1996 that priority should be given to election campaigning and all conferences would cease accepting resolutions and deliberating new policies. Yet important policy initiatives and changes continued to emerge from the core political leadership. With some initial reluctance by Brown, and particularly his advisor Ed Balls, the most important was the announcement on taxation and expenditure on 20 January 1997. Labour would not increase the basic rate of tax, nor would it raise the top rate of tax during the life of this parliament.

That time period was reassuring to business and to Middle England voters who saw this higher level of top-rate taxation as the thin end of a wedge which would affect them[39] and still had doubts about Labour's economic competence.[40] But it closed down a major source of extra income for social democratic national purposes. Brown and Blair also agreed Labour would stick with the public expenditure limits laid down by the previous Tory Government and continue Conservative Chancellor Kenneth Clarke's fiscal policies. This added to the heavy financial constraint. Within that constraint, any redistribution had to be tax adjustments which developed the acute disadvantage that they could be described as 'stealth taxes' by Conservative critics, and they avoided an educative debate over the principles of taxation and social justice.

Controlling policy change

The failure to consult the party on specific taxation issues was to be expected, but in the period of the election campaign other policies and tactics were being redefined and remade by Blair, Brown and Mandelson, although Brown and Mandelson were not fully cooperating together. Desperate for the election victory which had eluded the Labour Party for 18 years, the three acted without any perceptible regard for the reaction of the CLPs or the unions. Trade union leaders, including the TUC General Secretary, could not get any engagement with the process even where major issues which had been discussed for years looked to be in the process of change. Yet there was continuing consultation with business representatives, a situation which the TUC judged, with deep exasperation, to be yet again unprecedented.

Raising a substantial problem against a background of Labour Leaders' desperation to avoid difficulties, the *Daily Mail* blew up as 'a hit list' an article in a non-party publication, *Labour Research*, which had shown the extent of union support for the policy of recognition and gave a list of companies which might be affected. On what became known as 'Wobbly Tuesday', 25 March 1997, using this article there was pressure from the right-wing press, the Tories and the CBI. The union bogey looked as if it had been revived and a degree of panic ensued amongst the core policy-makers. To the dismay of the TUC, detailed policy on who would decide what constituted a bargaining unit in labour law was being made by Brown on the hoof, without technical knowledge or consultation. And yet the bogey did not have the expected effect. The immediate focus group's evidence was that the union issue 'was not yet hitting us'.[41] It was a finding that might have raised questions about the reality of the union bogey but it had to fit into the 'New Labour' mindset, particularly its increasing preoccupation with avoiding an adverse response of the CBI.

In the Leader's office, Blair had begun to discuss the idea of shifting the support level on recognition from 51 per cent of those voting to 51 per cent of the workforce. This was inconsistent with other Labour positions – including voting on devolution. But the inconsistency was waved aside. With little reaction going on in the electorate, the issue went off the boil before Blair needed to move. The manifesto of 1997 said: 'There will be full consultation on the most effective means of implementing this proposal.' But some ministerial and managerial insiders believed that Blair had, in effect, given a covert signal to the CBI over supporting 51 per cent of the workforce, a move also probably close to Blair's instinctive view that restrictive trade union laws here would make for the best industrial relations.

Agreeing the election manifesto
In the final formulation of the election manifesto there was discreet advance consultation of major party figures, and of trusted NEC members the day before the Clause V joint meeting of the NEC and the Shadow Cabinet on 27 March. At that meeting those who had not seen the 40-page draft were given 30 minutes to study the text. There were major continuities with the Road to the Manifesto document of 1996. Privately the advice was that votes at that meeting would not be welcome as they could be used by the party's opponents. Dennis Skinner moved various amendments which got no seconder.[42] At a time when election victory seemed within the grasp of the party there was no reaction to the fact that the manifesto said that 'We will build a new partnership with business', nor that there was no mention of a renewed partnership with the unions.

Equipping Britain for the Future
The importance of the business partnership was reflected in another extension of the management coup. A new business manifesto was created with its own distinctive narrative and policy emphasis, outside of party contribution, control or for many, even their knowledge. It was used as reassurance to business and also as a guide to the governmental implementation of party policy. *Equipping Britain for the Future* was launched on 11 April 1997. Tony Blair announced at the press launch that 'This is for us and for politics, a historic day'.[43] It was accompanied by an organised letter of business supporters for 'New Labour'.

In his introduction, Brown argued that, far from being in conflict, the interests of the Labour Party and the business community were in harmony. The later scholarly analysis of this business manifesto by John Edmonds[44] showed the extent to which the attempt to win business support by Labour Party manifesto phrases being redefined to make them more business-friendly also skewed the portrayal of problems. As Edmonds put it, the narrative here was that the past was not a joint failure but a failure of government in letting down business.[45] Flexibility of working hours, which in the party manifesto had encouraged practices to suit employees and employers alike, had been referred to as 'flexibility plus', but in the business manifesto there is no reference to flexibility plus or flexibility to assist employees. The document even announced one policy of (retaining) a Deregulation Taskforce which had not been mentioned in the party's manifesto.[46]

What could be found emphasised in Brown's introduction was a reference to the party's new Clause IV containing, he said, support for 'a dynamic market economy' – a formulation actually rejected by the NEC in 1995 but now in the party manifesto. The business manifesto did make clear that minimum standards of fair treatment at work were critical for good industrial relations.[47] But, there was a strong reassurance of not going back to the 1970s in industrial relations. As for the commitment to sign the European Social Chapter, that was put in a way which foreshadowed the restrictive role of the Labour government over European policies. It asserted that 'there is no appetite amongst other EU governments for significant new labour market legislation' and it was made clear in the face of any further European proposal a new Labour government would 'make sure the issues of employability and competitiveness are central to the decision-making process'.[48] Blair's driving force and his international ambitions were shown later in his stated intention that he would 'press the case for the rest of Europe to adopt the more flexible labour laws pioneered by Britain'.[49]

In the run-up to the election, a new shift in policy took place over privatisation which had not been discussed, let alone agreed, in the party and had not been in the party's manifesto. Brown, hemmed in by the refusal to raise income taxation and the need to build new sources of income, filled in a potential hole in the governmental budget by announcing the U-turn that privatisation of the national air-traffic-control system had become an option that could not be ruled out. The business manifesto also cleared the way to privatisation without the party bodies being told of it in advance. Public assets which had 'no further use' would be sold.[50]

Section 2: New Labour government, the unions and business

Pessimism uplift and offence

Many of the big union leaders woke up to the news of Labour's great election victory on 1 May 1997 with mixed feelings. They had worked, waited and spent their union's money for this day, year after year for eighteen years. They had helped get rid of the Tories, but they worried about what was now in store. As they met that morning they talked themselves into a mood of deep gloom, recalling the election-campaign shift in policy towards privatisation, the focus on labour market flexibility and the manipulative domineering ways of 'New Labour'. They were aware that there had been a softening in support for Labour from working-class and trade union members. As the Blair pollster Greenberg pointed out later, Blair had achieved what he intended but he had left a lot of traditional supporters less engaged and wondering where they fitted in the new politics.[51]

By this stage, most major union leaders had almost despaired of finding the way to a productive dialogue with the Leader. It was anticipated that he would be absolutely triumphant; the enemy Mandelson would come into his own, party management would reflect that, and all the anti-trade-union elements would be strengthened. The unions would gain little or nothing. The Byers 'fish dinner' threat to the union-party relationship might have to be faced. Although Blair met John Monks in Downing Street on 21 May there were no formal meetings with TUC union leaders until 4 September at the TUC Congress, whilst much publicity was given to the new links to business and the businessmen brought into government.

The cooperation of the unions in controlling inflation was rendered unnecessary by a policy developed by Brown and Balls in secret, transferring control of monetary policy to the Bank of England, so taking the government out of the economic responsibilities for setting the interest rate. The Bank's regulatory role was transferred to a tripartite system focused on the Financial Services Authority. Economic success encapsulated in 'the end of Tory boom and bust' became the foundation of electoral and business support and that became a driving force of party management. In the third term this form of regulation was found to be crucially inadequate but for the period of Blair's premiership, the new responsibilities, monetary arrangements and fiscal rules were made central to the reiterated public guarantee of stability with high and stable levels of economic growth and employment.

So dominant were the party's leadership duo and so great was the union leaders' pessimism in those first weeks of government that it had an effect of creating at least a temporary uplift when it became clear that the worst union forebodings were not to be fully realised. Against some resistance from policy advisors in No. 10, elements of the Queen's speech on 14 May indicated a commitment to fairness at work, restoring trade unionism to GCHQ, ending the opt-out from the European Social Chapter and moving towards the establishment of a national minimum wage, with the strong emphasis on employment at the centre of government policy. Other announcements in line with the manifesto told of implementing commitments. There was hope here of more accommodation from Blair.

The contact group arrangement between the party and the TUC was wound up, but in managing relationships with the unions and business Blair was to develop much more subtlety than anticipated, some of it influenced in the first term by the plurality of ministerial and No. 10 advice he had introduced on this. The commitment to fairness at work did go ahead, beginning a reversal of deregulation of Conservative governments. The complex and important details of the lengthy politics of this process and its relations with party management are brought together in the full analysis in Chapter 14.

Nevertheless, the main message of Blair's speech to the 1997 TUC was making absolutely clear the limits that 'We will keep the flexibility of the present labour market and it may make some shiver but it is warmer in the real world'. Much of this was not unexpected, but what was received especially badly was his patronising critique of trade union organisation to an audience which considered itself more informed than he was. 'Build unions which are strong and relevant, democratic and accountable' so you 'can be a true partner with government and business'. The most offensive comment was his 'I will watch you carefully to see how the culture of modern trades unionism develops'. This was said with no public acknowledgement whatsoever of what Monks was doing and no apparent appreciation of how the TUC had changed, all said in a tone described even by one leading union moderate as 'terrible – straight out of the public school headmaster's study'. It was hard to discern much respect in this speech. It sounded like spin to reassure business yet again. The change in affinity was marked by the fact that at no time in his period as Prime Minister did he, or any 'New Labour' politician, use this tone to the CBI, publicly challenge business to reform itself and prove that it was worthy to be part of a partnership.

Contact access and process

From December 1997, quarterly meetings with the TUC did begin, and from 1999 meetings had a secretariat of Brendan Barber, the TUC Deputy General Secretary, and Geoffrey Norris from the No. 10 Policy Unit, but still with no fixed advance date of meeting, no systematic agenda or follow-through. These early meetings were limited in their fruitfulness. Blair was as usual very skilful in his handling, now with the assistance of civil servants and an extensive array of aides and working in the historic and, for some in the unions, intimidating environment at No. 10.

The extent of business appointments to governmental positions (in line with a series of prior undertakings) was striking, and the TUC was under-represented in comparison. Yet they were much better represented now than they were under the Conservatives. Their biggest gain was in access to Whitehall departments. Though it was always variable department by department and dependent on individual Ministers in its effectiveness, overall it grew to be substantial. GMB officials, not noted for their unwillingness to criticise, said that by 2000 access and consultations were 'almost too much'.

Where they had access, this did have some effect on the detail of legislation because workplace expertise gave them some edge over civil servants. Within the TUC a similar point was made – that, over detail, the government was receptive to knowledgeable argument. The area most subject to productive relations and a shared set of values covered education, training and life-long learning, although the latter was plagued by huge administrative problems which interfered with all plans. In 1998 a Union Learning Fund with resources provided by government became part of skills agenda. Later, learning representatives were given a statutory right to paid time off to carry out their duties.

The government economic success and the union view

Blair's labour-market evangelism

Nevertheless, Blair's evangelical determination to become a force within Europe in favour of more flexible labour markets in conditions of globalisation marked a deep change from a TUC strategy established under Kinnock and Smith. That had emphasised using the European agenda to shift the British agenda towards what was seen as a modern social-market model. Now, some aspects of that model were seen in the Treasury as having become incompatible with competitiveness. Emphasised now was that rigid labour-market regulation impeded the facility for employers to hire and fire in reaction to market conditions; that produced burdens on employers, obstacles to job creation and to the capacity to innovate. Out of this innovation and competitiveness would come growth and from that more finance for progressive objectives. Defence of government policy within the party focused on the justice involved in providing for the third party in labour relations, and that was the unemployed.

A shift in opinion in Europe towards flexible labour markets, enhanced by Blair's backdoor influence from the UK, was then used to argue for the British party and unions to adjust their views on comprehensive employment rights. At a meeting with union leaders on 13 March 1998, Blair did not deny that a member of his staff had, in the previous November, contacted the office of German Chancellor Kohl to persuade German employers to break negotiations between the European TUC and the European employers federation over information and consultation, although he did apologise for not keeping them informed.

The TUC response

From the individual unions the main critique of the government's position emphasised the lack of full worker rights and the denial of their case on grounds of justice. Exceptionally, particularly from the TUC, came also a series of challenges to the broader government economic case. This was assisted in 1999 by an OECD review which found that employment performance of those countries with high levels of employment-protection legislation was no worse than of countries with less regulation. Weak productivity and low investment were the major British problems. Monks argued that France, Italy and Germany all had more-regulated labour markets but higher productivity than the UK and that well-designed regulation could be a spur to superior business performance and stimulate innovation.[52]

Running quietly underneath this TUC counter diagnosis was the pessimistic view that the government was impervious to argument here. Three explanations emerged from TUC staff and occasionally from union leaders and managers for this entrenched resistance. There was first the understanding that Brown was a talented Chancellor and running the historic 'end to boom and bust' gave him the confidence of a major success that reinforced his natural tendency to obduracy and a refusal to change. Second, the intellectual framework of the neo-liberal economy and 'the British model', with its emphasis on the City as international finance centre, had become an ideological hegemony considered to be the only modern view, spreading into and from economic journalists. Any changes must not replay, or appear to be replaying, the dreaded 'Old Labour' past, disturbing the appeal which was now central to government relations with the City and to the party's targeting in the marginals. Third, changes of the kind advocated by the TUC in strengthening union national representation could produce new problems for union relations with the government, and any strengthening could also make them more confident in responding to party management. That bogey may have been the major influence.

Criticisms of excessive boardroom pay made by the TUC and individual union leaders were sidelined. On neither prudential nor moral grounds was the greed of business directors and those working in the City to be a cause for interference by a government in terms of higher taxation or regulation. The danger of a financial oligarchy endangering democracy was not within the 'New Labour' frame of reference. The priority concern was that if inhibited or circumscribed these most enterprising risk takers, wealth creators and sources of revenue might lose motivation or even depart Britain. Avoiding this now became a central feature of Blairite identity and his party management, and it virtually ruled out of consideration any anxiety that lack of adequate regulation might produce damaging economic consequences.

Affinity and the No. 10 staff

In drafting the new Clause IV it had been made clear that the Leader did not want anything that could be seen as a critique of transnational corporations. Now it looked to some in the affiliated unions that the party's leaders were being pulled further to a closer alliance with potentially undemocratic business forces whilst within the party the unions were being deliberately weakened. On the other hand, Blair and his aides in the Policy Unit, its head David Miliband and the advisor on business Geoffrey Norris, saw a permanent party bias towards the unions which created a push for pro-union commitments. Norris believed that a 'people's party' implied an equality of consideration between the unions and the employers and he was adamant that, regardless of conference decisions, the unions had no 'right' to determine Labour Party policy and no right to veto the government's industrial-relations agenda. Blair and the Policy Unit also thought that the unions, with their continuing pursuit of rights, were failing to engage fully with the arguments about competitiveness, company effectiveness and the trade off with efficiency.

The Policy Unit staff took it to be their responsibility to correct for the union role within the party by becoming primarily the voice of business as party stakeholders. Although in principle they accepted the importance of justice at work they, the No. 10 press office and the Strategic Communications Unit were a persistent force influencing managerial filters to harmonise with business sensitivity and the realpolitik of riding the Murdoch tiger. In backstairs interventions, at the National Policy Forum and the party conference, they took this view into their management of policy outcomes and steered, usually successfully.

Cruddas, in contrast, working from the Political Office, laid far greater emphasis on the unions as defenders of workers' interests in an unequal employment relationship and also on the union pivotal and legitimate role in party management. He had mastered all the proactive intricacies of delivering for the Leader but took it as axiomatic that the management job could only be done well if it involved some important receptivity towards the unions and the workforce. He was also aware that, as one insider joke had it, Blair's instinctive and intellectual position was 'CBI plus'.

These difference of political and economic perspectives were heavily influential in the long battle over the Employment Relations Act of 1999 over union recognition and a wider canvas of other labour law reforms (see Chapter 14). All the way through, attempts to strengthen labour law and justice at work were viewed through sharply clashing perceptions of the legitimacies and inequalities of power. In radical moderniser 'New Labour' circles, it was said that the unions were in a 'privileged' position within the party sustaining an illegitimate inequality of power in relation to business representation. This became useful ammunition in contesting the unions' right to use the party's policy-making structures to establish a party policy binding on the leadership. But in doing so, it added to the disorientation and aggravation in the unions. These were organisations which had founded the Labour Party to counter the entrenched inequalities of British political life. They still axiomatically diagnosed this unfair social and economic power as the base from which differential political power had always sprung. They operated in a political world where increasingly, as Anthony Sampson put it, 'the landscape of power' was dominated by 'the masters of the market place'.[53] How were the unions privileged in the face of that reality? New Labour advisors did not want to recognise it.

Minimum wage

Implementation

The politics of 'New Labour' relations with organised labour and business became complicated by an attempt to build business receptivity into the agenda of limited reforms away from the Thatcherite agenda. This developed its most party-acceptable example with the delivery of the minimum wage. In June 1997, the first move in its delivery still shepherded by McCartney gave what the unions considered to be a victory, the choice as Chairman of the Low Pay Commission. Professor George Bain was an independent academic with sympathies for trade unionism, rather than an employer choice, which at one stage appeared possible.

But it became clear after much discussion that the TUC representatives and those of the CBI were quite far apart over the level of the minimum wage, with the TUC side looking for somewhat above £4 per hour and the CBI favouring nearer £3. Discussions were complicated for the Secretary of State who was having to fend off diverse ministerial representations for various exemptions, particularly pressure for a lower rate for young workers. Eventually Beckett won the argument for just one adult rate but there would be a lower rate for young workers. The Low Pay Commission recommended £3.60 per hour for adults rising to £3.70 by 2000 and £3.20 per hour for youth workers. Brown accepted the adult rate but the youth rate was reduced to £3 under his determined pressure when the national minimum wage was introduced for the first time on 1 April 1999. The argument with Brown continued over further phases of minimum-wage decisions of the Commission.

The TUC was disappointed with both the rates and the Treasury attitude, but as Blair had argued, the procedure did embed the minimum wage in British political and industrial life and at a rate which was shown not to cost jobs. That neutralised the opposition of the employers and eventually that of the Conservative Party. It became the jewel in the crown amongst the measures Labour was proud of in representing its commitment to justice at work. There continued to be some dissatisfaction in the unions, particularly UNISON, at the level of the wage, which was thought to err too much on the side of caution, low by international standards and without index linking. Nevertheless the wage increased roughly in line with earnings and later rose significantly in the more confident political climate of 2002 to 2003. Eventually the minimum wage became judged by the public as Blair's greatest success.[54]

Social partnership

The minimum-wage example also kept alive hope in the TUC that its success might also encourage a move from the government to a broader agenda of national economic and social partnership, embracing consultation and negotiation between business, the unions and the government. This became the terrain of a protracted low-key argument. For Blair, the TUC version of social partnership always remained a problematic conception. He could accept some role of tripartite institutions in implementation of government policy but not in its formulation where in most areas any talk to him of partnership tended to turn to dust, as the practice of Partnership in Power and the PLP Review showed. It was argued by his policy advisors that national tripartism involving the CBI and the TUC would not be fully representative of either the labour force or the business community. Corporatist government was said to take decisions over the heads of the public as a whole.[55] In particular, it could threaten the influence of small business, a dynamic force in job creation.

Yet forms of representation more open and appropriate to the new economy might have been developed were it not for the fact that the 'New Labour' founders were adamant that the unions must not 'expect to compensate for their loss of industrial influence by being given a privileged role at the cabinet table or in ministers' offices'.[56] In the Policy Unit at No. 10, when asked why they did not help the unions by bringing new institutions into being, the answer was 'Why should we?' In this they had the prompting and reinforcement of the CBI, who were strongly opposed to institutionalised national social-partnership arrangements, especially if imposed by legislative measures, although they could get involved in certain targeted areas of national cooperation on issues where there were common views on the best way forward.[57]

Leaving things as they were was also a potentially useful political mechanism for the government – a means of balancing claim with claim, and power with power, thus, at times, giving ministers extra room. Early in 2001 in a swirl of different currents in No. 10 it was even being said in the Political Office that it was perhaps useful having the unions there as affiliates, otherwise how else might they deal with some of the less welcome pressures from business? So, for this powerful amalgam of reasons, the national social partnership of TUC economic aspirations never came to fruition. To Monks's dismay, 'instead of a partnership approach ... we have ended up with a system that might best be called parallel lobbying'.[58]

Social partnership

Social partnership, management and party democracy
Yet, in spite of his major reservations about the union's involvement in national social partnership, the dangling carrot of possibilities continued to re-emerge or appear to re-emerge from No. 10. By 1999 Blair could be confident that nobody could now argue that the government was controlled by the unions, and he appeared to encourage partnership between the Government, the CBI and the TUC – Partners for Progress tackling the knowledge-driven economy. Possibly because of reservations by the CBI, this later turned into a DTI and DFEE conference 'supported by the TUC

and the CBI', and that was that. Under the pressures expected from the Exeter NPF, in July 2000 Blair floated the suggestion of more regular meetings and involvement of the TUC and employers' organisations. Meetings with the TUC did become more regularised but nothing substantial came of the idea of a social dialogue. Nevertheless, encouraging support in the election manifesto discussions of 2001, something called 'British social partnership' was placed on offer from No. 10. Again nothing came of it and later comments from the No. 10 Policy Unit were smilingly derisive about the concept.

Monks's view was that the whole parallel-lobbying process tended to encourage further distrust, adding to that regularly aroused by the media strategy and the serious politics practised by the hard school in Downing Street. The reaction also became a political game akin to the traditional British police advantage – a politics of seeking to win by appearing to lose or be treated badly. The government's swing back and forth led here to a political ping pong, giving something to one side then giving something to the other or even taking something from one side then taking from the other. In relation to the unions it could mean finding something to give, even if it was not what they were asking for. In this game of lament and ping pong, the TUC came to believe that stating their grievance 'helped to stop them doing things to us'. But the persistent loud clamour through media outlets, particularly that of News International Corporation, gave the business lament a decisive edge at key points.

The failure of the TUC to achieve what it regarded as rational political arrangements drawing on social cooperation meant that much more union attention came to be focused later on the role of more assertive Labour-affiliated unions. It thereby eventually caused Blair and the managers additional management problems. The affiliated unions had never relinquished their rights as affiliated organisations to share in the determination of future party policy including industrial-relations legislation, although that had normally been left to the unions' TUC role. They had also never conceded that they should share this party policy-making with the employers' organisations, let alone abdicating the role, and had never been consulted about any such development.

Closing policy-making and rectification of party representation

Having achieved an employment-relations settlement with the Act of 1999, Blair was determined to insulate the government from party pressure on future industrial and industrial-relations policy. The use of the party conference and the NPF by the CWU to campaign against privatisation of the Post Office was disliked intensely around the Leader – although not by the manager responsible for union liaison, Jon Cruddas. There should, it was argued by No. 10, be no discussion of amendments to labour law at the 2000 NPF and at the party conference. That was taken further. Privately the historically remarkable argument, put bluntly and pointedly twice by

Blair in meetings with union leaders in 2000 just before the Exeter NPF meeting and at a meeting of the JPC was, 'I cannot tell the CBI that the party conference has told me that I must do this'. It was not a position that Blair found able to impose, although the discussion of labour-law amendments was heavily constrained by the intervention of Norris, the No. 10 manager of CBI relations (see Chapter 10, p. 324).

Authority, social policy and the wages of spin

Taxation, public expenditure and the spin

It was an asset to the union relationship and to the management of the party that the Labour manifesto, suitably interpreted, with further policies in accordance with party values, were systematically implemented and underpinned by Brown's successful economic management and its effect on employment. Even though the main priorities of the unions were heavily work-focused, broad implementation of social-policy commitments mattered a great deal to them. The Sure Start scheme was established in 1997 and later brought together childcare, early education, health and family-support services for families with children under 5 years old, in the drive to tackle child poverty and social exclusion.

The minimum wage plus means-tested tax credits and, in 1999, the introduction of a 10p tax-band made work pay for the poorest of the workforce. Tax credits to help fund childcare was an assistance to working women. The target for overcoming poverty was hardened by a Blair commitment on 8 March 1999 to end it 'within a generation'. The windfall tax to finance the New Deal in combating youth unemployment became part of the developing Brown-led emphasis on creating a high level of employment as a means of reducing inequality. Employability became an extended joint concern of the skills-education and training agenda. Measures of rectification of the work-life balance continued. All this added to the sense of achievement of a fairer Britain and to the armoury of arguments used in party management. In 1999 Blair stressed the importance of partnership in government employment relations and announced a Partnership Fund to encourage it. That gave room and facilities for a union presence.

But a major problem emerged over the economic-political strategy. This had begun by seeking to address the lessons of the past where generous initial public expenditure had been followed by economic crisis and retrenchment. Now the government stayed within very tight public spending plans inherited from the Conservative Chancellor Ken Clarke. This strategy had been partly shared by Brown at the party conference of 1997.[59] At a time when there was a new realism about financial capability, it appeared to be generally accepted as the way an authoritative and straight Chancellor did the job. But Brown's speech to the TUC in 1998 gave no repetition.

Instead, although he had pledged in 1995 'no massaging the figures',[60] exaggeration of the increase in spending on the public sector became the substitute for the difficulties of persuasion of the people, the party and the unions. Introducing the Comprehensive Spending Review of July 1998, he declared: 'On the 50th anniversary of the NHS, the Government will now make the biggest ever investment in its future.' It was discovered later to be, as Rawnsley put it, 'funny money';[61] it was double-counted, and announced in July 1998 when the money would not start to flow until the following April. The spin also misled some in the government; it was not the quantum leap they thought it was.[62] The double- and treble-counting exaggeration was, it was said privately later in the Political Office of No. 10, 'in order not to disappoint the party'. But at a time when the media began focusing more and more attention on 'spin',[63] this was a self-inflicted wound especially in relations with those employed in the public sector and represented in the party.

The public sector: manipulation and reform

Jack Straw later privately noted about 'Gordon', that 'Fancy tactics . . . always catch you in the end'.[64] So it did here. Public sector workers from their direct experience became more quickly suspicious than others that the message of a huge input of resources was not accurate. The expenditure standstill for the first two years meant public sector investment was squeezed to a post-war low by 1999–2000. Prompted by the media, this led inevitably to the further undermining of trust and a cynical watch for the next spin. Blair's pollster Greenberg reported that not only were there public doubts over the NHS funding but they were beginning to think it was 'all spin'.[65]

A controversial headline-grabbing speech made by Blair on 6 July 1999 compounded the alienation. He complained of 'the scars on my back' from attempting to induce public sector reform in the face of a conservative workforce. Change in any sector is difficult, as Prescott publicly reminded him,[66] and much depended on what that change entailed, within what dialogue it was managed, and what trust was in play. Blair's speech did nothing to helpfully contribute because there had been no advance consultation and the complaint was not obviously connected to any recent immediate problem of which union leaders and some of his own colleagues were aware. His chief of staff, Jonathan Powell, later claimed that this was a remonstrance to the conservative civil service.[67] In the affiliated unions it looked very like cheap posturing to an audience of wealthy venture-capitalists at the expense of dedicated public sector workers. It was certainly not a sensitive prelude to cooperation in improving delivery.[68]

Problematic relations with public sector workers and with their representatives within the party were exacerbated by the new fervour in which the government expounded the virtues of the private sector and the failings of the public sector. It was reflected in the government turning away from any further public ownership and its willingness to implement a privatisation policy which had been supported by neither the TUC nor the party's institutions.

New turns in the unions

Readjustment

Dissatisfaction with the government was showing most in RMT, FBU, CWU, UNISON and the TGWU. But because the pressure was influenced by the attempt of the far-left organisations of the Socialist Alliance and Socialist Party to redirect finance to their own causes, they were more easily fought off. This push from the far left also helped to strengthen commitment to the relationship in 10 Downing Street. There were always some in and around No. 10 who would have liked to replay 1992–3, but Blair had by 1999 put the whole question of separation in the party-union relationship on the back burner. At the same time, the growing sense that the Blair government was not likely to radically change its positioning and methods led the pragmatic Monks to reluctantly adjust. Although still quietly pursuing as far as he could an independent cross-party strategy, Monks now turned more towards a TUC-plus-party strategy. In public he had given a penetrating reminder that 'If the unions bail out of the Labour Party who comes in? . . . the rich . . . but they always want something for something'.[69] He began privately warning off friends arguing for breaking the links.

This consolidation of the union-party linkage was also happening in another way. Just below the surface came new developments concerning the almost forgotten organisation of TULO. The TULO office was trying with some success to get No. 10 to work more closely with them in campaigning as a means of contact with sections of the party's core voters. It also sought a role in union policy coordination at the Exeter NPF in 2000. This was carefully managed into a Downing Street accommodation (see Chapter 10, pp. 323–5) but it was still possible to see it as the way forward in the future for a more assertive coordinated union policy role.

Business and a turn in friendship

There were even signs at this time that change might come from the government re-evaluating the way that the unions and business were regarded. The extensive fuel protests in September 2000 was feared, even at Cabinet level, to be a front for destabilisation of a Labour government by right-wing business forces. A sudden resolution of the dispute with the aid of the TGWU and the TUC brought the possibility of the Labour Cabinet re-recognising 'our friends' in the unions who had been judged by Alastair Campbell as 'being terrific' in the crisis whilst business 'was sitting on its hands'.[70] Problem issues relating to trade unions now barely registered in electoral terms, whilst the influence on government of company bosses and rich people had become an issue of public concern.

As early as 27 September 1998 by 59 per cent to 29 per cent a 2 to 1 majority of voters believed that the Prime Minister 'pays too much attention to company bosses and not enough to ordinary people'; 54 per cent to 23 per cent thought that 'rich people are buying political influence' from the Labour Government.[71] It was reported in 1999 that the British public was becoming increasingly cynical about big business.[72] Culturally significant was, as Donald Macintyre pointed out, that the villain of John Le Carré's novel *The Constant Gardener*, written around 2000, this time was a Blair donor.[73] Perhaps now, after the trigger of the fuel dispute, a major change in government attitudes towards the unions and business was in the offing? Perhaps that would change an important feature of party management? Continuing dissatisfaction and distrust now mixed with some new hopes that if a Blair government won a second full term it might feel more confident about its Labour identity.

The hope, articulated privately at that time by Clare Short, was that the un-rooted and pragmatic Blair, a consummate actor, might shift away from his subordination to presentation and the allure of business and find himself moving in a social-democratic and clearly Labour direction. Significantly, at the same time, a few of the Blairite inner circle also thought that the attendance of leading Brownites at a TGWU reception held at the 2000 party conference indicated a possible 'rebirth of Labourism'. For what happened in practice, see Chapter 15 and subsequent chapters.

Notes

1 *Independent on Sunday*, 1 October 1995.
2 'Building Prosperity: Flexibility Efficiency and Fairness at Work', p. 1.
3 *Guardian*, 11 November 1996.
4 Minkin, *Contentious Alliance*, particularly Chapters 1 and 2, pp. 3–53.
5 Peter Mandelson and Roger Liddle, *The Blair Revolution: Can New Labour Deliver?* Faber & Faber, London, 1996, p. 26.
6 Ibid. p. 22.
7 The late Jon Norton, a banker who had operated from the business side of building party support in the Kinnock years, emphasised the importance of Blair's early admiration of the rich in business and Brown's fear of them. Interview July 2006.
8 Colin Crouch, 'Coping with Post-democracy', Fabian Ideas 598, Fabian Society, London, December 2000, p. 47 and p. 68.
9 DO 3/10/97, NEC minutes 29 October 1997.
10 John William, Director of the New Local Government Network, *Renewal*, February 2002.
11 Tony Blair, speech to TGWU Biennial Conference, *Guardian*, 11 July 1995.
12 Minkin, *Contentious Alliance*, p. 84.
13 Ibid. p. 39.
14 *Observer*, 22 January 1995.
15 Minkin, *Contentious Alliance*, p. 28 and p. 38.
16 *Socialist Campaign Group News*, May 1995.
17 *Observer*, 13 October 1996.
18 TUC Congress Report 1995, p. 122.

19 *Guardian*, 5 May 1996.
20 Philip Gould, *The Unfinished Revolution: How the Modernisers Saved the Labour Party*, Little Brown, London, 1998, p. 266.
21 Telephone conversation after the meeting.
22 ICM/*Observer*, 1 October 1995.
23 John Rentoul, *Tony Blair, Prime Minister*, Little Brown, London, 2001, pp. 269–70.
24 *New Labour, New Life for Britain*, p. 14.
25 LPCR 1998, p. 11.
26 *Guardian*, 12 September 1995.
27 Gould, *Unfinished Revolution*, p. 258.
28 Ibid, p. 259.
29 Mandelson and Liddle, *Blair Revolution*, p. 224.
30 Gould, *Unfinished Revolution*, p. 255.
31 Noel Thompson 'That Stakeholder Moment: New Labour's Embrace of the Anglo-American Model', *Renewal* 11(4), 2003, pp. 37–47.
32 Reported in the *Guardian*, 30 September 1996.
33 Alastair Campbell and Richard Stott (eds), *Extracts from the Alastair Campbell Diaries, The Blair Years*, Hutchinson, London, 2007, entry 10 September 1996, p. 129.
34 *New Statesman*, 30 April 1998.
35 Robert Peston, *Brown's Britain*, Short Books, London, 2006, p. 279.
36 LPCR 1995, p. 9.
37 *The Times*, 13 June 1995.
38 *Guardian*, 30 December 1996.
39 Deborah Mattinson, *Talking to a Brick Wall: How New Labour Stopped Listening to the Voter and Why We Need a New Politics*, Backbite, London, 2010, p. 69.
40 Ibid. p. 101.
41 Alistair Campbell and Bill Hagerty (eds), *Alastair Campbell Diaries*, Vol. 1, *Prelude to Power*, entry 25 March 1997, p. 683.
42 'NEC Report, Clause V meeting', *Socialist Campaign Group News*, May 1997.
43 Labour Party News Release, 11 April 1997 quoted by Edmonds, 2006, p. 85.
44 John Edmonds, 'Positioning Labour Closer to the Employers: the Importance of the Labour Party's 1997 Business Manifesto', *Historical Studies in Industrial Relations* 22, Autumn 2006, final draft of John Edmonds.
45 Ibid. p. 9.
46 Ibid.
47 Ibid. p. 11.
48 Labour's Business Manifesto, *Equipping Britain for the Future*, April 1997, p. 13.
49 *Daily Telegraph*, 22 May 1997.
50 *Equipping Britain for the Future*, p. 5.
51 Stanley B. Greenberg, *Dispatches from the War Room: In the Trenches with Five Extraordinary Leaders*, Thomas Dunne, New York, 2009, pp. 218–19.
52 John Monks's speech to AEEU and MSF, TUC Press Release, 16 November 1999.
53 Anthony Sampson, *Who Runs This Place?*, John Murray, London, 2004, p. 372.

54 YouGov/*Telegraph*, 30 April 2007.
55 Mandelson and Liddle, *Blair Revolution*, p. 25.
56 Peter Mandelson, *The Blair Revolution Revisited*, Politico's, London, 2002, p. 26.
57 Adair Turner, Director General of the CBI, *The House Magazine*, 8 September 1997.
58 John Monks, *New Times*, October 1999.
59 LPCR 1997, pp. 28–9.
60 LPCR 1995, p. 11.
61 Andrew Rawnsley, *Servants of the People: The Inside Story of 'New Labour'*, Hamish Hamilton, London, 2000, p. 151.
62 An alert from Peter Hyman over a No. 10 paper on delivery, noted in Greenberg, *Dispatches from the War Room*, p. 225.
63 Margaret Scammell, 'The Media and Media Management', in Anthony Seldon (ed.), *The Blair Effect; The Blair Government 1997–2001*, Brown, London, 2001, p. 515.
64 Chris Mullin, *A View from the Foothills: the Diaries of Chris Mullin*, Profile Books, London, 2009, entry 13 March 2000, p. 86.
65 Greenberg, *Dispatches from the War Room*, p. 224.
66 *Independent*, 8 July 1999.
67 Jonathan Powell, *The New Machiavelli: How to Wield Power in the Modern World*, The Bodley Head, London, 2010, p. 72.
68 For a government-focused view see Michael Barber, *Instructions to Deliver: Tony Blair, Public Services and the Challenge of Achieving Targets*, Politico's, London, 2007, pp. 46–7.
69 *Tribune*, 1 May 1998.
70 Campbell and Stott, *Extracts from Campbell Diaries: The Blair Years*, entry 12 September 2000, p. 471.
71 ICM/*Observer*, 27 September 1998.
72 IpsosMORI website, 22 February 1999.
73 *Independent*, 9 January 2001.

10

Managing new policy institutions

Partnership in power

High expectations

The persuasion of the 1997 Party Conference to support the Partnership in Power document, explained in Chapter 7, aroused high expectations. The hope was that the future election manifesto would reflect not only the government view but the party's perspectives as conveyed through the documents, and (some assumed) a direct input into manifesto-making from the new institutions. As a result, the party would feel a sense of ownership. With close consultation, any policy gap between party and government would diminish. The government would avoid the mixture of antipathy and disillusionment. The focus in this chapter is on how practice measured up to expectations in relation to the new institutions, and what the role of the management was in this practice.

Deliberation and the new managerialism

The dual heritage

To understand these developments it is necessary to take a step backward and a second look at the politics and culture of the NPF. The coincidental conjunction of new deliberative processes and the election of Blair as Leader in 1994–5 meant that the political character of the NPF now had a dual development. There had been the stimulation of a culture of deliberation, amendment and mutual education which became the distinguishing characteristic of the NPF and excited considerable enthusiasm. However, Blair's private comments to party officials, and his welcome speeches to the NPF representatives, indicated that he saw it primarily not as a two-way process but as a one-way street of political education, making the representatives appreciate and confront the real policy choices as the leadership saw them – a vital role, especially facing the responsibilities and practical problems of governing.

After the Birmingham meeting in 1994, the forums held at Cardiff and Gateshead were relatively uncontroversial, but the Reading meeting, held in June 1995 and considered to be a major success, produced a new range of problems. As the worried Policy Director Roland Wales noted in a percipient document to the NEC later, at this Forum 'a number of issues

of concern arose . . . which . . . if they represent the beginnings of a different method of operation, might adversely affect the spirit and approach
which had proved successful to date'.[1] It became clear that his concerns
focused on growing interference by politicians in the NPF policy process,[2]
with Wales stating 'we were always under pressure'.[3] That experience
indicated that there would be no 'no-go' areas for managerial intervention,
whatever the ideals of the territory.

There was an inherent tension between Roland Wales's two-way deliberative model and Blair's one-way management model, and it left a dual
heritage. 'New Labour' politicians became the driving force behind attempts
at control and a search for policy managers who more closely shared the
same managerial perspective. The NPF, only briefly mentioned in the rulebook of the party, was open to creative democratic development, but it
was also vulnerable to creative managerial control. Partly because of frustration over the build-up of control and the decline of the NEC's role under
Blair's management, Wales resigned later in 1995 and was replaced by the
more-Blairite Matthew Taylor.

Robin Cook, who in November 1994 had replaced Sawyer, the new
General Secretary, as Chairman of the NPF, worked skilfully first with
Roland Wales then from 1996 with Matthew Taylor to appease the concerns. Facilitators generally did a fair job, as did the note-takers. And over
the years there was a remarkable absence of direct heavy front-bench
interference in the discussions themselves. But reports from the groups were
still sometimes subject to attempts at backdoor influence, and the extent
to which some politicians disregarded the forum before making pre-emptive
announcements began to provoke a critical private dialogue amongst forum
members about the organisation and management of the forum.

On one occasion, at Edinburgh in 1995, frustration led to an open revolt
in which there were some pointed contributions from those who viewed
the body as primarily an extension of party democracy. There was no means
of clearly assessing the full degree of support for any of the passionate but
comradely expressed criticisms. However, when news filtered through to
the Leader's office, the principal reaction from the Policy Unit fitted the
dominant mood of the managerial concern now growing in other spheres.
It was privately reported as not: 'how can we improve things?' but 'they
are not going to make trouble for a Labour Government are they'? This,
it became clear much later, was the voice of the future speaking.

It was, however, now recognised that there had to be more incorporation
of significant disagreements in the group reports, and votes might on occasions be necessary in the group and in the final plenary. The plenary was
to agree statements as amended, as a record of Forum views. But in May
1996 at an NPF meeting in Manchester, a brief reference to an elected
mayor for London in the document on English Regional Government led
to a discussion in the working groups of a Blair-favoured proposal for
elected mayors. There was an outright failure to represent the opposition

to that proposal in the report to the plenary session, a stage in a protracted policy battle.

Some final features of management have to be noted. Although the view that the forum ought also to discuss the electoral strategy had been forcefully expressed in the final plenary session at Birmingham in 1994, and although the Road to the Manifesto in 1996 was discussed without an amending process in June 1996, the major new elements of the Blairite strategy were not. After this meeting, the NPF was closed down until after the General Election. It meant that pre-election changes in policy on taxation, adherence to Conservative government spending plans, and the shift to privatisation did not go through the NPF. There was a long gap until the next meeting, in January 1998. This managerial record was rarely touched upon in the Party into Power discussions which had formulated a more central role for the NPF as though it were a free and regular assembly.

Partnership in power: the institution of subordination

Contrasting assumptions about management

In these Party into Power discussions it had been thought by some (but, as indicated later, not by others) that a strategy to minimise conflict by 'confidential advance consultations and communications involving the various party and political officers' would help draw the party and governmental views together behind the partnership, without the government dominating the whole process or the party seeking to impose itself as an alternative government. But the managerial interventions against which Roland Wales had warned and those revealed in the politics of the Party into Power meetings already reflected a syndrome of attitudes towards control and subordination that struck at the heart of partnership. This was reinforced by the fact that with the major exception of Mo Mowlem, Cabinet members had not been involved in the production of the partnership and felt little ownership of it. A few had attitudes towards the party and the unions that were particularly helpful (see below). Others, probably most, were very quick to see the process as simply a gesture, positive in itself but also a potential source of trouble unless kept under control. Impressionistic evidence suggested that only a few ministers gave the NPF their enthusiastic support in the partnership terms accepted at the party conference. The 'New Labour' version of party history motivated a determination not to be 'pushed around' by the party or the unions. The implicit 'what can you do for me?' message described by Mowlem, and the 'New Labour' management fixation on boosting the strong Leader, made his supremacy a central concern.

The closer coordination of policy supervision exercised through the policy directorate and its links to what was happening in 10 and 12 Downing Street continued to operate as it had done for some of the managers during the Labour into Power discussions, accepting the right of the government to dominate and the managers to control through whatever means were appropriate. Acting as police officers, some policy officials were so committed to the managerial interventionist role that did not just respond to ministers' calls for more protection, they ran ahead of them in their eagerness to show control. This tradition of management was later passed on to newer policy officials, less experienced and lacking political confidence, who were socialised into the controlling interpretation of partnership. Even those with reservations had to accept the culture. One later senior official began his uncomfortable account 'I'm not a control freak but it's more than my job's worth.'

Government advisors and partnership

Something had happened also to the government advisors which had never been discussed in Labour into Power proceedings, possibly because nobody thought about it. It seemed to be generally anticipated that any advisors in government could be integrated within the culture of Partnership in Power, recognising the usefulness of the new two-way process and the interplay of partnership influences. That turned out to be an unrealistic assumption, as the inherited model contract of the Special Advisors (Spads) indicated. It said that 'The Government may need to interact with the Party, *as it does with others*, to obtain accurate understanding of the Party's policy analysis and advice and to take full advantage of ideas from the Party'.[4] It was 'a legitimate role in support of the Government's rather than the Party's interest'.[5] Spads had the specific obligation 'to make sure that Party publicity is factually accurate and consistent with Government policy'.[6] The existence of such a contract, let alone its content, was never conveyed to the NEC and probably not even to the General Secretary. It was an understandable measure of protection of the non-party-political civil service, but in the development of the new policy-making process it had the advantage to No. 10 of fitting the one-way controlling version of Partnership in Power and 'what worked' for Tony.

The JPC composition and policy role is diminished

The management of the Joint Policy Committee was another major development that altered the envisaged partnership relations as the policy process began. The role of the JPC, co-chaired by Blair and Margaret Wall, was formally heavily strengthened and reasonably joint in composition. It was agreed in 1997 to have 18 members formally drawn equally from the NEC and the government plus a local government NEC representative. Within that composition, however, there were ten ministers. There were seven NEC non-ministers all of whom were senior trade union officials. Four – Jeuda, Jones, Prosser and Wall – had been very active in creating Partnership in Power. There were no GRA members. NEC representation remained the same throughout the first term except for the replacement of one retiring NEC union figure, Brenda Etchels, by another, Mike Griffiths.

The government side included Gordon Brown and were all senior in status. Frank Dobson and Peter Mandelson as they moved out of government were replaced by other senior figures, Steve Byers and Alan Milburn. The NPF membership was represented by three observers who were from the PLP, CLPs and unions. That observer status was changed after 1999 into full membership.

A party member reading the document on Partnership in Power (or even an advisor to it) might well expect the JPC to be involved in collective policy discussions, 'building on arrangements developed in opposition'[7] and with 'strategic oversight of policy development'.[8] It would be regularly and heavily involved in joint policy deliberations and decisions acting as a forum regularly reconciling any party and governmental tensions. In practice, the JPC met infrequently and was mainly attuned to the preparations for its role as 'the steering group'[9] and 'the executive of the National Policy Forum'.[10] Meetings took place for only one hour, normally before a Thursday Cabinet meeting, which was the only time to guarantee the attendance of ministers.

This was where it steered the rolling programme, where changes in the National Policy Forum process were initiated (by the Policy Director) and authorised, and where it mainly rubber-stamped the policy documents produced by the policy commissions. It agreed the timetable and subjects for documents of the rolling programme although in practice the driving role was played by the headquarters policy directorate working closely with No. 10. The JPC on the recommendations of the policy director made a judgement before each NPF about whether or not it accepted specific amendments proposed at the NPF. As these JPC meetings were 'consensus' meetings, no votes were taken, just voice indications – a feature which as will be shown had some importance.

Because there was an enormous range of such amendments, there was little time for discussions and even less for deeper policy exploration. A limited debate could take place but the normality was an unquestioned agreement to recommendations from the officials. Prior to JPC and NPF meetings, governmental positions were always subject to coordination organised through linkage between the ministerial teams (including special advisors), the Policy Unit in No. 10 Downing Street, No. 11 Downing Street and the Political Office. But on the NEC there was no prior discussion of policy at any time before the JPC or the NPF met, none were called by officials, and NEC members were inhibited at being involved in anything that looked remotely like a rebellious party caucus. Nor were there any detailed reports to the NEC of the deliberations on the JPC, just a limited note. Reopening detailed discussions was not encouraged. The JPC role as agenda managers of the NPF was also largely unaccountable to the NPF.

As a result of the governmentalised role of the party officials, their management reassurance of Blair, curtailment of the policy role of the NEC, the non-party prescription of the role of the Special Advisors, and the changed role of the JPC, a transformation had already taken place in the envisaged policy process before the new NPF ever met. In this phase of management control during the months before a ball was bowled in policy formulation, the party's collective independent role in formulation had disappeared and 'partnership' had become in great measure managed subordination.

Policy commissions

The diminished role of the JPC made all the more important the role of the new policy commissions. They integrated representation from the government, the NEC and the wider party, in a way which on the face of it again exemplified the jointness of the new spirit of partnership. There were three ministers from their particular areas of responsibility. There were three (non-MP) NEC representatives and two, later three, NPF representatives. As with the JPC representation, one was from the CLP representatives at the NPF, one from the trade union representatives and one from MPs. It had been assumed by optimists that the policy commissions which would 'provide a channel for communication and on-going dialogue between the party on the ground and the government'[11] would convey the party's input as well as that of the government representatives, and that it would seek a distinctive partnership approach. Yet that was not the predisposition, which was mainly the protection of government.

In any case, it would have been difficult to avoid here the same pattern of pre-eminence which had in the past normally characterised the role of the senior parliamentarians in working on NEC subcommittees and groups. They had the authority of acceptance of the right of policy-making initiative by the parliamentary leadership as a whole. They also drew directly or indirectly from the full-time expertise of government support staff and the resources which went with them. Teams around ministers, talented, knowledgeable and skilfully in command over the area of policy, were on the job on a full-time basis.

By contrast, as the AEEU had pointed out in its submission to Party into Power discussions, for such alternative positions to emerge required party resources and other forms of official support – none of which emerged. Trade union and local government representatives were better prepared and resourced than the CLPs, and in some areas could contest ministerial positions with a degree of specialist expertise, but in the limited form that it happened, it was contested by a government contingent at its strongest. NEC members on the commissions acted as individuals and with a restricted policy backup from party officials. This reflected the fact that what was understood to be the jointness of the new arrangements was in effect replaced by the coordinating management role of officials from both sides working to the government. The frequency, timing and length of meetings, the arrangements and rearrangements, sometimes at very short notice, were all determined by ministerial convenience. Commission members did not necessarily see submissions from the party which were dealt with by the party officials who gave advance information to ministers where necessary. The agenda followed ministerial preferences. Much of this was an inevitable acceptance of the special pressures on ministerial time and diaries. But some of it was confirmed privately later as deliberate defence of ministerial supremacy.

Partnership arrangements which involved joint convenors – one from the NEC and the other a senior minister, might have been expected to lead to a sharing of responsibility for chairing the meetings, the normality of similar arrangements. But NEC representatives, protective of status, were of varying capability and willingness to push. And it became the practice that chairing was normally taken by the senior minister, and if he or she was unavailable a junior Minister would handle it, even on occasions a Special Advisor. This dominance of the government departments, working normally with an element of supervision from Nos. 10 and 11 Downing Street, shaped the agenda and normally the outcomes. Coverage of immediate issues was virtually closed down unless it was an aspect of the documents which detailed and defended the government's policy, and here again the officials played their policing and protecting role.

It was not surprising that in this first term there was no case where weight of opinion on a commission changed a government position. The fluid nature of government policy-making contrasted markedly with the rigidities of those registered as party policy. Major adjustment of policy on the National Health Service or on transport simply outflanked and outdated party policy, including the future policies developed by the policy commissions. Exigencies of government might mean radical reversal of an agreed policy and last-minute second thoughts. Government policies changed sometimes after a new minister came in, regardless of the Policy Commissions' previous work and regardless of documents which had been authorised by the NPF. Government policy also sometimes changed on the eve of an election when the commissions had been closed down.

Perhaps this had to be judged by more limited criteria. The dialogue on some of these commissions did sometimes alert ministers to problems in aspects of their proposals and likely difficulties in arguing a persuasive case in the wider party. Also, the politics of the commissions were sometimes part of a wider movement of opinion, and strong opinion expressed here could become an element of the resources available to different individuals and groups within government. Taking again the policies on health, one example cited is that the shift in emphasis of Government policy towards preventive medicine in the years after 1999 was that the policy commission had a significant role in conjunction with others inside government.

The policy cycle 1998–9

In 1998 for the new Partnership in Power process the JPC agreed a policy cycle covering three documents, on health, crime and justice, and welfare in phase one, and six documents on Britain in the World, Democracy and Citizenship, Economy, Education and Employment, Environment Transport and the Regions, Industry and Agriculture, in phase two. In each case there would be a two-year process of consultation leading to an agreement on the final documents of phase one at the NPF held in July 1999 and of phase two at an NPF in July 2000. At those forums in 1999 and 2000 the policies reached the crucial stage where there would be votes not only on the documents but also on what alternatives might go as amendments to the party conference.

The policy documents

The form of the documents, as they emerged, was ill-fitting to the whole tenor of the discussions on Partnership in Power about the first year of policy formulation. They were not focused on 'identifying key issues and priorities and reflecting on currents of opinion inside and outside the party',[12] and there was little sense of preparing an agenda which would encourage a dialogue of creative shared involvement in determining the policies of the future Labour government. Instead, they took the present government position as the base to be defended against criticism and from which to attack the Conservatives. In noting future plans the documents were assertive rather than conjectural. They also varied in quality and form and were often very unstimulating, as though their reception was unimportant.

The NPF 1997–2001 and the cultural transformation

The new composition

The new NPF from a total of 81 in 1996 now had 175 representatives with a minimum women's quota of 72. The CLPs had 54 with a minimum women's quota of 18. There were also two each from 9 regional Labour Parties with a minimum women's quota of 9. These two regional representatives became in practice one CLP member and one affiliated organisation representative, usually from the unions. In addition, the trade unions had 30 representatives with a women's quota of 15. Local Government had 4 representatives with a minimum of 2 women. The Black Socialist Society had 4 representatives with a minimum of 2 women. Other Socialist societies had 3 representatives with a minimum of 1 woman. The Co-operative party had 2 representatives with a minimum of 1 woman. The government had 8 representatives with a minimum of 3 women. The NEC had 32 representatives with a minimum of 12 women. The PLP had 9 representatives with a minimum of 4 women. The EPLP had 6 with minimum of 3 women.

Managers and managing

Officials of the NPF

The NPF Chair held by Cook since 1994 was now an influential position with status. Ian McCartney was elected Vice Chair. After 1998, a second vice chair was to be elected who must be a woman. Margaret Wall was brought in by managerial consensus and then supported by the unions as one of theirs, despite some background misgiving about the degree of her closeness to the leadership.

The management process under Partnership in Power was complex and had to be closely detailed in its logistical and political timetables in a grid of meetings covering the period leading up to and at the NPF venue. The General Secretary Margaret McDonagh and senior staff were involved in organisational and political planning. There was a No. 10 management link to the unions organised by Jon Cruddas, and a network organised by Phil Wilson and Faz Hakim linking to the CLPs and supported by selected members of the Regional Liaison Teams (see Chapter 11, pp. 347–8). The policy directorate under Matthew Taylor continued its heavy involvement. In 1999 when Taylor moved to alternative employment, Margaret Mythen took on what became a more restrained and low-key role, but still subject to the influence of No. 10.

Tradition and management culture

In major respects the culture of the NPF as it had developed was ideally suited to the cultural change encouraged by Partnership in Power. Co-operation was highly rated; consensus was searched for, confrontation was generally to be avoided. With exceptional eruptions the NPF was generally receptive, uncomplaining and willing to 'move on'. The newly created procedures also added to the managerial requirements. Policy commissions now reported to the party conference through a document which included reports from the National Policy Forum. However, there were no reports back to the NPF on action taken in relation to its decisions. The whole PIP process involving national and local policy forums had no accountability mechanisms and there was no encouragement for progress chasing. Assisting the attitude of looking forward was the emphasis on submitting amendments which were future-oriented. Nevertheless, as it happened, so defensive of the government was the posture of the documents that openings for a verbal response on contemporary issues did emerge, even if such amendments were discouraged.

The feeling of riding the tide of electoral success and the enjoyment of the deliberative process encouraged a sense of community. That was also encouraged by the kind of CLP people who became NPF loyalists. Many either had worked for the party or for MPs or were working now for MPs, or aspired to be MPs. There was regular close linkage with a small group of significant party lobbying organisations including the

Campaign for Nuclear Disarmament, Socialist Environment Resources Association, First Past the Post and Labour Campaign for Electoral Reform. The managed continuities of membership sustained sociability, friendship and networking. The composition also added to the forces encouraging cooperation, a feature which could be turned into heightened manageability. Behaviour at the NPF drew attention and could evoke the approval of party managers and ministers who might be in a position to advance future careers.

To the traditions of the NPF there was also an important enhancement of the managerial cultural strand. Though this culture was hostile to all block votes as 'old politics', in practice it accepted the primary collective responsibility of government. All government ministers were in effect mandated by government policy and the 'New Labour' culture involved a determination to show all the time who was in charge in terms of voting at the NPF. The reality was that together with this collective responsibility of ministers the managers attempted also to create blocks of government supporters on the basis of a sharp cleavage portrayed as between loyalists and oppositionists.

Ministers and mobilisation

At the NPF, as at the conference and on the NEC, one major asset for ministerial and managerial dominance was the authority, determination and electoral appeal of a self-confident young Leader and the skills of the front bench; another was the developing organisation and expertise of skills of the managerial staff in the way that they added to or altered arrangements. Opening speeches by NPF officials, the Leader and others on the front bench were directed towards the electoral campaign and pride in the government's record of implementing the 1997 manifesto. Of 177 commitments 75 were 'already kept' and 100 'on the way'. Also, on key issues ministerial speeches in the lunch break set the tone before the later discussions. There was no restriction on the supportive government and party officials who could attend the NPF. This was all part of showing they were listening and taking the NPF seriously but it was also an addition to the influence being exercised in the informal periphery discussions and the audience for the plenary. Ministers still played a restrained role in the group discussions, but the position of ministers in the policy-amendments meetings with NPF representatives could affect the tone and could also be heavily reinforced by additional aids and advisors.

Not going back

Management of the CLP loyalist network

At the NPF, CLP representatives came, as before, without prior mandates. But that freedom has to be understood in the context of managed factionalism. A crucial feature of the politics of the NPF was that, though loyalist commitment was genuine, it was also organised and nurtured by the managers. A loyalist network had been initiated by Phil Wilson, who called for one person from each region to be the basis of the network and named his suggested list. The group changed over time, losing some members and gaining others but with a continuing core. Key figures included Jim Knight until elected to Parliament in 2001, Anne Snelgrove and Ann Lucas. The group also worked with Phil Wilson and the party officials to get 'good people' into positions at the NPF, building their own network for elections and activities at the party conference and in the regions.

From 1998 there were increasing attempts to ensure that the right delegates got there. As noted, OMOV was rejected for elections to the NPF, and hustings introduced in 1998 as promised were suddenly dropped, as the managers and loyalists liaison teams played an increasingly important and covert role. Wilson's view was that they 'were not seeking Blairite clones', just seeking to avoid those committed to opposition. The rationale of the loyalist group was their support for the Labour Government in contesting 'the oppositionists' and 'not going back'. But they resented being stereotyped as unthinking followers, and held the view, under increasing strain, that engaging with the leadership and the managers would be more productive than repetitive confrontation. Some at key points began to rebel on particular issues but, nevertheless, under pressure most were pulled into the managerial line and even deviants who broke, or were pushed from, the group kept up an overall pattern of loyal voting. They were huge enthusiasts for the NPF process with its distinctive form of procedure, dialogue and cooperative ethos. It gave satisfaction at the many small amendments in the programme even if they were without guarantee of manifesto commitment. It obscures a key feature of the political reality at the NPF to refer to the CLP representatives as having 'failed to organise as a group'.[13] If they had failed, it was that they had not organised independently from the first.

The CLP opposition: Grassroots Alliance

Their commitment was heightened in battle with the forces from the Grassroots Alliance (GRA) who were seen as the heirs of Tony Benn and the Old Labour world that had to be superseded. Given the elaborate partnership between partisan party officials and loyalists at the party conference where the main CLP elections were held, it was not surprising that the GRA was always a minority, but one that sometimes also reflected party opinion. At the first meeting of NPF in January 1998 it was reported that 'a quarter of the 27 constituency delegates will be from the alliance of left and centre groups opposed to the leadership line'.[14] There were said privately to be approximately 20 GRA supporters in 1999, but the maximum votes on the opposed resolutions was 15. Yet always there was a managerial worry that, with a 'New Labour' government facing many longer-term problems, the GRA would expand and cause serious trouble.

Some in the GRA also thought so, but their main preoccupation now was avoiding what was regarded as a leadership line of retreat from major past policies and principles. They were also gradually influenced by the NPF culture and their acceptance of the Partnership in Power spirit of 1997 in what they called for and how they acted. Their emphasis was on fairness and accountability in allowing the procedures to work.

Alternative policy positions

The most attractive feature of Partnership in Power to party democrats had been a commitment that in the second year of each cycle of documents, 'where the NPF was unable to reach a consensus view it would be the responsibility of the NPF to include alternative proposals representing different constituencies of opinion within the Forum and the Party as a whole'.[15] In the original discussions of Party into Power the assumption was that there would be two distinct processes. There would be one where the NPF decided whether or not they were in favour of or against particular amendments. These would become part of the policy document. There would be a separate process whereby a recommendation would be made by officials and the relevant policy commissions of the scale of minority support on the issue as indicated from the party submissions. That judgement would provide the basis for the NPF to give the party conference a policy choice it had generally not had before. The conference for the first time would be able to have separate votes on key sections and proposals.[16]

As with many other facets of the creation of PIP arrangements, there was a wrestle with logistical problems. The method now chosen and agreed through the JPC had the benefit of simplicity but also gave a considerable managerial opportunity. There was a single procedure of voting for or against an amendment which decided whether the forum favoured it, and also decided whether another amendment won enough support for it to achieve the status of an alternative position. To win this status of an alternative position it was agreed at the JPC November 1998 (following proposals of Taylor, the Policy Director together with the No. 10 Political Office) that an amendment needed the support of at least 33 per cent of the forum which must come from at least three of the seven sections of the NPF. There were many reservations expressed at the November NPF at this over-stringent requirement of the JPC and, having taken the pulse of the meeting, the acting Chair Ian McCartney referred the paper back to the JPC for more consideration. Eventually at the JPC of 8 March 1999 the sections vote was abandoned. Also, the requirement for a minority position was reduced to 25 per cent of those voting. There was, however, an important additional qualification in that the requirement also involved an absolute minimum of 35 members (20 per cent of the total NPF membership).

At the May JPC, Taylor also produced rules for the acceptability of amendments. It was proposed that amendments in its second year of consultation 'should seek to develop the existing position in the document rather than to overturn the substance of the document'.[17] This came under private attack from frontbenchers David Blunkett and Jack Straw, and others. It appeared to heavily circumscribe any amendments that proposed new policies. The judgement of Blunkett in his diary was, 'We're changing from a party riven and driven by dissent into a party that will tolerate no dissent'. It was 'not only unacceptable but politically inept'.[18]

It was not inept within the managerial code of 'what works' for Tony. It was an enthusiastic example of the reassurance and 'making sure' that had been going on for two years. Taylor still announced to the November 1998 NPF that there must be 'no parachuting of amendments' and the new wording given out read that 'amendments must accurately reflect the strength of feeling in the two year consultation'.[19] This appeared to amount to the same position as the one attacked by Blunkett and Straw. No such restriction was placed on the government, which was always in a position to parachute, as future meetings were to show.

NPF, NEC and JPC: the changing relationship

Meanwhile, there had been no indication that the constitutional responsibility of the NPF would change under Partnership in Power and no discernible demand for it from the party, but in an extension of the rolling coup over the NEC Policy Committee, in the NPF business session discussions at Warwick on 17 May 1998, Taylor made his announcement that the NEC had 'devolved its authority to the JPC'.[20] In effect, this made the NPF advisory to the JPC, not to the NEC. It was not challenged, perhaps because the NEC members had by now fatalistically accepted as irretrievable what they had never authorised.

NPF crucial meetings

Two crucial meetings dominated the policy-making process. One at Durham in 1999 and another at Exeter in 2000 would have votes on what amendments went to the party conference of 2000. They were similar in form and management but each also involved a changing mood and new elements of managerial activity.

1) Durham

Submissions and acceptance
On the lead-up to the Durham meeting in July 1999, where there would be votes, the managers in 1999 became affected by two fears fed by Blair. Would the extraordinarily complex process become unhandleable? Had they

secured enough controls? It did not decline into chaos but the considerable controls were further developed. Every party organisation had the right to submit its views to policy commissions and every NPF representative had the right to submit amendments to the policy document. This was part of its appeal as a means of ensuring participation in a process which might lead to a direct input into the final decisions made at the party conference. However, in these arrangements there was no procedure for local parties or policy forums to directly originate amendments, so the talking process at the local level never led to the satisfactions of the old conference amending process. Regional policy-forum discussions were reported to the NPF, but representatives there were given only two weeks to read all the submissions, understand the documents, draft amendments and obtain the agreement of eight other forum members. There was little time to do that and even less time to consult their CLP organisations, most of whom had no knowledge of what was being submitted in their name by NPF representatives.

The JPC as steering group

As 'the steering group of the National Policy Forum',[21] the JPC had become in effect the NPF standing orders committee but, unlike the traditional accountability procedures of the Labour movement, there was no formal appeal process to the NPF from its decisions. So although a business session at the NPF could sometimes make general representations and there could be informal pressure through the Chair, the JPC was largely a non-accountable body. Something similar was happening to the conference-arrangements committee relationship with the NEC and the party conference under Partnership in Power.

Only amendments which 'had arisen from the two year consultation' and had the support of eight members of the NPF were acceptable for discussion. New technical criteria emerged as controls with political effects. Amendments were said to be unacceptable if they covered more than one policy area, or were under the wrong heading. More directly, political amendments which were said to be not compatible with the new Clause IV or the 1997 manifesto were also ruled out.[22] Although a reference to these documents being 'two starting points' had been made in the Partnership in Power document, no advance warning or explanations were offered to the forum for their use as a basis for policing arrangements. Nevertheless, of the 225 amendments submitted only 21 amendments were deemed unacceptable and a further 26 were unendorsed by the JPC.

A practical procedure was introduced by which amendments might be made more acceptable. To avoid regular NPF confrontation and seek widest areas of agreement, those who proposed amendments which were not acceptable to the JPC were invited, accompanied by one supporter, to meet with relevant Ministers and advisory officials in order to consider the proposals. At this meeting an agreement could be reached on alternative wording which would be mutually acceptable. Within that process, some changes in wording were agreed but sometimes with a promise to examine or consider the proposal later. That might lead to withdrawal of the amendment. Without any agreement the amendment would be categorised as 'non-endorsed' and then went to a vote at the plenary session. These meetings had a flexibility which was welcomed as going past that of proceedings at the party conference, but at Durham some of these encounters were a daunting business with the two NPF members facing a phalanx of, at times, aggressive expertise and authority.

On the other hand, it did give representatives an opportunity they had never had in the past to secure minor verbal changes or some consensual concessions. Maurice Winstone refers to severely disabled people not being required to attend New Deal interviews.[23] Russell cited qualified commitment to end commercial planting of genetically modified crops and pledges to tackle domestic violence.[24] Potentially significant, there were three radical issues said by the NPF Chairman Robin Cook, in his opening speech at the NPF at Exeter in 2000, to have originated in the previous NPF process, on early action over fuel poverty, facilities for free nursery places, and dealing with loan sharks. Only the latter was controversial and important. (How it was later managed will be noted in Chapter 15, p. 480.) Very exceptionally, via some union pressure and UNISON cooperation with the managers and/or unusual links to government allies, some policy changes of greater significance took place (See below).

The unions and party management

To understand the party management here as in other spheres, it has to be related to the behaviour of the unions. They had a national and regional representation of up to 52. To this theoretically could be added the 12 members of the NEC trade union section, plus the Treasurer, but as they voted here as individuals, with a role definition that was heavily loyalist, they were more prone to vote for the government's positions. Party managers had no control over who came as representatives to the NPF from the individual unions. No elections took place, and there was little in the way of internal union publicity about the NPF. Representatives including those from the TGWU, and AEEU and MSF (later amalgamated with AEEU) were generally senior central party officials as designated by the General Secretary. Some General Secretaries themselves regularly attended, most notably John Edmonds of the GMB, and Derek Hodgson of the CWU. Bickerstaffe from UNISON left it to union officials more attuned to the partnership process and more aligned with the political leadership.

There was little in the way of internal union policy-making procedures specifically attuned to the new party arrangements, and union representatives were expected to follow union mandates on policy derived from their traditional internal representative systems. But the fluid nature of the

NPF procedures, and the lack of public openness, made it easier to loosen commitments and to find accommodation with the government if that was sought, and here they had more room for manoeuvre than at the conference.

Those in the unions who in 1997 had thought in terms of more inter-union cohesion to influence the process found unity between unions difficult to sustain and were always under pressure from the managers seeking to divide and rule any opposition. The cycle of policy-making was characterised by last-minute heavy union involvement, but with weak or no union coordination, it met heavy and well-coordinated last-minute party management to get the right outcome. UNISON contributed extensively from the start of each policy cycle and could with justification claim at the end to have made a marked contribution to party policy as represented in the draft NPF documents.

The atmosphere in the unions at Durham was to some extent affected by the way that two managers, Cruddas and McCartney, had been skilful in assisting the unions over the Employment Relations Act. The newness of the process also made most union leaders anxious to find ways of making it work, linked with a willingness of some of the unions to return to their old role as ballast for the leadership. A few union leaders, particularly Edmonds in the GMB, had talked of agreeing united union positions as they met before the Forum. But the unions quickly became divided as a result of managerial tactics plus some union leap-frogging to find a good insider position.

Union representation also became influenced by the absence of the most senior union leaders in three unions: UNISON, the TGWU and the MSF. These unions were led now by senior women officers who overlapped with the five-Margaret phenomenon on the NEC in promoting the loyalist momentum. From UNISON came Nita Clarke, Maggie Jones, Anne Picking and Margaret Wheeler. From MSF came Margaret Wall and Anne Gibson. Margaret Prosser, the party's Treasurer and convenor of the trade-union group, led the TGWU delegation.

Different forms of managerial influence over UNISON and the TGWU became pivotal to the politics in different ways. UNISON had always opposed the Private Finance Initiative with a two-pronged critique, first against what was regarded as economically flawed provision with exploitive and eventually greater costs and, second and more pressing, against different conditions of work between those inside and those outside the schemes. At this Forum through the role of Nita Clarke and Maggie Jones, PFI began to become subject to new deals. The UNISON amendment that 'Labour will ensure that PFI deals promote the interests of the NHS and allied staff, prevent privatisation of services and safeguard quality' embodied a concession over the terms of transfer of contracts from the health service for non-clinical staff in PFI schemes. Agreement on this proposal grew out of working in advance of the Forum with the Minister of Health Alan

Milburn and with the approval of Gordon Brown. It became a pivotal political arrangements in the sense that it locked the union into a loyalist role but also gained for them an insider influence. An inter-union tactical disagreement between UNISON and the GMB also began here over what was practicable to win. This also continued and fed into the managerial politics in the second term.

But a central and most controversial covert initiative here concerned the role played by the TGWU. Fashioning a modern welfare state was one of the essential challenges of modernisation, Blair had told the TUC in 1997. The TUC agreed and at a meeting with Blair on 12 December 1997 had called for a full debate with consultation on the issues involved. But there was deep resistance from the Treasury to making the consultative commitments. The policy document for this NPF said nothing about a full review of the welfare state. Nor did the Welfare and Pensions Bill, published in May 1999, agree to restore the pensions link with earning. The TGWU had an amendment down at the Durham NPF in favour of that restoration.

What happened next in the management of this issue arose out of the growing closeness between Gordon Brown and Bill Morris, who sat on the board of the Bank of England. At the eleventh hour, following a discussion with Brown, Morris instructed Margaret Prosser to withdraw their resolution on pensions and instead to call upon the government to 'lead a national debate on the future of the welfare state based on fundamental principles of social insurance, inclusiveness, redistribution and the promotion of equality'. Prosser was happy with the values involved and she had her own private doubts about the earnings link.

Following this initiative, other unions with amendments on restoring the link, including MSF, UNISON and more reluctantly the GMB, now withdrew in favour of the one from the TGWU. The unity that emerged was also natural for unions like USDAW, the AEEU (after putting down markers on proportional representation and manufacturing) and the CWU (after gaining assurances again on the Post Office). In the work groups discussing welfare, the TGWU proposal was said by a minister to involve a Beveridge-style enquiry. At the plenary session, Alistair Darling, the Secretary of State for Social Security, welcomed the TGWU amendment as the beginning of the national debate. The report of the NPF in 1999 read 'we believe that the government should lead a national debate on the future of the welfare state from first principles'.[25]

But with ministerial meetings with the unions taking place before the work groups met, the deliberative function of the NPF was downgraded. The working groups became simply a dialogue with no effect on the amending process which had already taken place. If representatives had not submitted amendments they were not involved in the decision-making about them. There was now no room for a plenary discussion of reports from the working groups, and the old process whereby they could be challenged and votes taken disappeared, not just at this NPF but at all NPF meetings whether they were final-stage voting occasions or not. In 1999, all the groups could do was focus on non-endorsed amendments. The sense that the groups had become downgraded because of private meetings with union leaders, from which others were excluded, became resented by CLP representatives.

Voting on amendments

The system by which amendments could carry into the documents against the advice of the leadership was a simple majority, but for amendments which could be taken as alternatives to the Party Conference, the 40 per cent threshold proved to be more of a hurdle than had been realised by many at the time this was first brought to the NPF. At Durham, there were 175 places for representatives under the rules. 133 actually arrived but only 90 were present at the plenary. It was then realised that the percentage required to force items on to the agenda of the Party Conference as minority positions was actually 40 per cent of those eligible and not just of those attending the plenary.

Plenary voting

It was never mentioned in Partnership in Power meetings or when the NPF commenced that the final plenary vote would be taken without a debate. There was also no right to speak on an amendment by the mover, a prohibition defended as a matter of time although time was found for a speech by a loyalist representative of the policy commission opposed to the amendment and then by a minister. There was even the pressure of the heckling of one GRA opponent by a minister during the vote, with no remonstrance from the acting chair who had just made his own appeal for unity. That was overkill because managerial manoeuvres had already produced an array of block votes, with the government and NEC votes united, the unions acting together and CLP and other loyalists organised into a block by the managers. This left the GRA CLP representatives isolated with their six amendments. All opposed by the JPC, they were voted down by overwhelming majorities.

The repeated promise had been that at the annual conference for the first time, documents 'will contain alternative positions ... (which) means that Conference chooses between different policies which have emerged during the consultation',[26] and such alternative options were 'a new right for members'.[27] Now in managerial practice there would be no such choice. Conference delegates would have to either accept or reject the policy document as a whole. Blair had told the 1998 party conference that 'trust is what Partnership in Power is all about'.[28] But, as shown, that turned out to mean only that it was good that the party trusted the leadership and that made them easier to manage. In that control and its manoeuvres, Durham with its reinforcing block votes came dangerously close to discrediting the whole exercise.

The description 'partnership' was not one that first came to mind to describe this relationship in 1999. It appeared to *Tribune* to be 'Undemocratic Centralism',[29] and was later likened in memory by the moderate Jeremy Beecham to 'Soviet style politics'.[30] A condition of the social-policy review promised at Durham that further explains the GMB backing for it was that it was thought to involve no further piecemeal policy changes until the debate took place.[31] From the governmental side the ministerial message was: 'We need to trust each other a bit'.[32] Later, the fact that he was 'sold a pup' exacerbated the already poor relations with Edmonds. He did not forget it. As with other expressions of excessive control, this was not the end of the story, as will be shown.

Members' representation and communication

Meanwhile, looking back at the various causes of dissatisfaction produced by the operation of Partnership in Power, the most striking was the treatment of ordinary members. Great emphasis had been placed on 'the members' party' and their contribution. The partnership dialogue would be with them. This, it was thought, would undermine the old culture of 'resolutionitis' and encourage a sense of ownership. Yet in practice the members lost the power to decide their representatives and the continuous dialogue turned into a thin, controlled and frustrating affair.

One acute problem arose from the virtues of the deliberations of the National Policy Forum. As a body meeting in private it discouraged grandstanding and encouraged a sense of internal community. It enabled ministers to confide in the audience without giving hostages to fortune in terms of exposure of internal divisions to mischief by the mass media. But the privacy was an obstacle to communication with the party's members who had none of the sense of participation in peering into the goldfish bowl of the party conference with the aid of media commentary. A few observers were allowed in but only with JPC approval, and the existence of this facility was not publicised. Hence there was considerable ignorance about the NPF representatives and their work. The process as a whole was more complex and less easily understood than the old arrangements. With many fewer representatives from the CLPs to the NPF and no direct electoral connection from each CLP, there was none of the ease of communication to the constituencies that had accompanied the role of delegates to the party conference, many of whom had traditionally spent the weeks after the conference touring the branches with reports.

There was an initial encouragement to a proliferation of local policy forums which would involve many members as possible. At the NEC away-day in October 1998 it was confirmed again that 'a high priority should be given to the policy forums and to feedback thereon'.[33] A problem which grew worse rather than improving was that the process was of members talking upwards with (at best) an acknowledgement and a statement of government policy but no dialogue of specific responses and with neither accountability procedures nor culture operating in a partnership with the grass roots.

Efforts in communications from NPF representatives varied but no central resources were provided for this purpose, not even access to constituency and branch addresses. From headquarters there was a general failure even to acknowledge – let alone respond to – the submissions.[34] Initial attendances at local forums were trumpeted as a sign of the popular support for the new arrangements. In 1999 the General Secretary said that 6,000 had taken part in policy forums, but that was judged by Jon Egan, an ex- party organiser, as fewer than ten per CLP and fewer than would have taken part in the process in wards and GCs. That was because of 'the failure to commit the necessary level of political and organisational investment'.[35] Later membership survey evidence was judged to show that participation in 1999 was greater than in previous policy discussions.[36] However, over time, as Russell describes, the discussions that did take place 'became concentrated in more traditional forums'.[37]

Post-mortem

There was much pressure on the managers and an urgent debate behind the scenes after Durham about the failure of alternative positions to emerge and the potential damage to the reputation of Partnership in Power. Discussions carried into the next National Policy Forum meeting in London on 30 October 1999. There was strong support for lowering the backing for an acceptable amendment at the NPF from eight representatives to two. But an attempt to lower the voting threshold for such amendments was rejected, as was an attempt by the managers to restrict the number of amendments to two per representative.

There was a special managerial problem, not shared with the NPF. There was too narrow a gap between the qualification for majority agreement and the qualification for an alternative position. As a result, in envisaging the presentation of a more open process they found difficulty in risking the emergence of minority positions without this tripping over into full defeats. That continued to be a problem, but there was now more willingness to accept minor defeats, especially defeats which could be retrieved later at the party conference or be avoided in the manifesto. That willingness was influenced by the declining party interest in Partnership in Power, the sinking membership and the loss of local activity.

2) Exeter

Background changes

The National Policy Forum held at Exeter in July 2000 was heralded by its Chair Robin Cook as 'designing the blueprint for the second term of a

Labour Government – building on the foundations of the first term'.[38] It was held against a changing political background. Criticism of the Government had begun to build up at union conferences. The threatened closure at Rover highlighted the lack of legislative protection for workforce information and consultation. At the same time the apparatus of control had come under increasingly fierce public criticism, particularly in relation to the London mayoral candidate selection.

There were some shifts of managing personnel now. Cruddas's position in No. 10 had been weakened by his role over the Employment Relations Act and he was less involved. Sally Morgan did some of the major advance planning and Lord Falconer, Ian McCartney and Geoff Norris were in the managerial lead for the Government on policy dealing with industry and labour law. Although comprehensive management would be retained, the command and control style of party management embodied in the abrasive domineering personal style seen at Durham was now viewed as a problem. Ministers were encouraged to show that they were listening. Some of the NPF members noted more eye contact and more smiles in meetings over amendments.

Unlike at Durham, the relevant policy-commission members were now included in the ministerial meetings. But the link to the rest of the party's policy-forum process was broken because, whereas in 1999 the NPF representatives saw what had been submitted from the regional parties, now they were not available unless NPF members visited the regional offices. It was a cutback for financial reasons, given that there were around a thousand submissions, but also reflected priorities about the partnership and became an additional permanent weakness.

Trade unions and coordination

Policy coordination and the No. 10 package

Arrangements for integrating the TULO organisation had not provided a policy dialogue with the leadership in spite of the original intentions of some union representatives in the NEC trade union review group. In 2000 came the first moves that would eventually lead to a more significant policy role for them. Encouraged by vigorous lobbying from an energetic new TULO liaison officer, Natascha Engel, Morris agreed that unions should try to coordinate their policy-document amendments through TULO in order to enhance the coherence of their collective policy input, although to what end was not immediately clear.

The TULO office was also trying to get No. 10 to work more closely with them in campaigning and communication. Important NEC union loyalists and the Political Office in Downing Street saw the possibilities of using this closeness for managing the coming NPF at Exeter. From the Political Office came a series of moves to ensure that the trade union coordination would in effect be taken over by a package of initiatives which would be offered by the government. The initiatives would involve pro-posals which received discreet support from a group of loyalist-inclined unions and which others were likely to favour, but the initiatives would be few in number and build on discussions taking place already with the TUC. The unions would also be told what red-line issues the government definitely would not find acceptable.

Just to make sure nothing went awry, unusually the Political Office tried to build into the NPF the role of the TUC rather than TULO which was considered less accommodating. The TUC was sounded out about submit-ting policy statements into the NPF party process and encouraged to be discreetly represented at the NPF in order, it was said, to give the policy deliberations some coherence which might be arrived at through Govern-ment-TUC discussions. At this stage also, this seemed to fit in with some new signals that Blair was moving towards national social-partnership arrangements. In a letter on 26 July, he proposed a more regular timetable of meetings, and alongside this was floated the idea of more effective dis-cussion involving the TUC and employer representatives.[39] Nothing came of it in terms of social partnership. As for reducing the role of the TULO and independent affiliated unions, after a tough negative response from some of them, the proposals were sidelined.

Blair grew increasingly nervous about what was shaping up at the NPF. He did not approve of the affiliated unions using Partnership in Power over anything which covered the conditions of work – an important area of CBI concern. At a meeting with the senior union leaders in Downing Street in the month before the Exeter NPF, Blair told union leaders bluntly that he could not tell the CBI that the conference (which followed the NPF) had told him what to do on these issues. At the JPC later he gave the view that they 'should not be discussing labour law at all'.

Once the political battle moved towards Exeter, pressure particularly from the GMB and the GPMU ensured that there was indeed a discussion of labour law, albeit one where past a red line there was no movement from the government side. More than at Durham, there were also regular union meetings to monitor and report about what was going on. These revealed, not for the first time, differences between different unions over how to respond to the package. A majority agreed that there should be no attempt to push further than where the government was by the opening of the NPF. The GMB's hard attempt to push the agenda, particularly on family-friendly policies, failed, so they voted for the existing package. The GPMU concentrated on trying to extend the Employment Relations Act to firms with fewer than 21 employees, but an agreement between Byers, the GMB and the GPMU was rejected on the advice of the Downing Street policy officer Geoff Norris. Essentially, as the voice of Blair-CBI, he over-ruled them. The GPMU then voted against the package.

The package covered information and consultation, national minimum-wage improvement, a fairness at work review, parental leave, in-work training, sectoral training, learning representatives, the partnership fund and the young-workers directive. They were carefully worded by No. 10 Downing Street so as to leave some room for manoeuvre and cause the fewest problems with the CBI. Some small adjustments were made as the consultations went on, and later two significant additions were added through the TGWU in the dialogue at Exeter, on transport workers' working time, and on the Agricultural Wages Board (see below), but it remained basically the package of policies proposed by the Downing Street managers in collaboration with loyalist unions. Of course the manner of it drove a coach and horses through the Taylor doctrine of 'no parachuting', but that was now ignored.

The huge number of amendments from UNISON had made them part of every issue. They were the most assiduous over the longer term in using the two tracks – through the TUC and through the party – and were also pivotal to party management tactics working closely with No. 10. They emerged from Exeter with an enthusiastic report on various positive outcomes including particularly acceptance of statutory learning reps, over which pressure from UNISON through the TUC was already leading to a degree of government acceptance. There was, additionally and separately from the package, a significant input over their major area of concern, drafted by Nita Clarke and Maggie Jones en route to Exeter. Acceptance was gained from the JPC that 'PFI should not be delivered at the expense of the pay and conditions of the staff employed in those schemes nor should it be based on the principle of a two-tier workforce.'[40] So UNISON gained the most in discussions with the government but also continued to assist as a wedge against union unity.

Negotiations had now become a feature of the culture at the NPF. Some in the leadership saw it as inevitable and some saw it as a helpful mechanism of accommodation. Others, however, were deeply resistant. They reacted to what they called an 'old politics'. Blair had always been unhappy at negotiating with the unions over policy at all. It was a contamination of the ideal of rational persuasion in policy-making. Yet management manipulative activity to control the politics of rational persuasion was acceptable if it ensured leadership supremacy, and block votes were acceptable if they were in support of the government. These priorities of management dominated other procedural considerations.

Generally the union leaders were at home in this culture of negotiation. As always and in accordance with previous attitudes towards priorities, there was no question of demanding it all. The TGWU at this forum was generally unwilling to push past the government position on labour law stated by the Friday that the NPF met. Their senior official and party Treasurer Margaret Prosser saw it in the context of general negotiation judged overall. 'We won't push on this if we can get that', particularly the reference to the extension of the working-time directive to transport workers. With the cooperation of the minister Larry Whitty, who had a partnership view of party and government relations, working with Joe Irvine of the TGWU secured a helpful verbal improvement.

More significant still was another variation in ministerial attitudes reflected in ways that issues were managed. On the Agricultural Wages Board, the Minister Nick Brown was sympathetic to the TGWU's opposition to abolition, a 'modernisation' which was being advocated from the No. 10 Policy Unit and the Cabinet office and supported by the employers and the CBI. Brown first ensured that abolition was simply one option rather than the government option. The draft of the policy document, influenced from the No. 10 Downing Street Policy Unit, met a furious response from the TGWU's agricultural workers' representatives at the Exeter forum. A meeting was held with ministers led by Brown, which came up with an amendment stronger than that originally put forward by the TGWU themselves and that became a resource in intra-governmental policy-making. Norris could not control everything.

The AEEU had priority issues which it was prepared to push vigorously in private but keeping a watch on the limits of the situation and with an eye to an overall gain rather than victory issue by issue. They had hardened their opposition to the elected mayor procedure with a clever amendment which stipulated that in the ballots to agree a mayor there must be a minimum turn out, on the same lines as for trade union recognition employment law. In the private discussions, the two ministers involved – John Prescott and Hilary Armstrong – were divided on this: the first against, the second in favour. As the AEEU position had been well publicised in the party, the union left the issue with the original neutral formula of the document. But the drive from Armstrong and the government in favour of elected mayors continued, and in the manifesto became a blunt commitment. As for electoral reform – another distinctive AEEU priority issue – the final 'compromise' of a review was more easily worded for ministers to accept it here and in the manifesto because Blair doubted that in the Cabinet there was a majority for electoral reform.[41]

These negotiations were very problematic in the eyes of many of the CLP representatives. The work-group deliberative process at Durham had been uneasily subordinate to the ministerial meetings and then to the deal over not discussing pensions. Now at Exeter it was further undermined by on-going discussions and accommodations between ministers and the unions which took so long that they delayed information to the workshops. Jim Knight, then a CLP representative, had an amendment on holiday rights but was not allowed in the meetings with the unions. Easily pilloried as union privilege, it was not a view of the unions that the Leader and the managers were anxious to contest.

Return to managing pensions

However there had been no implementation of the Durham agreement on the welfare state review. Various ministerial and managerial explanations were given for this non-event. It was an accident of 'too much on the ministerial agenda'. It was 'a failure of communication'. The debate 'did begin to take place, but through low-key contacts'. But pensions had become an even bigger public issue now as irritation festered amongst pensioners since the budget decision to uprate pensions by only 75 pence. Bad faith and a fix were suspected, particularly when it turned out that the issue of pensions was to be ruled out of order by the JPC at this Exeter NPF on the grounds that it had been decided the previous year. Brown's indication at that JPC meeting that he was opposed to a discussion on it at all this year was challenged by normally loyal union representatives. From the contributions that followed, it was assumed that their concerns had been registered but as was the practice, there was no vote. Later it was found that the agenda of the NPF was as Gordon Brown had wanted it.

There was a strong reaction from within the unions, even from officials who privately did not agree with the pensions-earnings link. Some of it was shadow boxing, but much of it was genuine concern and anger at the way the agreed partnership policy process had been subverted by the Chancellor and supported, as it turned out, by the Prime Minister. The procedural issue was even raised by Margaret Prosser after a speech that Blair gave to NPF representatives. The answer he gave was extraordinarily frank and revealing: 'We are trying to manage the party',[42] said as though that was sufficient justification. In the end the issue was only temporarily resolved by an understanding that it would be debated at the party conference on a contemporary-issues resolution, thus throwing the argument wide open to a major public confrontation.

Management and alternatives

Leaving the pensions issue to one side, in terms of their response to other resolutions the new situation gave the managers a dual task. They had to protect the government especially over issues considered important, but they also needed an overall outcome which legitimised Partnership in Power, including some alternatives which were not crucial but might receive enough votes to be sent to the party conference, ostensibly in the face of opposition by the leadership. Overall, 658 amendments had been received: 30 had been ruled out, 38 non-endorsed went before the NPF, of which 29 were defeated. The rest were accepted. Eventually after a series of plans had come to nought, by luck as much as managerial judgement, seven alternatives were passed to go to the party conference. Two, which the leadership could live with, were privately welcomed by the managers as alternatives extending New Deal grants for school repairs, and extending Sure Start programmes for preschool children into the second term of a Labour Government. One on lowering the voting age to 16 was regarded as very likely to be defeated at the conference. Four others were regarded as more problematic.

RMT, ASLEF and TSSA had gained enough support over a technical issue of rail safety to carry a minority position to take to the conference. Over House of Lords reform, in spite of ministerial resistance, some loyalists pro-reform broke with the managers to gain a minority position for the conference. Local government representatives, with highly developed expertise, realistic by nature but with some deep concerns over government policies, linked with CLP representatives who were also local councillors and secured some union support over the Education Local Government block grant. Here the influence of Jeremy Beecham defeated the appeals of the Minister Hilary Armstrong and gained an alternative position. The biggest ministerial problem was an amendment of some concern to the CBI raising the individual employer's responsibility and penalties for pollution. It was only narrowly defeated, so it went to the conference as an alternative position. Over all these issues, to varying degrees, the relevant ministers and managers had to shift their attention to the approaching conference. What happened to them will be shown in Chapter 11, pp. 359–60 and in Chapter 15, p. 480 over the manifesto.

Partnership and divergence of purpose

Creativity and management

Initially in 1996, one of the potential benefits of the new process appeared to be its openness to the creative identification of new problems, and the creation of new solutions. In 1999 Blair placed special emphasis on the wastage of the national creative genius of the British people.[43] Blunkett had encouraged the establishment of the National Council for Creative and Cultural Education. It was possible to envisage encouragement to a collective creativity in the party which would be a satisfying and unifying experience cutting across old alignments. But the 'partnership' process was not managed for a free flow of cooperative and iterative collective work. Horizontal policy communication between local parties had become discouraged and circumscribed. The early political education, well done in itself, was never attuned to ideas generation and then was seriously cut down for financial reasons: when this was replenished it was for education into electoral messages.

Evidence about the best circumstances for collective creative endeavour is that it helps if the initiating process is seen as being genuinely welcoming. It helps also if there is a freedom of communication, an absence of manipulation, a lack of fear of hidden agendas or forms of penalisation for deviance.[44] On all these counts management failed. Some aspirations in 1996 proved unrealistic in terms of the educational costs and the adverse effects of factional divisions, but they were crucially undermined by the way that No. 10 dominated formulation, by the way that members' representatives were subordinated and by the way that the managers policed the process. Police officers do not make good creativity mentors about anything other than how to do their own job. Creativity could have found much better facilitators.

There is always a difficulty in tracing the origins and interplay of ideas, but what is clear is that a headquarters list of 18 amendments noted after the NPF at Exeter as new ideas that had come through the process[45] was not persuasive. Some items were nonsense, as though David Blunkett had never thought about encouraging citizenship education or that Clare Short never considered primary education in the developing countries. It was suggested later that the idea of NHS Direct and Sure Start came from the local policy forums.[46] This is doubtful. The idea of the service appears to have emerged from a recommendation by Sir Kenneth Calman, the Chief Medical Officer, in his September 1997 report *Developing Emergency Services in the Community*. David Blunkett was confident that Sure Start came from a discussion between himself and Tessa Jowell.

Revealing about the politics of control was that one potentially significant new policy, the environmental personal culpability amendment of 2000, was hidden, and an important new diagnosis of the cause of a poverty problem, that of predatory lending (loan sharks) – specially emphasised by Robin Cook as NPF originality – went in the manifesto only after a late protesting push but in a form that was easily passed over and not easily pursued (see Chapter 15, p. 480). Instructive later also was the report from Powell of Blair complaining that in government all the new ideas came from No. 10 rather than the government departments. Powell's frank comment was that it was not helped by the No. 10 domination.[47]

Managed limitations and contemporary issues

The limitations of this policy process and its short-term value to the leadership can be seen across a wide agenda. Historically the party could pronounce its views before and during the governmental policy process as well as after the event. Now under Partnership in Power, as far as possible advance pronouncement by the party was prohibited. An emphasis on making sure of winning led to major policy developments being initiated without being brought into the process for debate and decision. Neither Partnership in Power institutions nor the PLP Departmental committee process (discussed in Chapter 13, pp. 419–21) were involved in the early formulation of what became the public sector reform policy around 2000–2001.

As for the steps leading to the invasion of Iraq, there was no party exposition, let alone detailed debate on Blair's Chicago speech, made on 24 April 1999, called *The Doctrine of the International Community*. There was, he said in that speech, a new need to qualify the principle of non-interference in the internal affairs of other nations and 'the most pressing foreign policy problem' was identifying 'the circumstances in which we should get involved in other people's conflicts . . . when and whether to intervene'. It might have been thought that given the pressing nature of the practical problems involved, opening up the discussion of intervention and its criteria could act as an essential education in the possible achievements and difficulties of this course of action, thus preparing the party and beginning to take the discussion into the public arena.

Yet in the draft National Policy Forum Report to the conference of 2000, there was only the briefest of references to 'conflict and rules for intervention' and it was not one of the items noted as 'given particular consideration by the policy commission'.[48] Privately the reason given by a key manager for this lack of consideration and emphasis was that it was 'non-controversial'. In retrospect, it is difficult not to see this as Leader and management seeking to ensure that any awkward questions relating to possible future interventions were not dwelt upon in the party. And the party was not in a position to prepare to deal with a Leader who proved to have, in Mandelson's later diagnosis, a tendency to 'a kind of tunnel vision' where Iraq was concerned.[49]

Shortsight and disillusionment

In the skilful managerial preparations, as in other forums and at other times, there was a short-term priority view of management imperatives which sometimes resulted in collateral damage and some unforeseen longer-term consequences. Initially enthusiasm led to about 800 party members putting themselves forward as candidates for the 27 CLP places to be elected for the NPF at the 1997 party conference. By 2000 there were only 41.[50] The decline was attributable to some disillusion with the whole process, and also the decline of membership and CLP activity. Durham in 1999 had for some in the unions deepened distrust and stimulated a reaction which led to the public conflict over pensions at Exeter in 2000. More long-term, though, in 2000 the package of other issues of union concern taken over by No. 10 under managerial supervision did the necessary job of forestalling a strong independent union input, but it also created an unanticipated precedent of tacit acceptance that TULO had a legitimate policy-coordination role. There was a development here which would eventually become central to the politics of union responses to management and what later became the Warwick Agreement in 2004.

Notes

1 NEC document PD38, 18 July 1995, p. 3.
2 Interviews with Roland Wales, Reading, July 1995, London October 1995 and Chicago, May 2000.
3 Ibid., July 1995.
4 'Advisors to Ministers', House of Common Research Paper, 00/42, 5 April 2000, p. 13.
5 Ibid.
6 Ibid.

7 *Partnership in Power*, p. 7.
8 Ibid.
9 Ibid.
10 NEC Committees, Task Forces and Panels, GS 2/11/98, NEC 17 November 1998.
11 *Partnership in Power*, p. 14.
12 *Partnership in Power*, p. 14.
13 Meg Russell, *Building New Labour: the Politics of Party Organisation*, Palgrave Macmillan, Basingstoke, 2005, p. 157.
14 *Morning Star*, 31 January 1998.
15 *Partnership in Power*, p. 18.
16 Ibid.
17 JPC May 1998, note on voting process and interview with Blunkett.
18 David Blunkett, *The Blunkett Tapes: My Life in the Bear Pit*, Bloomsbury, London, 2006, entry November 1998, p. 98.
19 My verbatim notes.
20 My verbatim notes.
21 *Partnership in Power*, p. 8.
22 Maurice Winstone, 'Filtering Out Democracy', *Red Pepper*, September 1999.
23 Ibid.
24 Russell, *Building New Labour*, p. 151.
25 NPF Report to the Party Conference, 1999, p. 85.
26 *Partners in Power, Newsletter of the National Policy Forum*, Number 3, December 1998.
27 Conference newsletter, *Partnership in Power*, a message from Tom Sawyer, General Secretary of the Labour Party, Monday, 1997.
28 LPCR 1998, p. 14.
29 *Tribune* editorial, 9 July 1999.
30 Jeremy Beecham, chairing a session of the 2005 Party Conference, my verbatim notes.
31 John Edmonds, quoted in CLPD Campaign Briefing, 28 September 1999.
32 Minister talking to a welfare work group, my verbatim notes.
33 GS 2/11/98 and interview notes on the away day, 27 October 1998.
34 Matt Coates, *Fabian Review*, September 1999.
35 *Tribune*, 15 January 1999.
36 Patrick Seyd and Paul Whiteley, *New Labour's Grassroots: The Transformation of the Labour Party Membership*, Palgrave Macmillan, Basingstoke, 2002, p. 24.
37 Russell, *Building New Labour*, p. 149.
38 My verbatim notes.
39 Letter from Tony Blair to John Monks (not supplied by Monks), 26 July 2000.
40 NPF Report 2000, p. 133.
41 Alastair Campbell and Richard Stott (eds), *Extracts from the Alastair Campbell Diaries: The Blair Years*, Hutchinson, London, 2007, entry 13 September 1998, p. 323.
42 My verbatim notes.
43 LPCR 1999, p. 58.
44 Derived from academic evidence submitted to the National Advisory Council on Creative and Cultural Education, 1998–9.

45 GS: 32/7/00, NEC papers, Report back from Exeter.
46 Hilary Benn and Meg Russell, *Rebuilding the Winning Partnership: Proposals for Labour Party Renewal*, pamphlet, June 2007, p. 10.
47 Jonathan Powell, *The New Machiavelli: How to Wield Power in the Modern World*, Bodley Head, London, 2010, pp. 79–80.
48 NPF Report to Conference, 2000, p. 2.
49 Peter Mandelson, *The Third Man: Life at the Heart of New Labour*, Harper, London, 2010, pp. 352–4.
50 *The Times*, 2 December 2000.

11

Managing the party conference

The intensification of management

Management organisation

Blair's first conference as Leader in 1994 had been less of a triumph than the skilful spin suggested. There had been not only the defeat over Clause IV but also an unpublicised defeat on composite 49 reaffirming existing defence policy by 54.2 per cent to 45.8 per cent.[1] His renewed doubts about whether many in the party were serious about winning the election were reported by Martin Kettle, a columnist close to the new leadership.[2] What then took place was indicative in method and purpose. Immediately following that conference, without consulting the new General Secretary or the staff of the organisation department, Blair called together a selected group, including Mandelson and other close insiders, to emphasise planning for future conference victories: 'Next year it must be five out of five' Blair is reported as saying by one official present.

There were two interrelated major concerns here. The first was that unwanted constitutional changes generated from below must be avoided, whilst securing the constitutional, organisational and policy changes judged essential to the 'New Labour' project. The second was a pervasive concern over presentation. The Leader must be seen to be in complete control of the party, and the many potential advantages of an event which drew so much media interest must be maximised. Avoiding a fractious conference, especially one where the leadership suffered a reverse, was essential. Getting out the right messages could give the party an electoral lift. One example quoted by Liam Byrne was that after the bitterly divided conference of 1981 the party had lost 10 per cent of its support. In the unifying conference of 1983 it gained 11 per cent.[3] The specific message of a good conference was contained, as it had been since 1985, in the changing key platform slogan. In future, management had, in the words of Peter Mandelson, to be conducted like 'a military operation' to 'defuse, discount, and eventually dismiss any vote against the leadership'.[4]

Planning delivery

In the past, the key managerial role had been played by the General Secretary, but after 1995 the work was delegated by Sawyer to two task forces.

One, concerned with organisational and administrative matters, was led first by Peter Coleman then David Gardner, with an organisational conference unit run for many years by Richard Taylor. The other was concerned with the politics of party management. This was run from the General Secretary's Office by Cruddas with Wilson, Hakim and (until he moved to the AEEU in 1996) by Tom Watson. They worked closely with McFadden and Morgan in the Leader's office. The group was augmented by others as required. It became a cross-departmental effort in headquarters.

Organising for victory each year had a long gestation. Delivering the conference meant initially envisaging the satisfactory final outcomes in collaboration with the Leader's office and shadow ministers and later the ministers. It then involved creating a 'real' agenda which would be taken in the conference (as opposed to the formal agenda of resolutions and amendments submitted by the CLPs and affiliated organisations). This would be constructed partly through instigation of resolutions and amendments, then by filtering the rest of the submissions though the CAC agenda-making and timetabling process, the tactical compositing of resolutions, and then the conference chair's scripted choice of which resolution to take (see below).

Unknown to the delegates or to the party at large this national and regional machinery covered a large canvas: summer seminars preparing the delegates, delegation liaison, delegates' questions, resolution and amendment instigation from CLPs and affiliated organisations, preparation of speakers, political-education workshops, NEC report problems, and liaison with NEC representatives on the CAC (a link stopped in 1998). Adapting management to the rise of the CLP vote in 1996 from 30 to 50 per cent involved an extensive local organisation and regional briefing on the eve of the conference (see below). Within and around the conference, managerial meetings could be a large-scale affair. On the Sunday evening prior to the start of the conference about 50 people were involved in the political-management planning meeting.

From 1995 onwards the conference appeared to be heading for major problems and possibly defeats for the leadership. The managers met a wide range of problems on policy. In 1995 these involved education/grant-maintained schools, Liz Davies, the minimum-wage process, Trident and defence policy. Instead, with total management success came a sense of celebration, and the view was confirmed that this was how it ought to be done in future years. Andy McSmith commented under a heading 'Ten–nil . . . and Old Labour was lucky to get nil'.[5] 'Disciplined and brilliantly orchestrated' was how Philip Gould described the conference.[6] In practice there was less coherence than that, with some things going wrong and having to be salvaged. Nearer to the mark was that, as McSmith revealed, Cruddas and McFadden became known then in party circles as 'the Lennon and McCartney' of party management – 'we can work it out'.[7]

In 1996 the final conference before election year looked especially tricky. But pensions, defence, minimum wage, rail transport, child benefit, education (selection again) – the expected big problem issues – were all dealt with without platform defeat. In 1997 lone-parent benefit, tuition fees, rail renationalisation and Partnership in Power were expected to be the difficult ones. But again, there were no defeats on any of them.

The process was not without its internal managerial aggravations and tensions, some of them between shadow ministers, the Leader's office, later No. 10 and the spin doctors, with some party managers in the middle. There were also some tensions within Millbank over who did what. The conference political task force operated semi-independently of the managing process in the General Secretary's office, and with the introduction of Partnership in Power came a reorganisation and further intensification of managerial activities (see below) and some new territorial and political tensions. At one stage the organisation task force was vying with the political task force for a political role. In 1999 and 2000 under a new General Secretary, the argument broke out again as the headquarters managers took more control but the No. 10 Political Office was still heavily involved.

Management organisation and the unions

Management and working with the unions
Whether voting weight of the affiliated organisations was 70 per cent as in 1994 or down to 50 per cent as from 1996, the unions – not the CLPs – continued to loom largest in the immediate priorities and focus of party management. Union relations were more important for the reasons that this political linkage had always been important. Regardless of the newly individualised voting arrangements at the conference in 1993, union procedures and culture committed the delegates of each union to voting together.

The managers had regular and, after 1997, virtually day-to-day contact over industrial and political matters with the unions; the conference planning was simply a natural extension. Although it varied union by union and officer by officer, being helpful to the Leader's office became part of a routine interaction. Even where the union and/or its senior officer was known to be uncooperative, there was usually somebody in the union hierarchy who could be more helpful, often the NEC representative.

Although the Leader and the managers did not know quite whom they distrusted the most – the unions or the constituency parties – initially it was the CLPs who were seen as the bigger problem, with the unions viewed as more likely to provide traditional stability. That role in limiting the political influence of the CLPs had another advantage. It was useful in deflecting criticism from the CLPs arising from their disappointment at being minor players in spite of changes in the voting weight.

Concentration of the union votes had always been regarded as a major asset for conference management in limiting the numbers of those directly involved in managerial discussions whilst raising the numbers being mobilised. Although all union affiliation declined after 1993 or in a few small unions remained stable, the concentration of votes on the union side continued. In 1993 NUPE had amalgamated with the Confederation of Health Service Employees (COHSE) and the non-affiliated National and Local Government Officers association (NALGO) to form UNISON and create a more weighty conference force. In 1994 the NCU and UCW amalgamated into the Communications Workers Union (CWU) and in 1995 the AEEU had amalgamated with the EETPU. By 1996 there were six major unions with over 200,000 affiliated members. The TGWU and UNISON each had 700,000, the GMB 690,000, the AEEU had 540,000, USDAW 258,000 and the CWU 252,000.

Union restraint and union divisions

Encouraging the managerial relationship with these unions was generally their role playing restraint, their understanding of the leadership's battle with the media and a traditional appreciation of the responsibilities of the political leaders, especially strong on the right of the unions. Whatever private supplication and sometimes criticism went on in advance of the conference votes, the most automatically supportive in voting were USDAW led by Garfield Davies, the AEEU led by Gavin Laird and Bill Jordan, then from 1996 Ken Jackson. The CWU was sometimes harder to pull into line, even led by Alan Johnson until 1997 when he became an MP and his position was taken by a maverick loyalist, Derek Hodgson. But it was normally one of the managers' rule-of-thumb positives for the party conference, as was also the GPMU, ISTC, MSF, RMT and TSSA.

Although John Edmonds remained irksome in his personal private challenges to Blair and where he thought necessary, Brown, and he was always looking to expand union leverage, the GMB also generally still voted with the leadership or helpfully remitted their resolution, until the battle over pensions, explored in Chapter 10. There was, as we have seen, some distancing by the TGWU leader Bill Morris reflected in his attitude towards the party's finance even though he was the chair of TULO. The uncertainties and divisions within the TGWU Executive Council lessened briefly just before and after 1997 as party loyalty became uppermost. Morris kept close links with, and on key occasions where the union mandate made it possible, responded favourably to Gordon Brown. In spite of his resentments at Blair's leadership, the TGWU majority, especially with Prosser as Labour's Treasurer and NEC trade union group convenor, prioritised a constructive, cooperative role in attempting to deliver support in the conference policy votes.

As on the NEC and at the NPF, UNISON politics at the conference each year was subject to distinctive internal relations around the commitments of the UNISON-Labour organisation and the priorities of the General

Secretary Rodney Bickerstaffe, already noted. At the conference he made some very effective and often critical speeches. Yet, in voting, he and the union attempted to be cooperative in the glare of conference publicity. In 1996 a UNISON emergency resolution on asylum and immigration management grievances, added to the public and CLP pressures for reform but was remitted on a technicality. In 1997 after a powerful two-pronged speech rejecting PFI ('a bad policy') and pointing up the creation of a two-tier workforce, Bickerstaffe agreed with the GMB's remittance to the NEC of the critical composite resolution No. 3 on public sector policy.

Bickerstaffe allowed room for the operation of Jones, the NEC representative and Nita Clarke, the Political Officer to secure some conference accommodations through their networking with the managers and other unions. He was also personally and politically close to RMT General Secretary Jimmy Knapp and to Prescott. Knapp was at times influenced by the Deputy Leader's signals to assist in some key conference votes and Bickerstaffe went along with that.

Blair's management and the 'good conference' meeting

It was a sign of the importance of the unions that regardless of increasing tensions and apparent distancing of the political leadership from the union leadership, remarkably, all the way through the period of opposition and then the first term of government, Blair called regular discreet annual meetings with six major union leaders just prior to the party conference, to urge 'a good conference' and discuss handling very problematic issues. This followed a pattern established by Kinnock and it marked an important stage in conference liaison with the unions.

These were not deal-making meetings and insofar as there were understandings and concessions over policy, these went through a separate informal managerial process. Blair's policy-making style in relations with the unions here was not one that invited negotiation. If he offered anything it was on a take it or leave it basis, as over management of the policies in the Road to the Manifesto document. In the 'good conference' meetings the unions invariably received nothing for their cooperation. If policy issues were raised in lament at all in these meetings Blair was adept at deflection, as 'we are already doing so and so', or 'we agree in principle but', etc. Most typical was his 'we cannot possibly commit ourselves to that' or simply and emphatically, 'we will not be doing that'.

Late on the Saturday evening after the compositing meetings had finalised the wording of the resolutions, there was also another significant follow-up meeting, this time of the inner circle of managers with the union political officers. This was especially valuable in eliciting the first collective responses to the situation in their unions in the light of what the Leader and managers were seeking. In some cases it was also a follow-up on the planning which had, with union support, produced the composite resolutions.

Agenda management: the conference arrangements committee

The historic role of the unions in party conference management was symbolised and reflected in the way that union representatives operated within the formal representative managers of the Conference Arrangements Committee, elected by the conference. The composition had been amended in 1993 after a recommendation of the NEC's trade union review group. It became five general section (effectively union) seats of whom two must be women and two from CLPs of which at least one had to be a woman. The committee continued to be chaired by a union representative from one of the five unions (at this time the AEEU, GMB, TGWU, UNISON and USDAW) represented by size and via a tradition of reciprocal voting.

The CAC was expected to be the servant of the conference and the voice of fair play. Historically in agenda preparation it had accepted items based on the number of resolutions submitted and then made a choice of acceptable and appropriate resolutions for discussions. The CAC had a range of genuine problems in managing the agenda fairly and had good practical reasons for taking a hard line on some exclusions. Much of what the committee did had been consensual, but it was always intricately linked to the party managers responding to the leadership.[8]

As indicated, the major key to conference management was the use of the agenda by representatives of the political leadership to assist the engagement of union allies. Generally (but not always) the committee was attuned to the leadership's managerial needs as mediated through the culture of 'a good conference'. That required some sense of a genuine clash of views, but also brought in wider political considerations either overtly or covertly. The committee under Blair was, as normal, heavily dominated by loyalists and discreetly prompted by its secretary – a senior party official. Also influential was the CAC Chair, head-hunted by the Leader's office to ensure cooperation. The Chairman during 1994–7 continued to be Frank Wilkinson, a GMB loyalist, and from 1998 was Margaret Wheeler, a UNISON Labour loyalist.

The traditional cultural pull towards the needs of the party leadership was reflected in the constitutional convention that NEC statements and documents went on the agenda automatically and had more authority than the resolutions. NEC rule amendments had to be tabled. But rule amendments from within the party were subject to one year's retention pending recommendation by the NEC and even then there had to be pressure at the conference to get them debated. Emergency resolutions, even if accepted as a valid emergency, could not be guaranteed time and, if it caused difficulties, the leadership's view of 'a good conference' often determined that it remained undebated.

On the CAC, some members could occasionally dig in their heels with another view of 'a good conference'. Especially was this the case in the rare occasions when trade union interests were thought to be seriously at stake and a resolution was backed by a significant weight of union opinion. Even then it was often finessed with some managerial agreement on the wording directing the resolution to an on-message target. The most sensitive case occurred in 1996 in the timetabling of an emergency resolution which defended the CWU in the postal dispute. It was unwelcome to the Leader but was handled diplomatically by the union without criticism of the Labour Leader and then skilfully buried by Campbell's media managers.

CAC and Partnership in Power

Under Partnership in Power from 1998 the tendency for the committee to operate as a sympathetic adjunct of the leadership was now further consolidated by the new culture of partnership defined as avoiding party–government confrontation. There was a new fixed round of policy-making which fed into the conference and involved the abandonment of the regular process of resolutions submission. There were new strict criteria to be applied to the small number of contemporary resolutions allowed. The criterion of 'one motion on a topic not substantially addressed in the reports to Conference of either the NPF or the NEC which has arisen since the publication of these reports'[9] left room for considerable interpretive scope which was used with political ingenuity and sometimes a degree of managerial effrontery.

'Substantively' was not to be understood literally. If a policy commission had made any reference to it, it could be ruled out of order by the CAC on the recommendation of party officials. The Secretary of State for International Development, Clare Short, told angrily in July 1998 how she had challenged a policy officer over the report of the Foreign Policy Commission which had said that one particularly controversial item had been discussed, making it ineligible to debate a conference resolution on it. No such discussion having taken place, she got it changed.[10]

The restrictions on the conference debating issues of immediate concern under the new policy-making arrangements were displayed particularly over moves towards privatisation. The policy change was never discussed by party institutions. By 1999 partial privatisation of air-traffic control was now in the legislative pipeline and referred to in a sentence in the commission report. It received thirty contemporary resolutions, three times as many as any other motion, but these were excluded on grounds that it had been discussed by a commission. Overall substantial numbers of contemporary resolutions were excluded but the figures were not announced. There was little that delegates could do in response. The CAC reported to the conference at the beginning of the session and often each day, but the procedures adopted in connection with contemporary resolutions after 1998 made it impossible to refer back the CAC report in relation to them. Voting for priority topics started before the conference opened because of the tight timing, and the CAC decisions thereby became irreversible.

Wheeler as the CAC chair was more inclusive than the previous occupant, Wilkinson, as the committee became more factionalised. The dominance of loyalist members of the committee was qualified by the unusual role of John Aitken of the TGWU, nominated to the CAC after an internal political move within the union in 1996. Although he was on the left, he had to be supported by both right and left as TGWU representative according to long-standing custom of reciprocal voting and representation by size. He was a close ally of CLPD who had one CLP representative, Doreen Cameron, elected in 1995 and then the left-wing MP Audrey Wise in 1998. Their combination resulted in several ties over crucial decisions, with some issues tabled but others not.

The election of Wise, an MP, created political room for a counter-attack by loyalist politicians. Both left-wing CLP representatives were defeated by two well-known junior ministers, Yvette Cooper and Stephen Twigg, in 1999. They were supportive of the office managerial position but also now more sensitive to the needs of the delegates for information and more open to calls for the CLPs to have a guaranteed share of contemporary resolutions.

Spin doctor Lance Price portrayed the unions as 'clearly out of order' and 'bending the rules' in forcing a debate on pensions as something which had gone through the NPF;[11] it was a typical instinctive anti-union line from No. 10. It failed to register that, as shown here, the spirit of Partnership in Power had been deliberately broken by the party leadership at the 2000 NPF. The evasive treatment of pensions and earnings strengthened the case for the value in having a contemporary resolutions procedure which would act as a safety valve. Attempts from the General Secretary to get the contemporary motion from the unions rejected in 2000 were repulsed by Wheeler, the chair of the CAC, backed by a CAC majority.

NEC and CAC: the change in communication

Here an important surreptitious change connected with the CAC should be noted. In the past, the NEC and its representatives had been in effect an appeal court against CAC decisions mainly acting as an instrument of the managers but also sometimes of NEC dissidents, adding a fresh voice on behalf of wider party considerations than the immediate managerial pressures. The convention had been that the NEC had one or two liaison members on the CAC as it approached the conference period. Also, just prior to the conference, the CAC went into the NEC meeting and sometimes faced a challenge to its planned agenda. One element of the managerial agenda of Partnership in Power was to change this pattern of communication in a way which protected managerial influence. Under the new Partnership in Power 1997 the two facets of conventional liaison with the CAC were abandoned, without any advance discussion by the NEC. It became now asserted that the agenda was purely a matter for the CAC.

Compositing

Up to 1997 the huge agenda of resolutions and amendments was reduced by the process of compositing. From 1998 the much smaller number of contemporary resolutions was also composited. In theory it was a neutral procedural device supervised by the CAC and helped by party officials. In practice as with so many procedures, there was a heavily political involvement, as was seen in Chapter 3 (see pp. 99–100). Historically this had always been the case.[12] An important element of the procedural advantage of the managers lay in the fact that if a resolution-holder refused to composite then there was no guarantee that the resolution would be called.

The creativity of this managerial process, as illustrated in 1993 on OMOV, lay in influencing the combination, exclusion and inclusion of resolutions or parts of resolutions which would fit the known commitments of trade union concentrations of votes so as to attain the product that 'worked'. The politics involved skilful suggestion amidst social pressure and the authority of officials. It could enable friendly union leaders to lose elements of their original position in the composite. Under 'New Labour' it increasingly also involved instigating resolutions which were formally part of the opposition to the platform but had damaging elements carried by supportive clued-up delegates who fitted into the tactical plans of the managers. It could as part of the composite ensure the neutralisation or rejection of unwanted decisions.

Perhaps the most important compositing politics took place in 1996 over the minimum-wage proposal. Ministers and managers wanted to ensure no commitment to the existing formula but to leave the final decision to a Low Pay Commission. Remittance was the favoured managerial target for resolutions which advocated the formula, but if it could not be achieved then help had to be given to supporters of change seeking arguments to disengage from their mandates.

It is uncertain whether what then happened had an element of good fortune or was perhaps a 'Maradona's-hand' of intervention. The printed composite resolution involved an uncorrected misstatement of the proposed minimum-wage formula. This had the crucial consequence that the TGWU and the GMB were given reasons not to stick with the formula at this stage. However, underneath this agenda-management the key was that the Blair position was winning a persuasive battle for union support at different levels in the unions. No union leader came to the rostrum to defend the formula, and opinion was moving behind appeals for unity on the central issue of winning a historic minimum-wage policy.

Agenda instigation

Much more than was realised, the conference agenda from 1995 up to 1997 became increasingly instigated by the managers. Instigation had been a managerial feature in the past, sometimes provoked by facing a group of what had been model resolutions sent in by a lobbying group – most typically, on party issues, the Campaign for Labour Party Democracy. But now the instigation was more comprehensive in its coverage. Managers privately estimated that at the extraordinary highly pressurised OMOV-battle Conference of 1993, about 30 per cent of the resolutions and amendments submitted by affiliated organisations and CLPs came in as a result of central prompting. By 1995 under the increasingly intensive management, this had shot up to around 50 per cent. In 1996 virtually all the resolutions actually tabled for debate came from instigated sources. As one key manager, worried about the future, put it, if they were not instigated there might have been no pro-platform resolutions on many issues.[13]

The instigation process started from the deciding what the managers wanted the conference to say and then finding a home for it. Instigation was first focused especially on those unions aligned with the traditional right who provided the most regular loyal assistance to the political leadership. But others, though more critical, could be relied on to see a common interest in the wording of resolutions. It was part of the expertise of managerial liaison with the unions that the managers knew whom to contact in anticipation of cooperation, teasing out the boundaries of union commitments and searching for whatever tweaking was called for in contributing to appropriate outcomes. The union political officers had their own pan-union network and from 1997 the party managers, particularly Cruddas, could use that linkage now increasingly organised through the GPMU.

As for increasing instigation through the CLPs, the managers worked to their own party contacts and then what could be done through other officials at national and regional level. The whips' office and its links to PLP loyalists were sometimes involved in getting resolutions in. The wording of resolutions would be done with an eye on the final form of the composite resolution that would be produced and placed before conference by the CAC. As with nominations, there was no obligation on the central managers to guarantee that the resolution had emerged through a properly constituted CLP process.

Union delivery

What the managers could do in delivering the unions depended on relations with each union and the ability of allied union leaders to deliver their unions in the light of their mandates. Each union had its own political traditions and policy commitment. Each took guidance from its senior official. But union leaders had varying degrees of effective authority and control over their delegations. Much depended on salience of the issue to the union membership and the weight of opinion amongst the active members. Leaders of several unions, particularly the UCW (later CWU), TGWU and MSF in opposition, all faced periods of unstable support in their delegations, and most others had their problematic moments and issues. Each union also had its subtle differences in the way those at or near the top related to the management around the Leader. Union representatives and officials could be privately more accommodating than their union's formal position, and there was an important role in some delegation meetings for prominent loyalist NEC representatives who also played a party managerial role.

The subject of pensions precipitated important interventions which led to the bypassing of the union resolutions. In 1996 Barbara Castle and the retired union leader Jack Jones, now leader of the National Pensioners Convention, had built up a considerable momentum of support behind re-linking annual pension increases to rises in average earnings as well as bringing back a state earnings-related pensions scheme. In reply, a full review of pensions policy was promised by Gordon Brown and, in the negotiations, Jones also gained the inclusion of the National Pensioners Convention in the discussions. Jones's action followed his old concerns, assisting pre-election unity on the one hand whilst attempting to advance the policy agenda on the other. Under his influence and that of Bill Morris, the TGWU agreed to support the NEC pensions statement. In conjunction, UNISON agreed to move from its opposition and to abstain. However, the promised review did not report till after the 1997 conference and failed to deliver what the union leaders and the pensioners lobby wanted.

More unusually, in Opposition, there were occasional issues which provoked tension between some old-hand Shadow Ministers and different managers in the Leader's office. In 1995 the abolition of compulsory competitive tendering in favour of 'best practice' in local government procedures was pushed by UNISON, supported out of conviction by the Shadow Minister, Frank Dobson, and given background support by Cruddas, despite some gritty reservations from the media managers. It did gain NEC and conference support.

In 1997, the NEC was pushed by the Leader to urge remission of composite resolution 26 from TSSA, which supported the return of railways to public ownership and total opposition to privatisation of the London Tube. Remission was supported by 16 votes to 9. Amongst the 9 were representatives of GMB, GPMU, RMT, TGWU, TSSA and UNISON. That seemed to indicate a likely defeat for the platform on a resolution moved and seconded by the rail unions. But Prescott argued powerfully that financial priorities for 1999 could not be set now and, privately, gave guarantees to the rail unions about their immediate priority, safety protection. That was accompanied by acceptance of the emergency resolution from ASLEF on rail safety and followed by TSSA remission of composite 26. Encouraged by the TSSA and with no protest from the RMT, UNISON came into line.

In government, defence policy produced important issues which divided the unions on priorities. Some unions – AEEU, ISTC and MSF – wanted a positive statement about defence diversification and the maintenance of the British defence industry. There was also an argument which was to loom larger in the years to come: 'If we expect them to risk their lives . . . we have a duty . . . to ensure that they are provided with the best military equipment'.[14] Those arguments, carefully managed, won the day against what was described as 'arbitrary one-sided' disarmament decisions,[15] carried in CLP resolutions to cut defence expenditure and scrap Trident. Straight policy deals at the Conference were unusual but the dropping of UNISON support for the decommissioning of Trident was helped by an offer from the government securing the unions' representation on the committee dealing with PFI. The UNISON delegation was encouraged to ignore its mandate and move behind the leadership.[16]

Management and the CLPs

Preparing the new regime

The redistribution of votes that first gave CLPs 30 per cent of the vote in 1993 and then 50 per cent in 1995 stimulated new intensified managerial moves to influence the CLP delegates. From the party's national machinery working through the regions, a managerial organisation had emerged, integrating with the Sunday evening socials set up by Whitty before his departure in 1994. There was an extensive organisation of effort to win CLP delegates' support. However, this should not be represented as a 'redefinition' of management,[17] especially without defining what that management was. The purpose of management was the same everywhere – organisation to produce outcomes in accordance with the management definition of the party's interest, normally as constructed by the leadership. In that process it was subject here as elsewhere to the codes of the culture of party management which were described in Chapters 4 (pp. 136–40) and 5 (pp. 162–3).

CLP delegates: who were they?

As with the affiliated organisations, delegates were appointed in accordance with the size of the membership under the rule of one delegate per first 750 members then one for each 250; normally most CLPs could send only one delegate. The rule change of 1991 clarified in 1993 made it an obligation that CLPs send a woman as delegate at least every alternative year. Ironically in the light of Blair's furiously critical attitude towards the rule noted in Chapter 5, this change reinforced the obligation to rotate male and female representation each year[18] and made management easier.

In 1994, 57 per cent of the 654 CLP delegates were women – a record in that feature, and in 1995 because of the rule it was estimated by party officials that approximately 80 per cent of delegates were first-timers – probably a record since the party was founded. This enhancement of the turn-over of delegates, and the greater presence of the inexperienced, made the CLP delegates less knowledgeable about past behaviour, rules and practices, and requiring new assistance in understanding the way that the conference worked.

This supportive educational process was also an opportunity to encourage a constructive role and amenability in awareness of the role of the media mischief-makers. New delegates were in general impressed with the sense of occasion. Although it was never in the rules, historically the general belief in all the attending organisations had been that the delegate was there to implement the mandate of the organisation that sent them. Advice from the party officials had always been (correctly) that mandating was not part of the constitution and delegates could not be penalised for disobeying a mandate. However, the way that this was expressed by officials after 1997 was taken to indicate that mandating was inappropriate. It then became the encouraged folklore that 'you are not allowed to do it'.

So, although it never disappeared, mandating decreased especially as the absence of any detailed advance agenda under the new arrangements meant that there was less incentive for local parties to discuss what was likely to happen. Local policy forums had no discussions focused on the party conference. The link between local political decision-making and the conference was broken, and the delegates were more open to new communication and new influences.

Attendance

Overall, as far as one can ascertain from limited information from party officials, there was a decline in delegates sent from the CLPs over the first term of government. It affected primarily the minority of CLPs whose membership entitled them to send more than one delegate. Some of this decline may be accounted for by a period of financial stringency, some of it by the reaction of the more Northern regions to repeated use of venues on the South coast. There was a notable shortfall of CLP delegates from Scotland, said to be because devolution gave Scotland powers which made the British party conference less important to them. In 1998 only 23 of 73 Scottish CLPs were represented.[19] Some of the decline may have been another sign of disillusionment with the way the conference was managed. Whatever the cause, the decline lowered representation in the NPF elections, adding to the case for reform of that procedure.

Voting with their bums

In general CLP delegates had, in the past, been assiduous in their conference attendance, glued to the debates. But, by the late 1990s, many delegates did not stay in their seats the full time. The party conferences became seen as more of heavily managed PR events and fund-raising tools[20] with the conference hall surrounded by a massive army of paid promotional stalls on behalf of various organisations and lobbyists. It became increasingly expensive for ordinary party members to attend. Symbolic also was that the security arrangements turned the conference areas and hotels around it into an almost impregnable zone. Both contributed to a sense of diminished importance of the delegates. To some extent they were even encouraged to be absent by the organisational events put on whilst the conference was sitting. In the past, the party's training sessions for improving facets of party activity had been confined mainly to lunchtimes. These events were interesting and effective, particularly on campaigning, whereas the debates in the hall, with carefully chosen speakers and reiterated themes, often became boring. With votes now held at the end of the day rather than immediately after debates there was also less pressure for delegates to stick around during the day.

The undermining of the tradition of delegates attending consistently made them less aware of what was going on and what was being said. When votes were taken abstentions were not recorded and the votes were announced in percentage terms for and against. Thus the organisation that could keep 'the right people' in their seats at the time of voting could be much more important than it used to be under the old pre-1993 voting system. After the Leader's speech, people were often gagging for a coffee and apt to stay talking about the speech in the cafes. This was particularly significant because the debates and votes on organisational and constitutional issues were taken after the Leader's speech.

CLP attitudes and moods

The initial problem for the managers in winning policy votes in the CLPs section, and the limited influence of 'New Labour' on the party at large under Blair, is made clear by the valuable studies of Seyd and Whiteley. There was some shift in attitudes closer to Blair's policy positions amongst the new members after 1994 but the difference from existing members was smaller than often thought over the touchstone issues of free markets, public ownership, attachment to trade unionism, defence expenditure, nuclear weapons, high public expenditure and high taxation.[21] Amongst the members generally the biggest shift in attitudes had taken place in favour of tough policing policies towards crime[22] and against extending public ownership on principle.[23] But privatisation had miniscule support amongst new or old members[24] and simple majorities of old and new members were in favour of returning privatised enterprises to the public sector.[25] Majorities of new and old members were uncritical of high income tax.[26] There was strong opposition to nuclear energy even amongst new members[27] and a simple majority of them were opposed to British nuclear weapons.[28]

In the most striking of overall findings, Seyd and Whitely found that 'Grassroots support for collective intervention in the market, redistributory strategies and strong trade unionism remained consistently strong and belies any notion of successful New Labour takeover of the party'.[29] In a significant shift in members' attitudes between 1990 and 1999 there was a drop from 57 to 37 per cent in those wanting policies adjusted in order to capture the centre ground.[30] This was a problem for the managers which, insofar as they picked it up, justified getting the delegates away from the influence of the local parties and under their own managerial influence.

Still, there had always been a strong loyalist and realist tradition in the CLPs as well as robustly critical radical forces. Although the networks of the traditional right were ageing now and had lost some of their organised local strength, the solidaristic attitude and loyalties could be aroused in local parties by encouragement to atavistic reactions against what were considered repeated 'oppositionists' who failed to see the bigger picture and 'move on'. The 'New Labour' victory in 1997 particularly aroused a practical realism about financial constraints. There were 'priorities' and 'you can't do it all at once' effectively became the managerial messages. To that extent, Mandelson's view that 'the new party's instinct is to be their ally'[31] was correct. But there were other forces at work.

Regional liaison teams

The managerial message carriers became very well organised. In 1995, the first year of extended involvement of the regional party organisation in managing the conference, there was some uncertainty about whether it would work and from some an anxiety about the propriety of it. But the extent of the success – all votes supported the leadership – led to considerable enthusiasm in the party machine and a keenness to be part of the managerial action. The job gained prestige and became seen as an asset in reputation and advancement.

Following this success, at the instigation of the national centre, each region created a regional liaison team of less-senior party officials and trusted loyalists to handle the management of the regional delegates. Their objectives were every year the same, to ensure complete victory for the leadership and to organise the elections of suitable loyal candidates for the National Policy Forum. Prior to the conference there was a national meeting of the one person from each regional staff who was responsible for 'the politics'. They received the line in steering the delegates on key organisational and policy issues which was then passed down to the regional liaison teams.

The primary initial task, then, was one of intelligence in relation to the list of delegates. What was the political position of each delegate likely to be and what effect would this have on the voting of the conference on key issues? More particularly, what did individual delegates feel strongly about, which ones might be moved in support of the leadership even if doubtful now, and how might they be persuaded and by whom in the region? The delegates list was also graded in terms of their capability to liaise and speak in support of the leadership.

The whole process became consolidated with Labour in Government. Regional officials grouped delegates into categories A, B, C and D in terms of voting reliability. Keeping the As and Bs informed and in support and ensuring that they voted was the key to winning. Approaching the uncertain Cs with the most appropriate arguments and repeated approaches, and through the most appropriate contacts, was also an important part of the task, and with that also a nursing which assisted in building up their sense of obligation.

After 1997, at least one meeting of conference delegates was called in the summer in each region prior to the conference to help the delegates by introducing them to the procedures of the conference and to give advice on various practicalities, including getting in to speak and preparing the speech. This meeting also provided an opportunity to begin the reiteration of the importance of having 'a good conference' and especially an awareness that the media were constantly looking out for divisions.

CLPs and national persuasion

Information about the delegates was conveyed also to the national managers, making it easier for them to know how to approach those carrying resolutions from their constituencies. It involved giving favourable interpretations of the leadership's policy commitments, specifying the difficulties and appealing for patience and loyalty, perhaps with intimations and assurances about what might happen in the future. It could also involve an invitation to meet the relevant shadow minister or, later, minister with, possibly, a breakfast meeting. It might on occasions involve movement back and forth between delegates and political leaders to illustrate and at times genuinely reflect responsiveness, if only in a limited way. Over time the central managers developed a code which obliged them to show respect for the delegates in what they said and did, but over issues of greatest concern there was the occasional report of heavy intimidating pressure by regional managers desperate to deliver. Repeated dissidents in category D could find themselves at the receiving end of what they regarded as bullying.

Although there do not appear to have been any cases where policy was initiated or changed simply because of CLP representations at the venue, as at the NPF, CLPs could combine with those of other forces particularly the unions to secure limited adjustments or parallel concessions. And here also CLPs were elements in a network of moving influences which sometimes interplayed with the internal disagreements and changing views of ministers and managers. Over what was called the primary purpose rule, which barred entry into the UK for people married to British citizens, following pressure from UNISON and TGWU and other unions, from CLPs and also from the constituency and local party of Jack Straw the Shadow Home Secretary, the rule was dropped quickly after Straw became Home Secretary in 1997. Without changing the general thrust of policy,

immigration and asylum issues even evoked at times a managerial cooperation in adjustments (see below).

Some CLP representatives were linked to effective pressure groups
with contact networks across the party and the unions. Protection of the
environment on occasions gained enough CLP support to threaten defeat
for aspects of government policy. That did not happen, but in 1997 a
composite resolution 22 moved by SERA urged a review which would lead
to phasing out of the reprocessing of nuclear waste. Unusually, this was
accepted by the NEC although No. 10 was not entirely happy with it.
In practice the policy became submerged in practical problems and never
implemented.

Conference internal communication

Alongside the changing voting weight of the different sections, and the new
procedures of Partnership in Power, the most significant change was in the
pattern of internal communications. Although some old features including
fraternal addresses remained, communication was reorganised and redirected
so as to increase the influence of the managers and the leadership, a feature
noted already in the covert undermining of communication between the
NEC and the CAC.

Outside the hall in the past, organised by a wide range of Labour Party
tendencies, interests and policy positions, was an extensive range of fringe
meetings. In the continuation of this fringe under Blair, there was no evidence of decline in party debate during the Blair years. Indeed the managed
predictability of some of what went on in the hall may have stimulated
more argument outside it, and some managers thought that that was how
it should be. However, with the conference itself now beginning not on
the Monday morning but after 2 pm on the Sunday, and the introduction
of Saturday and Sunday regional party events, there was an increase in
managerial mobilisation before the conference, some difficulties in booking
venues and a reduction in the size of attendance at traditional fringe events.

Sunday morning before the conference officially opened, traditionally
the first meeting of a prominent opposition group from the left took place
under different names, speeches were made and tactics openly discussed.
In 1996 the Grassroots Alliance took over the Sunday morning slot with
the same spirit of open conspiracy backed by information on conference
management, supplied in booklet form by the tireless Pete Willsman. Their
meetings varied in size at around 80 to 100, much less than it was under
the last Labour government. Around 50 to 70 people from the traditional
right in the party, who kept their identity in the Labour First organisation,
had a private meeting on the Sunday morning. In a subdued way, they
lamented some government attitudes but mainly went through the agenda
noting the problems for the leadership and urging support. Other pro-
government public meetings were called as necessary.

Conference delegates had also for years been bombarded with leaflets and literature from different organisations as delegates made their way into the conference. Many of these were political day-trippers seeking to influence events from outside the Party. There were always also internal Labour Party groups including the Labour Coordinating Committee, before it closed down, and the Fabian Society magazine. The most regular were the daily broadsheets of the Left groups, particularly the familiar 'yellow pages' of CLPD. This gave news usually critical of the leadership but also performed a service of giving the delegates information on the previous day's decisions and advising them how to vote on what was coming up today. After Partnership in Power, this was now in effect challenged by another piece of assistance to delegates in counter-insurgency: communication from the party organisation was strengthened. In 1998 a conference newsletter sometimes called *Conference Brief* and later *Conference: the Newspaper* (or *Conference Daily*) was produced. The policy unit in the hall produced its own daily information service to delegates with an official view, daily policy briefing with a précis of key speeches.

Regional liaison teams at the conference

The operation of the regional liaison teams varied at the conference, to some degree depending on the style of the regional organisers. London region particularly had a reputation for heavy pressure on the delegates in terms of which way they should vote. In other regions the persuasion was normally softer and more discreet. The conference regional events, organisational and social, were important places for the regional liaison teams to move around, explaining the leadership's decisions and elaborating tactics and arguments, spread round those delegates known to be supportive, A or B. The senior public representatives in the regions joined in the operations – urged by the managers at the parliamentary end to play this role. Aspiring MPs or junior ministers earned kudos by assiduous management activity.

On major issues mobilisation of loyalist MPs was also done nationally in a London meeting preparing the ground for the conference and assisting the managerial process. The national and regional outcomes fed into the central organisation, usually with Phil Wilson as coordinator. By the time the conference opened the managers centrally as well as regionally knew all they needed to know about each delegate and a sophisticated management system was in place to communicate with the majority of delegates and urge specific votes on each issue. The view grew that, as a senior (perhaps over-confident) No. 10 manager put it: 'If we can get to them first we can get them'.

By 1999 or thereabouts, in a break with years of traditional differentiation, the regional officials as well as the liaison teams were sitting with the regional delegations. 'Just resting or sorting out arguments over seats' was the explanation, but the fact was that there was now an influential presence: leading the applause could produce its own inhibitions upon dissent. If delegates needed on-the-spot advice the managers were more than willing to give it to them. It added to the situational pressure of constant inclusive attention.

Elections to NPF

Following the managerially influenced decision of the Party into Power discussions the conference was also the location of the election of a majority of the CLP representatives via nine regional groupings. For the conduct of the conference elections it was announced to the NEC in 1997 that the conference would also be the venue for 'regional hustings for National Policy Forum elections on the Sunday evening as part of the regional delegate briefings'.[32] But NPF elections, which the Partnership in Power document said 'would be made more transparent',[33] became more controlled and manipulable as a result of the partisan communication of central party members of staff to the regional liaison teams informing them who had voted and who had not, thus assisting their job of further getting the vote out. Even so, the open clash of positions and ideas which is normally the essence of democratic contest did not fit into managerial priorities under the delivery ethic. In subsequent years the hustings were abandoned without advance announcement.

Where the managers had strongly disapproved of 'oppositionist' or 'difficult' candidates, special efforts were made to try to ensure that they were defeated, but it was not possible to shift some candidates with high reputation and a high work rate. In Yorkshire the private view of a leading official was that a GRA minority representation made the whole thing look more legitimate anyway. Some NPF loyalists were adamant that they did their own basic work and were critical of the efforts of the machine, but this attitude could also be a useful contrivance to cover the extraordinary dominance of the managerial organisation in creating and sustaining the loyalist organisation.

Communication: conference speeches

In the conference debates there had always been a communication asset for 'the platform' in that the last word was given to those from the NEC, replying to the debates with speeches substantially longer than those which had been made from the floor. They could not only argue the NEC's response to the debate but, until the replying procedure was changed after 1997, also interpret the resolutions in qualified ways, politically convenient as seen from the platform. Apart from the conditional rejection of NEC reform in 1995 noted in Chapter 6 (see p. 188), the eve-of-conference meeting of the NEC, which agreed its attitude to conference resolutions, did not go against the wishes of the Leader after 1994, and therefore neither did the NEC wind-up of the debate.

NEC members had always had a strong presence in platform speeches but after the introduction of Partnership in Power in 1998, on the initiative of the General Secretary,[34] in the marketing of the party, primacy of platform contributions was given to speeches by Cabinet members. Since the mid-1980s the centrality of the NEC had been visually altered to bring to the fore those who would make the best impact on TV. This caused regular friction over the implied loss of status of the NEC. By 2000 there were two platforms – an NEC platform at the side and a small changeable operational platform in the centre which held the chair, General Secretary and a variety of NEC and non-NEC people, some of whom were preparing to speak.

It became taken for granted that major parliamentary leaders spoke from the platform with more time than others. Other ministers frequently backed them up, in speeches fitted into the debates to boost support at appropriate points. They were also in effect supported by loyal CLP representatives from the National Policy Forum presenting reports covering the different commission areas. Guest speakers could also be brought in to showcase practical aims and achievements and exemplify the transformation of lives, sometimes recounting a relevant experience in support of the government's position.

With rare exceptions, an MP did not become a front-bench spokesperson without command of rhetorical skills as well as mastery of a case and a capacity to handle large meetings. These speakers were almost always effective, with some of them raising waves of spontaneous applause which drew coffee-drinking delegates back into the hall. Their contributions were attuned to what would enthuse and please the delegates as well as the wider public audience, sometimes announcing new initiatives, leaving delegates feeling well disposed, enthusiastic and at times inspired. Blunkett, Brown, Cook and Prescott could make speeches of a force and quality which almost invariably received a standing ovation. There was always plenty of servicing for them, sometimes advance prompting at the regional meetings. The place on the timetable could sometimes influence the reception. Immediately after lunch was the time to avoid with constant movement, slowly coming to life as the hall filled.

Though rarely did speeches, even those of great quality, turn debates there were exceptional occasions. It is possible that the vote of the CLP delegates on education policy was decided in 1996 in the hall in a battle between Blunkett the Secretary of State and Hattersley, speaking from amongst the delegates. At the end of the debate, Blunkett produced a very powerful speech, holding the audience in his grip. At one point he told them in reply to Hattersley's call for an end of selection, 'Watch my lips. No selection either by examination or by interview',[35] and the following year, Blunkett repeated 'no more selection'.[36] The statements were later heavily criticised by Hattersley as not consistent with what was happening under the Labour government. 'Lies, lies, lies, Mr Blunkett – selection really does mean selection'.[37] But at the time it was accepted by the managers that Blunkett 'won the debate'. Much less contentious was one highly unusual and impressive case in 2000 of a brilliant extempore winding-up speech by a Minister, Geoff Rooker, over pensions. It may well have boosted the majority in the CLPs for the government (see below).

The apparatchiki clap

Nevertheless, making sure was always part of the Blairite managerial psyche. A carefully choreographed cheering 'people's welcome' to Blair in Downing Street in 1997 was organised by party managers and included many party staff. In 1996 for the first time, groups of party officials were put in the aisles at the conference to lead the clapping during speeches by Shadow Ministers. The activity was obvious and, at the time, an expression of invulnerability. Simon Hoggart writing in the *Guardian* noted that 'They can be spotted by the way they stretch their arms in the manner of an angler boasting about his fish, then slamming them together to create a sound similar to the battle of Monte Cassino'.[38]

In addition to the press derision, some on the front bench also pointed out, in irritation, that it got in the way; they needed to know what the party was feeling. That this consideration had not weighed much in the balance for the party managers was indicative of one of their acute weaknesses. Too much control could hide party opinion, making the leadership insensitive to the state of the party and vulnerable to sudden explosions of anger (see below on the 1999 revolt). Comprehensive strategic clapping in debates was dropped the following year. But it reappeared from time to time as party officials suddenly emerged to clap loudly from the back and side of the halls at key points for favoured speakers. This 'Monte Cassino' clapping could be very intimidating and at times influential.

On three mornings a week, conference debates were replaced by policy seminars held in private 'to give delegates the opportunity to discuss policy in detail with ministers and policy commission members'. Seminar sessions took the form of brief speeches followed by question and answer and some discussion. Potentially it gave ministers the chance to more fully engage with delegates and open out the issue with more candour. Some sessions worked very well, others were one-way streets. A lot depended on the style of the speakers and their capacity for openness and cooperative inclusiveness. Mowlem, Darling and Blunkett were said to be particularly good at it.

Projecting the Leader's supremacy

'You are not the government's audience, you are actually part of the show', Blair told the 1998 Party Conference.[39] This beautifully ambiguous comment was even more significant in the light of the politics of the Leader's speech. It was formally billed as the Parliamentary Report, but the essence of the report – that it could be questioned and if necessary referred back – had long since disappeared. It had become primarily a party celebration of its own identity and of its Leader. Leaders spent a long time before the conference preparing these speeches and were almost invariably seen as triumphant. No Leader had had a difficult reception for his speech since Gaitskell in 1959 met critical interruptions.

That was not enough for Blair's managers. From 1995 the central managerial aim was to project the Leader as the supreme and acclaimed force within the party. 'Presidential' superiority was boosted, if necessary, by taking some of the best bits from proposed speeches of ministerial colleagues. It was reinforced also by preventing anything disturbing his superior status. For many years it had been the custom that two long-serving old party members received merit awards and would make speeches just prior to that of the Leader.

This established an atmosphere of jovial community and an exemplification of commitment and service to which members responded. It was also sometimes very moving. However, it also exemplified a historic continuity which was not a 'New Labour' message. And nervous managers could not guarantee what the experienced obstreperous characters might say in a friendly and amusing way which was shared by the audience. In 1996 the merit awards were pushed from this prime spot to the end of the week's agenda and later the speeches were abandoned. Their original high-spot was replaced by an enthusiastic video which in government came to be accompanied by loud thumping music, in which the managers encouraged a happy-clappy and at times excruciatingly embarrassed audience to join in the wild zombified build-up to the entry of the Leader. As he said, they were 'part of the show'.

Blair was a naturally fluent speaker with or without a written prompt. He had an unerring ability to choose the right word, tone and timing. But, after the initial formidable if misleading speech of 1994, his soundbite-riddled speeches took on elements of the artificial, becoming what Tony Wright MP called 'confections addressed to the TV'.[40] However, to ensure a continuous tumultuous reception from the hall, marked copies of the Leader's speech were handed to about 30 favoured figures from the regions stationed in the delegations around the hall. The text was underlined with indicators at key points. The officials all clapped or laughed instantly and appropriately at these points. Groups of likely supporting visitors were also given favoured places in the hall. For the platform party, groups of loyal presentably representational faces, guarded by their regional officers, were invited from the visitors as well as the CLPs. They had a hidden coordinator encouraging them to clap at key points. This was socially difficult to resist and part of the signal to the hall to join in. In that sense they also became part of the show.

Blair's great strength on these occasions after 1997 was that he was the man 'who has taken us into power'. Implicitly or explicitly, his case to critics was underpinned by understanding that, as Blair put it in 1998, 'the choice you have got is not between the Labour government of your dreams and the Labour government you have got, it is a choice between the Labour government you have got and a Tory government'.[41] In the video before his speech and in the speech itself there was a growing litany of achievements. The Leader's performance and the managers' skill was in drawing out a pride, enjoyment and fulfilment in sharing, however vicariously in the collective party sense of 'our party' and 'our government', successful and doing good over the years in major achievement and in a hundred small ways.[42]

What could not be discerned from this theatrical display and its clamorous reception was any ambivalence, let alone heckling opposition. Yet for many in the party, supportive attitudes lived uneasily alongside a sense of discomfort about Blair's trajectory and the symbols of what he regarded as important. Blair evoked a complex mixture of feeling which included admiration, some disappointment as well as gratitude, and also, even on the most militant traditional right of the party, a nagging concern over what might be being lost.[43] Robin Cook later diagnosed the response of his CLP as being aware of Blair's successes yet with a dawning realisation that he did not share many of the values that brought them into the party: 'regretful rather than angry'.[44]

Floor contributions

There was a decline in floor contribution from the CLP representatives after 1997, from 208 in 1997 to 165 in 1998, as more time was taken up by ministers, NPF reports and guest speakers.[45] Initially, in 1998 and in 1999, this change was balanced to some extent by Blair's question-and-answer sessions. Boldly and impressively, these were taken in public and with no management of the delegates who wished to speak. An uncontrolled selection produced 15 CLP representatives all to one degree or another not fully on message. The atmosphere was friendly; Blair was, as usual, hugely engaging and got his various priority messages across. Around the hall later delegates were enthusiastic and appreciative of the procedure. Lifted by this, nervousness about it amongst most managers disappeared, albeit with some reservations from those who thought that it left too much room for the unexpected. In 2000 the slot was passed from the Leader to Alastair Darling to take questions about the controversial pensions policy before the debate.

These uncontrolled question-and-answer sessions ran much against the trend of floor-speaker control. The predetermination of some floor speakers had often been an element but was now much more rigorous.[46] With the rise in the CLP vote after 1995, the management of contributions to debates was judged potentially significant in influencing their votes in a way that normally did not apply to union delegates. The proposers and seconders of resolutions, in effect, with managerial encouragement chose themselves at the compositing meeting, and there was room for some advance planning and influence by the managers through the earlier managerial instigation of resolutions. Otherwise, the choice of speaker in each debate was the formal responsibility of the conference chair who changed in each session.

Nevertheless, behind the scenes there was one official doing the preliminary selection on the basis of advice from other managers. All delegates wishing to speak were requested to attend the delegate-support office and indicate the topic and content of the speech. Potential speakers were categorised on the basis of information provided by the regional liaison teams. Assistance in drafting was then offered.[47] Within the hall the speakers were then coordinated by a member of the managerial task force. Speakers from the unions were arranged separately but with much less direct individual control by the managers. If a major union General Secretary wanted to speak then usually that was that. The chair and his/her advising official Andrew Sharp and later Greg Cook had indications of the names of speakers to be called, their location in the auditorium and the means of recognition.

There was often great pressure from delegates to allow them to speak in key debates, and complaints that this or that section or group of CLP delegates were not being called. It was impossible to satisfy everybody and sometimes the complaints were unreasonable or special pleading. At other times it was very reasonable. After a row in 1995 between the chair and an over-aggressive manager doing the hall preliminary selections, the chair's responsibility was reaffirmed and a change was made in the hall manager. Strong chairs could make up their own minds but there was a tendency to follow guidance. Even within that guidance there were always some noncontentious criteria of fair balance between the conference sections and between men and women, and always need for advice on those with special experience who could make a unique contribution on an issue. There was also the need to promote parliamentary candidates and sometimes give publicity to individuals standing, with the backing of the managers, in elections such as for the CAC. Not all these choices met the agreement of all the managers.

But partisan management steering in the big debates was the normality. One official, closely involved, asserts that from information available to them it was tactically possible to follow a known opposition speaker with an effective supporter of the leadership and to know who were the most ineffective and unpopular of the potential opposition speakers who might be chosen. Shaw notes that over the 2000 pensions debate all CLP speakers backed the government line yet there was considerable if mainly anecdotal evidence that the pensions-earnings link had broad support in the CLPs.[48] Where they generally found difficulty was in avoiding key opposition speakers. In 1996 the attempt to prevent Hattersley from speaking in the education debate failed. And although some of the managers would dearly have loved for Barbara Castle not to speak in the pensions debate of 2000, they accepted the inevitable.

With so many new CLP delegates now at the conference, a speechwriting unit whose purpose was to give advice and assistance to delegates with their speeches was a helpful initiative, but after 1998 there was an increased emphasis on utilising the party's sound-bites and slogans for media consumption. The most monotonous was in 1999, repeating the mantra of 'the many not the few'. One result of this was to make parts of the speeches excruciatingly boring and to arouse at times audible groans from some delegates. It did not help create a cooperative attitude. On the other hand, boredom also had the effect of highlighting the excitement of hearing senior front-bench speakers and especially the Leader's speech.

Voting and instigation

Partisan steering did not end with the debates. Voting was done by show of hands where the result was assessed by the conference chair or, under the conditions laid down by the CAC, by cards which were counted by official tellers. Asking for a card vote was formally done by a voice from the delegates but there had long been occasional contentious responses from the chair. That continued after 1995 with much depending on what the advance managerial preference was, who was in the chair and who was demanding the card vote.

Managerial excess and miscalculation

Lone parent benefit

The strong commitment to stay within the Tory spending plans had been an integral part of the political strategy of seeking to reassure floating voters and the business community about the prudence of Labour's economic management. Its implication for benefits had not been spelt out in detail. When the party was in opposition, shadow minister Harman had been asked whether a future Labour government would implement regulations proposed by the Conservatives to reduce, by up to £11.25 per week, the benefit of new lone parent claimants for income support, housing benefit or council tax. She had said no. But in government Brown was determined to push the cut through, emphasising the dual economic-political message of prudence and control. Although heavy control could make the public less aware of the party's internal differences, it could also desensitise the leadership to the developing party opinion and signs of an approaching storm. On this it is illuminating to trace the early management in 1997 of the important issue of cuts in lone-parent benefit.

The preparation for the victorious 1997 Conference involved the assistance of loyalist UNISON officers whose resolution on lone parents, which became composite resolution No. 6, emphasised child care and encouraging single parents back to work. Acceptable to the leadership, it became the centrepiece of the conference debate. Composite resolution No. 10, which specifically opposed cuts in lone-parent benefit, was taken off the agenda by the managers after it became clear that the delegate would not be remitting it. No reference to that resolution, or to the benefit issue, was made in the replying speech by the minister, Harriet Harman.

With no voice in the conference debate a momentum built up outside the conference. The delegate with composite 10, Jenny Rathbone, had attended the Labour Women's Action Committee tea party (not as docile an event as it sounds). There she met Annie Marjoram and Audrey Wise MP, LWAC leaders who became organisers of the PLP revolt. After the failure to take the resolution, Rathbone met with Alice Mahon MP, who was later reported to have 'won massive applause at Tuesday's Tribune rally' about the issue.[49] Tribune rallies were written off by the confident managers at this point, but the cause now had lift-off with an added grievance directed at the government's suppression of debate.

Rathbone, it turned out, had been a producer of BBC *Newsnight* and had wide media contacts. The media briefing by opponents of the measure which started at that point continued after the conference, yet the party's media managers, anxious not to give the dissent publicity, refused to supply spokespersons for *Newsnight*.[50] As one minister involved explained wistfully years later about the conference management of this issue, 'We had always got away with it'. As will be shown later, that proved also not to be the case here when it came to the management of the PLP in the Commons. The managerial politics of showing that there was no dissent at the party conference contributed towards a much bigger PLP revolt than had been anticipated (see Chapter 13, pp. 411–12).

Partnership in Power, procedural revolt and the loss of Brown's economic policy

Under Partnership in Power, the resolution-based conference was largely (but not completely) superseded by a rolling programme with amendments that had first passed through the NPF. The promise of alternative positions which could be voted upon at the conference had been central to the support won for the new arrangements of Partnership in Power. But the controls over this procedure and the pressures of majoritarian loyalty at the NPF left no decisions for the conference of 1999. The final version of the Partnership in Power document had, as noted, lost the right of reference back of first-year documents but, in the rush to persuade the delegates, an unqualified facility to reject parts of the report had been confirmed by Mowlem replying for the NEC to the debate in 1997.[51] It was also confirmed by the General Secretary in his post-conference document, *Implementing the New Policymaking Process*.[52] The conference could refer back to the JPC relevant sections of the report which were 'felt not to represent the views of the party'.[53]

Accordingly, articulate CLP delegate Claire Wadey from Brighton Pavilion sought to refer back sections of the economic policy first-year consultation document referring to PFI. This perfectly proper procedural challenge led to great confusion and nervous agitation on the platform. Eventually, under pressure, a reference back was carried of the whole economic document. More uncertainty followed and this was then superseded by a second vote in which the document was declared carried, although with many abstentions. Officials then declared that the vote would be rerun in the morning. There was some quiet enjoyment by Downing Street managers at the loss of control by 'Millbank' but they immediately got to work on the union delegations: 'You can't leave us with no economic policy.' Overnight the unions agreed that they would not rock the boat.

The next morning Margaret Wheeler gave the CAC explanation to the conference that first-year consultative documents could only be accepted or rejected in full. She also gave the important judgement that second-year documents could be amended by alternative positions (of which as we have seen there were none) or, she added, 'it is possible effectively to amend documents by contemporary resolutions' (of which again there were none this year).[54] On this basis and with the unions focused on getting the business through, the document was overwhelmingly carried on a motion to support the CAC report. Subsequently however, as will be shown, contemporary resolutions were not regarded by the managers as having the authority to amend documents.

NPF alternatives

In 2000, an alternative from the NPF on lowering the voting age was opposed by the leadership and easily defeated. Four more problematic alternatives from the NPF had to be managed through the conference. The more controversial alternative on House of Lords reform favoured a chamber with a majority of elected members. The unions did not regard it as a priority and were susceptible to the argument that they should not get bogged down in percentages, elected or appointed. The traditional right, with its majoritarian loyalist tradition, saw an elected Lords as an impediment to an elected Labour Government.[55] With this combination, managers found no difficulty in producing a rejection of the amendment. On funding in education the alternative amendment 'based on a block grant with specific grants to encourage innovation and pilot new ideas' was regarded as too committing and met a different kind of fate. It had never been established who owned the alternative resolutions from the NPF, the mover at the NPF or the NPF itself, given that it had decided its alternative status. The uncertainty was, as often, an asset to management. The amendment was suddenly withdrawn by the mover following discussions with a minister. Other local government representatives were very disconcerted.

Two other issues which had been alternative positions, the rail-safety system and the pollution of the environment, were much more tricky and dealt with accordingly. On rail safety the RMT argument could be said to be essentially technical and about timing, and as a safety measure it was likely to be carried whatever the political leadership said. So it was not contested and a hand vote carried overwhelmingly. The result was buried as far away from media observation as possible.

The most important was over environmental pollution, where the alternative position coming from the NPF was to press for higher fines for companies who polluted the environment and to 'consider introducing penalties for directors as we have done with health and safety'. The workshop report at Exeter said that 'the principle of holding polluting directors personally responsible for the action had widespread support'. But the No. 10 Policy Unit was unsympathetic to various aspects of the environmental campaign which constrained the market. They were not in favour of penalisation and the proposal involved various legal complexities. Crucially, in this pre-election period, they were more than normally anxious not to stir up the CBI. An extraordinary clever multifaceted cover-up therefore ensued at the conference to avoid the defeat.

The NEC representative speaking from the platform was not told that he was replying to the environment debate, thus there was no direct reply from the platform one way or the other. The amendment was treated as agreed so that no vote was held on it. No reference was made to it in any report to the press and the Minister for the Environment, Michael Meacher, was not made aware of it. What the spin doctors made of it was the same as what they made of the rail-safety amendment. The media was told that the leadership had won on all alternatives. Even a very enthusiastic national party official responsible for the propagation of support for Partnership in Power did not know any different.

Contemporary resolutions on policy

The rules

The contemporary resolutions procedures still aroused strong hostility from the Leader, the General Secretary, initially Sally Morgan, and some of the NEC loyalists who became the most hostile. There had been no specification in Partnership in Power of a limit on the number of such resolutions which might be tabled for debate. In practice it was later privately agreed between the managers and the unions that there would be a limitation. Both Sawyer and McDonagh preferred none at all but if there had to be resolutions, then just two. There was some pressure for eight from the unions and others. Four became the compromise. In 1998 four contemporary-issues resolutions were instigated by the unions, and four became 'the rule'.

But there was never any central encouragement for CLPs to submit such resolutions and the tight criteria created by the Policy Director, backed by No. 10, positively discouraged it. Many resolutions were ruled out of order and their content not reported to the conference. Since the ballot for contemporary resolutions got under way before the first session of the conference, nothing could be done by the conference to challenge an exclusion. In 1998 Margaret Wheeler reported to the conference that over 200 resolutions had been received, but by 1999 this had sunk to 141 resolutions. There were hopes in headquarters and No. 10 that under these conditions the procedure would drop away entirely, especially as the CLP organisations were never directly informed of the resolutions which had been received, no amendments were allowed and there was no formal procedure of response.

For Cruddas, managing relations with the unions, it remained a useful device for showing increased sensitivity, moving issues along, smoothing relations and/or affirming a supportive position for the government. Indeed it became the tacit understanding that union contemporary resolutions would be produced each year in cooperation with Cruddas at around the time of the TUC. By agreement with the managers, the unions voted together in the priorities ballot and always secured the chosen four union issues, submitted by the four major unions, none of which in this period caused a problem in the No. 10 Political Office. There was some tension with the medium- and small-sized unions which could not get a look-in and even more so from CLPs. Their resentment, directed at the unions, became part of the range of arguments from those managers who were opposed to the contemporary resolutions procedure, adding to their campaign for abolition. Criticism of union dictatorship gained a new momentum. Yet what was illuminated in practice in the way the facility was used were the limited priorities of leaders of the big unions. And they did not attempt any constitutional changes that would have strengthened them or limited the party leadership.

The Post Office campaign and contemporary resolutions

Policy-making over the Post Office was unusual and long-lasting in its tensions. Unconstrained advocacy of his union policy against privatisation by Derek Hodgson, General Secretary of the CWU, continued in all the relevant venues. The campaign was all the stronger because it had public support. Also, privatisation as a policy had not been in the 1997 manifesto, and had never been argued for by the leadership in a party forum. Mandelson, whom Hodgson found 'straight and prepared to listen', decided it should be kept in the public sector. Brown and Mandelson then became involved in a long private argument over the technicalities of commercial freedom within the public sector, with Mandelson heavily spun against by Charlie Whelan.[56] To helpfully keep up the pressure at the conference of 1998, Hodgson protested from the floor of the conference that his members were 'sick and tired of spin and leaks' on the Post Office. Some of the delegates welcomed it mistakenly as a rebuke to Mandelson.

In the autumn of 1999, endeavouring to ensure that opposition to privatisation of the Post Office was debated and supported once again, Hodgson demanded that there should be five not four contemporary resolutions. Margaret McDonagh's derided statement to the NEC about the number – 'It's a rule but it isn't written down' – made perfect sense within the agreement between the managers and the union leaders over the number of contemporary resolutions. In the end, after Hodgson had mobilised support across the NEC, the CAC accepted five. As it happened, the Post Office topped the priorities ballot so the extra place was not needed. The leadership and the NEC found it politic to accept the resolution, given the scale of support from the wider party.

Yet what was also clear is the extent to which the other contemporary resolutions which went on the agenda in 1999 were an accommodation involving the No. 10 managers with the unions in instigating a positive agenda. Thus, the UNISON-led resolution congratulated the Government on the Good Friday Agreement in Northern Ireland and attacked the opportunism of the Conservatives. The resolution on the European Working Time Directive moved by the TGWU and supported by MSF was used to reiterate policy and publicly confirm assurances about the scope of the adoption into British law given by the Secretary of State at the TUC. The resolution from the AEEU on the knowledge-based economy welcomed a recent Prime Ministerial announcement of a tripartite conference on partnership. As a consensual concession to the CLPs the resolutions on poverty were all from CLPs supportive of the government – including one which came from the local party of the General Secretary, Mitcham and Morden. All this was more a managerial device operating with support from the unions than any union dictatorship.

More pressure built up for reform of contemporary-resolutions procedure but it now came from two different directions. Some came again from the managerial abolitionists but also, in 2000, CLPD attempted to create a constitutional ruling that there be eight priority issues: the top four from the CLPs and the top four from the affiliates. It was a move deeply resisted by the managers, and the NEC followed suit. It was argued to be a divisive proposal but it also presented a challenge to managerial control. The CAC now began a long series of discussions leading to a compromise outcome in 2002.

Contemporary resolutions on party organisation, and the NEC report

Historically, the resolutions on organisational and campaigning issues which were submitted each year could contain important proposals or indicators of dissatisfaction with the management of party organisation. They could also form part of a movement for constitutional change which became successful in encouraging pressure from below. As noted, the rule change embodying Partnership in Power went through the conference of 1997 with the fulsome promise that an NEC Report would offer options and alternative proposals on organisational and campaigning issues, and would be subject to a much longer debate. As it now appears, this was simply another managerial ploy and the procedural choice never materialised.

The report was part of the managerial agenda of the political task force managing the conference. What was discussed on the report was influenced by the rubric of 'moving on' in avoiding post-mortems on difficult issues, especially on issues which were connected with government policy. Debating internal party issues, including NEC constitutional amendments, depended on the extent of internal pressures from managers and loyalist NEC representatives. If managers were expecting opposition and criticism, supportive comment would be organised with the NEC speaker as usual having the last word. But there was an element of the haphazard in these sessions. An adroit delegate could find some room on the organisational reports which covered finance as well as organisational issues and some rows were impossible to contain, notably the party's angry reaction to the levy on CLPs to fund the European elections, after the members' role in selections had been restricted; that finance issue turned into a widely critical session. Nevertheless, this was not a big managerial concern as it took place in front of empty press seats and out of sight of any interested TV coverage.

As one of their contemporary issues on party organisation, the party bodies had the right to submit one constitutional amendment. But here the old controls survived. These were filtered through a process which laid down that all constitutional amendments must be referred to the NEC for a year. They then made recommendations to the next year's conference, at least in theory. But the amendments were not timetabled by the CAC. A campaign had to be mounted to ensure that this happened. Once voted on, such a rule could not appear on the agenda for three years unless the NEC required it. Building up a broad party campaign was made more difficult because the now reduced agenda of resolutions was no longer circulated to CLPs for amendment well in advance of the conference, and horizontal political contact amongst CLPs had diminished.

The big conflict: contemporary resolutions and pensions

From early September 2000 there was pressure – particularly on Rodney Bickerstaffe proposing a resolution from UNISON – to follow his union's previous behaviour and seek to help the platform in some way to avoid a defeat over pensions. He attempted to find his way through by standing out for the union position but with a resolution carefully worded so as to leave open the possibility of acceptance. The UNISON policy proposal was 'an example' of how to ensure the integrity of the basic state pension. His priority objective was to keep up the pressure to get the pensioners a better deal in the light of its decline as a percentage of GDP since 1997. Some of Blair's staff were prepared to accept the UNISON resolution couched that way in order to avoid a defeat, but Brown was adamant he would not do it.

Instead, an Economic Policy Commission statement on pensions in accord with government policy was taken to the JPC for its support. It reaffirmed the government's commitment to the basic state pension as the foundation of pension provision. It outflanked the critics by its emphasis on putting pensioner poverty first and announcing the plans for raising the Minimum Income Guarantee. And it announced the introduction of a pension credit to help pensioners with small savings or small occupational pensions.

This was followed by a highly unusual procedure by the ministers for dealing with the critical UNISON resolution. The compositing meeting was recalled with Brown and Darling in attendance. The majority there were persuaded to accept remittance,[57] although by convention the decision to remit or not was in the hands of the mover not the meeting. In the event, in the hall Bickerstaffe refused to remit. After the debate the resolution was carried by 60.21 per cent against 39.79 per cent. The unions had supported the resolution by 84.17 per cent to 15.83 per cent but the CLPs had voted 64 per cent to 36 per cent against. It was argued with some justice that the leadership had won the debate and it was declared that Blair and Brown would ignore the linking of pensions to earnings, although years later both he and Blair eventually moved behind the policy.

There were interesting ramifications to this result. It had been understood by managers that Blair would get a personal lift from the public if he 'took on' the unions. Yet party focus groups before the conference found a resentment against arrogance and certitude[58] and a *Times* focus group showed Blair's major conference speech had met a very unenthusiastic public response.[59] There was a recovery in the polls after the conference and with it a reluctant private temporary acceptance in No. 10 that the party might be being rewarded by the public for its passionate concern over the pensions issue. It was even said that Blair accepted that over the pensions grievance the party had a right to take it up and he would have apologised for the 75p uprating 'if Gordon had not objected'. Still, in November, Labour's lead had dropped again and Greenberg's polls found a 'breathtaking' 60 per cent of those polled said that Labour (presumably meaning the government) was 'getting too arrogant and out of touch'.[60]

Meanwhile, the conference defeat for Blair and Brown aroused an immediate managerial reaction especially amongst those who were against having contemporary resolutions at all. The case for the procedure was rejected because 'We are not going back to the politics of smoke-filled rooms', as though there were no smoke-filled rooms of the politicians and managers managing and the Blair and Brown behaviour at the NPF had never happened. In familiar 'New Labour' mode they went on a counter-attack, 'we are going to have to look now at union policy-making', a regular threat when things were not going their way, sometimes accompanied by instigated media support. Yet, moving into the pre-election period, cooler heads prevailed, the atavism subsided and the agenda of the NPF was settled so as to avoid recriminations and keep policy discussions minimal.

Never lost for an opportunity, the managers also saw another face to this conference defeat that was more reassuring and useful. In Opposition and in the first term in government, the CLPs had not been as docile in voting as they were sometimes made to appear. Even at the pre-election conference in 1996 there had been votes on the rights of the disabled and on the reacquisition of public utilities where according to the managers a majority of the CLPs voted against the platform. But now victory in the CLP section over pensions was presented as 'the party' speaking, giving the leadership, it was said 'the moral high ground'.

However, even on this year's voting, this was not quite what it seemed. Over the alternative position on sanctions against environmental polluters, the strong support for environmentalism, with no difference between old and new members,[61] the strong lobbying through the Socialist Environment and Resources Association, the mood shown in the NPF workshops, the narrowness of the vote against it at the NPF (61–57), and the overwhelming hand vote in the Conference hall, all indicated that a majority in the CLPs voted for it against the leadership's preference. On rail safety also it is almost certain that, if it had gone to a vote the leadership would not have been supported by a majority of CLP delegates. Nevertheless, after this, card votes were, if possible, avoided unless they looked like producing the result that could be presented as the voice of the party members fighting the unions.

Accommodation and insulation

In 2000, a contemporary resolution moved by the TGWU over asylum-seeker vouchers had strong backing in the CLPs as well as some unions. Under pressure, Home Office Ministers agreed to a review and immediate action over the 'no change' rule operated by shopkeepers. With that assurance which the Home Office had been initially unwilling to give, the TGWU agreed to remit its contemporary resolution. Pressure from Bill Morris was crucial to the shift but Faz Hakim from the No. 10 Political Office was adjudged by insiders to have been a significant liaison figure. In 2001 the new Home Secretary David Blunkett, after signalling a change of mood, abolished vouchers for asylum seekers.

Insulation

But management normally created considerable insulation against pressure on the parliamentary leadership and the follow-through which might have kept up that pressure. Remitted resolutions at the party conference went now to a policy commission not to the NEC; so formally did any resolutions agreed by the conference, but no special action followed as a result of a conference decision. They just joined the rejected resolutions and the multitude of unanswered submissions. What happened in 2000 also illustrated that resolutions passed by the conference against the leadership's preferences, even those which had gone through the Partnership in Power process, were not automatically reported to Ministers and were not obliged to be in the next party document even though they were 'party policy'.

In 2001, the report from the environment, transport and regions policy commission made reference to rail-safety protections systems but only after the NEC representative of the RMT, Vernon Hince, had protested against its exclusion. Extending the systems did go into the manifesto although without specification of its form. As for the environmental-pollution resolution, the same report to the conference in 2001 talked only of policy to 'help' and 'reward' companies in relation to emissions, not of sanctions.[62]

Accountability and the end of history

Various firm commitments substantive and procedural had been made from the platform at the conferences of the Blair years, including about the precise operation of Partnership in Power. They could be referred to, in principle, by reading the past verbatim annual conference reports. These had been regarded as a contribution to Labour Movement history and an essential accompaniment to party accountability. Under Blair, the practice became that a verbatim report was only produced after the following year's conference and not advertised for sale, although it was possible (until 2003) for a determined scholar to purchase a very late copy. Needless to say, as with other management activity, nothing of this change was put to the NEC for approval. Many people by 2000 thought that a verbatim conference report no longer existed, but the managers always had it when they needed it.

Notes

1 LPCR 1994, p. 189.
2 *Guardian*, 22 October 1994.
3 *Progress*, Autumn, 1996.
4 Donald Macintyre, *Mandelson: the Biography*, HarperCollins, London 1999, p. 315.
5 *Observer*, 8 October 1995.
6 Philip Gould, *The Unfinished Revolution: How the Modernisers Saved the Labour Party*, Little Brown, London, 1998, p. 281.
7 *Observer*, 8 October 1995.
8 The history and politics of the CAC is examined extensively in Minkin, *Party Conference*, especially pp. 66–83 and pp. 320–1 for the period to 1976, and it is also covered intermittently throughout Minkin, *Contentious Alliance*, for the period to 1990.
9 Rulebook, 1998, Clause 3C2.3.
10 Clare Short, interview.
11 Lance Price, *The Spin Doctor's Diary: Inside No. 10 with New Labour*, Hodder & Stoughton, London, 2005, entry for 15 September 2000, p. 252.

12 Minkin, *Party Conference*, pp. 66–76.
13 Private evidence from managers in the Partnership in Power discussions.
14 Bob Elson, AEEU, LPCR 1997, p. 137.
15 *Tribune*, 25 September 1997.
16 *Morning Star*, 13 October 1997.
17 Meg Russell, *Building New Labour: the Politics of Party Organisation*, Palgrave Macmillan, Basingstoke, 2005, p. 210.
18 Labour Party Rulebook 1995, Chapter 3A, Clause b, p. 14. The previous formulation of this rule had been a recommendation 'should'. It now became 'must'.
19 Ann Black, NEC away-day document, 9 October 2001.
20 Peter Oborne, *The Triumph of the Political Class*, Simon and Schuster, London, 2007, pp. 82–3.
21 Patrick Seyd and Paul Whiteley, *New Labour's Grass Roots: The Transformation of the Labour Party Membership*, Palgrave Macmillan, Basingstoke, 2002, pp. 50–9, and information on new members derived from data supplied privately by Patrick Seyd on attitudes towards union affiliation to the party.
22 Seyd and Whiteley, *New Labour's Grass Roots*, p. 62.
23 Ibid. pp. 51–3.
24 Ibid. p. 52.
25 Ibid.
26 Ibid. p. 59.
27 Ibid. p. 67.
28 Ibid. p. 57.
29 Ibid. p. 59.
30 Ibid. p. 61.
31 Peter Mandelson and Roger Liddle, *The Blair Revolution: Can New Labour Deliver?* Faber & Faber, London, 1996, p. 211.
32 DO 1/10/97, NEC Minutes, 3 October 1997.
33 *Partnership in Power*, p. 11.
34 Partnership in Power: Implementing the New Policy Making Process, GS: 3/10/97, NEC minutes, 3 October 1997.
35 LPCR 1995, p. 147.
36 LPCR 1996, p. 111.
37 *The Times*, 15 February 2001.
38 *Guardian*, 4 October 1996.
39 LPCR 1998, p. 14.
40 Quoted in Hugo Young, *The Hugo Young Papers: Thirty Years of British Politics – Off the Record*, edited by Ion Trewin, Allen Lane, London, 2008, p. 480.
41 Q and A session, LPCR 1998, p. 11.
42 Focus groups' response to Labour Commission, in 2006, conveyed privately by Stuart Weir, an adviser to the process.
43 See on this John Golding, *Hammer of the Left*, Politico's, London, 2003, pp. 371–3.
44 Robin Cook, *The Point of Departure: Diaries from the Front Bench*, Simon & Schuster, London, 2003, p. 122.
45 *Campaign Group News*, October 1999.
46 Eric Shaw, 'New Labour in Britain: New Democratic Centralism?' *West European Politics* 25(3), 2002, p. 155.

47 Ibid. p. 155, fn 40.
48 Ibid. p. 156.
49 Labour Left Liaison 'Campaign Briefing', 2 October 1997.
50 Mike Marqusee, 'A Revolt Against Benefit Cuts', *Frontline* 14(26), 27 December 1997–9 January 1998.
51 Mo Mowlem, LPCR 1997, p. 27.
52 GS:3/10/97, NEC Minutes, 3 October 1997.
53 Ibid.
54 Margaret Wheeler, LPCR 1999, p. 49.
55 'Labour First', 24 September 2000.
56 Macintyre, *Mandelson*, p. 417.
57 Mark Seddon, *Chartist*, November/December 2000.
58 Greenberg, *Dispatches from the War Room*, p. 234.
59 *The Times*, editorial, 29 September 2000.
60 Stanley B. Greenberg, *Dispatches from the War Room: In the Trenches with Five Extraordinary Leaders*, Thomas Dunne, New York, 2009, p. 234.
61 Members have been concerned with post-materalist issues through the decade; and on this there was no difference between members recruited post- and pre-1994; see Seyd and Whiteley, *New Labour's Grassroots*, pp. 68–9.
62 National Policy Forum Report, 2001, p. 76.

12

Managing candidate selection

Changing selection procedure and management

In 1995 candidate selection became another major area of tightening management control. There was a clear shift away from the national managerial culture which operated under Kinnock and Smith. That had emphasised the non-intervention of party officials in the freedom of constituency parties to make a selection, apart from in by-elections. Candidate selection was also now at the sharp end of the new pressing concern to encourage effective candidates high in ability, and the projection of the party's new modern centre-ground image, shedding off-putting associations with the past. This was given additional motivation by the fact that the PLP, like the party at large, continued to have a centre of gravity to the left of the Leader. The political character and positioning of candidates for the coming elections could be crucial in deciding the degree to which the new PLP would be supportive and disciplined in relation to a Blair government. It would also provide the pool from which would emerge potential Blair ministers.

Blair and his office began demanding to know from the national and regional staff in 1995 what they were doing to ensure that 'the right people were coming through' in the target seats where the party had a good chance of winning. It was made clear to the 'political organisers' that this was a test of their organising ability crucial in pursuing the party's urgent interest. In practice, the calculation of the number of target seats proved to be highly cautious and the 1997 landslide affected seats that nobody dreamed would go Labour. But for the moment that was only a fantasy. The priority was for the right candidates in the right targets.

There was another pressure, that of time. The regional managers were fighting against the clock in responding to the demands of the job and faced some new frustrations. One immediate problem was that some of the winnable seats had been nursed already by candidates in the Smith era, and even some from the Kinnock era. Then there was the new problem of OMOV. The old system before the introduction of OMOV had in some regions been a means by which the leadership and the regional officials managed outcomes with their union allies. OMOV brought into the ballot members who otherwise had little or no direct contact with the party organisation. With it came a sense of wider ownership of the outcome.

But it proved to be harder for the management to do the fixing job that was expected of them because 'You cannot make them do something if they do not want to'. That was true, but it still left room for organisational management skills and it put pressure on for discreet mechanisms to be brought into the pursuit of delivery.

The new managerial drive

In the new management of selections under Blair, a landmark case came at Swindon in 1995 in the contest between Jim D'Avila, a union shop steward who had fought the seat in 1992 and Michael Wills, a TV producer who was close to both Brown and Mandelson. Wills won the selection but D'Avila, supported by his union, alleged postal-vote irregularities and challenged the decision in the courts – a highly unusual course of action. On 18 March, the Judge, although directing the party officials to write a more impartial report and finding that the ballot should be rerun, conceded that he had no power to compel that rerun, an important statement of the limits of appeal to the courts.

It was highly unusual for selection conflicts to go on appeal to the NEC, but such were the issues and feelings raised by this case that not only did it go to the committee but the arguments divided the Leader and Deputy Leader about the candidate and about the process. The NEC rejected a second ballot by only 14 votes to 10. Then, under the Leader's prompting, it interviewed the candidates and imposed Wills.[1] Around the Leader the process had aroused some additional frustration at the problems they faced in this facet of changing the party, accentuating their concern for getting in the right people. It also strengthened the view that to do this should not be held back by following the letter of the rulebook in every case.

Managerial interventions

In exploring and assessing that response, it is as well to repeat here Eric Shaw's earlier judgement that it is 'impossible to determine with any precision the extent of regional organisers' influence over selection decisions'. But as he himself illustrated, it need not preclude us making the effort to understand it better especially as seen through the evidence of managers and ex-managers. As conveyed in interviews, the consensus view about intervention was that the party's interest was generally served best in being seen as doing the job fairly and in doing so building up a capital of trust which could be used for other purposes. The regional office was, however, expected to have its informed view of who was best supported as capable and suitable to the constituency and to a future 'New Labour' government. Normally their intervention was limited to networking with loyalist allies within the party about the quality of a favoured candidate, giving advice to the candidate and linking him/her to those networks and various key players and opinion formers.

Under Blair, in the case of potential candidates who might, it was thought, be damaging to the Leader's objectives, the key legitimising assumptions of the operation of the Leader and party managers was that they 'were not looking for people who would vote against and bring down a Labour Government', and they must seek to protect 'the people' from problems caused by the party coming under the wrong influence. In contrast to the virtuous triangle of good relations between the people, the party and the parliamentary leadership, if there was a problem on the horizon in candidate selection it was thought to be the misrepresentation of the people's wishes by the party not its leadership, and especially by its left-wing public representatives. Managerial control was therefore morally justified in impeding that potential misrepresentation. Stopping somebody was generally easier to achieve than making sure a managerial favourite succeeded, but it did not cover all eventualities. The biggest unusual political deviation from this in the marginals was in Hayes and Harlington where John McDonnell, who was always going to be a leading left-wing critic but was also an impressive candidate, won the selection for the seat he had so narrowly failed to win in 1992. Anne Cryer, also an impressive candidate, recaptured the Keighley seat previously held by her husband.

The managerial codes and delivery

As with other aspects of Blair's party management, if managerial control produced effective short-term delivery there was less incentive to dwell on other potential costs of the new character of the management. The way that under Blair attitudes changed towards rules and the realpolitik of 'serious politics' is relevant here. As an entry point we can draw from the experience of one of the party's big political figures, Charles Clarke. Coinciding with the new pressure from the Leader's office, and the new definition of the role of officials as political organisers, Clarke (who from his experience in Kinnock's office understood candidate-selection issues) became angry at the way that some of the selections were conducted where he himself was a candidate. He had secured one rerun at Newham after complaint (although the second contest there did not advance his position). In a private letter to the General Secretary on 28 September 1995, headed *Fairness not Favours*, he made a robust and comprehensive attack on the way that the Labour Party was now run and in particular the way that candidate selection was operated.[2]

Key managers who have seen the letter judged it to be misconceived in its focus on the role of the NEC, over-the-top in its totalistic characterisation and simply wrong in his own case. But there was no denial that it gave a revealing summary of potential control points and procedural devices and did highlight some of the techniques admitted by managers to be in use after 1994. Early partisan provision of membership lists, for example, did happen and was a factor in success if the organisation and energy was there to follow it up. However, with good local connections the provision of membership information could come also from a range of sources other than party managers, including the CLP officers and the MP and MEP. In an aggressive counter-attack it was even said by different senior managers that any candidate who was not resourceful enough to get hold of a list was *ipso facto* 'useless', so it continued to be a significant element of the managers' arsenal.

There was also an ex-managerial acknowledgement that the trade union levy-plus scheme could be used in cooperation with the party for late recruitment to boost favoured candidates, although this procedure stopped after 1997. Under Blair, postal votes were permitted without having to prove good reasons for not attending the vote. Canvassing and collecting postal votes whilst assisting and advising did happen, in contravention of the rules. In 1997 Assistant General Secretary David Gardner did attempt to stop it, but with regional managerial assistance it started again. It was also pointed out by managers defending the practice that this help could be given by anybody and it was not unknown for regions of a union to second an official to assist a union-connected candidate. As for prejudiced constitutional interpretation which assisted or obstructed candidates, this had long been an element in the politics but managerial critics now pointed out that, as in other managed areas, within this culture there were fewer constraints than previously. Linked and of broader relevance here was the Charles Clarke view of party officials 'acting as judge and jury in relation to any concerns raised by a local Constituency Party or individual members without any semblance of due process'.[3]

For the observer, as for Clarke, in tracing new attitudes there are dangers in making generalisations about behaviour. Generational differences had some influence, with Smith and Kinnock appointments less interested in broadening the activity. There was acknowledged to be a traditional practice of informal managerial mentoring of favoured candidates, but those officials influenced to some degree by the older National Agents Department mores were more careful in drawing the line at anything which could undermine trust in the process whilst recognising that lines of behaviour were drawn wider by others. As with the period of the Shaw study, whether and how it operated did depend on the individual, and there were initially some significant differences in the responses of officials to the attitudes emanating from the centre. Some managers were more natural controllers than others, or more ideologically driven, or more seduced in an area where delivery earned kudos and boldness gained the Leader's respect for delivery.

Targets and receptivity

In candidate selection, as with other target areas of management, the shift in policy attitudes at the grassroots towards 'New Labour' positions was nothing like as great as had been hoped. In some seats, many activists remained heavily critical of Blair and 'New Labour', causing some leadership supporters to complain publicly about the difficulty of being selected.[4] Yet the very existence of 'New Labour' with its swing away from traditional positions and its reputation for control did have the effect over time of weakening the organised left wing current at the grassroots. Though even loyalist constituencies liked to see some independence of mind, the accumulating changes in the party made an openly consistent left-wing identification less comfortable and the Blairite-looking candidate appear more appropriate. The desperation of the emphasis on winning reinforced a longer-term tendency for CLPs to go for 'a winner', even if their political stance was not four-square with that of the CLP. To the surprise of many, this had been found to be the case even during the Bennite period.[5] In this respect, in the marginals, constituency opinion and managerial perspectives found much in common, and the network through managerial allies could find a more receptive audience than policy preferences indicated.

Complications in management could also arise from the multiplicity of managerial and politician pressures. Though it was a regional responsibility, that did not stop other interventions. The Leader might express a firm personal interest in a candidate, especially in target seats. There could be some disagreement between headquarters and a strong Regional Director. Brown might be in the contest by proxy. The Deputy Leader and the Chief Whip could be involved, as could other regional parliamentary big names. McDonagh as General Secretary might have one view; the Political Office in No. 10 might have another. Candidate selection was a way of building up the obligations of the favoured, and it was also a process which could reinforce or set off national-level rivalries which prejudiced working arrangements on other issues.

OMOV had added to the momentum towards the selection of local candidates with established personal connections. Local understanding and first-hand experience told increasingly, but the quality of candidates as national representatives could not be guaranteed. In contrast, rising stars from any area had an appeal amongst some members in their own right but also as heightening the status of the constituency. Within the CLP, heavy-handed interference from outsiders could be counterproductive, increasingly so by the end of the first term in government.

Not every attempt at influence by the managerial organisation was done well, and the best-laid plans which relied on interpersonal communication and avowed commitment could go wrong. In some areas the party managers were criticised as not very good at this placement. In others the managerial role after delivery was exaggerated to win kudos. Energetic, attractive and impressive candidates prepared to work became their own best managers. Examples are privately cited by officials of a favoured candidate being defeated in the selection, although these examples given by party officials are couched in terms of being exceptional.

One such case to which managers refer came in March 1997 at Bethnal Green and Bow. Although generally a Labour loyalist, Oona King was not the management's preferred candidate. That was Claude Moraes, who was thought to have a better appeal in a strongly Asian constituency. That may have backfired, given the complexity of Asian politics and the varied mix of the constituency. There was, according to King, also some resentment against the idea that a candidate was being imposed.[6] As for her broad appeal, in her own words, in a hall 'vehemently anti New Labour' she had the attraction of 'drifting away' from 'New Labour' at that time.[7] She was also herself an attractive articulate candidate from an unusually mixed ethnic background who was said to have given a very good performance.

By-elections

In by-elections the NEC had responsibility for preparing the short list. Normally the NEC by-elections panel had a majority who knew what the political management job entailed. The Leader's office was always consulted and the Leader himself might offer a firm view. Those who were on the short list were generally those who performed well or were 'known to be good' – a judgement which left open considerable discretion, especially as 'New Labour' suitability was involved. Favoured candidates could be helped by the choice of those with whom they would be competing. There were skilled ways of framing the list by picking weak alternatives including perhaps a token woman or by keeping off serious local contenders who had known constituency strength.

These considerations did not always mean that the favoured candidate carried the selection. In the Dudley West by-election selection in December 1994, Jacqui Smith was considered the ideal candidate and had the Leader's support, but she was defeated by Ian Pearson, an able local candidate who was also a Blairite. He carried the seat with a record swing of 28 per cent in the first Labour by-election victory under Tony Blair's leadership. A sharp conflict over suitable candidates for a by-election took place on a different basis over the Paisley by-election in 1997, and it happened 'off-stage'. Pat McFadden, a Scot from the Leader's office, had an understanding that he would have Blair's support, but another Scot, Douglas Alexander, had the support of Brown. After a tussle between the big two, McFadden was asked to withdraw. It was an outcome which added to concern in No. 10 that Blair should stand up against what was said to be 'Brown's people colonising the party'.

The judgement of 'New Labour' suitability could backfire significantly. In the first by-election after the 1997 General Election, at Uxbridge, a Conservative majority of only 724 seemed a relatively easy target for 'New Labour' given the surge of public enthusiasm that followed the Blair General Election victory. David Williams, who had fought the General Election as the local Labour candidate, was removed by the NEC by-elections panel with the explanation that Williams was not suitable as by-election candidate. In a ballot between two alternatives he was replaced by Andrew Slaughter from Hammersmith. It was, as Blunkett noted in his diaries,[8] 'a grave error of judgement' insulting the electorate, giving the Conservatives a cause over a non-local candidate and dividing the local Labour Party. The Conservatives increased their majority from 724 to 3,766. There was then a rush to distance the Leader from the selection decision. Yet Blair had said at one point that 'What matters is that we have somebody who is thoroughly New Labour and is a supporter of mine'.[9] That, it turned out, was more of a problematic judgment than it seemed, and not only in Uxbridge, as will be shown.

Women's representation and positive discrimination

Blair first conference coincided with an NEC statement agreeing positive discrimination policy in selections. Whilst supporting an increase in women's representation in Parliament, Blair was not happy with the mechanism involved. Yet the weight of support for it proved strong, and the party agreed to support a policy of all-women short lists in the selection of parliamentary candidates in 50 per cent of vacancies in Labour-held seats and 50 per cent in the most winnable marginal seats, as a means of providing a sharp boost in the number of women MPs. With some skilful handling by the party officials, the regional 'voluntary consensus' meetings to decide which CLPs should have the all-women short list generally proved more manageable than had been thought.

The process of short-listing in 1995 was initially entirely local and hence less controlled by the party machine. This accounts for the developments in the target seat of Leeds North East where the CLP, having gone for all-women shortlists, selected Liz Davies after an impressive performance. She was associated with the aggressively left-wing *Labour Briefing* and Blair, who knew her, reacted strongly, and became an initiator of the NEC's refusal to accept her candidature. This decision received an unusually bad press even from commentators normally unsympathetic to the left. She was described by Michael Jones as a 'Human Sacrifice on the altar of Labour's new conformity' facing a 'bag of accusations' which included the charge that she was a temperamental 'oppositionist'.[10] But she won an open contest in Leeds North East. After an appeal to the party conference the NEC's refusal to endorse was upheld. In the letter to Sawyer already cited, Charles Clarke considered the handling of this case to be 'simply . . . political prejudice'.

Shortly after this, in 1996 pressure on the leadership to drop all-women short lists mounted following the Leeds Tribunal decision where two male members of the Party, Peter Jepson and Roger Dyas-Elliot, won a case against the Party which judged all-women short lists a breach of the Sex

Discrimination Act of 1975. There was a fierce reaction within the party, but the NEC agreed that it was too near the General Election to make an appeal which could be concluded before the election.[11] This led to a procedural change from all-women short lists to a prescribed 50–50 gender balance for seats in which members were retiring. It proved to be no great boost to women. In the end only four women were selected in the 40 seats from which members were retiring, and six of these had been women.[12] Still, a record 101 women Labour candidates were elected in 1997.

Late selections and parachuting

Alan Howarth, a Conservative MP who defected to Labour in October 1995, had failed in two selections at Wentworth and Wythenshawe even with the Leader's backing, and he had advance rebuffs in other constituencies. Howarth was included in the selections process for Newport East in 1996 after the sudden announcement of the resignation of Roy Hughes who had already been reselected. Following a discussion with Blair, he had given up his seat and later received a peerage. For the NEC short-listing a strong ISTC union candidate was excluded and a major effort was made involving key CLP people being invited to No. 10 before the selection vote; Howarth was selected in an OMOV ballot in March 1996.

Around the Leader an urgent sense of the need to get high-calibre candidates with talent into Parliament was assisted in 1997 by some obvious last-minute 'parachuting' of candidates into seats which suddenly became vacant. Five MPs retired late and three others retired very late. With the exception of one of them, Willie McKelvey, who did not want to go into the Lords and retired on health grounds, all the others were made peers in an exercise organised from No. 10. In the Leader's office they saw it simply as another form of problem solving. Others saw it 'a bit iffy' for modernising radicals. Anthony Howard commented later 'Sleaze may be too harsh a term . . . but there was something unattractive about this negotiation'.[13]

The NEC in January 1997 agreed that all selections after 1 February would be short-listed by a late-selections panel. The politics of this short-listing resembled that of by-election politics in that it was a serious attempt to find good candidates, but the judgement also had a 'New Labour' political dimension. Those especially unacceptable were kept off and the choice of companions on the short list could be advantageous to the favoured candidates. But all had to perform well on the day to get on the short list, and some short lists were more open than others. The mix of control and openness was pronounced in the late selection for Pontefract and Castleford. In the short-listing, three candidates – one a Yorkshire council Leader, another a neighbouring councillor with close links, a third the very articulate union national official Jack Dromey – failed to make the short list for different reasons. But, after a high-class performance the final run-off was very open and the seat went to Yvette Cooper rather than Hilary Benn who had been favourite.

In three very late selections the procedure was more abbreviated. Five candidates were called for interview by the panel for three seats suddenly available in Dudley East, Hull East, and Kilmarnock and Loudon. The Leader's preferences were made known to the panel. In Kilmarnock and Loudon, the only one of these three seats which did not become vacant through what was effectively a peerage replacement, there was an informal sounding of the local party opinion with some indication of who might be the candidate. Des Browne, a Leader's preference, got that candidature. In Hull East the postal workers union leader Alan Johnson was personally sounded out by Blair with an offer of a safe seat.[14] He wanted, he told Johnson, people from different backgrounds, and Johnson was also a talented loyalist moderniser voice. He was parachuted into Hull East by the selections panel after the election was called and the MP Stuart Randall stood down. The constituency party executive committee accepted the recommendation of the selections panel. Randall later went into the Lords.

However, in Dudley East, vacant after John Gilbert was given a peerage, Charles Falconer, the Leader's preference and a close friend, failed to make it to the earmarked candidacy because the selections panel reacted to his candid attitude towards the practicalities of the job and his views on education. The Leader's second preference, Ross Cranston, divided the committee but they eventually went for him. Since the Dudley recommendation was changed, the CLP executive committee was called together to agree it. Falconer became Blair's first life-peer appointment in 1997.

Labour in government and new representation

The National Parliamentary Panel

Within the drive for modernisation there was a particular attempt to encourage equality of opportunity, increasing the number of women and ethnic minority candidates, and to improve the professionalism of candidates. These all gave a new legitimation to a more interventionist central role and closer steering by regional party officials. But it also expanded the room for arguments over priorities, and at times tensions with the local parties where receptivity towards gender and ethnic equality was variable. In terms of gender representation the idea of a national panel received a particular push from the enforced abandonment of all-women short lists and then the fall-off in the selection of women candidates. But as always there was another managerial dimension to this interest in new procedures. As a form of potential political trouble-shooting to produce 'a good outcome', proposals for a National Parliamentary Panel became more urgent after Liz Davies and the Leeds North East result.

Through the Panel which began its work systematically in 1999, most potential candidates would in future have to be vetted for acceptance on it. The exceptions were that trade union and Cooperative Party-backed candidates continued to have acceptance on the Panel without going through a party interview, although the party had to verify the quality of individual panel systems of affiliated organisations. The new panel system had strong party support in the consultation, providing that CLPs remained free to nominate from outside the panel, which became the agreed position. The aims of the process, as presented to and accepted by the NEC, were first to provide a training framework, second to broaden the diversity of candidates in terms of ethnicity, gender and occupation, third to deal with the implications of the industrial tribunal decision, and fourth to improve the services to local parties and potential candidates.[15] It was seen by its proponents as an idea which had worked well on a local level for years and as an obvious means of guiding the new drive to professionalism and effectiveness.

As expected, there was a concern that this panel might be used as part of the increasing management control over those coming into the PLP. Studying its purpose and drawing from comments of one of the managers involved, the national expert in this field, Byron Criddle, described it as aimed principally at 'a more professional screening process'[16] with the intention of 'weeding out the charlatans', securing more women candidates, and generally improving the quality of the candidates.[17] He also noted, however, that it had the understood intention of eliminating candidates who 'appeared not to have a pragmatic line on policy disagreements' or 'who could not avoid sounding divisive and combative if disagreeing with party policy' or 'showed an unpreparedness to listen to the whips'.[18] The 886 applicants became 681 on the panel.[19]

In a later discussion with me, one senior official involved in organising the process contested an accusation that they were trying to produce 'Blairite clones'. There was 'a light touch approach' with an acceptance of a wide range of views to 'a certain point' with political control working in 'only a tiny number of cases'. In an acknowledgement of the new counterpressure coming from accusations of control freakery, the point was made that 'If control freakery had been the dominating motivation 60 of those accepted would not have got on'. My conjecture is that some of this lightness of touch may have been a way of embedding the procedure, but the 'certain point' was still a signal of unacceptability which added to the influences in local selections weakening the position of some potential candidates from the left.

Candidate selection, union membership and the union role

There was one major feature of the party rules which went against the surface flow of pressure for reform of the union position. In the extensively rewritten rulebook of 1995 the obligation to be a member of a bona fide trade union as a condition of membership was still included (in terms 'if eligible' as recommended by the Trade Union Review Group in 1993).[20] And, as before, those obligations were also specified as a condition for nomination or selection as a parliamentary candidate.[21] That helped consolidate the trade union position within the new PLP after 1997. Virtually everybody was a member of a trade union, although that said little about the union role in candidate selection.

There, following the row over the Swindon selection in 1995, the position of the unions, already partially weakened after the introduction of OMOV, appeared to be threatened by 'New Labour's' aggressive party management seeking candidates who would disassociate its image from that of the unions, whatever their formal relationship. The loyalist AEEU saw themselves as being 'carved up by the Blairites'. After the union, which had long prided itself on moving people from the shop floor into Parliament, found that source beginning to dry up as did other union groups, the AEEU became more systematic in organising their own panels and introducing their own candidates through it.

Under its Political Officer – Tom Watson and then Peter Wheeler – there was a reorganisation of its political influence. This tied into the changes at the top of party headquarters with Margaret McDonagh, first as Deputy General Secretary and then as General Secretary, working much more closely with the traditional right and its organisation Labour First. Under Ken Jackson the union now pushed for encouraging the inclusion of manual workers in the improved social representation agenda. This was backed by other unions and also by Jon Cruddas in the Political Office and Chief Whip Nick Brown. In 1998, as part of a package of selection procedural change, it was supported by the NEC Organisation Committee without question. It looked like a major breakthrough.

But rectifying this particular social distortion was never regarded as a priority by headquarters, and the Blairite focus continued to be extending the party's social base and public representation to the middle class with candidates who exemplified the shift. Within the AEEU itself there were different views on the priority to be given to drawing in the manual working class given that it could involve a long haul of encouragement and nurturing. Even Ken Jackson who supported the shop floor emphasis was more encouraged by party managers to see the value of attempting to win friends of the AEEU amongst high-flying candidates with strong connections to the party leadership.

The major twist in this effort to gain more manual working-class candidates was that the better organised union panels came to be seen increasingly as having a special advantage to Blairite middle-class candidates in term of nomination rights in the selection process, a clear Labour movement identity, and the fact that association with their chosen trade union meant that another challenger from that union was very unlikely in particular contests. As a result, to get into the PLP, many with only a formal union background began to find a more emphasised advantage in their union membership. It was easy to see selections as the powerful unions getting their candidates in, but this gave little indication of the real strength of their union identification or the degree of push from a particular union.

In organisational terms, where a union was motivated, it could provide some support for the donkey work and was well placed to take advantage of the nomination rights providing that it could get the right candidate with a wider appeal. Knowledge of the party in a town, city or region could rival or be superior to that of the regional office. Independent union networks could involve more trust. But the fact remained that the unions were not strong enough at local level to take full advantage of their opportunities. In particular, union delegates to CLPs were weak in number even in areas of relatively high affiliation. Nor was the replacement for the sponsorship procedure, constituency development plans, a significant factor in selections.

Union strength had traditionally been boosted by inter-union arrangements agreeing an apportionment of seats to particular unions so as not to challenge each other's seats. Yet the national 'done-deal' put together at a party conference often did not hold locally, and there were few union easy victories, even for a strongly motivated and hardworking union-backed candidate. The AEEU working with the machine and with a broader range of candidates did better after 1997. But the CLPs with an increasing middle-class composition tended to judge winning candidates as those coming from their own social class and, with encouragement from the managers, that Blair model view of a good candidate also extended to some seats where the manual working-class composition was stronger. Even Tom Watson, a mature-student graduate from a working-class background and a skilled organiser seeking the West Bromwich seat, was said later by a national party official involved in selections to have found it hard going and required their assistance to win the selection for 2001. Perhaps that was simply a competitive claim to superior fixing abilities.

Mandatory reselection, the union role

However, union influence developed in another way, surprising in the light of Blair's 1992 crusade for OMOV and attempts to evict the unions from candidate selection. In the revolt of the Campaign for Labour Party Democracy, mandatory reselection had been aimed at securing the greater accountability of MPs to their constituency parties. That had been weakened somewhat under Kinnock, by the party conference agreeing to an OMOV ballot of members trigger-mechanism which could reselect a sitting MP for the candidature without going through a time-consuming and attention-preoccupying full reselection procedure. This was altered coming up to 1997 when the trigger mechanism was made two-thirds of nominations by party units and two-thirds of all affiliates who have made nominations. The measure in effect quietly ditched the ballot, but at the time aroused little controversy.

In 1998, an NEC consultation of the party found the idea of a trigger mechanism still appeared to have 'general acceptance',[22] but a majority of CLPs favoured an OMOV ballot for such a mechanism.[23] In spite of this, the NEC working group stuck with a nominations procedure inclusive of the affiliates, and as also taking less time and effort by the CLP and the MP. On that basis it was strongly defended by amongst others Chief Whip Nick Brown. But now the percentage needed for constituencies to avoid a full reselection contest was reduced from two-thirds to 'a majority' and it was to be decided on the views of an overall majority of nominating organisations. In many seats the unions had an overall majority of the nominating organisations. These moves also fed from the managerial view that on a local level the major problem of management would come from the constituencies whilst the unions would still act as a stabilising force in selections and reselections. Unions from the traditional right like AEEU and USDAW always saw it as their business to defend local party stability on loyalist grounds, and local unions had a tradition of defending the sitting MP, affected also by their reluctance to start a competitive war of eviction which might damage their own union representation.

And MPs, even if deviant on particular issues, developed a range of local friendships and in various ways gave years of supportive assistance to their parties and members. They were generally highly skilled in dealing with critics. On the General Committees there was always a deep awareness of the dangers of adverse media reactions to a local civil war arising from attempts to deselect. There had also been a decline of the organised left at the grassroots which might have spearheaded some removals. All this meant that the pressure on MPs through mandatory reselection was not as great as it might have been, and outside of peculiar personal circumstances MPs were now very safe. Later, following the Leader's damaging reputation for control freakery, strengthened by what happened over Livingstone in London (see below), the avoidance of deselection became a wider managerial concern lest it was portrayed as stemming from No. 10 attempts at further control.

New selections, new management and the public response

Candidate selection under the Blair Government was subject to a range of new selection procedures covering different areas of constitutional reform. Selection procedures changed for the European Parliament. British institutional innovations led to involvement of the party in selections and leadership elections after devolution to Scotland and Wales. In London selections for the recreation of a London authority with a directly elected mayor also became subject to new party involvement. All of these were managed in such a way that they brought heavy internal party controversy.

Management control at this time was regarded as so instrumentally important and so publicly virtuous that it dwarfed consideration of potentially damaging party consequences. The result at Uxbridge did nothing to diminish confidence that by controlling to ensure that with Blair's personal backing and 'New Labour' identity, candidates would win public support. The axioms of party management did not allow for the idea that anybody associated with the left of the party might launch from outside the party an independent revolt against such controls and receive public backing. Managerial assumptions were so deep-rooted that it was not in the framework of managerial calculations that their own management might become a significant and sustained electoral negative. Yet one after another, these assumptions came to be challenged, in events and developments which had a major impact.

Europe

The most radical change produced by a combination of procedural reform and party management was in the political complexion of the European Parliamentary Labour Party. The problem faced by the leadership was that the EPLP had loose internal discipline and its centre of political gravity was well to the left of the new Blairite leadership in attitudes towards Clause IV and the party's policies. It was also, oddly enough, much more Euro-sceptic. The EPLP, elected under a British system of first-past-the-post, was the largest national party delegation in the European Parliament. Changing the method of candidate selection might reduce some Labour representation but (it was thought) not dramatically, and it offered a way of changing the composition and culture of the EPLP thus securing greater coordination of the national and European parties and increased party discipline.

A commitment to PR for the next European elections in 1999 was inserted into the General Election Manifesto of 1997 even though there had been no formal party agreement. As was learned later, this was part of a deal done by Blair with the Liberal Democrat Leader Paddy Ashdown during the 'progressive alliance' phase. The party managers thought that it would be introduced in 2004 after a Bill during this parliament. But it was brought forward by Blair to 1999, thereby providing an earlier opportunity to manage 'the problem of the EPLP'.

There was to be a regional list system of PR for large multi-member constituencies. The procedural mechanisms within this were the subject of considerable managerial disagreement. The Home Secretary Jack Straw wanted regions big enough to provide a hurdle too large for the BNP to get representation. Party officials Coleman and Gardner favoured constituency-based lists, but were overruled by Downing Street. The insistence on a closed-list system, in which public preference played no part, was a Headquarters insistence. Their view was that 'We can't have party representatives fighting each other in public'. The system backed by both Lord Whitty, responsible for coordination with the European party, and Wayne David the EPLP Leader was a useful mechanism of 'what works' in party management producing the desired internal outcome.[24]

Unlike the development in Westminster reselections, under this system there were no protective trigger mechanisms for incumbents. There were membership ballots for the nominations in order to ensure wide support for the regional list, but OMOV was abandoned as a mechanism of allocating candidates to places on the list. This was in spite of the OMOV option being the one supported in the consultation exercise. Allocation was made after interview by selection boards which comprised the General Secretary, five NEC members, two other members nominated by the NEC and three variable regional people. Each board was heavily influenced by NEC loyalists and by the push to get a new and more cooperative EPLP. In the final allocations most left-wing critics were not allocated to winnable positions on the lists. The official view was that the final result was a fair judgement of abilities. But the private managerial view was that this was a necessary 'political operation'.

Accompanying the new ideological composition of the EPLP were new arrangements which linked the EPLP much closer with the national Labour Party and with ministerial policy-making. The relationship was eased and cohesion strengthened. That was the success of the management process and added to leadership confidence about what could be done in changing the party with determined effort. On the other hand, it also showed the unanticipated party and public electoral interaction in a campaign marked by a lack of party workers and large-scale abstentions. In the European elections of 1999, Labour's 62 seats were reduced to just 29. There was a warning here from the backlash of dissatisfaction in the party both with the selection process and the top-down management of the election. But, as noted in Chapter 8 (see p. 254), the managers focused on other explanations.

Devolution and coordination

Overlapping with the European process was the birth of a new National Assembly for Wales and a new Parliament for Scotland, also to take place in 1999. Devolution was a new experience and produced new anxieties for a leadership and management already obsessed with avoiding loss of control. Party management was seen as the corrective which preserved British Labour's national unity. But there was never full agreement on how far this central management should extend into candidate selection.

Scotland MSPs and the Canavan case

For the form of Scottish selections the NEC devolved its role to the Scottish Executive Committee. The new procedure was overwhelmingly supported at the Scottish Labour Party Conference. A system of pairing constituencies, agreed by the Scottish Executive, secured gender equality without much controversy, marking a significant advance in women's representation. For the selections, potential candidates were to appear before one of a series of vetting panels to judge on their suitability to stand for the party. The procedure was based on an employment model which, it was thought, would avoid cronyism and seek the best-qualified candidates, taking into account equal opportunities guidelines. It would exercise rigorous scrutiny of everybody. The Scottish Leader Donald Dewar emphasised that they were looking for the qualities of people, not their point of view.[25]

But Shaw located a covert criterion of 'sufficient loyalty' to the party[26] and anticipation of the management of the Scottish selections was not helped by an article in the well-informed *Financial Times* which suggested that the party hierarchy had plans to use procedures like these in order to deselect Westminster MPs with dissident views.[27] Consequently, the Scottish party was described on the left as in uproar at candidate exclusions, noting how many from the left were excluded.[28] In reality, the outcome overall was a mishmash of political results following diverse interventions in the interviewing panels and unanticipated outcomes with many different thing going wrong. 'A complete mess' was one leading manager's view. As the *Guardian* noted, 'Widely respected figures or senior figures with a long track record of service'[29] did not get on. Murray Elder, advisor to Donald Dewar over selections and much else, was himself not approved as a candidate. The feature that caused intense controversy, and gave it greatest significance in terms of the national party management, was the fact that left-wing figures Denis Canavan and Ian Davidson, two would-be candidates for the Scottish Parliament who were already Westminster Labour MPs, were refused entry onto the list.

Canavan was a veteran critic of the Labour leadership who had poor relations with some of his colleagues. Unusually the three-member panel which interviewed Canavan (a panel decided by the Scottish party office) was chaired by the Selection Board Vice Chair and fellow Westminster MP Ernie Ross. As it happened, he too had a difficult relationship with Canavan. His panel meeting was later described by Canavan as 'an interrogation rather than an interview'. Party officials privately confirmed later that the meeting was conducted in an unsatisfactory way, giving grounds for an appeal. The same was thought about the interview with Davidson. There was a common view that over Canavan this had been a set-up but there was disagreement about its political source. A well-attested version of why this happened was that it was 'a Scottish thing' with influence to keep Canavan off initiated from Scottish Leader Donald Dewar following what was said to be a long-standing feud. However, a source close to Dewar asserted that from the earliest discussions with Dewar, Blair had been in gung-ho mood and happy to see Canavan excluded in the way he had in mind for Livingstone in London (see below). A national party official confirmed that, given his views, Blair did not need any persuading in relation to Canavan.

Both Canavan and Davidson saw it as 'an ideological purge of the Left'.[30] Canavan, but not Davidson, made an appeal. Party and Downing Street officials in London became sufficiently worried by the transcript to hold a special meeting on the issue to see if they could steer away from the panel decision. But because of the pending party appeal by Canavan, and what was said to be a reluctance to cause offence to the Scottish leadership, it was left to the established Appeal Committee. They voted to uphold the decision. Canavan then decided to break with the party and fight the by-election at Falkirk as an independent – a course of action which, when taken in the past, had led to political marginalisation. But there was huge enthusiasm for his cause, and on 6 May 1999, he secured a 12,000 majority. The only previous Labour Party case like it in modern times was that of the octogenarian S.O. Davies in Merthyr in 1970, but then there had been no broader political or factional element to Davies's victory. Canavan on the other hand made it a protest against Labour Party centralisation and authoritarianism. The result could be read as a huge warning that control over the party could be control over the people's choice, and in spite of the government's lead in the opinion polls it could provoke an electoral revolt. Here was yet another warning which was disregarded.

The Leadership of Wales

In general, selection for the Welsh assembly did not cause any of the factional ructions which were exhibited in Scotland and very few criticisms of the management of the process other than over twinning to ensure women's representation (see below). There were no complications about Westminster MPs sitting on any of the panels. But the election of a new Wales party Leader was to provoke uproar. The Welsh Secretary Ron Davies resigned suddenly following an embarrassing episode on Clapham Common. The most popular alternative amongst Welsh Party members was Rhodri Morgan, who had been Davies's opponent in his election.

It has been suggested that the principal designers of the crisis which now developed were those who controlled the machine in Wales,[31] the Wales party and particularly its leading union officials.[32] But as a senior party official directly involved glumly recalled, nobody could stop Blair's decision to impose Alun Michael and to stop Morgan, of whom Blair had a variety of doubts that made him unacceptable, and Blair's commitment to Michael was made in a private conversation before internal opposition could mount. On this kind of issue Blair had the confidence that he had (almost) always succeeded. It was a decision taken not only regardless of Morgan's popularity in Wales but of the evidence that the party in Wales was already smarting over a variety of cross-cutting resentments – as party officials well knew.

After the Euro-selections there had been deep resistance to the imposition of candidates in the selection process – particularly Lyndon Harrison, from Lancashire not Wales. As one senior party official described it in

October 1998, 'Wales just went woosh – they are pissed off with us'.
Twinning to secure a fair representation of women also proved much less
acceptable in Wales than in England where there was considerable friction
with Secretary of State Ron Davies over the issue. An influential speech by
John Prescott carried support for twinning at the Wales Labour Party
Conference but on a vote of only 51 per cent. It also needed a strong push
from London headquarters whose representatives David Gardner and Diana
Jeuda won acceptance of the procedure from 20 of 40 constituencies with
16 opposed, a result which indicated their diplomatic skills. But there
remained resentment against the London impositions and the exclusion of
some key male candidates, and opposition to one constituency 'dictating'
to another in the consensus process. These grievances, added to some
historical resentment against 'London' control, raised the level of political
dissatisfaction outside the party as well as in.

It was in this atmosphere that Blair sought to impose his will over the
election of the Wales Leader. He had some enthusiastic anti-Morgan
supporters in the party in Wales who worked closely with London. In
the process the commitment to OMOV (already quietly dispatched in
Partnership in the Power and disregarded over European selections) was
now publicly shed in the most controversial of circumstances. It had been
said by Blair's allies in 1996 that he had 'little sympathy with the old right
– deal-making and fixing votes with the trade unions',[33] yet all that was
brought back to dominate the members' view. The Wales party (on which
much was later blamed to protect Blair) accepted a task force recommendation to use a three-way electoral college split. Blair now claimed
misleadingly that it was the same system that elected him in 1994, although
in that election the unions had an OMOV ballot from which their votes
were split.

Here there was no such agreement and no attempt to secure one. Most
unions did not ballot and the votes were not split. Where a minority of
unions did hold an OMOV ballot they backed Morgan by 3–1. As Lance
Price, working in Downing Street at the time, put it later 'we feebly tried
to maintain that it was not an old-style Labour stitch-up using union block
votes, but of course that is exactly what it was'.[34] Thus, what emerged was
not only a result in which the constituencies voted one way and the unions
voted another but one in which it could be plausibly claimed by Nick
Cohen that 'Morgan won every democratic vote in the Welsh Labour
movement, but lost the rigged election'.[35] Studies of these processes reveal
a range of examples of manipulation, official partiality and rule-breaking.[36]

Michael's victory had swear-provoking adverse consequences for the
Wales results in the Euro-elections and denying Labour a majority in 1999
Wales Assembly elections. Michael did not last long in office. He resigned
on 9 February 2000. Six days later, Rhodri Morgan was elected unanimously
and unopposed as First Secretary of the Welsh Assembly. Blair later
admitted that Morgan was a good and loyal Minister. The collapse of Alun

Michael's position came too late to encourage Blair into a rethink of his management of Ken Livingstone's attempt to become the elected Mayor of London – although again it is doubtful whether anything would have deflected the Leader.

London and stopping Ken

The Wales leadership debacle did some damage to Blair's reputation as a straight politician, especially in Wales, but not with the same national public awareness as the battle in London over Ken Livingstone. He had been the Labour MP for Brent East since 1987 but before that, as Leader of the Greater London Council from 1981 to 1986, had been a major figure on what the right-wing media labelled 'the loony left'. He was a bold innovative figure using the GLC as a left-wing base from which to attack Thatcher. However, he came to be seen by the Kinnock and Blair leaderships as epitomising the dark forces that had damaged Labour's electability, a symbol of the Old Left. He was regarded as personally untrustworthy and an inveterate oppositionist bound to come into public conflict with the Blair Government, of which he was a regular critic. For Blair and most of the other leading figures it was a case of 'we are not going back to that'. The commitment to a new Greater London Authority, which would replace the old GLC abolished by Thatcher, produced an acute problem. How was he to be stopped?

The problem and the system

A large body of opinion in the London Labour Party did not want a directly elected mayor and neither did Livingstone himself – who wanted the post indirectly elected by the new GLA. But the directly elected mayor fitted the Blairite ideological model of effective leadership and that model was driven. Although Livingstone had a strong claim to have the qualities and experience necessary for the post, virtually the whole Blair Cabinet and not a few of Livingstone's ex-colleagues were united in seeking to stop him. However, he had considerable party support and, as some managers much later acknowledged, many in the electorate had moved away from the unflattering portrait of Livingstone painted by Blair and his colleagues. A huge majority of the public in London thought that it would be 'wrong' for the Labour leadership to stop him from standing.[37]

The problem of what to do about this became a long-running background issue around Blair. The Leader, determined though he was in his objective, prevaricated, or as might have been described later, he dithered over the method. Neither politicians nor managers could decide for a long time how best to defeat Livingstone. To be helpful to the Leader, many joined in the calculating game of what to do. Various scenarios were offered. The biggest decision was over whether Livingstone should be excluded entirely on the grounds of his political unsuitability. Others thought this was clumsy and he should be allowed to stand but that the authority of the Prime Minister, the skills of media management, and the famed Millbank campaigning machine could be used to get the right result. Meanwhile the difficulties of getting a suitable candidate to stand against him added to the uncertainty about what to do. Blair's first preference was for a businessman 'star' but none emerged and none of the likeliest Labour politician 'winners' wanted the job. Attempts to force a decision on the procedure were fobbed off for a long time. Loyalists were told, 'Tony doesn't want it'.

At one point, unsuccessful attempts were made to get Mo Mowlem to stand as the personality most likely to defeat Livingstone in a straight contest but she demurred. Meanwhile Nick Raynsford had put his hat in the ring as the loyalist candidate and Glenda Jackson had also announced her entry into the contest. But the situation suddenly changed when Frank Dobson, who had turned it down earlier, decided to run after great encouragement from his friends. He was now seen as the likeliest to beat Livingstone. Raynsford withdrew. Then it transpired that Mowlem might now be prepared to stand but Dobson refused to withdraw. Jackson' s relations with Millbank deteriorated badly when she complained of clumsy briefing to force her to withdraw. She stuck to her decision and as the contest wore on she added to the anti-control freak voices and the fierce public reaction against the manipulations of the organisers. Frank Dobson never did attune to the tactics carried out on his behalf and made it clear he too was opposed to blocking Livingstone.

What happened in this situation typified much of Blairite party management and the politics of 'what works'. The story is too full of twists, turns and a multitude of managerial partisan practices for justice to be done to it here, but the key points are essential in confirming attitudes toward management, rules and winning. It tells also of the problems and the damaging consequences that emerged when Blair's form of management was revealed day by day and week by week under the harsh public spotlight.

The battles and their consequences were partially affected by the territorial competitiveness and personality conflicts between the party headquarters and the Political Office in No. 10. Candidate selection played some part in the tensions. The by-election in Wigan on 23 September 1999 was a classic safe-seat battle and the No. 10 Political Office favourite was Jack Straw's Special Advisor, Ed Owen. But party headquarters and other national figures pushed their own candidates. The end result was that it went to a local, Neil Turner, who was not the candidate of any of them although he was a Blairite loyalist. Labour retained the seat although with a greatly reduced majority and a turnout of just one in four voters. The tensions over this process added to the niggling relations at the party's national level.

It was assumed that if Livingstone was not be blocked by administrative-political means the selection of the London candidate was almost bound to be by an OMOV ballot of party members. That had been the expressed wishes of the London Labour Party and was widely supported at national level. The OMOV arrangements had been consolidated to the point that, with No. 10 approval, a paper was prepared on those lines to be taken to the NEC at its meeting on 12 October 1999. This was suddenly dumped as the long private discussions on 'the way to stop Ken' took a decisive new turn.

The pragmatic case made against just blocking Livingstone was that it would make Blair look both afraid and authoritarian and would rile many party members. It would be best if he went through a procedure that could work in producing the right outcome. How was that to be done? The decision to move to an electoral college of a particular form was developed in Downing Street, not Millbank, and came from an unusual alliance. The initial suggestion came from memos from Jon Cruddas in the Political Office and also from Ian McKenzie, special advisor to the Chief Whip. Cruddas was looking both to keep Livingstone in the contest and to bring in the unions (his area of responsibility in terms of party management). McKenzie thought that going back to the form of the Leader's own election procedure would add to the acceptability of the process. At the same time Philip Gould had done a study of party supporters which indicated to him that Livingstone could be stopped via the wider college.[38] Blair's Political Secretary Sally Morgan was then won to the argument and Blair was persuaded that this would 'work'.

As it emerged from these discussions the college was equally divided in three sections between individual members, affiliated organisation, and a third section of public representatives which comprised 57 London MPs, 4 London MEPs and 14 GLA Assembly candidates, but it did not include London councillors amongst whom a substantial number of Livingstone supporters could be expected. That section looked particularly manageable given the small number involved and the fact that the GLA candidates would themselves be subject to a selection-panel vetting process.

The first that most members of the NEC knew of the extraordinary volte-face over procedure was after the trade union group meeting on the Monday evening prior to the NEC which would formally make the decisions. Primed by the convenor, Margaret Prosser, the group gave full support to the proposed procedure. Anything that kept the unions in the process was welcome and it looked likely to produce a widely based NEC agreement. So it proved. At the NEC meeting a 20–4 majority went with the proposal, with Ian McCartney a powerful voice in favour.[39] The GRA advocated OMOV in line with London Labour Party policy, and Dennis Skinner joined with them to question the legitimacy of the composition of the section of public representatives.

The sudden emergence of this electoral college was instantly viewed outside leadership circles as a 'stitch up', a deliberate fix to stop Livingstone. And the NEC agreement on the procedure did not stop a further bitter internal conflict over whether Livingstone was acceptable as a candidate.

A vetting panel of NEC and regional figures looked at one stage likely to block him after Livingstone had refused to be bound by all the manifesto. Eventually amidst considerable acrimony, he gained a place on the short list, after Blair had come round to the view that simply blocking Livingstone at this late stage would result in 'real damage to ourselves'.[40] It was now becoming clear to the political leaders that this was an even bigger problem than had been anticipated.

Helping Frank

McDonagh had never been a supporter of the electoral college for London nor was she consulted on it. She had favoured simply preventing Livingstone from standing as the Labour candidate and facing the political battle over it. That had been one school of thought in 10 Downing Street as well as headquarters before the late change of procedure. Now, because of Blair's prevarication, no plans had been made even about the most basic of decisions on when the selection would take place, and how it would take place. It fell to McDonagh to try to establish the procedure in these circumstances.

In Campbell's diaries there is a note of a meeting with party people from Millbank where he said that 'it was important that there be no chicanery and we had to play by the rules'. That, it must be said, was the formal position. With the party's (and Blair's own) credibility on the line, and a Livingstone victory seen as a potential disaster, the instructions to headquarters from the Leader were that 'Frank has to have everything that he needs'. As some officials described it later, the interpretation put on this by the party officials followed their past understanding of management and of what Tony meant. McDonagh threw all her unrestrained and energetic weight into the campaign. She held her own independent planning meetings of 'her people' from the Millbank office driving forward the campaign.

Everything was done on the hoof. The rules were being developed or changed as the campaign progressed and in accordance with the same political criteria used in producing the electoral college. It was all about 'stopping Ken'. The closing date for nominations had been delayed to give anti-Livingstone campaigners more time. Influenced by the same consideration the date of the ballot was also delayed with ballot papers sent out on 26 January and the closing date 5 pm on 16 February.

Neither No. 10 nor Millbank could afford to be seen to get openly involved, and Dobson was even given campaign instructions from No. 10 which included distancing himself from the Prime Minister.[41] Behind the scenes, it was a different matter as the No. 10 team joined in the campaign for Frank and against Ken, pulling out all the stops. Oona King MP reports refusing a direct request from the Prime Minister, backed by an intimidatory Sally Morgan, to intervene against Livingstone.[42] The Downing Street press office sought to orchestrate a media campaign against his party candidature.[43] The spin operation from No. 10 and party headquarters sought to remind people of Livingstone's past as they had done with Rhodri Morgan.[44] Blair, with Prescott and Brown, held public meetings in London at which implicitly Livingstone was attacked. Yet what they projected simply added to the distrust of the spin. The General Secretary had agreed the circulation of two statements per candidate, but there were repeated expressions of party concern over the scale of the Dobson mailings and the phone calls received from his camp. These began to enrage some of those in receipt of them. It felt as if their homes were being inundated by the detested spin.[45]

The biggest row came over the availability of lists of names, addresses and telephone numbers of those involved in the ballot.[46] These were made available to the Dobson camp via, it was said, the request from an MEP, Claude Moraes, to a London-based party official of the EPLP and thence to Millbank. McDonagh denied that they had themselves initiated the supply to Dobson but had responded to a legitimate request from the MEP who had the constitutional right to membership lists. Dobson himself complained to Millbank and told them that all the candidates must have the list but that 'The party wouldn't do it'.[47] Eventually in the face of an enormous public clamour and another clear own goal over this process, in the first week in January 2000 the lists were provided by the Euro MPs Clause Moraes and Richard Balfe.

There was a contested attempt to regulate intra-organisational balloting arrangements. The late decision to include the affiliated organisations, the complexity of tactical assessments, the lack of consistent procedural values and the general lack of trust between the unions and the party management made it virtually impossible to gain agreement. There was nothing in the rulebook which directly applied to affiliated organisations operating in a mayoral electoral college. So, at its November meeting, the NEC agreed that the unions would make their own decisions with votes cast either as a block or in proportions. The procedural discussions continued as things moved messily towards the hotchpotch of politically discredited Wales-type arrangements.

The AEEU had received much of the blame in Wales for not balloting and not splitting their vote. The situation they faced in London now angered them particularly, as they had never favoured elected mayors. Officials of the union argued later that in the London case the General Secretary, Ken Jackson, had expressed his support for balloting and a splitting of the vote at the first TULO meeting following the announcement of the college. Bill Morris for the TGWU had said that though they might ballot he could not deliver the union's Executive Council for the splitting of votes. The GMB did choose to go on its own with a ballot and split votes. It went Livingstone 67 per cent, Dobson 19 per cent, and Jackson 13 per cent. USDAW did the same. Theirs went Livingstone 60.5 per cent, Dobson 22 per cent, Jackson 17.5 per cent. Although most unions balloted and overwhelmingly the unions voted for Livingstone, most did not split their votes.

The fact that Millbank and No. 10 were seen as working flat out for Dobson made brokerage from them over the union procedures futile. Everybody was doing the tactical sums. As the campaign developed, various efforts were made. McDonagh attempted to persuade Rodney Bickerstaffe of UNISON to agree that they all split votes (which she thought would advantage Frank) but he too had done the calculations and in any case refused on grounds that he could not instruct the London region. Later, AEEU officials said that they had still been prepared to ballot members and split votes but 'the powers that be' said 'no, it will damage Frank if the others don't do it'. So they decided to back Dobson on a collective vote of their London Labour Party General Committee delegates.

The tactics of argument over decision-making spread into other organisations. The South London Co-op, the largest non-union affiliated organisation in that area, voted Dobson after failing to ballot. Labour Students was a particularly easy target of Millbank influence; they were affiliated as a socialist society to the London Labour Party but unlike other affiliates the officers had to sign a document which pledged them to accept the line management of the national party officials. The organisation was denied a ballot and, according to a leading student representative, their votes were cast with national party officials looking on to ensure that they supported Dobson.

London members of three affiliated unions – ASLEF, MSF and RMT – who might have been expected to vote for Livingstone were prohibited from participating on the grounds of a failure to pay party subscriptions by the due date of 31 December 1998, although their subscriptions were normally paid late and they had always had full membership rights before. An appeal to the courts by MSF members was turned down on the grounds that the fees should have been paid in accordance with rules not precedent and there was no automatic entitlement to participate in the elections. What was remarkable in the Wales and London cases was how limited were the legal challenges. This was in part a reflection of the reluctance of the party members to involve the courts. But also, as Ewing has pointed out, although there was a record of the courts applying the rules of natural justice to discipline and expulsion cases involving individual members of parties (leading to a tightening of party discipline procedures) the courts remained reluctant to extend the reach of these principles in the context of internal party government.[48] Here declarations relating to legality were tempered by acceptance of party autonomy, and party management had a degree of immunity.[49]

The financial arrangements for the extended campaign also raised serious questions. In spite of the 1994 NEC decisions over restrictions on internal campaign expenditure, this had not been strictly applied. As local selections had shown, finance could buy a lot in terms of publicity but also in some cases in the employment of canvassers. Now, late into the contest, a limit was placed on expenditure per candidate of £60,000 (based roughly on £1 per member in London). To the Jackson and Livingstone camps this was seen as an advantage given to the Dobson campaign because their resources did not match his. But to the Dobson camp this was regarded as over-restrictive. After requests for clarification, it was made clear publicly from Millbank they would take a 'generous' interpretation of the rules.[50] Even so, there were some controversial judgements, with costs of the meetings of Blair, Brown and Prescott not added to Dobson's expenses because 'they were not specifically about the Mayor'. The fact was that there were huge problems of policing any financial arrangements – particularly third-party expenditure favouring a candidate. This raised again important and unresolved issues for all internal Labour contests, including candidate selection, NEC elections and subsequently leadership elections.

Public attention to the controversial development of the process was drowning the policy focus on which it had been thought that they could put Livingstone on the defensive. Insiders reported later that so badly was the campaign going that panic was beginning to affect the management of the process, now taking place in a cauldron of growing public and party resentment against the manipulation. Normally loyal supporters began to drift away. Senior managers in headquarters and Downing Street now talked of friends who were 'all voting Ken'.

Frank's aggravation

Some of these efforts to 'help Frank' caused Dobson himself increasing aggravation. He was reported later to be furious that the electoral college was set up in a misguided attempt to help him.[51] It was 'messed up from start to finish'.[52] The party management was obscuring his natural sense of fairplay and rousing that of the public. Managerial behaviour was off-putting to some of his potential supporters, provoking a variety of well-publicised and proliferating complaints. Jackson and Livingstone submitted dossiers of complaint of impropriety and partiality in the selection contest to Union Security Balloting Ltd. These complaints were well reported in a media now overwhelmingly hostile to 'the stitch-up'. The *Guardian* gave an analysis of 'Labour's 10 top ruses to stop Ken Livingstone'.[53]

Complaints also stretched into the selections for the Greater London Assembly which took place in panels followed by a top-up list. In this suspicious atmosphere everything was liable to be judged a Millbank fix. Davies in her study focused, as did others on the left, on the fact that those excluded by the panels included prominent left-wing figures.[54] Those managing the London party selections argued strongly that they were conducted reasonably and were not partisan. As with other panels at other times, it seems not unlikely that whatever political judgement was involved in their decisions in these tense times was then integrated into their perception of a candidate's ability. It is important to register that it was privately boasted later by a leading figure involved that when one board decision was judged to have picked a politically 'wrong' person, an attempt was made from headquarters to get the decision reversed but it was fought off.

In the end, after Jackson votes had been redistributed, Dobson won the selection by the narrow margin of 51.53 per cent to 48.47 per cent. After this redistribution, individual Labour Party members voted Livingstone 19.966 per cent, and Dobson 13.367 per cent; the unions voted Livingstone 24.003 per cent, Dobson 9.330 per cent. The MPs, MEPs and GLA candidates swung the contest, voting 28.829 per cent for Dobson and 4.54 per cent for Livingstone. In a narrow sense it was a victory for management of the electoral college and the tactics of composing the third section. But in a broader sense the victory went against the Leader and against the party management because it was, as Mullins wrote in his diary, 'a result that stinks'.[55] Only 15 per cent of Londoners accepted that the college result was fair and 61 per cent favoured him standing as an independent.[56]

On 6 March Livingstone announced, in spite of his previous commitment, that he was indeed standing as an independent. With a huge lead in the polls it was only a question of how far he could hold on to it. In the end, the official Labour candidate Dobson got 223,884 votes and failed to make the final run-off. In the final stage, Livingstone beat the Conservative candidate Steven Norris by 776,427 votes to 564,237. Moreover, Labour had only a very narrow lead in the party list vote and even trailed the Conservatives in the constituency contests for the Assembly by 1 per cent. It is reasonable to assume that significant damage was done by the split in the party and its much criticised management. Important reverberations followed within the party. It is the interconnectedness of hidden managerial developments and responses to them that we find much that is new and significant in this study. From events in London, a range of reactions and new management initiatives can be discerned and followed through. (See also the continuation of the analysis in Chapter 15, pp. 470–6.)

Sanitisation success and the search for the Blairite?

Cowley and Stuart were right to contest the idea that 'only Blairite clones make it to the Commons'.[57] And it went too far to argue as did Dominic Wring, David Baker and David Seawright that 'Labour candidates are increasingly chosen by Millbank'.[58] Nevertheless, there had undoubtedly been an increased managerial role in selections. As Assistant General Secretary David Gardner put it, 'We are a broad church. But we also want candidates we can rely on to sustain Labour in power.'[59] In that objective they got near to what they were after in avoiding most whom they would classify as 'oppositionists', although it was never completely achieved. That shift was also affected by a deep decline of the organised left at the grass roots.

Peter Riddell informed us that Blair's staff had come to realise that he was 'not very good at using the levers of power and influence' in looking after 'his own people' in terms of parliamentary seats compared with

Brown.[60] Peter Wilby took the view that 'he had little interest in using power and influence to place 'his people' in parliamentary candidacies.[61] These judgements hold some truth in that, unlike Brown, Blair did not normally prioritise pursuing advancement for his staff especially if it extended the area of conflict with Brown. Over McFadden v Alexander, Blair simply walked away from the row. However, if 'his people' is taken to mean people generally aligned with him, Blair had a considerable influence on candidate-selection management either indirectly or, in the big cases, directly on the job. Blair's record of selection management in Uxbridge, Europe, Wales and London, and initially his comfort with Falkirk, were huge successes in terms of Blair's immediate selection objectives.

But, as with so much else about Blair's party management, the assumptions about public responses proved weak, there were damaging side-effects and there were unanticipated consequences. Uxbridge and Falkirk were lost and there was a very poor electoral outcome over Europe. Severe damage was done at the time to the party's electoral position in Wales and London. The methods used in London particularly, following on from what happened in Wales, became a public education into the politics and ethics of 'New Labour' party management and of another face of the 'straight guy' Blair. Historically, the occasional hard managerial practices in the party had been justified as a means of holding back unrepresentative minorities. In Wales and London, managerial practice had turned into a means of control over British democracy and the British people.

Under the pressure of Blair's urgency, the OMOV procedure, a crusade of Blair in the period leading up to 1993, became disposable in favour of a more secure means of party management, backed by a 'what works' array of techniques. Together with the managerial criteria used to establish procedure for NPF elections, these episodes illustrated yet again that peculiar absence of firm procedural values which became the hallmark of 'New Labour' politics.

Accommodation and Reforms

The state of the London party was described by insiders as 'near meltdown' as Livingstone was elected. McDonagh was sensitive to the scale and depth of the reaction; there was no purge of Livingstone supporters and, given the threats that had sometimes been hurled about, there was surprisingly little authoritarian vindictiveness. (For a contrasting story see Chapter 18, pp. 615–16 for the expulsions of party members following the loss of Blaenau Gwent in 2005.) Under the fierce attacks on 'control freakery', at the NEC on 25 January 2000 there was a promise, from a now defensive management, of a review of procedures for future mayoral elections and a review of their conduct. The *21st Century Party 2000* highlighted the need for selection procedures which were 'open, transparent and fair'.[62]

Steps were taken to change the rules on the availability of names and addresses to all candidates for selection. So much controversial unofficial supply had taken place, with party officials involved, especially in the European elections and over the London mayoral election, that it was deemed unpoliceable and a vulnerable target. Party officials in 2000, with McDonagh's agreement, decided to make lists available for everyone at a reasonable fee, but only after the short-listing stage. This did not stop advantageous early supply from a range of local sources, including party officials.

Selections for by-elections and the next General Election continued during and after the London battle. For reasons more fully explored in Chapter 15, but particularly in the light of public reactions, a new managerial emphasis was placed on avoiding the charge of 'control freakery'. Both on the NEC, as shown in Chapter 8 (see pp. 380–1), and in reselections, the unions became the local ballast preserving the status quo. There was also a new restraint in short-listing for the by-elections. Over the selections for Annisland, Preston and West Bromwich some of the candidates would not have survived the short-listing in the early days of the managerial juggernaut. 'We would have wacked them off' said one manager with a penchant for US gangster language. However, none of the short-listed candidates was absolutely unacceptable. In the case of West Bromwich, one short-listed candidate who met some managerial opposition won selection and the seat. The other two seats went to managerially approved candidates.

In candidate selection for the 2001 election McDonagh's view was that favoured candidates who wanted seats should do the work and insisted that retiring MPs should make their announcements early so that full selections could take place.[63] Again there was restraint by the managers in seeking to avoid public opprobrium, although this did not impede the management when their actions were not available to public scrutiny. Although Downing Street connections to the potential candidate were no longer popular, things were made easier by the further decline of the organised left – inhibiting 'some talented left-wing bolshies' from joining or staying in the party and reducing the number of those seeking selection. The Blair middle-class persona proved to be very acceptable even in parties in working-class areas. The fact that they included Chris Bryant described by Sion Simon as 'a 38-year-old openly homosexual, Blairite ex-vicar, who lives in Hackney and works for the BBC'[64] who won in the Rhondda, was seen as the party's recognition of talent and also a sign of Blair's growing support in these selections.

The Leader and direct involvement after London

In practice, after the London affair it also became publicly harder for Blair to be seen to be directly involved in selection fixing; parachuting particularly linked to a publicised offer of a peerage was now avoided or used with more nervous discretion. However, one case stands out indicating still the strength of managerial influence. Amongst all the preferences being conveyed from the centre to the regions in the period leading up to the 2001 election the top of Blair's priority list was Shaun Woodward, a prominent defector from the Conservative Party. The managers were finding it difficult because of not only Woodward's background but also the restive mood in the CLPs and the embarrassment of the claims that MPs were being offered peerages to retire. There was a fear that the issue might tarnish the Labour pre-election campaign. Eventually, late in the session, St Helens became available after the MP Gerry Bermingham unexpectedly announced his retirement. Shaun Woodward still had to go through a selection process with a short-listing.

To help on this the management process went into higher gear. Woodward was put on a favourable short-list which sidelined awkward opponents including the most able and popular of the alternative candidates, Marie Rimmer, the town's council leader. The word went out from the centre to build support in the CLP. Some unions including the GMB initially would not play ball but there was a crucial favourable response from the AEEU with which Margaret McDonagh had strong links. Eventually with a very low turnout of party members Woodward won by four votes after second preferences were counted.[65] The retiring MP Gerry Birmingham was not given a peerage (up to the point of writing).

As for his departing staff, Jon Cruddas and James Parnell made their own arrangements and managed their own campaigns for the seat – the general pattern from No. 10 after 2000. But there was an exceptional case of David Miliband, the head of Blair's Policy Unit. He did not quite fit Blair's plans for a 'New Labour' radicalisation of his staff in 2001 and Miliband wanted to leave No. 10. It was indicated to headquarters that the Prime Minister wanted a seat for him. McDonagh was again given the task of fixing it. In North Shields there would be an NEC short list after the incumbent David Clarke suddenly retired. Miliband, an impressive candidate, might well have got a seat elsewhere after some work but the condition of the North Shields party gave him added attraction. There had been a long history of internal conflict and it was said that there was a need for a broadly acceptable and diplomatic candidate. He was selected and Clarke became a peer in June 2001.

In target seats the candidates generally conformed to what the CLP as well as the party organisation thought would make for candidates who could win the seat. But two problems emerged. The first was that those with a business background seeking selection were few and got no systematic special push or support even though making the PLP more representative in that respect was considered desirable. In 2001 only 8 per cent of the PLP was drawn from business.[66] The second was that the managers found that identifying the likely parliamentary behaviour of the candidates could be difficult. 'Blairites' in this period varied from Mandelsonians (not many of them) to redistributive and constitutional radicals and civil libertarians, and included many who were primarily party loyalists enthused by being part of the drive for another Labour victory. It also included some whose façade of Blairite commitment moved as interest took them, a feature described by one manager as Odoist – shape-shifters.

Further, defining Blairite candidates could not keep up with national and PLP political developments as Blair and Blairism changed over the years. Peter Mandelson in a fascinating echo of his grandfather Herbert Morrison's 'Socialism is what a Labour Government does', argued at a Labour Party Conference fringe meeting in 2000 that Blairism was what a New Labour government did.[67] Given that definition and the second-term sharper movement away from the party's centre of gravity over both domestic and foreign policy, problems of party management in the PLP were bound to increase. Criddle's summation in the Nuffield General Election study of 2001 was that the leadership had 'sanitised the process of candidate selection'.[68] But sanitisation had limits and as far as it went, would not be enough. Although the aim was consistently to assist the management of the PLP, there was no more consistent total control here than in any other sphere of managerial operation, whatever methods were tried.

Notes

1 NEC minutes, 24 April 1995.
2 Letter Charles Clarke to Tom Sawyer, 28 September 1995.
3 Ibid., point 9, p. 4.
4 *Independent on Sunday*, 17 September 1995.
5 John Bochel and David Denver, 'Candidate Selection and the Labour Party: What the Selectors Seek', *British Journal of Political Science*, 13(1), 1983, p. 58.
6 Oona King, *House Music: the Oona King Diaries*, Bloomsbury, London, 2007, p. 61.
7 Ibid. p. 65.
8 Blunkett Tapes, August/September 1997, p. 37.
9 Derek Draper, *Blair's 100 Days*, Faber & Faber, 1997, p. 203.
10 *Sunday Times*, 1 October 1995.
11 NEC minutes, 31 January 1996.
12 Byron Criddle, 'MPs and Candidates', in David Butler and Dennis Kavanagh, *The British General Election of 1997*, Palgrave Macmillan, London, 1997, p. 195.
13 *The Times*, 8 July 2003.
14 Alan Johnson, BBC, *Desert Island Discs*, 12 October 2007.
15 Minutes of the NEC Development and Organisation Committee, 22 July 1997.
16 Byron Criddle, 'MPs and Candidates', in David Butler and Denis Kavanagh, *The British General Election of 2001*, Palgrave Macmillan, London, 2001, p. 185.
17 Ibid. p. 186.
18 Ibid.

19 Ibid. p. 187.
20 Rulebook, 1995, Rule 2 A.6(b).
21 Ibid. Rule 4 A.9.
22 NEC document, *Labour's Future: Keeping a Strong Voice in Parliament*, 1998, p. 14.
23 Ibid.
24 William B. Messmer, 'Taming Labour's MEPs', *Party Politics* 9(2), 2003, p. 215. For critical views on the process see 'One Leader – All Votes'. Ken Coates MEP and others, Independent Labour Network, November 1998, especially Henry Pepper, 'Confessions of a Selector', and Lord Evans of Parkside, 'Confessions of a candidate'.
25 Eric Shaw, 'The Scottish Labour Party under devolution', paper to the Elections Public Opinion and Party Group of the Political Studies Association, Cardiff, 2003, p. 4.
26 Ibid. fn 9.
27 *Financial Times*, 6 May 1998.
28 *Socialist Campaign Group News*, July, 1998.
29 *Guardian*, 30 June 1998.
30 Ibid.
31 Kevin Morgan and Geoff Mungham, 'Redesigning Democracy: The Making of the Welsh Assembly', Seren, Bridgend, 2000, p. 129. The study is very informative, as is the very witty Paul Flynn, *Dragons Led by Poodles: The Inside Story of a New Labour Stitch-up*, Politico's, London, 1999.
32 Steven Fielding, *The Labour Party: Continuity and Change in the Making of 'New Labour'*, Palgrave Macmillan, Basingstoke, 2003, p. 139.
33 Peter Mandelson and Roger Liddle, *The Blair Revolution: Can New Labour Deliver?* Faber & Faber, London, 1996, p. 36.
34 Lance Price, *The Spin Doctor's Diary: Inside No. 10 with New Labour*, Hodder & Stoughton, London, 2005, p. 78.
35 *Observer*, 21 November 1999.
36 There are a wider range of examples in Morgan and Mungham, *Redesigning Democracy* and especially in Flynn, *Dragons led by Poodles*.
37 NOP for *The London Evening Standard*, 27 April 1998. In November 1998 a survey for the ITV programme *London Tonight* found 91 per cent saying that they wanted Livingstone to stand. Mark D'Arcy and Rory MacLean, *Nightmare: The Race to become London's Mayor*, Politico's, London, 2000, p. 50.
38 Ibid. p. 101.
39 Ibid. p. 99.
40 Alastair Campbell and Bill Hagerty (eds), *Alastair Campbell Diaries*, Vol. 3, *Power and Responsibility*, Hutchinson, London, 2011, entry 3 November 1999, p. 153.
41 Price, *Spin Doctor's Diary*, p. 198.
42 Oona King, *House Music*, p. 114.
43 Nicholas Jones, *Control Freaks: How New Labour Gets its Own Way*, Politico's, London, 2001, p. 108.
44 Price, *Spin Doctor's Diary*, p. 52.
45 This was the angrily conveyed experience of London Labour members and supporters who talked to me.

46 Paul Lettan, a volunteer worker for Dobson, gave a detailed critical view of his own experience of the party machine's supportive practices in *Tribune*, 7 January 2000.
47 The NS interview: Frank Dobson, *New Statesman*, 31 January 2000.
48 K.D. Ewing, *The Cost of Democracy: Party Funding in Modern British Politics*, Hart, Oxford, 2007, pp. 74–5.
49 Ibid.
50 *Guardian*, 25 November 1999.
51 Frank Dobson, NS interview, *New Statesman*, 31 January 2000.
52 Ibid.
53 *Guardian*, 24 February 2000.
54 Liz Davies, *Looking Glass: A Dissenter inside New Labour*, Verso, London, 2003, pp. 74–5.
55 Chris Mullin, *A View from the Foothills*, Profile Books, London, 2009, entry 20 February 2000, p. 77.
56 CM/*Evening Standard*, 21 February 2000.
57 Philip Cowley and Mark Stuart, *When Sheep Bark: The Parliamentary Labour Party 2001–2003*, Paper presented to PSA Public opinion and Parties conference, 2003, p. 7.
58 *Guardian*, 9 November 1999.
59 David Gardner quoted in *Tribune*, 9 October 1998.
60 Peter Riddell, *The Unfulfilled Prime Minister: Tony Blair's Quest for a Legacy*, Politico's, London, 2005, p. 29.
61 Peter Wilby, *Guardian*, 5 May 2007.
62 *21st Century Party*, p. 39.
63 *The Times*, 12 December 2000.
64 *Daily Telegraph*, 26 June 2000.
65 *Independent*, 14 May 2001.
66 Criddle in Butler and Kavanagh, *General Election 2001*, p. 203.
67 Peter Mandelson, *Independent* fringe meeting, Labour Party Conference. Monday 25 September 2000. My notes.
68 Criddle in Butler and Kavanagh, *General Election 2001*, p. 205.

13

Managing the Parliamentary Labour Party

Old problems and new attitudes

Rebellions, opposition and 'not going back'

The landslide of June 1997 gave the Blair government a huge parliamentary majority of 179. Even with this majority, the PLP was always likely to be a problem for 'New Labour'. Parliament was the arena where party activity was under maximum daily media scrutiny and where the government's standing was regularly tested. An obsession with the electoral dangers of being portrayed by the press as divided produced a desperate need to show that 'we have changed', reassuring the floating voters and particularly the business community that the party's leaders were fully in control of the party. The PLP under 'New Labour' would not be allowed to go back to the rebellious ways of the PLP under Wilson and Callaghan, nor would it follow the example of the Conservative dissidents, 'the bastards', who made Major's term of office such a bumpy ride.

Survey evidence showed a significant change in the values of the Parliamentary Labour Party, particularly on many of the traditional touchstones of socialist values between 1992 and 1997, yet the PLP was still to the left of Blair.[1] And it was recognised by PLP managers that fully committed adherents to Blairism in the PLP – who could be described as Mandelsonian Blairites – were a small minority amongst those who had been elected MPs prior to 1997. Further, a study by the Philip Norton-inspired Hull Centre for Legislative Studies showed that since 1992 almost 70 per cent of the PLP had rebelled against the party line at one time or another. More than twenty times, 38 MPs had voted against the whips' instructions in the House. The conclusion was that 'Tony Blair has more bastards than John Major'.[2]

It was hoped that managerial influence over candidate selection would turn the factional balance of forces and, as shown, Blair's personal interest in the loyalty of the target-seat candidates was made clear to the party's regional directors. Nevertheless, although Blair and the managers proclaimed huge victories in the party, there remained a concern that the positive votes for Clause IV, and especially the Road to the Manifesto document, hid policy tensions which challenged claims that the party was ideologically united. Private conversations between the managers and Blair found him, and some of them, doubtful about how far the party had changed. This strengthened the search for more and new managerial control and for creating a climate that would make dissent more difficult when Labour formed a government.

In the period after 1994, on occasions when backbenchers broke ranks publicly, Blair had muttered angrily to loyalist NEC members and senior party staff about 'what we have to do with these people'. In June 1996 after a complaint about Blair's authoritarianism by the MP Paul Flynn, Blair was only restrained from acting immediately by reminders from Donald Dewar, then the Chief Whip, Prescott, Morgan and Sawyer, that disciplinary action would probably exacerbate the situation and show the party divided before the election. Campbell, who had successfully spun public warnings that there would be 'new powers to get MPs to toe the line in government',[3] personally thought the threat of action over Flynn had been 'daft'.[4] As the stories of new powers took off Blair realised that the spin had been a mistake.[5] But he continued to play with various proposals for 'new disciplinary powers to deal with the real bastards in the PLP'[6] whilst managers in the House continued to shy away from the problems which might be caused by authoritarian overkill. There were no sanctions applied for not following the whips' instructions. The Hull study pointed out there was instead a propensity to move to free votes rather than confrontation.[7]

The MP Harry Barnes, proud to be second on the list of major rebels compiled by the Hull study, was complimentary: 'In 10 years, I have not had a dicky bird said to me by Whips or Ministers to seek to control. Does that not show that there is a great deal of tolerance within the Labour party?'[8] The skill of Campbell was in persuading the media not to notice the occasional dissent here or elsewhere, by smothering it with loud notes of Blair's supremacy over a disciplined party. Yet Mandelson and Liddle, voices of the Blairite future, had given an emphatic message it would not go on under a Labour government. 'Troublemakers and extremist groups will get short shrift'.[9] The party was not going to be allowed to 'go back'.

When the unexpectedly large Labour majority brought in MPs from outside the target seats, including some whom few people had heard of, Mandelson sent out an order that all regional organisers be contacted to find out the 'potentially troublesome new MPs'.[10] A national party official was given the job of keeping tabs on them and their local parties. In various warnings and remonstrations, it was made clear to MPs that they were expected to abide by party policy, give full support to the government and be energetic ambassadors for it. Mandelson and Liddle had lamented the appearance of a weak and powerless Parliament,[11] but this voice quickly became subordinated in practice to the demands of strong leadership and the message of unity and discipline.

The 'New Labour' PLP

In general, this message met a receptive audience from the huge Labour intake. There was joy at being back in government, enthusiasm about what lay ahead and awareness of the ever-present dangers from hostile media. It was also helpful to discipline in the PLP that the front bench under Blair became a much larger entity than in the days of the last Labour Government. The payroll vote was regarded as 'an essential parliamentary tool and the bigger the better'.[12] Its size was constrained by the Ministerial Salaries Act but ways were found round, especially through the rise in number of the PPSs bound by collective responsibility. The convention that Ministers did not sign early day motions now extended to all of them. The front bench was now approximately 180 out of 418 Labour Members.

Given all these factors, what happened to and from the management of the PLP after 1997 was in one major respect entirely predictable. During the first term the government secured majorities for all its legislative proposals. It had been found in the Hull study that during the last Labour government 1974–9 there had been a remarkable increase not only in PLP dissent against the government but also in the number of Labour MPs dissenting on each occasion. Now it was found by Cowley when the PLP did break ranks, 'they did so in sizeable numbers',[13] but 'we have to go back to 1955 to find a parliament with fewer rebellions by government backbenchers'.[14]

Yet important things were happening unnoticed by observers of this cohesion in House votes. Influenced continuously by wider party managerial developments, behind the scenes there was a range of important conflicts and revolts within management itself. This had continuous impact on what was going on, and what was not going on, in the House. It gives us another perspective on the politics of the PLP as it developed in the three terms of Blair's premiership.

New integration

An important but often overlooked contribution to the managerial politics of the PLP was the new integration of the PLP into the Labour Party. Russell diagnosed that since their loss of sole voting rights for the Leader the PLP now had a more independent existence.[15] In reality, as her own work indicates, under Partnership in Power the PLP was for the first time represented on the NEC and on the National Policy Forum. These required new PLP elections and produced new political interconnections. In addition, to some surprise, because of a change which had been lost sight of since being introduced in 1980, the Parliamentary Committee of the PLP now had a direct representation on the Clause V meeting that produced the general election manifesto.

Added to this, the new managerial culture pursued with considerable vigour delivery of and control over united and collective campaigning activity throughout the party. Millbank became recognised for its assiduous attempts to keep the whole of the party 'on message' responding to the media-management task. All this provided reasons for what was happening to management within the central party organisation, becoming of greater significance for the management of the PLP. The observer of party management in the PLP has to dig into the deeper managerial developments in the House and also to keep an eye on their linkage to the wider canvas of internal Labour politics and changing public opinion.

The PLP managers and management cultures

Standing orders and whips

It had been long accepted that if the party was to be an effective political force, its actions must be coordinated. The primary responsibility of MPs was set out in the code of conduct which was part of the standing orders of the Parliamentary Labour Party. That recognises rights of conscience – but within limitations. 'While the Party recognises the right of Members to abstain from voting in the House on matters of deeply held personal conviction, any such intention should be intimated in advance to the Chief Whip. This does not entitle Members to vote contrary to a decision of the Parliamentary Committee.'[16] MPs in the whips' office were responsible for ensuring that individual MPs were shepherded in support of the decisions of the Shadow Cabinet then Cabinet. They favoured a form of democratic centralism – discussion before decision; complete party unity after it. Defenders of the role and responsibilities of the whips' office saw them as an expression of Labour's collectivism, and also of the party's connection with the people through the electoral mandate. In that sense the whips' office was judged to be, as one whips' office representative put it, 'the corner stone of democracy'.

The PLP officials and institutions

In academic and media coverage, management in the PLP was normally seen almost solely in terms of the activity of these whips. Perhaps understandably, given the difficulty of access and the public interest in parliamentary whipping, these other managerial arrangements have been under-explored, indeed barely covered at all even in the work of Cowley.[17] Here, in examining PLP management, the shepherding function of the whips is not the primary focus. The whips' role on issues of discipline, communication between the government and backbenchers, and the protection of the operation of the parliamentary party took place within a shared authority and a wider pattern of party management. Examination of that shared authority brings us into a hidden managerial conflict over the principles and forms of party management and the relations between party centre and PLP management. It involves the joint and at times conflicting activity of the Parliamentary Committee, which was the executive authority of the Parliamentary Labour Party, the PLP meeting, and in its most serious disciplinary form, the NEC of the party. Ultimately, within the Labour Party, the power of using significant sanctions against dissent was held by these other institutions, not by the whips' office. In that plurality arose the potential for important differences affecting managerial politics.

The Secretary of the PLP

In understanding what happened within these managerial arrangements under Blair, not to be underestimated was the role of the other parliamentary party officers. Historically a long-serving employee of the party, the Secretary was chosen by the NEC. Alan Howarth had been appointed under Kinnock in 1992, just prior to Smith becoming Leader. Although a personal friend and supporter of Blair and a believer in collective discipline, he was far from being an instinctive authoritarian. He had come through the period of the 1974–9 Labour government with a strong belief in the need to improve receptivity on both sides of the government-PLP relationship, and he shared the view that it was important to give the parliamentary party a positive involvement in policy-making. As manager of the PLP office, he had a staff of nine.

They were, however, part of the wider party organisation and financed by the central party office. Their staffing was determined and, in some aspects, administratively supervised from there. Howarth and his officers came under pressure from headquarters over their priorities, especially political management and electoral campaigning where the PLP was seen as a problem in terms of its old civil service mentality, therefore lagging behind the modernisation in the central party. PLP officials felt that they needed to protect the PLP's autonomy and had a more respectful attitude to rules, procedures and consensual flexibility than had developed in party headquarters.

Chair of the PLP

The post of Chair of the PLP had often been important, particularly at crisis points in the relationship, and it had normally been held by a consensual figure. Clive Soley's background was regarded as on the soft left of the party. He saw the party as having changed substantially since 1983 and was privately critical of the central 'command and control' management as being generally unnecessary and unhelpful. He too sought an inclusive approach, thinking it futile to attempt to suppress dissent. Because the members of the PLP were highly motivated and politically skilled, they provided an immense opportunity as policy-makers and ambassadors. He made clear that 'In principle, we need MPs to have more power and influence'.[18]

At the same time, Soley also shared the view that the disunity of the last Labour government had 'led to similar electoral disaster' to that of the Major government.[19] This combination of views produced a difficult balancing act with at times a precarious line to walk. As with Howarth and the PLP staff, Soley was protective of the traditional claim of autonomy of the PLP and defensive of the rights of MPs. But he occasionally took a leading role on television defending the government – an activity which, in the eyes of some MPs, undermined their sense of him acting as their advocate.

Parliamentary Committee

The Parliamentary Committee of 1997 consisted of fifteen members, with six elected backbenchers, four ministers appointed by the Prime Minister, one back-bench Peer elected by the Labour Peers Group and four ex-officio members, the Leader, Deputy Leader, Chair of the PLP and Chief Whip. Like the PLP it normally met weekly. As 'the executive authority of the Parliamentary Labour Party',[20] its functions included 'dealing with the Business of the House and in Government maintaining an effective two-way channel of communication between the Government and Back-benchers in both Houses'.[21] An element of that communication involved making regular reports to the Parliamentary Party and giving a written report, circulated with the weekly communication from the whips' office known as *The Whip*.

Amongst its other duties, the committee was involved in a regular dialogue on general strategy for dealing with discipline, and shared some of the disciplinary functions. Normal practice was that the Chief Whip made a report to the Parliamentary Committee, usually in general rather than in specific terms, on any problems he or she had had with individual members. Under the code of conduct, disciplinary actions of the Chief Whip had to be reported to the Parliamentary Committee.[22] And it was very significant that over voting it was stipulated only that the House members could not vote contrary to the decisions of the Parliamentary Committee;[23] no mention was made of the PLP, the Leadership or the whips.

Whips and the new regime

In 1997, the appointment of Nick Brown as Chief Whip and George Mudie as the Deputy Chief Whip, both ex-union officials with a background of working with the union traditional right, reinforced expectations of disciplined authoritarianism. Nick Brown had a reputation as a robust fixer of Shadow Cabinet elections. He believed that 'The ability to act together in concert is, and has always been, the corner stone of Labour movement power'.[24] Norton reported that Brown took compliance as given and 'exhibited an air of quiet menace'.[25] This was not the image others including regular dissidents encountered during his term as Chief Whip, although for some on occasions in the past it might have been a recognisable feature.

Brown was now more influenced by Kinnock's emphasis to the whips of his time on the importance of less coercive management and more self-control. He was keen to differentiate his own behaviour from that of the heavy whips' operation in the regime of 1974–9, which he thought helped poison the atmosphere. His view was that reasoning was far more useful than bullying because that built grievance and undermined good will. The PLP could now only be run by consensus and the build-up of two-way cooperation as a habit of mind. Millbank's present role he saw as heavy-handed and clumsy, but he was not averse to using procedural means to limit the success of the left-wing Campaign Group.

The whips after 1997 did have the advantage of some new rules and processes. Suspension was reintroduced into PLP rules, but rather than this being an instrument of new authoritarianism, what Brown and Mudie wanted was an extra option which avoided the swift escalation from repri-mand to expulsion. At this time, it was primarily focused on individual behaviour which did not involve dissent in the House. Suspension had to be reported to the Parliamentary Committee, which had the power to extend it whilst the colleague was under investigation.[26]

The most serious action, withdrawal of the whip, which was expulsion from the PLP, could be decided upon by a meeting of the PLP 'at which prior notice of motion had been given by the Parliamentary Committee'.[27] In this way again the Parliamentary Committee shared disciplinary initia-tion with the whips. Further, as the role of the whips extended discreetly into other aspects of political management including in relation to the conduct of elections in the PLP, the Parliamentary Committee's responsibil-ity for liaison with the whips extended into supervision of these activities also, as we shall see.

Parliamentary Committee composition

The general political perspective of this committee was highly influential in shaping the culture of party management in the PLP. As a result of a voting procedure by which each MP had to vote for at least three women, and because the huge infusion of women into the PLP were well organised in restricting their nominations, there was a preponderance of women on the first Parliamentary Committee elected in 1997. Chris Mullin was the only man elected. The women were Charlotte Atkins, Jean Corston, Ann Clwyd and Sylvia Heal who were all, at this stage, when the style of man-agement was established, associated with the soft left, and Llin Golding who came from the traditional right. In 1999 and 2000 the famously independent Andrew MacKinlay, and Colin Pickthall from the soft Left, replaced Chris Mullin who had become a Minister and Llyn Golding, making it marginally even less receptive to authoritarian discipline.

Crucially, there were no incoming members who might be classifiable as Mandelsonian Blairites. In representation it was close to the centre of gravity of the PLP. In attitudes towards party management, there was always an element of liberal Blairism in the PLP, especially notably in the work of Dr Tony Wright whose ministerial ambitions fell foul of his principled independence. He became chair of the influential Public Administration Select Committee. Also, significantly, there was a body of opinion amongst the new women in the PLP who sought a new style of politics that rejected the macho and the confrontational.[28] Although the PLP was the most party-oriented group of legislators in the House of Commons, only 19 per cent at most had a role conception that ruled out rebellion.[29] This contrasted sharply with the rhetoric and drive of the Millbank managerial style.

Influence of the Parliamentary Committee

By 1999, as tensions rose in the PLP, the Parliamentary Committee came under fire as not being effective in following through the policy positions of the PLP. In a special report to the PLP on 24 February 1999, Mullin acknowledged the scepticism but argued that it was a useful body. The PM had attended an average two out of three meetings and the committee, he said, had not shrunk from raising contentious issues and forcefully delivering their views.[30] But how influential it was over policy issues remained a moot point. Because of Mullin's deep expertise and interest in the security and intelligence services, their accountability gained from the strong representations by the Parliamentary Committee and an annual PLP debate. Over fox hunting, the committee was one of several locations where the government was pressurised with eventually some success. On miners' compensation, determined pursuit by Ann Clwyd led to Blair asking for regular reports on progress and in the manifesto meeting that was further strengthened by Dennis Skinner.

Otherwise over policy there was little to show. Concern over a lack of policy influence led Andrew McKinlay to seek more opportunity for the committee members to consult in advance and then to meet the leadership with its own agenda. This was contested by Soley who warned of the dangers of creating a 'them' and 'us' situation and argued that the current system worked well in providing a means of communication yet avoiding the exacerbation of divisions. However, the important point here is that the committee was at its most influential over procedural and party management matters – some of which had much wider significance, as will be shown below (see p. 413).

PLP meeting

The weekly meeting of the PLP included all Labour representatives in Parliament. Thus the Labour leadership had built-in support from the front bench within the meeting. The agenda was dominated by immediate parliamentary preoccupations. For a period under Smith 'The Political Situation' had moved up in importance. But under Blair 'The Political Situation' was relegated to the final place on the agenda. With Labour in government the topics for discussion were chosen by officials and led off by ministers, occasionally by Blair. Given the huge wave of enthusiasm and his warning of not giving ammunition to the enemy, Blair hoped for PLP meetings which were low-key gatherings operating within a supportive consensus and playing a subordinate role to the government. It was indicative of his attitude that his office had to be reminded by the PLP Office that under the constitution there had to be a special meeting of the PLP before the Queen's Speech was written. The meeting was held but Blair did not attend and the NEC was not invited, in spite of the constitution.

However, there was nothing low-key about the PLP meeting which covered the early contentious issue of changing lone-parent benefit (see below, pp. 410–11). There were 18 MPs from all sections of the party allowed to speak on the issue at the PLP meeting. Only 6 spoke in favour, 18 against.[31] Later meetings of the PLP were never the scene of such widespread dissent. They were often not very well attended and regarded by the managers and by critics as not very effective in accurately expressing PLP opinion. Loyalists regarded adverse responses as often posturing by noisy unrepresentative minorities. Dissenters, on the other hand, were critical of what they saw as a loyalist phalanx working to a script prepared by the whips.

PLP officers and the whips did not accept the criticism that the PLP meetings operated under tightly scripted control. But management did take place as an extension of the role of the whips in keeping in constant dialogue with loyalist supporters, arming them where necessary with the best arguments on key issues. When the pressure was on, loyalists were 'teed up' to come with an eye on boosting morale through supportive even congratulatory contributions as they were in the House, with continued awareness that the PLP meeting was virtually a public arena of conflict. The media waited outside in the corridor to pick up stories. Meetings were very leaky with regular briefings from officials and sometimes unofficial briefing from the critics.

When Blair was due to speak, which he did four times per year on average, the pressure was particularly strong to get the right response from the meeting through a potent combination of receptivity, the Leader's performance and the managers' prepared setting. At the least, efforts were made to organise a loud noise of enthusiasm, which would show the waiting and listening media outside the door the degree of unity behind the Leader. He personally approved of that kind of organisation, even though in action he was almost invariably a commanding figure with a capacity to seize control over the meeting by the conviction and force of his arguments, especially his focus on priorities to which MPs instinctively responded. His authority was also boosted by the regular generation of pride felt in him as conqueror and master of the old enemy across the House floor.

Special pressures built up by 1999, after adverse results in the European elections of June 10 led to much criticism of the campaign and the method of producing candidates. That led in response, on the NEC, as noted in Chapter 8, to what amounted to an organised deflection of the party reaction. In the PLP, three meetings in succeeding weeks which followed these European elections began with the Chair, Soley, refusing an immediate debate in view of the media interest in the meeting but promising that Blair would speak at the next meeting and that the party headquarters would produce a paper on the results. Blair did address the next meeting and was followed by one speaker after another supportive of the leadership. The third meeting was introduced by a defensive Margaret Beckett, the campaign coordinator, and by the General Secretary Margaret McDonagh, who was followed by an optimistic headquarters analysis from a party official, Greg Cook. His contribution was followed by mainly critical speakers. In an experience sometimes cited by severe critics of the atmosphere at the PLP, the first of these speakers, Harold Best, gave a robust response, drawing a comparison of the party member with the character of Boxer in *Animal Farm*. He was shouted down – a spontaneous response in the view of officials but one which could be tactically anticipated, given Best's militant frankness.[32]

Subsequently, the PLP Chair Clive Soley decided to ask the regional groupings for their comments and to hold a meeting of two representatives from each to discuss their experience of the Euro elections rather than relying on the PLP meeting. The officials also tried to find ways in which to come to terms with criticism of the agenda of the PLP meetings. One improvement was the introduction in 1999 of what were called 'Soley days', when the agenda of the meeting was proposed by members of the PLP, not the officials. But by now those with policy doubts did not always turn up to express themselves even on contentious issues where they might have taken on the relevant minister.

The absence of voting at these meetings added to the sense of dissatisfaction by some critical MPs anxious to maximise pressure. Although the standing orders retained the provision that colleagues could table motions and amendments for the PLP, and there was provision for votes, this was not encouraged. By custom and practice, for a resolution to be accepted on the agenda of the PLP there had to be agreement by the Parliamentary Committee. Three resolutions were submitted in the first term but none was accepted. The committee was reluctant to change the atmosphere of the PLP to something more adversarial with entrenched and embittered positions, and foresaw a flood of resolutions with no clear criteria for acceptance or rejection. Their response was also part of a broader managerial discouragement away from a culture of resolutions in the party and a defensive determination to avoid open registration of criticism which could be used by the media against the government.

Lone parent benefit revolt

Dealing with the issue of a cut in lone parent benefit became a significant landmark in the early management politics of 'New Labour' in government, and had major consequences. For Blair and Brown, showing prudence and control on this was all the more important because the left-wing Campaign Group appeared to them to be the driving force of a limited opposition. They, the usual suspects, had to be faced down and publicly pulled into line some time or other, so why not over this early issue and now? The breadth and scale of the emerging revolt had been neither anticipated nor appreciated as it began.

Why there was this lack of anticipation became a sore point with mutual attribution of blame between No. 10 and the whips' office. The view of the Chief Whip and his Deputy was that there was 'a low-key build up' in the PLP. Opponents, it was said, were late in signalling their opposition; only on the day before the parliamentary summer recess did Audrey Wise MP table a critical EDM which was supported on that day by eighteen others. 'Once it became apparent' that there would be a problem they had, they said, tracked it closely and accurately, but their warnings were ignored by Ministers. Privately, 10 Downing Street was to complain later that they had not been made aware by the whips of the early strength of feeling about lone parent benefit.

But seeking an explanation takes us back to the conference politics covered in Chapter 11 (see pp. 257–8). It was Downing Street managers with strong ministerial backing (and possibly at Treasury insistence) who had ensured that the lone parent benefit issue was managed off the conference agenda and into the margins of managerial attention. In 'fixing it' at the conference in the way they did, they thought that the issue had been 'consigned to the dustbin', as one very senior Minister later described it. And behind the fixing was an important contributory mindset. The common view at leadership level was that in the euphoria of the General Election, voting in the Commons would be 'no problem when it came to the vote'.

Those who organised early opposition to government policy on this issue became convinced that pushing it off the agenda at the conference had been counterproductive for the government in that neither the political leaders nor party managers appreciated the danger till the momentum of opposition was well developed. As Annie Marjaram, one of the key opposition organisers, described it, their opposition and organisation in effect went 'off the radar' of the party and media managers. The government case had not been heard at the conference whereas the dissenting case had been heard loudly on the fringe. The managers in the House were not expecting the force of the revolt, whilst the dissenters were focused and organised with links to the media. It was clearly a contribution to the scale of the problem. When the conflict built up in and around the House and the managers attempted to catch up with the opposition, that early failure of managerial perception and operation had put them at a disadvantage.

The problem was reflected in some internal tensions between No. 10 and the Treasury over what flexibility should be shown. And there was disagreement over tactics between them and the whips' office who were seen in No. 10 as being 'all over the place' in terms of what should now be done. That was not surprising given the concerns and reservations of the Chief Whip and his deputy on encountering what was found to be the strength of PLP sensitivities over the issue. A major problem was that a measure which could be presented as hitting the most vulnerable caused great concern even among MPs who prided themselves on their loyalty. And the government's proposals appeared to have some inconsistencies in encouraging welfare to work. If those on welfare took a job and it folded, they became new claimants and subject to the cuts. Reassurances about the future were important but left more doubts than ministers and managers expected. A reasonable judgement of the debate in the PLP and in the House was that the ministers had failed to convince many of those who were worried over the proposals. In the vote on 11 December the government won by 457 votes to 107, but 47 Labour MPs voted against, and although abstentions are not recorded there was a substantial number, estimated by Cowley as at least twenty.[33] The scale of the revolt was an enormous shock to both No. 10 and the Treasury.

The barking dogs that did not bite

What became important for the future was that there was also a second revolt. It has been suggested by Cowley that once the size of the rebellion became clear all threats to discipline MPs were abandoned.[34] Yet the scale of the rebellion was an added incentive to make a greater public show of the firm smack of control. As one Downing Street advisor noted, Blair's belief and resentment was that public opinion had not been opposed to the policy until the critics took their position; this was an additional point in favour of immediate disciplinary action. PLP officials became aware that Blair and Brown, although sometimes varying in their tactical response throughout this conflict, were now signalling a hardening of their united positions about taking disciplinary action. Gordon Brown's first widely reported response was telling Soley: 'We'll get those bastards.'[35]

But they did not. The striking feature of this whole episode was that the barking dogs did not bite. There were no disciplinary measures against dissenting MPs other than a light reprimand. No new disciplinary regulations were promulgated. Years later it was this point to which some control-minded managers looked back as the great failure as they sought rectification. There were always those in the leadership, amongst party managers and amongst loyalists, who regretted the loss of major sanctions and, as will be shown, this was far from being the end of that battle.

Why then, was there no significant disciplinary action now? Most important was the contribution of the non-rebels in the robust post-mortem. Under the standing orders, the Chief Whip could not move over serious sanctions without committee support and in practice the agreement of the back-bench representatives. The lone parent benefit issue had been discussed three times on the committee before the vote, but calls for delay or change were unavailing. After the vote their overwhelming view was very unsympathetic to the government's actions, expressed strongly along the lines of 'how did we get into this?' and 'don't put us in this position again'. That mood affected many in the PLP.

Labour's new women MPs had voted overwhelmingly in support of the measure and Cowley's researched view was that the new female post-1997 contingent were half as likely to have rebelled in House votes as the new male contingent.[36] But that does not address what appeared to be their significant influence on the second lone parent revolt, against disciplinary sanctions. That does seem to have involved a reaction against inappropriate political practice, a rejection of the macho confrontational and an aspiration to do politics differently. This current of thought justified and reinforced the propensity of women PLP representatives on the Parliamentary Committee to reject strong disciplinary sanctions, especially over an issue on which many loyalists had such deep reservations. Many of the female non-rebels had already made their position clear personally to the Chief Whip, agreeing to support the government but emphasising their dismay and distress.

His personal reaction in taking account of the post-revolt mood of the PLP was that it had been a lousy issue to make the test of a new disciplined party. Repressive management sanctions now were likely to create a worse situation for the whips and future party management. He rejected or evaded the leadership duo's private calls for sanctions. Privately Sally Morgan on behalf of No. 10 had promised rectification of the cuts the next year to persuade them to support the government. Clive Soley had done the same. That now became the common priority.

Trade union group reorganisation

There was something else going on here – or rather, not going on. The liberalism in responding to revolt was also reinforced by changes in the union relationship with the government. The historic collectivism of the trade union manual worker PLP representatives had in the past acted as the ballast on behalf of Labour's political leaders. Now, there was a significant continuing change in the social composition of MPs in the House towards white-collar occupations and at 13 per cent in 1997 the manual-working-class element of the PLP was the lowest ever.[37] Now also, Cowley found no difference between the propensity to dissent of the different manual-worker/higher-educated social groups.[38] That is explicable in the light of the New Labour changes described in this study, and of the feeling amongst the remaining manual-worker unionists that this was not quite 'our party' as it had been before.

The larger unions had separate group meetings regularly to represent the interests of their members: GMB 89, TGWU 87, MSF 80, UNISON 58, AEEU 18, as also did UCW, USDAW, GPMU, ASLEF and ISTC (a cross-party grouping). Direct relations with Whitehall after 1997 had contributed to a longer-term decline in the work of the individual groups, and only the GPMU and MSF together with GMB over Remploy closures had notably effective operations in the House in this period. It began to look as if they and the collective union group of the PLP were permanently weakened.

Yet coinciding with the revolt over lone parent benefit and its immediate aftermath was an approaching battle over union recognition legislation. (See Chapter 14 for a full analysis.) Its importance and wider 'New Labour' behaviour had the effect of stirring the unions to a renewal of their organisation in the PLP in order to find a new leverage over the government. Under the code of conduct of the PLP, though MPs' groups could only come into operation with the permission of the whips, the individual PLP trade union groups and the collective trade union group, which predated the Labour Party, had never been subject to regulation.

Initially, there was some concern in the unions that reorganising in 'the backyard' of such a supremacy-conscious Leader might be seen as too provocative. The strong business-sympathetic elements in Downing Street were said to be twitchy when they first got wind of it. A revived and reorganised PLP group ran contrary to the managerial agenda and the media presentation of the affiliated unions as 'under control'. But the reorganisation was in the end undertaken without asking permission of No. 10. More remarkable still, it even operated also in close contact with a minority of supportive managers (see Chapter 14, p. 444). The fact that the trade union group was organised to dissent against crucial features of where Blair was heading, or appeared to be heading, had the effect of constraining support for sanctions from what had been a past underpinning of the disciplinary tendency. The whips recognised it but within the strategy of the media managers did not publicly acknowledge it. Observers, including Cowley, did not register it.

Benefit reform postscript

There was an important postscript over lone parent benefit. At meetings of Downing Street representatives with special advisors the following week, the No. 10 people were said to be obviously listening in a way which some saw as both new and significant. Later, the lone parent decision was widely considered to be an error 'attributed within the Treasury to a particular right wing official and to a rare misjudgement on Brown's part'.[39] His later policy amounted to 'a generous rectification'.[40] Indeed, by the following spring, generosity towards lone parent families appeared to Cabinet Minister Blunkett as 'anything goes'.[41]

Whips and shepherding skills

Nearer the end of the parliamentary sessions would come what proved to be a decisive battle over sanctions against dissenting MPs. For now, much revolved around the traditional skills of the whips and individual Ministers. This is a subject extensively covered by Cowley. Here it is necessary only to give a brief résumé, but fitting it into the broader analysis offered of management politics. The traditional skills were augmented by improvements in the general provision of helpful communication making for cooperation. These included a *Daily Briefing* of party and ministerial information on a range of topics and a *Weekly Briefing* which contained the whip document of advice on supportive action and coverage of major issues. In addition a new PLP resource centre made available a store of advice, research and data which was well thought of by MPs. More controversial was the pager operated from headquarters which assisted in making MPs more informed but was also a means of keeping the MPs on message, and in line with the whip. It became a symbol of central control.

In confronting the possibility of dissent, the first task of the whips was an assessment of the size and significance of the dissent. There was then a focus on tracking its development and locating its supporters. This was followed by dialogue and a series of tactical moves whittling down the support and avoiding maximum unity of the opposition. This generally involved a degree of detailed policy adjustment and perhaps promises for the future which did not compromise the main thrust of the policy. The offer of a meeting with a minister was very useful in an attempt to finesse and adjust policies, possibly with suggestions of future re-examination. As the revolt developed, it was important to have some sensitivity to movements of opinion amongst 'the touchstones'. These were judged in the whips' office to be 'the more reflective types, specialists, those normally very loyal but suddenly uncertain, the prestigious and the influentials'.

Reception of the traditional call to loyalty was boosted by party patriotism which generated a desire to see the party winning and by avoiding the disunity that helps the opposition. Whips never stopped reminding MPs of what happened to the Labour government in the past through disunity, and what had happened to Conservatives under Major. There was a more particular appeal focused for many on not damaging the Leader as vote-winner, particularly in the seats newly gained in 1997. There were reminders of what they owed to him. For most Labour MPs uncomfortable with open rebellion, most of the time these were potent appeals alongside which tactics had to be flexible and focused on the individuals, what s/he wanted, feared, or worried about.

The aspiration to gain individual advancement in a hierarchical order was never far from consideration for most MPs and until after 2003 (when an extra salary was given to Select Committee chairs) virtually the only career path was through a front-bench position. That path was regularly drawn attention to. On the other hand, ex-ministers could be much more difficult to deal with both in terms of their expertise and the lack of patronage now available. Tough talk was a regular feature including at times from some whips threats and warning, but whips varied in style and generally were much less personally threatening than their reputation suggested. Responsiveness and reciprocation from MPs drew from a similar syndrome of supportive features evident in the other party institutions. There was a new realism in relation to practicality and particularly financial constraints, a weakening of the organised-left opposition, a general aversion to being classed as an 'oppositionist', and a growing sense of being part of an achievement in economic policy and the delivery of the manifesto.

The Lords

What happened in the Commons interacted with what was happening in the Lords and produced new consultations and complications. In the Lords, management had distinctive difficulties because there was a built-in majority who were not Labour Party representatives, and even for Labour representatives there was a loose discipline with a thorny problem of ensuring attendance. Although there was a separate whips' office and peers were expected to follow directions, the Labour Peers Group did not even have standing orders until 1995 when a Lords whip, Baroness Gould, wrote them. Still there were no effective sanctions against indiscipline in relation to voting.

Awareness of this led the irritated No. 10 managers to seek more life peers who would make their future activity in the Lords more of a priority. Parachuting just prior to the General Election involved retiring MPs who had been experienced loyalist work horses. Similarly the peerages regularly awarded to retiring leading union members of the NEC produced an increase in loyalists from there. Technically all Labour members of the Lords were members of the Parliamentary Labour Party and eligible to attend its Commons meetings. That appears to have strengthened the volume of loyalist support there. Not until November 1999 did a House of Lords reform bill abolish hereditary peers, with a small group of exceptions elected within the Lords.

New managerial aspirations: the PLP review committee

Meanwhile, it was a crucial feature in the development of the Blair style of governance that the listening and now partially adjustive mode of ministers following the post-lone parent shock, never fully accommodated to the formal consultative arrangements agreed by Blair before he moved into government. Those arrangements became lost to the view of commentators and academics as they became one of the 'New Labour' unmentionables. But there is much to be learned from this experience and the long struggle it involved. Alongside the regular authoritarian noises-off in 1996–7, there had been new aspirations for a more constructive relationship between the PLP and the government, comparable to and interacting with the development of Partnership in Power.

In 1996, in anticipation of election victory, a Review Committee on the relationship between the Parliamentary Labour Party and the next Labour Government had been set up under Doug Hoyle, the Chair of the PLP. Its broad-based membership included the Deputy Leader John Prescott, the Chief Whip Donald Dewar, and the frontbencher Mo Mowlam. There were three backbenchers, Bridget Prentice, Andrew Bennett and John Garrett. The Secretary was Alan Howarth. It produced in November a document titled *Preparing for Government*, which had a practical vision of what should be involved in the policy-making dialogue. This drew heavily from the Horam Report of 1976, which had received the formal support of both the government and the PLP at that time.

Different views had emerged about the value of the Horam venture. A memo from Frank Barlow, Secretary of the PLP, noted in 1979 at the end of the Labour Government that before the dissolution the committees were badly attended and now the PLP needed to be persuaded that they were not a waste of time.[42] Drawing from his historical research, Tim Bale warned that Ministers do not take kindly to having to explain themselves in advance.[43] However, Norton had also noted that some of the committee chairs saw the committee's role in more successful terms.[44] And Howarth's own investigation of the problems of the operation of the Horam recommendations saw the variations in success he had uncovered, linked particularly to the differences in attitudes and activities of individual ministers. That was taken as a sign of the possibilities of a constructive proactive relationship. The most effective was judged by Howarth to be that of employment with Secretary of State Albert Booth, although this may have been unusually influenced by being in the territory of the government-Party-TUC Liaison Committee and by the coordinating role of Michael Foot as Deputy Leader, enthusiast for the role of the backbencher and engineer of government-party-union unity.

From the Horam report, the PLP Review Committee adopted the obligation upon ministers to cooperate with the PLP in early policy formulation. Clause K 12 of the Standing Orders of the PLP read: 'The guiding principle shall be that except in exceptional circumstances, backbenchers will be consulted before major policy decisions are taken. In the case of legislation there should be an absolute obligation on ministers to consult relevant Departmental Committees as soon as possible, and certainly early enough for views to be taken properly into account.' The clause was very precise about government obligations. It was 'expected that three times a year, normally in October, January and after Easter, Departmental Ministers will send the Chairs of the Departmental Committees a memorandum briefly outlining the major policy areas and activities their Department will be concentrating on over the next three months'.

Leadership cooperation and control

There was always a question to be raised as to how this strand of the philosophy of *Preparing for Government*, like its Partnership in Power counterpart, fitted into Blair's strong leadership style and the managerial culture which emphasised leadership control. Nevertheless it progressed, and when the group's unanimous report emerged in 1996 it appeared to receive support from the leadership as a whole. This was helped along by the advocacy of John Prescott, who was a consistent and determined supporter. It was also helped by the fact that the cooperative philosophy of the document was expressed in terms of rights and responsibilities and included in an extension of the code of conduct a new clause which stipulated that MPs had the duty 'to do nothing which brought the Party into disrepute'.[45]

Unfortunately, but in character with 'New Labour' news management about controlling discipline, this code of conduct was announced by the Leader's office well before the publication of the cooperative aspects of the report of the Review Committee. It was described as being plans to give the whips greater powers to enforce a 'code of conduct' on MPs.[46] The authoritarian spin drew attention away from the participatory departmental committee proposals and its broader view of the role of the PLP. Not for the first or last time, the spin doctors had produced a successful media-focused exercise with damaging intra-party side-effects.

That exercise became a cause of concern to members of the Review Committee, as likely to evoke unjustified distrust and hostility in the PLP. A similar experience had taken place the previous month around the Party into Power committee meetings following the Sawyer interview. John Prescott let it be known publicly that he was angry that this presentation of the PLP review was undermining his efforts at PLP unity.[47] When it was debated in the PLP in December 1996 there was a strong response about this 'disrepute' clause from many critics and it produced a clever amendment on tolerance from the MP Dennis Canavan.

Being anxious to gain consensus and counter the suspicions, Donald Dewar the Chief Whip and Alan Haworth produced their own amendment, which Canavan decided to accept. In a separate section it now read: 'These duties shall not be interpreted in such a way as to stifle democratic debate on policy matters or weaken the spirit of tolerance and respect referred to in Clause IV of the Labour Party Constitution'.[48] There was an important indication here of different schools of managerial thought in dealing with dissent (again similar to what happened in the Party into Power discussions). One was the top-down voice of suppressive management control; the other was a sharing voice of dialogue and encouragement to cooperation and self-control. Whilst the latter won out, over the code of conduct formalities, the role of the former, for public consumption, set another tone which affected receptivity in the PLP and denied the proposals the enthusiastic new start that they needed.

Dialogue and departmental committees in practice

After the shock of the lone parent revolt, followed by an improvement in consultation, the philosophy and practices of the two-way communication envisaged by *Preparing for Government* might have been replenished and come into its own. The departmental committees arrangements of ministers, whips and backbencher volunteers under elected chairs had been set up in June/July 1997. In meetings of the chairs and of the Parliamentary Private Secretaries at No. 10, on 10 and 17 July, there had been an emphasis on giving the committees early involvement in policy-making, a positive role in a two-way process. Blair had made an encouraging speech at the first meeting of committee chairs in October 1997. That had raised hopes amongst PLP officials that it would get lift-off. In his diaries, Blunkett reported a good discussion at Cabinet about involving backbenchers (although, in a canny note, he was uncertain about what would come of it).[49]

For the system to operate successfully it required a well-resourced and additionally staffed system, up-and-running quickly, backed by strong and sustained support from the party's headquarters. It required also a consistent drive from a committed Leader. Failure in either of these might encourage any ministerial backsliders, allow problems to fester and discourage the participatory enthusiasm. This seems to be something near what did happen in practice. The PLP office staffing was initially reduced and then reviewed at a crucial early point in the potential development of the departmental committees. Much of this was to do with the usual post-election shortage of funds. But there were also some unresolved managerial tensions in relations with Millbank – a feature which, as will be illustrated, recurred time and again.

Headquarters placed a much greater emphasis on the party's campaigning role. Attempting to share in detailed policy-making or scrutiny appeared an indulgence and, worse, it might interfere with the momentum and cohesion of government policy-making whilst strengthening centres of opposition. In January 1998 a report on PLP staffing from the headquarters finance department was rejected by the Parliamentary Committee and had to be rewritten. The committee took the view that the headquarters report was addressed to what Millbank thought MPs should be doing. The real question, the parliamentarians argued, was what do MPs need in order to do the job envisaged by the PLP Review Report?

A limited increase in staffing did eventually take place but of the nine members of the PLP staff, three at most and often fewer, acted as departmental committee officials as well as doing work on the regional groups. There were never enough of them nor were they equipped with the policy expertise that would have given them the drive to cope with the lack of cooperation they encountered. At a later stage, the solution to the problem of resources was suggested from headquarters to be joint staffing with the

Millbank policy directorate to which the PLP staff would report. This might have given an extra boost in numbers and policy expertise. But from the PLP side, admiration of aspects of Millbank professionalism was mixed with concern that the PLP would be taken over by their priorities and their version of 'command and control'. The problem here had much wider ramifications. There was, as was described later by the Chair of the PLP, 'a clash of cultures'[50] in party management and with it a threat of the subversion of the PLP policy role. Given what had happened in the quiet choking off of the NEC Policy Committee role in 1997, these fears were real enough.

The drive to make the Departmental Committees work drew much less enthusiasm than had been signalled from the Prime Minister and the No. 10 Political Office. There were two reasons for this. The first was that, as already noted, relations with the civil service over the personnel and protocol of the incoming government had its points of friction. Sharing policy formulation with the PLP went outside the normal assumptions of government, and special advisors had inhibitive limitations placed on their party activities. These limitations might have been challenged by a modernising and hugely authoritative new Prime Minister as too narrow a preoccupation. After all, Callaghan had thought it legitimate in principle and Blair had not himself questioned it on those grounds. But given the other tensions he was reluctant to use political capital in Whitehall by throwing weight behind this arrangement.

Perhaps the major consideration was that here as in the wider party Blair and his aides were really pursuing supremacy not partnership. Four years later, it was candidly but privately made clear that around Blair they had been very sceptical about the proposed arrangements and that there was an element of 'false pretences' that Blair simply 'went along with it'. The 'New Labour' mindset produced the usual tendency to turn partnership into what one senior minister referred to later, ruefully, as 'the supporters club'. The limitation of the cooperative ministerial response was illustrated by the stark fact that by 1999 only one department, Health under Frank Dobson, had taken up the standing orders prescription to lay its plans for the year before the committee. And only two departments, including that of the Deputy Prime Minister, had involved themselves in drafting and inviting papers.

There were practical problems on the ministerial side similar to those that faced Partnership in Power but here with more immediate effect. A body of ministers found sharing with each other, not just in interdepartmental relations but even within the same department, an irritation in terms of time and an externally determined focus. This and the fear of feeding the political opposition stories of disputes through the 24-hour media, tended to dominate other considerations. Also, on the PLP side judging by their reported comments there were those who seemed ill-equipped or unwilling to make meetings work in the new way envisaged, and saw them in terms of the normal routines – lists of speakers, topic for discussion and so on.

Overall, the new arrangements never gained credibility and impetus in terms of the ambitious objectives of the Review report. In 1999 a confidential inquiry was launched by PLP officials.[51] This was so critical of ministers that it was suppressed and then heavily amended. Discreetly worded, the enquiry report eventually said that the committees were 'working steadily' and 'an opportunity for dialogue' but there were a variety of problems including times when committees were sidelined by ministers. A later reflective document by Clive Soley noted wistfully that 'many MPs felt that 'the government has not involved them in the policy-making process as well as it might'.[52]

Attendance varied department by department. In the best around thirty might be the average, others could have an average of fewer than a dozen. The numbers shot up when something very controversial was involved or there was trouble brewing. To that extent, the committees provided a regular and potentially useful channel of communications alongside other channels. But overall the feed into, and from, the departmental committees at an early stage in policy-formulation, did not provide anything near the sense of shared policy ownership and the transformation of the culture of the government-PLP relationship that had been the aspiration.

Conflicts within management

The culture clash as counterpoint

The culture clash over the priorities surrounding the financing of the departmental committees had a wider significance. The development of management in the PLP was at times heavily influenced by a reaction to excessive management at the party headquarters and/or the intention to move the PLP in that direction. There were discreet but firm rebellions around the Parliamentary Committee beginning from the outset of the Blair government. Voting and signing motions in the House gave only a partial and at times a surface view of dissent in the PLP and of the constraints on party management.

At the heart of this was the managerial culture described in Chapters 4 and 5. The new definition of the role of party officials as 'political organisers' was not shared by Howarth, Soley or his successor Jean Corston. Howarth saw himself and his staff as civil servants of the party. For him it was 'a badge of honour'. His defence of the standing orders of the PLP in this phase he saw as a protection against abuse. Margaret McDonagh, first as an assertive Deputy General Secretary from July 1997 and then General Secretary from October 1998, in common with others in the party machine after 1994 was derisive about the term 'civil servants' when applied to party officials, seeing it as a constraint on the energetic pursuit of the party's goals.

The reputation of Millbank for control and its mode of operation became part of the background awareness of MPs, reaching its height towards the end of the first term in government when 'control freakery' became a major issue. But from the first, anxiety amongst PLP officials and back-benchers on the Parliamentary Committee drove them to assert quick defences and a differentiation of behaviour that fed off regular private conflicts over managerial conduct. In 1997 representations to the PLP over the financial obligations of MPs to the party led to a significant confronta-tion when the Chief Whip and the Chair of the PLP sent a message to MPs repudiating any suggestion 'that the Office Costs Allowance might be used for purposes other than those for which it was provided'.[53] McDonagh contested this interpretation of what she had suggested and thought their interpretation of the proprieties was wrong and too restricted; it reflected that unreasonable caution which sprang from 'a civil service' mentality. Judging by their use of the Short money, it was said that the Tories had few such inhibitions.

The attempt to create a more politicised and committed party machine drawing in all available resources to secure delivery did not stop at the border of the PLP. In the document *Partnership in Power*, it had been argued that MPs should play 'an ambassadorial role for the government within their local parties and communities and feeding back the views of local members . . . ministers should make time for local campaigning and meetings with local party members and public representatives'.[54] Taking this up with enthusiasm, Millbank senior staff sought to boost the party work of MPs. This included efforts to integrate their campaigning role into influencing party opinion as well as influencing the electorate. There was a constant critique from party officials of the lack of effort and priority given by some politicians to such activities. It was a permanent frustration and a frequent lament that these MPs would not do the party work, indeed would not do enough campaigning work generally in spite of four differ-ent parliamentary committees to organise campaigning.

The Parliamentary Committee accepted that there was a problem and that the party organisation had a case. At one stage the Committee criticised the whips for their unwillingness to give time off from the House. Evidence produced later indicated that absences from the House promoting the party's cause in marginal constituencies produced a better result than the national trend in 2001 General Election.[55] On occasions, the impatience of Head Office led to a conflict over the priority of party organisational and election work in relation to other work in the House. In November 1998 the Parliamentary Committee complained about the party headquar-ters arranging, without consultation, meetings of MPs which clashed with the regular weekly meeting of the PLP.[56] In January 2000, one official of the PLP working to the departmental committees was taken away for elec-tion work at short notice without consultation.

Also significant was the concern amongst PLP managers that they should not be pulled into wider intra-party conflicts influenced by central party managers that might compromise their own internal relationship. This was brought out over Canavan and Davidson in the Scottish selections. It was discussed in the Parliamentary Committee in July 1998, where Davidson's critique of the process was accepted by the committee but they could not interfere with the results. They did share the Chief Whip's view that in future MPs should not be members of panels involving the reselection of their colleagues.

Taking power from the whips: NEC elections

The development of Partnership in Power arrangements not only integrated the PLP into the national party processes in a new way, it opened up new balloting arrangements and invited potentially new divisions and new dimensions of control. For the first time in 1998 the PLP would elect its representatives on the NEC. With headquarters and No. 10 emphasising the need for a loyalist majority on the newly elected NEC and, as noted in Chapter 8, with some bitter recriminations over managerial behaviour, an argument broke out over the practice by the whips of utilising pre-printed nominations forms, supporting their favoured three-person slate of candidates in the new PLP elections to the NEC. The three nominees – PLP Chair Clive Soley, European Socialist Leader Pauline Green and Anne Begg – were elected with 259, 247 and 207 votes.

What was later acknowledged privately to have been an organised attempt to avoid any possibility of Socialist Campaign Group members getting on the NEC, kept off Dennis Skinner, who received 182 votes. Under the old arrangements, Skinner had been elected to the CLP section of the NEC for many years. When the Partnership in Power arrangements had been introduced, indications were given by John Prescott and (less explicitly) by Blair's office that they would support Skinner's election under the new procedures.[57] The rejection of Skinner now seemed an even more unsavoury fix and/or a snub to the Deputy Prime Minister. The aftermath here was very important. In a party getting increasingly irked by the manipulation of procedures in different forums, the action of the Chief Whip was badly received.

At Parliamentary Committee meetings on 20 May, 27 May and 3 June 1998 it met a series of robust challenges, from members including Prescott and Soley, which moved from the inappropriate action of the whips to the challenge, 'Why were the whips involved in processes like this at all?' The Chief Whip, in a remarkably candid statement of his position, was not prepared to accept that he had done anything improper but agreed to think further about it. The Leader made clear that he was 'interested in the outcome', and thought it would be bizarre if 'the party' (i.e., the party managers) were not involved at all. One contributor thought that it had been damaging to the Prime Minister, stimulating the joke that OMOV had been replaced by OLOV – one Leader, one vote.[58] After further private discussions with the Deputy Leader, the Chief Whip accepted that he had made a mistake about the nominations in this instance.[59] A line had been drawn, adding (for the moment) to the constraints on the Chief Whip and inferentially the Leader in the management of the PLP.

NEC Elections and holding off Millbank

There was a further consideration affecting attitudes towards the management of party elections for the NEC under the new arrangements for Partnership in Power since 1998. After representations in a letter to the General Secretary on 4 June 1998, it was confirmed that the votes in these elections would be by secret ballot and held at the party conference. But the managerial reputation of Millbank and the fact that the secret ballot papers were numbered led to complaints from MPs who believed that names of voters could be traced. McDonagh argued, not unreasonably, that numbered ballot papers were a normality of balloting arrangements – an insulation of the process against fraud. But in the light of the deep distrust which increasingly accompanied much of the activities of central Blairite party management, it led to some bitter arguments. In the end the numbers were all snipped off by the PLP Secretary. As a result, the procedure the following year moved to a postal ballot conducted by Unity Balloting Services.

Reshuffles and continuities

It is tempting to read the reshuffles and appointment of the Chief and Deputy Chief Whip in this period in terms of the Leader's preoccupation with party management. Nick Brown and his deputy were heavily criticised in No. 10 over the management of the lone parent benefit revolt. The fact that Nick Brown was a 'Gordon Brownite' was given in part-explanation for the generally poor working relations between Chief Whip and Leader. His replacement in 1998, Ann Taylor, had as the Leader of the House been critical of Nick Brown's style of management, and coming from the traditional right was expected to move into an improved working relationship with Blair and a more disciplinary regime.

But the replacement of Brown by Taylor did not function well. The Monday meeting with Blair was later declared by the Political Office to be 'useless'. The dissent continued although, as under the previous Chief Whip, there were no defeats for the government. The biggest u-turn forced on the Chief Whip and the Leader was not by dissidents opposing the whip but by the PLP demanding a whipped vote. Repeal of Section 28 of the Local Government Act prohibiting promotion of homosexuality had been in the manifesto. It was a party commitment which ought to have been subject to a three-line whip but Blair at one point had agreed with Ann

Taylor's suggestion of a free vote. Taylor came under fierce criticism from John Prescott and sections of the PLP and had to back down.

Apart from dissent, attendance also became a growing problem, some of it by MPs prioritising the nurturing of political support in the locality. Given the size of the government's majority some backbenchers disagreed with the heavy shepherding. The situation was liberalised by the new Chief Whip for a while but there was a further relapse to increased absences without permission. As for the expectation of a new stricter disciplinary regime, it did not happen. Defenders of Taylor later explained this in terms of the liberal precedent set by Nick Brown and how difficult it was to row back to more control from the refusal to act after the lone parent benefit revolt. Whips' office disciplinary records on individuals had not been passed over from Brown to Taylor. 'They should have had their heads on poles' was a view attributed to Taylor's special advisor Ian McKenzie on the regular dissidents. The Nick Brown camp on the other hand did not accept that their regime was unchangeable if that was the will of the Chief Whip but that she had rightly realised that an authoritarian response would create major problems. A relevant background consideration was also that increasingly the wider context of arguments over control had an effect in strengthening defensive PLP sentiment. This was not a party receptive, nor later an electorally receptive atmosphere in which to launch a new disciplinary regime.

In 1999 in a less manipulated contest for the PLP representation on the NEC, Skinner was elected together with Helen Jackson and Clive Soley, producing a strengthening of the independent voices over party management issues at the centre.

Tensions over the elections for the National Policy Forum were eased by the lack of interest shown in the NPF by most of the Socialist Campaign Group, who regarded the forum as a subversion of party democracy. In 1999 there was a whips' office list but it was managed in a low-key way and resulted in a big spread of votes from top to bottom of the winning team. At this stage, the PLP was in various ways not geared up to the full participation in Partnership in Power. PLP representatives to the NPF even had to make an appeal for MPs to read the documents and feed views to them but they received a limited response. Afterwards, they gave a brief report to the PLP but there was no energetic debate. For the moment the politics of PLP representation at the NPF was considered unimportant.

MPs, sanctions and the operation of the NEC

In Chapter 8 it was noted that the atmosphere was such that a potentially crucial attempt to further boost parliamentary sanctions and discipline over MPs following a report by the Chief Whip to the NEC in 1999 detailing 'unauthorised absences, abstentions and votes against the whip', failed to produce the expected outcome. Here it is important to note the parliamentary origins of these managerial difficulties and manoeuvres. The partially sub-merged context has already been noted: differences between schools of management, a culture clash between central management and the manage-ment of the PLP, and the regular pressure and raising of temperature from the spin of media managers responding to the Leader's attempt to show control and supremacy.

Over the Chief Whip's report, Downing Street sources had been reported as warning that whilst one-off rebellious votes on 'matters of conviction' would be tolerated, 'repeated dissent' would not.[60] A pattern then developed in which, alerted to the threat and at times exaggerating it, opponents of more sanctions in the PLP made complaints to members of the Parliament-ary Committee who in the light of their common concern about Millbank management sought reassurance. In this they were assisted by the campaign in the mainstream Liberal-left press already hostile to 'control freakery'. An *Independent* editorial was headed 'Blair unleashes the party heresy hunters'.[61] A *Guardian* editorial headed 'In the grip of Millbank' called for the party to 'loosen up'.[62] Led by Clive Soley, the Parliamentary Com-mittee made clear its opposition to the idea that any sitting MP would face deselection because of his/her political views.

Chief Whip Nick Brown reiterated that the information to CLPs would be purely factual in relation to parliamentary performance and particularly job attendance. His primary objective in matters of discipline was to do something about the lazy and those who in other ways did not take their obligations seriously. Deselection he did not regard as part of the PLP's disciplinary process. David Gardner, Director of Organisation, now felt that he had to make clear to the PLP that the headquarters view was that the report would contain 'only information that was already in the public domain'.[63] The NEC would interview a sitting MP 'in exceptional circumstances only on the recommendation of the Chief Whip, and CLPs would be able to select the candidate of their choice in line with party rules'.[64] The new Chief Whip Ann Taylor made clear to the Parliamentary Committee that she too accepted that the report by the whips would be purely factual. But as she was expected in the PLP to produce a new hard line on dissent, the pressure mounted even on this, and MPs were given a right to see and challenge the accuracy of what had been reported about them.

Nevertheless, in the whips' office, the Political Office in Downing Street and at headquarters there continued to be a view that some warning shots must be fired against a few regular dissenters, perhaps excluding 'say, three of them' from their reselection in order to establish more control for the second term when the majority might be smaller. It was hoped that at least there would be more sanctions over regular absentees. Yet by the time that the whips' report was ready in 1999 the managerial handling of the Livingstone affair in London was beginning to add to a control freak reputation which was now adversely affecting the Leader. Consequently, even action against bad attendance might be publicly misunderstood and be counterproductive in terms of the reaction in the PLP and the public.

Here the politics of the NEC described in Chapter 8 is further explained. The spin from Millbank by this stage was now publicly reassuring. 'Left-wingers can relax' was the message.[65] Treading softly, in the Chief Whip's report, the record of each MP was stated in fairly anodyne terms and made no recommendation for action by the NEC. But behind this a discreet political understanding had been reached between the Chief Whip and the General Secretary (with covert support from No. 10) that when it came to the NEC such action would be initiated via the agreement of the NEC trade union group which had so far generally worked closely with the General Secretary.

Yet because there was such a public risk in operating through the much criticised Millbank, so furtive did this attempted plot become that there was uncertainty about who was supposed to do what. One key loyalist member of the NEC trade union group was apparently told by the whips' office that it was a matter for the whips' office alone; the implication appeared to be that they should do nothing. It was not surprising then that the existing doubts of a majority of the NEC trade union group were reinforced, nor that when the tactics became clear to the PLP representatives on the NEC, as has been shown it sank against the strong opposition expressed by Soley and Prescott.

Significance

The total failure of these tactical manoeuvres point up once again that PLP management can only be understood against the wider managerial politics of the party, especially 'the culture clash' and the wider reaction of party and public against 'control freakery'. The Political Office in Downing Street could only think of seeking to strengthen the sanctions available to whips when the No. 10 influence was hidden, and the whips in practice behaved the same way. Again it illustrated also that the management of the PLP was much more pluralistic than a focus on the whips suggests. The PLP officials, representing Parliamentary Committee back-bench opinion and supported by the Deputy Leader, were unhappy with the possibility of outside intervention in the PLP, especially if it was led by the icon of command and control.

Cowley has argued that voting-record circulation did not work because CLPs if anything were 'on average marginally to the Left of the MPs' on most questions and CLPs more likely to be urging revolt'.[66] But, as shown, the use of the voting-record procedure as political leverage had already been undermined within the confidential confines of PLP management and then on the NEC. Cowley's evidence from MPs also notes that in some constituencies where the local activists were putting on pressure to toe the line, MPs were complaining that the original source was Millbank.[67] That had been true ever since 1997 via the managerial network. But slowly

recognising the unexpected counterproductive ramifications of heavy management, the No. 10 aides began to accept the media priority of avoiding
the accusation of 'control freakery', and here Blair had the wisdom to
operate his reverse gear. In a development undreamed of in 1997, by the
turn of 2000, the managers working with the unions found themselves
using the reselection trigger as a protection not just for loyalists under
threat but for dissidents also. Protecting both left and right it therefore
further liberalised the position of MPs without announcing it to them or
the public.

Blairite management and the disciplined party

Few would have argued with Rawnsley's view that 'In the Blairite conception of parliamentary democracy the role of New Labour MPs is to sustain
the Government. New Labour did not get elected by licensing dissent, and
it is not going to be re-elected by encouraging the habit now. This is an
article of faith with the Prime Minister'.[68] Given the accuracy of that characterisation, it was understandable that commentators of various kinds
should fail to notice the absence of heavy sanctions and over this the weakness of the whips. In practice, as we have seen, it was not as Cowley put
it, that 'they could not rely *solely* on coercion' to retain cohesion[69] but
that they could not put into practice at all a key element of the armoury
of 'coercion'. Further, the reselection trigger influenced by the unions was
now a protection for loyalists and dissidents. This was the big story. MPs
gained a more assured freedom whilst the whips were thwarted and had
to be more discreet even over some guidance powers. Had these developments been described to a group of Blairite managers in 1994 the reaction
would probably have been one of horror and trepidation, fear about a PLP
descent into internal anarchy producing a media-fest as a result. Yet for
the moment, the high level of disciplined self-control over voting behaviour
in the House held.

That liberalism could not be publicised for fear of encouraging further
dissent but also because of its possible threat to the image of Blair the
supreme controlling Leader. On the other hand, neither could Blair benefit
from the liberalism as much as it might have been helpful, as he began to
be blamed for 'control freakery'. As a result it may have looked, as Andrew
Marr argued in January 2000, as though 'The Commons has become a
dull whipped chamber, short on independent minds'.[70] On the left it was
even thought that there was 'tightening discipline'.[71] Many shared those
views.

Yet the important point here was that the chamber was not the only
forum of decisive conflict in the House, and there were some very independent minds within the managerial conflicts responding to opinion in
the PLP. Here as with other sites and forums of party management there
was a crucial struggle over what kind of Labour Party management there

should be. That went on virtually unnoticed throughout the three terms of Blair's premiership. There was a neutralisation of what was seen as potential impediments to Prime Ministerial supremacy over policy formulation through the departmental committees; that was a major victory. But there was never a victory for imposed disciplinary party management. In that battle over sanctions it was the most authoritarian position, not the PLP, which had been brought quietly under control. The full significance of these developments was to become more apparent after 2001 and then after 2005.

Dissatisfaction and reassurance

Dissatisfaction

The 1999 campaign in Kosovo generally impressed the majority of the party and divided the left but it also raised an issue which was to come even more to the fore in the second term. The style of running the government was described by *Guardian* columnist Hugo Young as that of 'Commander Blair' 'playing it tough' in refusing a vote on the adjournment.[72] Blair continued to be much admired in the PLP for his despatch-boxing supremacy over the opposition, but there was also some frustration over the Leader's policy-making style and the limitations of the role played by the party's backbenchers. Another columnist, Jackie Ashley, referred to Labour MPs' 'resentment at being taken for granted and at the initiatives which came out of the blue accompanied by the torrent of spin'.[73] That was the very problem that *Preparing for Government* had sought to overcome.

In addition there was a criticism, not normally publicly articulated but one which could be picked up from MPs' private remarks, that the Blair No. 10 operation had managerial attitudes which were deeply off-putting. The pollster Peter Kellner spoke to a cross-section of normally loyal backbenchers who had been enthusiastic Blairite optimists. The PM was 'blamed for being increasingly remote, and for surrounding himself with arrogant apparatchiks who hold backbenchers and the wider party in contempt, who bend the truth and who bad-mouth Ministers and MPs they don't like'.[74]

There were also now a growing number of ex-ministers making their experienced voices and criticisms heard. Some 'wannabe' ministers were beginning to wonder if they would ever be taken inside and expressing their frustration. These became a grumbling addition to the offensive against the style of party leadership and to the increasing interest in modernisation of the House. Prominent senior Labour backbenchers who were members of the Liaison Committee of the Commons made the charge against the government of disregarding Parliament, as they called for a strengthening of Select Committees and a weakening of the powers of the whips over their composition.[75]

Blair, however, was not 'a House of Commons man' and never became one, although he had to take account of it. He did not bother with making comradely tea-room appearances, rarely participated in debates and his voting record was the worst of any modern Prime Minister.[76] It was in part that he was a careful guardian of precious time in the light of the government's majority, but he was also expressing his special supremacy in the role of premier. This became seen by critics as sending a message about his low regard for Parliament. Though he had not opposed the Select Committee on the Modernisation of the House of Commons set up in May 1997, and various changes had taken place to improve the working arrangements of the House, he was also never an enthusiast for a Commons modernisation which constrained a Labour government – his government. Margaret Beckett, who became Leader of the House in 1998, although often appearing more open to argument, felt the same about defending the government.

That view was a natural reaction of many Labour loyalists, but within the party another mood was also developing. Evidence of growing PLP dissatisfaction came first in the election of a new Speaker on 23 October 2000. Sir George Younger, a Conservative, was seen as the government's preference but much Labour support and victory went to Michael Martin, an 'old Labour' MP from a working-class background with strong union connections. In November the boldly assertive Andrew McKinlay challenged Soley for the post of PLP Chair; McKinlay made it clear that he was not so much standing against Soley personally as seeking to shape and mould a role for this important office because Britain was 'inexorably moving towards a presidential style of government'. In his view the PLP Chair, therefore, needed to be like a US-style 'caucus leader'.[77]

That became more a marker of deep unease rather than a proposal which gained him electoral impetus. The main challenge came not from McKinlay but from Tony Lloyd, an ex-Minister and leading figure in the PLP trade union group. Soley carried the first ballot and, with covert organised whips' support, defeated Lloyd in the final ballot, but only by the narrow margin of 184 votes to 178. That was remarkable and indicative. Soley acknowledged that in his managerial role he might have got the balance wrong in the last six to nine months.[78] But perhaps even more significant than the result was that those who had first alerted the Prime Minister to the danger to Soley's position found Blair reluctant to hear it.

Reassurance

Blair and the No. 10 aides thought that an accusation of 'not listening' was unreasonable and was not to be taken too seriously. In 2001, in the Political Office of No. 10, the most recent example given was over Parliamentary Committee opposition to the abolition of Community Health Councils where Blair was reported to have said, privately, 'We'll have to give a bit on that one'. However, as it happened, though delayed it was enacted after the General Election. The mood in No. 10 as before was influenced by what they had overcome, by the created image of Blair's supremacy and also by the discreet security of the procedural insulation against removal of the Leader. Managing officials at headquarters did not regard it as their job to facilitate disunity and still less to encourage revolt. So, another extension of the rolling coup, not mentioned by officials in the Party into Power discussions or announced subsequently, nor registered by commenting observers, was that the nomination forms for leadership elections would no longer be automatically circulated to the PLP each year and, since 1997, succeeding General Secretaries had neglected to send out the forms.

At the close of 2000, in relation to PLP management, Blair's aides thought that they were doing rather well. Attention was drawn to the strong base of support in the House. Although between November 1999 and November 2000 there was an increase in rebelliousness and a notable increase in the number of MPs prepared to break ranks, it was still, as Cowley pointed out, from a high base of cohesion.[79] The rising numbers involved in dissent were still small in relation to the huge majority. The Socialist Campaign Group, seen as the main potential factional opposition, was limited in size, poorly organised and weakened by a declining organised left at the party's grassroots. It was also circumspect in attempting to oppose some policies without appearing 'oppositionist'. Against that background, the fact that attempts to seek more sanction-backed control over PLP absentees and dissidents had floundered did not seem so significant. Defeat in the Commons or even being pushed to a narrow vote victory appeared for the moment to be highly unlikely.

What decisively reinforced an element of complacency in No. 10 was the Parliamentary Committee's repeated concern about publicly squabbling cabinet ministers, particularly Mandelson and Brown over Europe. This was expressed very strongly about Mandelson's comments made to a business audience on 16 November 2000. The committee's reaction was judged in No. 10 as specially significant in revealing the PLP's priority about unity. As Blair said, reflecting on the past with one of his aides, 'It just shows the difference'. The whips' office was not apparently signalling any other message than reasonable reassurance about the PLP. Around Blair it was, therefore, considered unlikely that in the second term there would be a major upsurge of rebellion, even though 'the most cohesive parliamentary Labour party for a generation' might, in the heading of a contemporary Cowley article, 'huff and puff'.[80]

Notes

1 Pippa Norris, 'New Politicians? Changes in Party Competition at Westminster', in Geoffrey Evans and Pippa Norris (eds), *Critical Elections: British Parties and Voters in Long-term Perspective.* Sage, London, 1999, pp. 22–43.

2 Philip Cowley and Philip Norton with Mark Stuart and Matthew Bailey, *Blair's Bastards: Discontent within the Parliamentary Labour Party*, Centre for Legislative Studies, Hull University, 1996.

3 Alastair Campbell and Bill Hagerty (eds), *Alastair Campbell Diaries*, Vol. 1, *Prelude to Power*, Hutchinson, London, 2010, entry June 30, p. 484.

4 Ibid., 1 July 1996, p. 485.

5 Ibid.

6 Ibid., 10 July, p. 493.

7 Cowley and Norton et al, *Blair's Bastards*, p. 32.

8 Hansard, 26 June 1997, col. 990.

9 Peter Mandelson and Roger Liddle, *The Blair Revolution: Can New Labour Deliver?* Faber & Faber, London, 1996, p. 231.

10 Derek Draper, *Blair's 100 Days*, Faber & Faber, London, 1997, p. 9.

11 Ibid. pp. 187–9, also pp. 203–4.

12 Jonathan Powell, *The New Machiavelli: How to Wield Power in the Modern World*, Bodley Head, London, 2010, p. 142.

13 Philip Cowley, *Revolts and Rebellions: Parliamentary Voting under Blair*, Politico's, London, 2002, p. 231.

14 Phillip Cowley and Mark Stuart, 'In Place of Strife? The PLP in Government, 1997–2001', *Political Studies* 51, 2003, p. 317.

15 Meg Russell, *Building New Labour: the Politics of Party Organisation*, Palgrave Macmillan, Basingstoke, 2005, p. 279.

16 PLP Code of Conduct, Item 3.

17 Cowley, *Revolts and Rebellions*, which covers the period from 1997 to 2001, has no coverage of the crucial internal party managerial operations and conflicts of that period.

18 *Tribune*, 20 June 1997.

19 Ibid.

20 PLP Standing Orders, Item F12.

21 Ibid., Item F12 (iv).

22 PLP Code of Conduct, Item 4(a), (b) and (d).

23 Ibid., Item 3.

24 Nick Brown, *Fabian Review*, August/September 1996, p. 2.

25 Philip Norton, 'Parliament', in Anthony Seldon and Kevin Hickson (eds), *New Labour Old Labour: the Wilson and Callaghan Governments*, Routledge, London 2004, p. 204.

26 PLP Code of Conduct, Item 4(d).

27 Ibid., Item 4(b).

28 Sarah Childs, *New Labour's Women MPs: Women Representing Women*, Routledge, London, 2004, pp. 144–65 with Philip Cowley and pp. 180–94. Many of the new MPs were keen to criticise MPs' aggressive and confrontational style (p. 181).

29 Cowley, *Revolts and Rebellions*, p. 106.

30 PLP minutes 24 February 1999.

31 Derived from minutes of PLP, 20 November 1997.

32 Derived from minutes of the three PLP meetings and interviews with party officials and the MP Harold Best.

33 Cowley, *Revolts and Rebellions*, p. 27.

34 Ibid. p. 150.

35 Tom Bower, *Gordon Brown: Prime Minister*, Harper Perennial, London, 2004, pp. 261–2; Andrew Rawnsley, *Servants of the People: The Inside Story of 'New Labour'*, Hamish Hamilton, London, 2000, p. 115.
36 Cowley, *Revolts and Rebellions*, p. 117 and (with Sarah Childs), pp. 127–47.
37 Byron Criddle, 'MPs and Candidates', in David Butler and Dennis Kavanagh, *The British General Election of 1997*, Palgrave Macmillan, London, 1997, p. 165.
38 Cowley, *Revolts and Rebellions*, p. 115.
39 William Keegan, *The Prudence of Mr Gordon Brown*, John Wiley, Chichester, 2003, p. 290.
40 Ibid. p. 262.
41 Blunkett Tapes, April 1998, p. 76.
42 Frank Barlow Memo: 'The Subject Groups and Organisation of the PLP in Office', 8 June 1979.
43 Tim Bale, 'Managing the Party and the Trade Unions', in Brian Brivati and Tim Bale (eds), *New Labour in Power; Precedents and Prospects*, Routledge, London, 1997.
44 Philip Norton, 'Organisation of Parliamentary Parties', in S.A. Walkland (ed.), *The House of Commons in the Twentieth Century*, Clarendon Press, Oxford, 1979, p. 45.
45 PLP Code of Conduct, Item 1(d).
46 *Financial Times*, 25 July 1996.
47 *Observer*, 11 August 1996.
48 PLP Code of Conduct, Item 1(d).
49 Blunkett Tapes, week beginning 24 November, p. 55.
50 Clive Soley, 'The PLP: a New Structure for a Second Term', 18 June 2001, Para 2.2.2.
51 Report of Work of Parliamentary Labour Party Departmental Committees, June 2000.
52 Soley, 'The PLP: a New Structure', Para 2.1.
53 Statement by the PLP Chair and Chief Whip, 5 June 1997.
54 *Partnership in Power*, p. 13.
55 Ron Johnston, Philip Cowley, Charles Pattie and Mark Stuart, 'Voting in the House or Wooing the Voters at Home: Labour MPs and the 2001 General Election Campaign', *Journal of Legislative Studies* 8(2), Summer 2002, pp. 9–22.
56 Letter from Clive Soley to Margaret McDonagh, 19 November 1998.
57 In the NEC meeting agreeing the Partnership in Power arrangements, 30 July 1997, Prescott said that he would be 'campaign manager for Dennis'. Support for Skinner was also thought to be Blair's own position after Sally Morgan's favourable comments in the final PIP Convenors' Group meeting.
58 Minutes of Parliamentary Committee, 3 June 1998.
59 Interviews with party officers.
60 *Financial Times*, 6 May 1998.
61 *Independent* editorial, 25 May 1998.
62 *Guardian*, 19 May 1998.
63 Minutes of NEC Organisation Committee, 18 May 1998, and also what is understood to be his contribution to the PLP meeting, 4 June 1998.
64 Ibid.

65 *Guardian*, 9 July 1999.
66 Cowley, *Revolts and Rebellions*, p. 113.
67 Ibid. p. 112.
68 *Observer*, 7 June 1998.
69 Cowley, *Revolts and Rebellions*, p. 179.
70 *The Observer*, 23 January 2000.
71 Ray Winstone, *Red Pepper*, 5 April 2000.
72 *Guardian*, 20 April 1999.
73 Jackie Ashley, *New Statesman*, 20 January 2000.
74 Peter Kellner, *Evening Standard*, 3 July 2000.
75 *Shifting the Balance: Select Committees and the Executive*, document of the Liaison Committee of the House of Commons, March 2000.
76 Phillip Norton, 'Parliament', *The Blair Effect: The Blair Government 1997–2001*, Little, Brown, London 2001, pp. 54–5.
77 *Guardian*, 28 June 2000.
78 BBC News Online, 4 December 2000, Soley interviewed by Nyta Mann.
79 *Independent*, 18 December 2000.
80 Ibid.

14

Employment relations, representation and party management

Whitehall, Westminster and the politics of implementation

Here, still following the politics of party management, as in Chapter 13 the focus is on Westminster and Whitehall and centres on the Labour Party's commitment in the 1997 general election to a statutory right to trade union recognition. Arising out of this and other manifesto commitments came, in 1999, the Employment Relations Act, which embraced the agenda of labour law and work-life changes noted in Chapter 9. The intention here is not to examine the various legal and legislative complexities of the Act, nor is it to attempt a comprehensive detailed examination of the process as a study of policy-making. It is to provide from that process a case study of the influence of the party, and particularly party management-connected activities, upon the implementation of a vital area of government policy and business relations under Blair.

The priority of implementation

For the unions this was an issue of the highest priority following a long period of decline in membership and recognition since 1979. For Blair it was the opportunity for a landmark change in the character of industrial relations. His view was that relationships at work needed to move away from their old class-conscious adversarial forms and move towards a partnership. Legislation that guaranteed minimum standards of fair treatment in employment relations would help change the culture by introducing decency and fairness in a way which did not add much to the bargaining power of organised labour. It would 'leave intact the main changes of the 1980s in industrial relations and enterprise' and would not damage the ability of an employer to run an effective business. That would create a new industrial-relations settlement which would be reasonable and workable[1] and draw a line under the issue of industrial-relations law.[2]

There were always other political considerations, electoral and managerial, to what was being sought and what was not, in the process of policy-making. In his own election statement for the post of Leader, Blair had declared that strong, democratic and accountable trade unions are at the heart of a healthy democracy and a productive economy.[3] But he and most of those close to him were very uneasy at the thought that they might reawaken an industrially 'over-powerful' trade unionism. This might threaten industrial stability and was bound to cause political problems in influencing the future electoral role of the CBI and in stimulating the antagonism of the Conservative-supporting press.

The reaction of the News Corporation of Rupert Murdoch was a particular concern because of their hostility to the return of trade unionism in their operation at Wapping. The last thing Blair wanted was legislation covering his territory that would dramatically damage the attempts to persuade Murdoch that Labour was 'literally a new party'. A consistently strong private view in No. 10 was that 'we can't upset Murdoch before a General Election'. Because, in the nature of things, elections were never far away, his acceptance of any settlement especially in his area of vested interest was always an important consideration.

There was another dimension to Blair's concern about a settlement. He was particularly averse to the unions using the party as a means of pulling the pendulum of industrial power further and further in favour of organised labour. What they saw as an expression of the historic character and purpose of the party, he saw as a characteristic that he needed to manage and radically change in a way which would attempt to make business feel like stakeholders within the party.

For this it was necessary to be seen to act in a way that business regarded as reasonable in implementing the manifesto commitments and thereafter to avoid future party commitments on labour law unless agreed with the employers. The TUC saw some merit in this seeking of consensus, particularly if it acted as a precursor to a new social partnership which involved the TUC, the CBI and the government, but the view in Congress House was that such a settlement could only be stable if it was based on rectification of the major union grievances. Neither the TUC nor the affiliated unions were happy with Blair's claim that 'The changes that we do propose would leave British law the most restrictive on trade unions in the Western world'.[4]

Issue management and party management

Moving forward

In 1997 the union leaders, depressed by the consistent accommodating attitude to business, saw Blair's sensitivity to employers as likely to dominate his perspective on everything to do with the unions and their claims, including the policies that had been placed before the electorate. They would not have been surprised to find that there were other conditions placed upon them before government action. There were some grounds for this. David Blunkett's fraternal speech to the 1997 GMB conference included an enthusiastic welcome for a white paper on employment rights which he thought had already been announced. This was met by an angry private objection from Blair that it would only be on the basis of the unions agreeing to change their internal structures (a complex process which could last years) even though the manifesto had laid down no such preconditions.

Yet, this was also accompanied by another signal embodied in the political views of the three senior people he chose initially to implement and advise on the new legislation. Each had a deep belief in the legitimacy of union affiliation, and had a historic contact with union grievances. Whilst moving with Blair towards the fusion of fairness and flexibility that was to characterise the 'New Labour' competitive economy, they were to the left of Blair in their developing views of what would constitute a fairer balance in the world of work, perhaps to a degree which was not so apparent to Blair at the time of their appointment.

Margaret Beckett moved from the Shadow position to become Secretary of State for Trade and Industry, and was given overall responsibility for the new employment legislation. As spokesperson on Health when Labour was in Opposition she had been very effective and earned praise from both Blair and business. She was also the most experienced Minister, having served in the previous Labour Government. Ian McCartney was made Minister for Employment Relations within the Department of Trade and Industry. He had been an active trade unionist since leaving school at 15, and had some natural sticking points. But he too had earned praise from Blair for his discreet and skilful work with both the TUC and the CBI on the minimum wage. Jon Cruddas, now Deputy Political Secretary in the No. 10 Political Office, had been an adviser to Blair on employment issues when Blair had that portfolio. His past and present role in liaison with the unions, as already noted, made him at times the most important coalface figure in party management, especially in the skills of fusing control with accommodation. All these had long-established union sympathies, although now working within the Blair agenda. It meant that although enthusiastic supporters of union affiliation were a small minority within 10 Downing Street they developed a skilful linkage of party management with union liaison which had a useful double edge to it.

In an extraordinary new pattern of politics around the Prime Minister, laying primary emphasis on the importance of building relations with business, the Downing Street Policy Unit made initial attempts to persuade Blair to leave this whole policy agenda to one side for the moment. But reminders from the DTI Ministers and Cruddas about the damaging reaction of the unions and the party, forced into the Queen's Speech on 14 May a commitment to 'fairness at work'. Limited as it was, this reference, together with the promise of a minimum wage and the return of union rights to workers at GCHQ, was significantly better than the pessimistic union leaders had anticipated. Nevertheless, with argument still raging in No. 10, not until 4 September, following discussions with Beckett, McCartney and Cruddas, did Blair tell them at the TUC that the government would be bringing forward a White Paper in the new year to include union recognition.

Blair management and advice

In the first phase of discussions on the main details of this legislation the TUC preferred a negotiation between themselves and the CBI which would be chaired by a Labour Minister. The CBI rejected that and Blair then made it clear to the TUC that he wanted the social partners to reach maximum agreement between themselves, in order to 'narrow the gap'. It was Blair's general perspective that the real interests of labour and business were not fundamentally opposed and that partnership was best attained by as much voluntary action as possible and with as high a degree of consensus as possible. The discussions could be kicked off with the unifying issue of abolition of the 'check off' system – a Conservative Government measure which required three-yearly reauthorisation of employers' deductions from the pay of trade unionists for trade union subscriptions. This legislation was regarded as a burden by both employers and unions.

Blair also did not want to be put in the position of immediately choosing between the TUC and the CBI and he did not want any limitations on his own freedom of action. There was no Cabinet committee on this legislation and the Cabinet was kept out of detailed discussions as far as possible. When the issue was raised there, on 11 May, Blair told them that the CBI and the TUC were talking and he wanted them to talk more. At no stage in the long process that followed was there any encouragement for the Cabinet to develop a collective position. On the grounds that he did not want anything to go on in the Cabinet which could be reported externally as 'a split', bilateral meetings were held with key Cabinet members before the formal Cabinet meetings to manage the discussions.

This all conforms to the model of the quasi-presidency and Blair's supremacy over his party. But, as will be shown here, it is misleading to imagine as was often the case that policy-making in this highly controversial area involved a hierarchy of relations in which the powers behind the Prime Minister were unusually harmonious and acted as a unified chain of command with clear terms of reference steering a homogenous government. Stephen Byers whilst Shadow Minister for Training and Employment had been given the task of preparing the main outlines of the new labour laws. But at that stage there was some political reluctance around the Leader to produce anything which might draw too much public attention to the issue. Also, unlike under the previous Labour Government, there had been no TUC-Labour Party Liaison Committee influencing the detailed preparation of the legislation in Opposition. The result was that there was nothing resembling a blueprint, and the basic commitments of the manifesto left much room for ministerial creativity and manoeuvre, especially as Blair was not the kind of manager who gave clear terms of reference to his staff.

Those officials who dealt with the conflicting perspectives of unions and business were expected to develop their own responsive relationship with each in order to stroke and nourish the constituency which would have to accept the settlement. That had to be, as a pivotal No. 10 manager put it, 'one which the CBI would not kick up about and the TUC would be unhappy but would grudgingly accept'. The fact that this might involve a degree of double agency in behaviour was generally accepted as the only way to operate. The reassurance for business was especially important because business was the historic outsider to the Labour Party and a Labour government and it was judged essential for them to feel part of both. Attitudes towards the trade unions were both more restraining and more complex. They were to be treated publicly as having no 'privileged' advantage in relation to the party and no special role in relation to government although in practice, because they remained integral elements of party organisation and party campaigning, there was always a party management concern about their major reactions to what was going on in government.

The double face of party management

As noted in Chapter 5, the two key officials were Jon Cruddas, responsible for liaison with the unions, and Geoff Norris with the same responsibility for liaison with the employers. In the roughly categorised politics of Downing Street both were regarded as 'party' people with, as it happened, a high degree of respect for each other. But they had different views on the party, the unions and business and were in more or less permanent conflict over the content of the proposed legislation. Some of this was an inevitable product of dealing with their different clients, but it was also a product of a difference of conviction and role.

A central feature of Cruddas's role, as we have seen, involved not just day-to-day relations with the unions but particularly the fixing of the party conference and the National Policy Forum where McCartney was also a significant managerial figure. This dual role of Cruddas was important as was the fact that behind the role was a man with deep convictions about changing the condition of labour. He operated, however, with the understanding that Blair's gut instincts on issues connected with the unions were significantly to the right of his own and close to the CBI's position on future labour law. The push from the party on employment issues became part of his armoury of argument.

Cruddas had the wording of the manifesto to draw upon and also a composite resolution No. 12, moved by the GPMU and agreed at the 1997 party conference in October. This was in line with the TUC position in its 1997 policy statement *Your Voice at Work* and had been engineered by Cruddas in cooperation with the unions. In the internal No. 10 politics this was Advantage Cruddas. Norris in contrast saw himself as responding to what Tony really wanted. On this he worked closely with Jeremy Hayward who became Blair's influential Principal Private Secretary. Norris's private description of the business manifesto of 1997 as 'the longest reassurance note in history'[5] tells only part of the role that he played. In practice, it allowed the pro-business network within No. 10 to work to a separate agenda and nuances close to Blair's instincts and positioning, but constructed by Norris himself, as were the subsequent business manifestos.[6] Advantage Norris.

Other important voices in Downing Street and the Cabinet Office weighed in, supporting a hard line that the Government must not 'cave in' to the unions and must keep business on board. Peter Mandelson, Minister without Portfolio in the Cabinet Office, had a background role all the way through the production of the White Paper. Campbell was the major guardian of the media strategy, which was heavily attuned to removing the association with the bad old image of trade union power and pragmatically very sensitive to the industrial position and media response particularly of Murdoch and News International. Phil Basset, in charge of Strategic Communications Unit, had as a labour correspondent favoured a separation of the party from the unions. Media inputs into the policy conflicts were often touched by the hands of these communications operators and strategists. A similar but more spasmodic input came later from and via the laments of union voices in the party, the TUC and the PLP trade union group, some planted by more union-friendly party managers.

Over the proposed legislation there were many points of agreement on objectives. Recognition would be part of a substantial agenda of partnership, fairness at work and work-life reforms. As McCartney put it, 'We take a wider and more balanced view of labour market flexibility than our predecessors. We favour flexibility based on minimum standards and security of employment.'[7] But in practice, what was the minimum, what degree of security and what conditions of flexibility? There was room for continuous substantive argument around this in the white paper and then over the legislation. Beckett and McCartney as ministers continued to keep channels of communication open to the CBI. Norris kept similar contact with the TUC. But in great measure this became at key points a battle between primarily 'union-sympathetic' and 'business-sympathetic' forces, as both sought to gain advantage for their primary constituents. It has been noted by Roger Undy that 'restructuring of the old Department of Employment dispersed and weakened the influence of civil servants with expertise in the field' and may have strengthened the role of No. 10'.[8] But the steering of the DTI by Downing Street was complicated here by the fact that alliances and shared perspectives at times passed though institutions rather than reflecting the influence of one administrative group or institution over another.

McCartney, who was throughout a major source of policy initiatives, sought to expand the implications of partnership and to get a wide range of commitments of different kinds in the document. This included, with enthusiastic support from Beckett, the filling out of the 'family-friendly' working practices which was a commitment in the manifesto. This development had been associated in the Labour Party with Anna Coote, Patricia Hewitt and Harriet Harman, now Secretary of State for Social Security. It had also been pushed at national level by women's officers in some of the unions, notably the TGWU, MSF, USDAW and UNISON, and in the TUC office. But it was not generally a priority concern of male union leaders and had also to take account of the manifesto proviso that 'There must be a sound balance between support for family life and the protection of business from undue burdens'.

Together these broad agendas produced a wide range of controversial and technically complex issues in the formulation of government positions. McCartney, working closely with Cruddas, had the expertise, infighting skills and at times aggressive push to drive forward. Beckett forcefully fronted their agreed position and eventually drafted authoritatively and defended the note which embodied the basis of the White Paper.

Blair and policy implementation

Blair and the policy-making style

Blair did not have too many fixed positions, and his decision-making style on delicate issues involved caution and a strong element of judicious pre-varication and procrastination at odds with the image he cultivated. Policy-making at times became a crab-like process of questioning and listening to representations and the conflicting advice from his own staff, making a slow circling of the evidence, acting on occasions as devil's advocate, assessing costs and benefits. The circumlocutory line of march was tentative and adjustive with frequent lurches to one side or the other, then swift movements back as he faced many occasions of advice from strongly conflicting perspectives. Being a man responsible for a hundred other concerns, he had time to move into dialogue on the issue only spasmodically and was necessarily reliant on others to carry the detailed work forward and to keep him well informed.

One result of all this was that in this policy-making area there was often a high degree of uncertainty about where he stood. At any one stage Blair's position was just a snapshot and could be misleading to those outside Downing Street participating in the dialogue. It was at times a source of deep puzzlement as well as irritation to the TUC which preferred the more formal and clear process it was used to, with papers and arguments for and against. It was a new feature of Labour government and movement politics that they did not know quite how to engage with. It appeared to sway back and forth in a way that seemed to obscure the sources of influence. The bemused state at the TUC combined with the distrust of Blair's methods of party management and their reaction against the usual media messages by spin nods and winks indicating where the Prime Minister was leaning.

TUC and CBI: disagreement and procedural values

Preliminary discussions between TUC and CBI did come to some agreements including the abolition of 'check-off'. They accepted also that new arrangements were needed for recognition, that recognition should be on the basis of voluntary agreement wherever possible and that new statutory procedures would require an effective infrastructure and a new independent representation agency to administer the recognition procedure. But on 8 December 1997 the talks were concluded with a joint statement that laid out the areas of disagreement as well as agreement. Thereafter, the process was handed to the DTI Ministers to manage, but with both camps in No. 10 keeping a watchful eye over developments.

Three key disagreements were to dominate the politics of the period leading up to the white paper, *Fairness at Work*, published in May 1998. The CBI believed that to assess the level of support for collective bargaining there should in all cases be a requirement for a ballot, with a threshold involving a majority of all relevant employees before recognition was granted. In this provision, abstentions would count against. The TUC in contrast favoured the normal democratic practice of a majority of those voting. They also favoured automatic recognition where a union had majority membership in a bargaining unit. The CBI was opposed to automatic recognition. The CBI also wanted small firms with fewer than 50 members to be exempt from the legislation. The TUC rejected any exemptions because it would disadvantage and be an injustice to millions of workers.

At a meeting in December 1997, Blair was pressed by union leaders to deny that he had already done a deal with the CBI over the threshold for recognition. He made no clear response but said that 'in the first instance' it was a matter for the DTI team. Cridland, interviewed later by Edmonds, insisted that in Opposition they had not gone too deeply into the detail but ensured that 'the mood music' was right.[9] Beckett thought that Blair was determined to have a threshold, and by the new year there was a strong rumour that Geoff Norris had told the Engineering Employers Federation that Blair favoured the CBI position. Cruddas and McCartney operated on the assumption that a general understanding had been reached and they knew where Blair's instincts lay, but they attempted to give themselves room for manoeuvre as the discussion went on.

The CBI argument was that a threshold was justified in an industrial environment where a small minority could force an apathetic majority into joining unions. The unions and their supporters noted not only that that a threshold was loaded against the unions but that it ran against normal democratic procedure. As John Monks put it, 'If it is good enough for electing MPs then it is good enough for union recognition'.[10] At one stage the support of the Secretary of State for Scotland Donald Dewar was gained in arguing against the threshold on the grounds that it had potential implications for devolution. Blair was unmoved. In this pragmatism, he was consistent with the general inconsistency of 'New Labour' procedural values.

Trade union group management and the Parliamentary Labour Party

Into this and other conflicts came a new organisational input involving another aspect of union-party relations, the reorganisation of union representation in the House of Commons. In tracing its significance we have first to note that the TUC had been attempting since 1994 to broaden union influence across the parties, even possibly setting up an all-party group on trade union affairs – a development seen by John Healey in 1997 as about five years off.[11] Moving on a different track, in 1996 John Mann the TULO liaison officer, Bill Morris the chair of TULO and officials of the existing PLP trade union group sought to strengthen their joint operation and link it more closely with the union role in the Labour Party, but this for the moment made little impact.

Now, in the light of fears aroused by the shifts in Labour policy just before the general election, the search for more union influence on government quietly intensified. Union leaders including Edmonds and Monks became determined to explore the possibilities of an energetic trade union group which would provide a pressure group 'in Blair's back yard' in order to take effective action in relation to a Labour Government. But whose baby would it be? Would it to be an extension of the TUC's new non-party strategy and the beginnings of a new parliamentary pluralism – with the group potentially open to all parties? Or would it be a recreation of the Labour-committed group of affiliated trade unionists focusing on the intra-party battle in relation to the government? One piece of evidence which pointed in the direction of the latter was a survey of MPs which found only 9 per cent in favour of the unions ceasing to be formally affiliated to the Labour Party. Of those opposed, six out of ten 'strongly' opposed ceasing affiliation.[12]

In the event, the initiative was seized by the GPMU under the leadership of General Secretary Tony Dubbins. This was the union which (as SOGAT) had in 1993 initiated the birth of TULO as a party liaison organisation. In 1996, the union appointed a new Political Officer, John O'Regan, an experienced official with a broad non-factional Labour Party-oriented approach to strategy. The PLP trade union group secretary also changed in 1996, bringing in Gerry Sutcliffe, a GPMU-sponsored MP who was an innovating and very subtle political operator, over the years acting as both poacher and gamekeeper. He became chair of the group in January 1998, and Ian Davidson became its secretary. It had a permanent working secretary, Sarah Merrill, also of the GPMU. Though keeping close relations with the TUC it was made clear that this was a Labour Party group.

In November 1997, the anxious mood amongst union leaders and in the PLP about Blair intentions facilitated a second major change in the organisation of the unions. There had been no executive committee of the trade union group, simply the officers. Now a new form of representative structure was created. It involved regular meetings of an executive (sometimes called 'coordinating') committee with representatives from each individual group of trade union MPs to bind in all the unions – the TGWU, GMB, UNISON, AEEU, USDAW, MSF, CWU, GPMU, RMT, NUM, and more loosely ISTC, which unusually had a cross-party group. This was an entirely new form of PLP-union organisation.

This group was also significantly different in composition from the old. Taking advantage of the obligation upon MPs that all should be members of a union, its member meetings were now made open to all trade unionists. There was a conscious attempt to turn it away from its past dominance by manual-worker males. For the first time in its history there was a good attendance of women at the group meetings. Though the left was well represented, the group leaders made determined effort to position it as speaking for the mainstream of the party. The group must not be defined as endemically oppositionist and it must be non-factional.

Alerted to the possibilities of this new organisation, some in Downing Street were unhappy at a strengthening of the trade union position but such was the unity of the unions that a destabilising counter-attack against it was not viable. In practice Downing Street officials with close affinity to business were faced not only with a fait accompli but with an independent organisation working discreetly with sympathetic pro-labour managers, Cruddas and McCartney. Whilst avoiding a Downing Street takeover, the union group leadership attempted to keep good relations with Blair in spite of the policy criticisms. Good relations were kept also with the whips' office where it had some strong supporters.

The first open meeting of the new group was on *Fairness at Work* and addressed by John Monks on 25 November 1997. It was attended by only around twenty people including the officers and it was very low-key. But in the next two months, after it appeared that Blair was going ahead with commitment to 51 per cent of the workforce and not simply a majority of participants, there was a huge change. A second members' meeting, organised via a meeting of the new coordinating committee of the group, got 140 with 100 apologies – it was said. This was probably inflated for PR purposes but it was unquestionably substantial.

The breadth of the attendance was also impressive. It came from all sections of the party including many old hands but also a significant presence of the 1997 intake who were normally categorised as Blairites. (And, it was said, not all of them were spies.) The continuing scale and composition of the meetings of the trade union group indicated that union recognition and the democratic issues involved in it had become something of an identity issue for many in the PLP. Later, members also reported that

MPs enjoyed coming to these meetings which drew upon a residual sympathy for workers with a legitimate claim to rights. These were issues on which even some new Blairite MPs felt 'justifiably Old Labour', as one of them put it. This was of major significance in a PLP where the manual workers and ex-union officials were a slowly decreasing component. Seeing the sudden flowering of the group the ex-Leader Neil Kinnock commented to John Monks, 'The trade union group has always been a sleeping giant'. That was true, but it needed organisation and a motivating and unifying issue to get it on the move – and was helped by having a friend or two in significant government positions.

Through Gerry Sutcliffe the chair of the group, who kept close contact with Cruddas, McCartney, and MP Frank Doran who was PPS to Ian McCartney, the group was able to get access to information on the background political conflicts over the legislation, giving them indications what issues to press about, what arguments might be useful. The size and atmosphere of group meetings was conveyed to ministers and upwards to the Prime Minister. One of Blair's two PPSs, Bruce Grocott, was sympathetic to the union position, attended all the group's meetings and reported back to Blair on the strength of feeling all across the PLP. Another Blair PPS, Ann Coffey, came away impressed with the meeting of March 1998 that was determined not to allow the CBI to dilute the party position. The presence of new loyalist MPs was also conveyed to Blair.

The organisation and form of these meetings had another significance in party terms. There was always a regret at Congress House that the TUC's rational re-launch strategy had fallen foul of the prejudices and tactics of the 'New Labour' Blair leadership. For their part, some in the Labour affiliates watched the TUC with an uneasy eye. Might it yet be taken towards the cross-party strategy? Yet the PLP group's activities now further encouraged the TUC to move back to seeing the Labour link as essential to the TUC's relations with a Labour Government. And what was also important was the extent to which the TUC now helped forge the unity and effectiveness of the group.

Monks in collaboration with the Group officials and assisted by Isobel Larkin, the Parliamentary Officer and Sarah Veale, the Senior Employment Rights Officer, played sophisticated roles in underpinning and assisting the work of the union group including its representation to the government. The group were kept fully informed by Cruddas and McCartney, who encouraged the unions to work together through the TUC. In the light of past divisive experience the exercise was remarkable. Even the ultra-loyalist and at times militantly independent AEEU did not break away. Nor did UNISON, whose officers had in these years a marked propensity to work towards a private accommodation with the political leadership. Skilfully briefed, the group became the united voice of the unions and in great measure the voice of the PLP itself on employment-relations issues. Managing the group became a crucial part of the politics of PLP management.

Democracy, party and management

As we have seen, behind the controlling management of Partnership in Power was the fear of a great divide between the new Labour Government representing 'the people' and a Labour Party taken over once more by the ghosts and monsters of the past. Yet here was an issue (and not the only one) where the people and the party were generally of the same disposition. A poll found 77 per cent of the public agreeing that if a majority of staff chose to be represented through a trade union, employers should be required by law to negotiate.[13] On a very specific point, a survey found that 51 per cent supported the TUC position of a simple majority of those who vote in a ballot, whilst 39 per cent supported the position advised by the CBI – a majority of those eligible; there were only 10 per cent 'don't knows'.[14]

In the PLP all the indications were that the overwhelming majority were sympathetic to the TUC position and to what it understood as the spirit of the party manifesto. A straw poll of new MPs showed more than 90 per cent support for the TUC position.[15] A later survey of MPs for the TUC also showed that more than 90 per cent of Labour MPs supported the TUC position rather than that of the CBI on four crucial issues within the proposed legislation. A remarkable new indicator was that new MPs were slightly more pro-TUC than old ones.[16] There was no indication of support for the Blair position of even-handedness towards the TUC and CBI in the various discussions taking place in the PLP and its committees. Warnings of this intra-party mood were conveyed to the Leader by Clive Soley, Chair of the PLP, by the Parliamentary Committee meetings and by the Chief Whip.

Up to 13 members of the Cabinet had privately indicated to Monks their sympathy for the TUC position in a series of dinners held in the spring and summer. To the *Sunday Times* 'Cabinet sources' had indicated that ministers were 'set to revolt on union rights' and 'at least seven Ministers were demanding a Cabinet debate'.[17] But no such debate took place and maybe none was demanded; Monks was always pessimistic about the tendency of politicians to posture. There was always a problem in Blair's control over the proceedings of the Cabinet over the big issues of labour law. According to Powell later, the practice was that Sally Morgan rang round Cabinet in advance to find out their views, sometimes passing on advance information on Tony's responses[18] but collective registration of the preferred direction of travel was avoided.

The movement in crisis

Between February and April 1998, the pessimistic mood in the unions and the PLP over union recognition was made worse by media reports of Blair's personal attitude to the union leaders. One particularly damaging article in *The Times* by the journalist John Lloyd painted a revealing portrait of the personal gulf between Blair and the unions in an article titled 'Blair has no time for the unions'. He described how Blair would much rather be talking to businessmen than 'this lot' (the TUC). 'Their ideas bore him. No general strategy, no big ideas; no technology. No TV channels; no newspapers. No private jets; no Tuscan villas'.[19]

Discreetly, for the first time since the whole issue of separation or divorce had been raised to public prominence in 1992, some of the most senior leaders began to think in terms of doomsday scenarios. Edmonds privately captured the predicament. 'We have a party policy. We must be able to defend the fundamental interests of our members. What's the use of the relationship if we can't do that?' They thought initially in terms of a new non-cooperative relationship with the management inside the party, but what exactly that would involve was not clear. It seemed to Morris that Blair's position was so committed to that of the CBI and so much of a 'sell-out' that it must only be a prelude to 'an attempt to force the unions out of the party'.[20] The situation was further exacerbated on 16 March by a No. 10 confirmation that the Labour Government would oppose the production of a new EU directive which would require employers to set up new consultation procedures with the workforce.[21]

Yet in spite of what was understood to have been the signals from the Leader via the Byers fish supper threat, noted in Chapter 9 (see p. 283), there was no evidence that Blair now wanted to accept, let alone promulgate a separation. This had little to do with union money. The poll evidence and discussions within the PLP indicated with even more clarity than in 1992 that a fundamental split with the unions would also produce a fundamental split in the party – from top to bottom. Though at grassroots level in the party the middle-class composition had grown, support for 'powerful trade unionism' at 74 per cent was exactly the same in 1999 as it had been in 1990.[22] Majority support for the party-union link continued to be supported by a majority of the membership active and inactive, including the new members.[23]

What had been a dangerous possibility had now become an approaching reality. The fracture would give the right-wing press a field day. Separation would also damage the party's organisational capacity just when it was becoming clear that the individual membership was in fast decline. And what effect would this all have on the trade unions after such a bitter separation? How would this help moderate elements in the TUC and a new employment-relations settlement? Monks's own position might come under threat given that the trade union left had reformed into a new organisation to 'Reclaim our Rights'. The stark fact was that there were far too many costs. As had been warned in the past, a bitter disputatious separation led nowhere useful.[24]

Monks and tactical accommodation

The paradox was that things became so bad on 19 March 1999, after a very hostile meeting between Blair and the union leaders, and on a day when the TGWU and the ultra-loyalist AEEU pressed the TUC for the first special Congress for twenty years, the shock of it led to some renewed attempt to 'cool it' and find some way through. There was a new spurt of diplomatic discussion between the TUC, union leaders, ministers and 10 Downing Street but nothing satisfactory emerged. Blair remained adamant that the CBI would not accept less than 40 per cent, which was probably true but was also not discouraged by his own responses. His view was also that it was as far as he could go in presenting this to the public. This was much more doubtful.

Monks, very conscious of the impasse over the 40 per cent, now seized the initiative after a very pessimistic appraisal. He considered that too much militant public agitation from the unions might make it even more difficult for Blair to compromise, indeed cause Blair to react against it. For him, dedicated to 'presenting trade unions as a constructive and reasonable force in society',[25] becoming an open warrior was a road to disaster for the unions. His view was that this was all leading to a fundamental confrontation which Blair could not afford to be seen as losing and therefore the unions would in the end find themselves backing down. Blair would then simply impose an across-the-board policy close to that of the CBI.

The TUC tactical concession and the response

On 21 April, led by Monks, the TUC General Council, whilst affirming that it believed that a simple majority should be sufficient, agreed that 'to move things on . . . there could be a case for specifying a minimum yes vote'.[26] Thus 30 per cent of those working in the bargaining unit would have more merit than 40 per cent, which would be unreasonable and unworkable. It accepted also that there could be a case for the exemption of very small firms with 'say ten employees or under'.[27] The decision was heavily attacked by the left and by some individual union leaders. At the Scottish TUC particularly, harsh things were said about making such a concession on an issue that had been the central focus of the CBI campaign. Blair now let the PLP trade union group officials and some of the Cabinet Ministers know that although he would be insisting on the 40 per cent, he would give the TUC as much as possible appreciating the strength of feeling. But again he did not want a Cabinet discussion on it before it had been agreed.

Blair was particularly fearful of the danger that the PLP might take a stronger position than that of the TUC. As he told one Parliamentary Committee meeting in early May, that would be a political disaster, pushing the CBI back to the Conservatives and losing CBI cooperation. It might also fundamentally damage the management of the PLP as the government moved towards the next election. In the dialogue within Downing Street the Prime Minister and his advisor Norris now became anxious to see what concessions could be made to the TUC. As a result, at one point it looked as though the TUC's fall-back position of 30 per cent had been accepted, but in the dialogue between Blair and Brown which some saw as Brown digging in, it hardened up again to 40 per cent. Under pressure from the Parliamentary Committee now came a promise of a review of the 40 per cent of the workforce 'after a reasonable period' if it proved to be unworkable. Later, when the oddity of just reviewing one element was recognised, this turned into acceptance of a more general review. Another concession made to the TUC at this time to help them digest the 40 per cent was agreement that if there was already a union membership of 50 per cent plus 1 in any bargaining unit there would be automatic recognition,[28] although later that became heavily qualified.

A concession was made by Blair in another area of major disagreement. Blair had accepted the CBI case for small-business exemption and the importance of small business in economic growth, but after the CBI had moved their position on what constituted small business down from 50 to 30 employees he lowered it further to 20. Still, in contrast, in other countries there was no parallel exclusion of workers in small firms from the coverage of workplace-protection laws.[29] It involved around six million workers. For them there was to be no guarantee of 'fairness at work'.[30] One consequence of the politics of this protracted focus on the 40 per cent and the exemptions for small business was that it produced more space and a favourable time for Cruddas and McCartney to press for other parts of the employment agenda and work-life issues with backing from the knowledgeable TUC staff who were all on top of all the details. Blair was persuaded to confirm agreement to a TUC proposal by which an employee had the legal right to be accompanied during grievance and disciplinary hearings by a fellow employee or a trade union representative whether the union was recognised or not.

Fairness at Work White Paper

There was some quiet satisfaction in the DTI that the draft white paper of Fairness at Work turned out better than they had at one stage feared. From the pro-business lobby in No. 10 on the other hand, Beckett was subject to a quiet but sustained counter-attack of last-minute phone calls about the changes 'that Tony wants'. At one point, deeply suspicious about this, Beckett insisted that she would only take 'what Tony wants' in person and otherwise would refuse to sign the document. This background conflict continued right up to the white paper going to the printers. According to the DTI ministers, some of its tensions can be discerned in the difference of emphasis between Blair's own introduction which stressed 'the most tightly regulated labour market of any leading economy in the world', and elements of the document itself. But in any case there was an awareness that the battle about what would be in the legislation was far from over.

The final version of the white paper was welcomed by John Monks as injecting 'much needed balance in the UK labour market'.[31] Bill Morris gave it 'Two cheers only',[32] but that was more than he had expected to be giving it. In the journal of the Labour left, *Tribune*, the package was seen as 'victory for union supporters in the government over hawks'.[33] It was said by the *Guardian* editorial to be a 'modest re-balancing of the axis of power between employer and employee' but still 'a surprising victory for the workers' given the advance publicity;[34] in that paper Larry Elliott saw it as 'a significant shift in the balance of power between capital and labour'.[35]

Contrasting strongly with Conservative legislation, there were procedures for union recognition and an automatic right to that recognition where there was majority union membership. There was also a series of new individual rights including a reduction of the qualifying period for protection against unfair dismissal from two years to one. A maximum limit for awards on unfair dismissal was to be abolished. A member had a right to be accompanied in grievance or disciplinary hearings. Although restrictions on strike action remained as they were under the Conservative legislation, workers sacked for engaging in lawful official industrial action would now have the right to complain of unfair dismissal to a tribunal. As expected, ending of the check-off would be brought into effect by an order under existing legislation. Improvements to the work-life balance included an extension of maternity leave to 18 weeks, an enhanced right to parental leave and a right to reasonable time off for family emergencies. The government also proposed to make the blacklisting of trade union members unlawful.

The TUC in its official response as expected called especially for improvements over the 40 per cent threshold for recognition ballots, the exclusion of small firms and the qualifying periods for employment-protection rights. Nevertheless Monks was anxious that a TUC conference on the White Paper held on 24 June should be positive, and he was helped in this by an impressive performance by McCartney urging the unions to realise what they stood to gain and to ditch their 'victim culture'. Following eighteen years when the unions had been severely legally constrained and disempowered, there was enough here to head off the more rebellious although a body of union opinion remained unhappy over the limitations.

Checks and balances

Responses

After a sensitive private intervention by Mandelson,[36] Campbell's media operation in No. 10 had been encouraged to give Monks room for his enthusiastic defence of what had been achieved. However, that enthusiasm, the message from McCarthy for the unions to end their victim status and the general welcome for the white paper on the union side made the pro-business media and then Blair worry that the unions had gained too much. In particular, a *Financial Times* editorial on 22 May 1998 that described the result as TUC 6 CBI 4, was seen on the pro-union managerial side as a steer and stir from pro-business managers in Downing Street. Assisting the momentum, it was followed by a provocative *Sunday Times* report that several Blairite Ministers believed that the pro-union ministers 'won too many concessions'.[37]

Mandelson comes to the fore

Their opportunity came after Margaret Beckett was replaced by Peter Mandelson in July 1998. He was well known for his business-sympathetic views, his lack of enthusiasm for the union role within the Labour Party and his view that the TUC had had too much power over the last Labour Government. Since 1997, as Minister without Portfolio, he had already been involved in this legislation and had crossed swords with Margaret Beckett. Immediately he replaced Beckett, employers were reported as facing him with a barrage of demands for 'sweeping changes' in the Fairness at Work reforms.[38] The CBI's Director General expressed their most serious concerns as the abandonment of the ceiling on unfair-dismissal compensation, giving employees the right to be accompanied by a union official in grievance procedure, and the proposal for a procedure for automatic union recognition.[39] According to his biographer Macintyre, Mandelson was determined to recover some of the ground which Blair thought had been conceded to the unions.[40]

He was very adroit about it. John Edmonds, who was not a natural fan, revealed in an interview with Steve Richards that 'Peter went out of his way to ask the TUC to see him immediately after he was appointed . . . to reassure us that the "Fairness at Work" white paper was government policy and that people who thought he would automatically side with the employers were wrong'.[41] Mandelson assured the TUC Congress, 'You will always get honesty from me. No more spin, honest'. And he took the unusual line of understanding and appreciating rather than criticising the unions. They were 'a force for good in society' and 'a voice of direct workplace experience in public policy-making'. They had made 'huge efforts to modernise'. In a remarkable diagnosis he asserted that the relationship of employer and employee was by its nature a fundamentally unequal one: one which could be exploited by 'unscrupulous employers'.[42] At the party conference Mandelson drew attention to the record of ruthlessness of the Tories in seeking to weaken the already weak at the workplace. It was a situation which, he promised, Fairness at Work 'I personally guarantee, will correct'.[43]

But shortly afterwards, with the conferences out of the way, Mandelson wrote that in order to safeguard jobs, fairness-at-work legislation had to be introduced in the 'most business-friendly way'.[44] Amongst the issues which were said in the media to be under business pressure for re-evaluation was the introduction of a new proviso that employees would have to be union members for a fixed period to be counted for automatic recognition. Within the government, the forces ranged behind the Mandelson business-friendly adjustment were now seen by the union side as overwhelming and led by another close friend of Blair, Charles Falconer, who became Minister of State in the Cabinet Office at the same time as Mandelson was made Secretary of State at the DTI. In the PLP and at the TUC the unions began gearing up for a long rearguard action through the rest of the legislative process.

Uncertainty and conflict

In an atmosphere of deep uncertainty, the unions made no formal moves to use party policy-making machinery to register the union view but as noted, on the NEC, trade union voices could be heard expressing alarm over reports of possible retreat from the White Paper. McCartney dismissed the reports and asserted that the spirit of *Fairness at Work* would be adhered to. Blair endorsed his comments. To McCartney and Cruddas the concerned voices were not unwelcome in the battle going on.

Mandelson talked frequently with the officers of the PLP trade union group and was invited to the PLP Group on 4 November. He told them that whilst he wanted to offer the CBI some comfort and reassurance in the details it would not be at the expense of hindering the effectiveness of the legislation. The main planks of the White Paper would all be in the bill. However, in reply to the discussion, he then made a very emotive and counterproductive point, 'I've no intention of doing a Barbara Castle'. This reference to the government retreat over the White Paper *In Place of Strife* back in 1969 in the face of opposition from the TUC and the PLP was interpreted as a bad sign and exacerbated the alarm.

On 17 November at a meeting of the TUC with the Prime Minister, Cruddas and Norris, the TUC side began by expressing great resentment that the political agenda was dominated by CBI concerns and that none of the TUC points were being considered. They complained also that the CBI was putting forward new points that they could not comment on and had to read about in the newspapers. In reply the Prime Minister made an unnerving central point that 'everything was still in play' and, getting down to the details, his reply to the TUC's request for reassurance on key points was regarded as not very satisfactory.

The meeting was followed by a series of what one pro-CBI participant referred to as 'spats' but what a pro-union participant called 'brutal confrontations', in Downing Street and at the DTI, over the details of the proposed changes. Mandelson developed a reputation in Whitehall for his impressive skills as a minister, but in these employment-law conflicts McCartney had the support of senior civil servants, a shrewd sense of the politics and complete command over the detail. Further, he and Cruddas had close links with the unions as party managers and were in a superior position to report on the likely reaction there. They had, by this stage, developed a comprehensive strategy which linked the role of the unions in party management with a view of modernisation and an important place for the gains made through *Fairness at Work*. Part of this strategy involved a new bi-monthly journal *Unions Today* launched at the 1998 TUC and aimed at winning support from trade union officials and activists.

Mandelson did seek to improve relations with Monks and with the officers of the PLP trade union group to head off a back-bench revolt. He also sought to counter McCartney's control in the office by seeing civil servants privately, although his success is contested. McCartney at a later stage in the process won some victories responding to claims of 'what Tony wants' by negotiating them directly after insisting that he saw the Prime Minster personally.[45] In a very fluid political situation it was not just the TUC which was uncertain about Tony's position. Mandelson was seen by some of his allies as becoming uncertain how far adrift he himself was of Blair. This series of arguments led at one point to a serious falling out between McCartney and Mandelson. McCartney felt powerful enough to make a threat of resignation. Weighing in the balance here was the senior party manager Sally Morgan's view that it was crucial that he be kept on board in reassuring the party in the country.[46]

Confrontation with Mandelson

Insecurity or faulty tactics may account for what happened next. John Monks was reinvited to readdress the PLP trade union group on 1 December, and Mandelson was also invited to be on the platform, although he gave indications that he would not be attending. To the surprise of the group Mandelson then made a sudden appearance at the meeting whilst John Monks was speaking. According to detailed private reports, he stood there in a manner interpreted as an attempt to intimidate. Eventually he agreed to speak. But his five-minute contribution was sarcastic in tone towards Monks and embarrassingly out of touch with the meeting. He was received in silence whereas Monks (who had been getting stick before Mandelson arrived for not being hard enough) got loud applause.

Whatever its purpose, Mandelson's behaviour here was seen as counter-productive, reminding the audience of one of the things that they disliked about him. His performance became part of the folklore of the trade union group. Some thought that it marked such a reverse for the Secretary of State as to have an immediate direct effect on the development of policy, but this is doubtful. What does seem clear from officials in Downing Street – both pro and con the union position – is that it became, as one acute Mandelson ally described it, 'emblematic' of the PLP capacity to cause difficulties for the government. It is probable that the continuing PLP pressure and the concern for future management added to the creation of an atmosphere where the retreat from the White Paper was less than the CBI wanted.

Union pressures and Party management

Before and after the Mandelson event, Blair was becoming increasingly concerned at the divisions on the issue and the possible further deterioration in party unity – perhaps with alienated trade unions linking themselves to grassroots party activists and the party left. He was concerned also that this had now all been dragging on for over a year. There were unhelpful press descriptions of the operation of the unions involving (it was said) holding Tony Blair to ransom over Labour's finances. In an article by journalists Graeme Wilson and Tom Baldwin, a statement from Bill Morris that it would be difficult to motivate members to back Labour in elections was headlined by the *Sunday Telegraph* as 'we'll stop your election funding'.[47] There was certainly an unwillingness in TULO meetings to discuss extra finance and future affiliation levels till the legislation was finalised. This could be read both ways. It was interpretable as a warning signal of suspended judgement about whether future requests for finance would be met favourably, or it was a respect for propriety.

Far more significant than finance were the party management implications. The AEEU was not prepared to be helpful in backing the management tactics in contesting Rhodri Morgan as the Leader of the party in Wales whilst the threat to the White Paper 'consensus' remained. Eventually the union lined up behind the Prime Minister in defence of Alun Michael but for a time there was reluctance to help in resurrecting this 'stabilisation' role that he wanted. The message which was coming to the party managers from loyalists was simply 'Get it sorted'.

Mandelson's perspective and the changes in policy

Near the culmination of the consultations, at a meeting of the Secretary of State with the TUC on 2 December, Mandelson argued for the TUC to have some perspective. In 470 responses to the White Paper, the employers wanted none of it; nevertheless the government was proceeding as intended. The White Paper contained 29 proposals or issues for consultation. There was only one where the government did not intend to proceed – zero hours contracts. It was his and McCartney's view that these were best dealt with in other legislation concerning the minimum wage and the working time directive. Mandelson had rejected the dropping altogether of automatic recognition and that employees would have to be union members for one year to be counted towards the 50 plus 1 per cent. Also some changes had been made which were welcomed by the unions and were not in the White Paper. ACAS terms of reference were to be amended to give it a more proactive role in improving industrial relations. He promised that there would be action on the employment-agencies regulation. As a result, he said that the CBI was 'not happy'.

Nevertheless, the outcome published on 17 December did show further movement towards meeting employers' concerns. Accompanying attendance at grievance and disciplinary hearings had been made subject to a code of practice and restricted in what was covered. Automatic recognition now had 'an element of Central Arbitration Committee discretion' concerning three qualifying conditions which could lead to a ballot being ordered 'in the interest of good industrial relations'. The White Paper proposal of abolishing a cap on compensation for unfair dismissal was dropped, although it would now be at a higher level than at present and index-linked. In the white paper, no time limit had been specified for the protection against dismissing employees taking part in lawfully organised industrial action. The CBI had pushed for it to apply only for the first four weeks. The government then said six but then moved to eight in response to TUC representation backed by McCartney. That was to be a running sore for years until a further change to 12 weeks was introduced in 2004. On employment agencies there were no proposals.

Union and party pressures, including the activities of the sympathetic party managers, had probably fought off or diminished potentially greater reverses. Judged by one leading authority, the outcome after amendments still constituted 'a major step forward for trade union and employee rights in UK workplaces'.[48] The message from the TUC and from Cruddas and McCartney was that something very significant had been won. A labour-sympathetic journalist Kevin Maguire reinforced that message in imploring the unions to see what they had gained. 'The unions should be grateful and now move on'.[49]

Rupert Murdoch and News International Corporation

There was, however, one issue where the trade union-Labour Party influence had met special resistance and left a particularly aggravating political legacy. Since the first discussions of recognition in opposition, Rupert Murdoch had been heavily involved in these processes both directly and as a member of the CBI recognition committee. News International Corporation's own employees were in a company-approved staff association not recognised as a trade union. Murdoch wanted their position protected and with no return to strong competing multi-unionism at Wapping. Managers recognised that Blair had reached some understanding with him. The main point about the so-called Murdoch clause para. 35 was that a general immunity from the recognition procedure was granted for employers who recognised a trade union, whether independent or not. Such protection for employers' staff associations had not been there either in the Conservative Industrial Relations Act of 1971 nor the Labour Government's Employment Protection Act of 1975.

A new opportunity to raise the issue of recognition in these companies came when there was publicity surrounding a *Private Eye/Independent* story that News International Corporation's political activities were being advised by lobbying firm LLM Communications, who had well-publicised access to the government. The lobbyists challenged the story, but in the minor furore this aroused it was possible to secure a new provision for employees to trigger a ballot to seek de-recognition of management-sponsored staff associations. This went into the bill in January 1999 after Mandelson's resignation and just before it went through the Commons.

But the legislation still involved substantial and complex hurdles for the unions. Unions had to seek de-recognition of an existing staff association then recognition of a bona fide union. Where an association was already recognised, whether it was independent or not, 10 per cent of the workforce had to request a ballot through the Central Arbitration Committee. The unions had no access to the workforce in the ballot – that was a matter between the employees and the company. For de-recognition, in the ballot there had to be a majority of at least 40 per cent of the whole workforce. If that was achieved an independent union seeking recognition had to commence a new process again seeking 10 per cent then a majority of the 40 per cent of the workforce. McCartney later saw the legislation as crafted to avoid inter-union disputes over recognition and with hurdles which were necessary for the unions to show that they could sustain their membership. But the new provision left much room for Murdoch's skilled lawyers. The TUC regarded the procedures as 'impossibly complex'.[50] Tony Dubbins the print workers union leader complained that what he called 'Rupert Murdoch's protection racket' made it extremely difficult for independent unions to gain a foothold'.[51]

The legislative process and the party connection

Mandelson to Byers

On 22 December Mandelson was forced to resign over an undeclared loan from another minister, Geoffrey Robinson. He was succeeded by Stephen Byers, a man generally seen as from the same political stable. However, Byers had begun to reassess his attitude to the unions, accepting the case that they brought more to the party than they took away. He was also influenced by a growing concern over the lobbying activities of business and had come to see the unions' role within the party as a necessary counterweight to business influence over government. In the summer he had already appointed Gerry Sutcliffe as his PPS and now attempted to build a good relationship with Ian McCartney, an old adversary but somebody whose handling of the portfolio he was now broadly happy with. They had weekly meetings but knowledgeable though Byers was, a political genius would have found it difficult to keep up to speed with developments in this immensely complex area. The main political, intellectual and tactical arm-wrestling passed elsewhere as the political battle mounted yet again.

Labour interests and business interests

In March, Blair was still meeting business criticism of increased regulation, and at the same time he was being alerted to a new concern that in the battle between managers the pro-union side was too skilful. Cruddas aroused more suspicion as a committed union supporter, and there was an accusation that McCartney and DTI civil servants were going further than their brief. There were intimations in the media that the new Employment Bill was to be watered down.[52] Lord Falconer, working closely with Norris, was given an enlarged remit of talking to the CBI, listening to their concerns, trying to massage their support for the legislation and keeping Blair aware of who was doing what. Falconer was a first-class lawyer but McCartney was a first-class political operator more adept at infighting. He retained the support of the DTI civil servants and consolidated his channels of communication to Blair.

In the journey through the procedures of the Commons and Lords, at the request of McCartney, after discussions with Monks and Larkin, regular Monday evening briefings were arranged with a team of trade union parliamentary and political officers whilst the bill was in the Commons standing committee stage. These were convened by the TUC with Frank Doran, PPS to McCartney, acting as the coordinator. It became a contribution to the Labour Party input partly because poor relations with the Liberal Democrats were affected by McCartney's pro-Labour tribalism but mainly because the Liberal Democrats on the standing committee were judged as unimpressive and not pushing on the major union concerns. The purpose of the meetings was two-fold: to keep the unions informed about progress and the timetable but also to enable the unions to feed in technical skill and knowledge as well as to voice misgivings. They were not policy-making meetings and managed to avoid the temptation to re-fight old battles.

Towards the end, Monks, in a lament that was also now in effect playing the Labour Party card, made the public accusation that Blair was treating the party's loyal traditional working-class voters like 'embarrassing elderly relatives'. The accompanying claim that heartlands support for the party was therefore being eroded was not given much open credence in the No. 10 Policy Unit, but it was said at the TUC to have given McCartney more room for manoeuvre in securing some very small final tidying up 'the dots and commas' in arguing his case with Falconer and Norris. At the end of this process, with the legislation settled and coming into force on 27 July 1999, the view on both sides at the end of this was that McCartney had conceded nothing new of any substance at this stage and even gained some marginal improvements.

Significance and political repercussions

The unsurprising feature of this intense politics was the historic success of Blair at the zenith of his power working with a weak collective Cabinet and assisted by a Policy Unit and No. 10 allies here acting as the voice of business as party stakeholders. The legislation disappointed union aspirations. It was heavy on detail over collective rights but lacking in substance, and there remained heavy legal constraints on industrial action. Under the small-business exemptions of firms with fewer than 21 employees, more than a fifth of the labour force were excluded.[53] The proportion of the workforce under part-time and temporary contracts, a growing area of the labour force seen by the government as essential to flexible labour markets, was not covered by this legislation. In spite of the promise of a review the outcome met Blair's firm intention to draw a line under changes in industrial-relations law. It illustrated the major limitations on union claims in an area they traditionally thought of as where a Labour government represented the claims of labour. But it was heavily influenced by the perspectives of neo-liberalism and by business-media pressure. In sections of the unions, that media role was especially deeply resented.

The influence of News International and its courtship by Blair fed an increased union sense of operating within an unfair political system. Other problems of democracy had been highlighted by this legislative process. Polling indicated that over the terms of union recognition the electorate had more support for the TUC position than that of the CBI but that was not allowed to be decisive. A freer flow of the collective PLP view might well have produced another outcome. The same applies to the unregistered collective Cabinet opinion.

Still, what has been noted here was an element of 'New Labour' distinctiveness influenced by party values and party management considerations. A significant pluralism within management linked most managers to Blair's priorities including close links to the CBI, whilst other managers were linked to party and union constituencies which they responded to but also primed. This extraordinary and lengthy conflict within Blair's management, involving an element of genuine institutionalised pluralism within the quasi-presidency, was in part a deliberate and constructive Blair arrangement. But it was also influenced by the variety of union responses including the governmental role of their allies, especially Cruddas and McCartney and, in a contrary role, at one stage an intervention of tactical accommodation by the TUC. The 'pro-union' managers even assisted (for the moment) the operation of a reinvigorated PLP trade union group working within a pro-labour PLP culture showing here (and later through TULO) that even within Blair's ascendancy, the affiliated unions always had some capacity for renewal of their policy role.

As a result, although the legislation was more limited and restrictive than many in the unions wanted, it also gave them more gains than they had feared at the beginning of the exercise. Pressure in the PLP and concern for its future management probably ensured that the retreat from the Fairness at Work document was less than the CBI wanted. The gains then became a party management resource used in planning to secure union accommodation on other issues and in different forums. The conflict also indicated how fatuous were suggestions that a Blair Government facing trouble from the unions could manage the situation by declaring a referendum and precipitating a divorce from the unions. The Byers 'seafood dinner' solution in 1996 – if that was what it was – had minimal party support and its political costs would have been enormous to the point of all-round destruction. Blair saw that and at the point where separation was most likely to be fruitful did not push for it. Support for the old separatism and confrontation of 1992 never died, but for him and some aides and allies, it now became more of a privately shared nostalgia, waiting hopefully for a new indirect opportunity.

The protracted internal managerial conflict here actually strengthened the ties between the unions and the party. Since the re-launch of 1996 the TUC had placed a continued emphasis on the possibility of a broad-front union political representation. In this crucial parliamentary battle the broad-front strategy had given way to the party strategy and new links to the PLP trade union group. At the same time, the long battle had not, as Blair had feared, forced the CBI into the arms of the Tories. Experience of the fruitful dialogue, a continuing level of employers' involvement that had surprised the CBI,[54] and strict limits around the Employment Relations Act, brought them, and Murdoch, amicably closer.

Notes

1 White paper, *Fairness at Work*, CM 3968, May 1998, section 4.20.
2 *Fairness at Work*, foreword by the Prime Minister.
3 Tony Blair, *Change and National Renewal*, 1994, p. 12.
4 *The Times*, 31 March 1997.
5 John Edmonds, 'Positioning Labour Closer to the Employers: the Importance of the Labour Party's 1997 Business Manifesto', *Historical Studies in Industrial Relations* 22, Autumn 2006, Edmonds final draft, p. 7.
6 Ibid.
7 Speech to GPMU Conference, 12 June 1997.
8 Roger Undy, 'New Labour and New Unionism', *Employee Relations* 24(6), 2002, p. 642.
9 Edmonds, *Positioning Labour*, Edmonds final draft, p. 6.
10 *Tribune*, 20 March 1998.
11 *The House Magazine*, 8 September 1997.
12 Harris Research Centre, fieldwork 13 March and 9 April 1998, cited by Peter Kellner, *New Statesman*, 3 July 1998.
13 NOP/TUC 29 to 31 August 1997.
14 ICM/*Guardian*, 28 May 1998.
15 *Sunday Times*, 5 April 1998.
16 Connect Public Affairs: a Survey by BPRI Panels, 'The Position of the TUC and CBI on Union Recognition', 22 April 1998.
17 *Sunday Times*, 22 March 1998.
18 Jonathan Powell, *The New Machiavelli: How to Wield Power in the Modern World*, Bodley Head, London, 2010, p. 69.
19 *The Times*, 13 February 1998.
20 Morris, *New Statesman* interview, 13 February 1998.
21 *Guardian*, 17 March 1998.

22 Patrick Seyd and Paul Whiteley, *Labour's Grassroots: The Politics of Party Membership*, Clarendon, Oxford, 1992, p. 53.

23 Patrick Seyd, 'New Parties New Politics?' *Party Politics* 5(3), 1999, p. 307. Also unpublished data on new members supplied by Patrick Seyd from the Seyd and Whiteley study of *New Labours' Grassroots*: 2002, covering the period 1990–9.

24 Minkin, *Contentious Alliance*, p. 650.

25 *The House Magazine*, 8 September 1997.

26 TUC Update: Union Recognition Campaign. John Monks, Introduction to the text of a document presented to the Prime Minister for his meeting with union representatives, 27 April 1998.

27 Ibid.

28 This proposal is understood to have emerged initially from a meeting between Ian McCartney and TUC officials David Lea and Peter Mitchell in response to concern at the new assertiveness of left-led unions.

29 K.D. Ewing and Anne Hock with a foreword by Brendon Barber, *The Next Step: Trade Union Representation in Small Enterprises*, Popularis, Kinston on Thames, 2003, p. v.

30 Foreword, *The Next Step*, by Brendan Barber, General Secretary, TUC.

31 *Financial Times*, 22 May 1998.

32 *Voice of the Unions*, July/August 1998.

33 *Tribune*, 22 May 1998.

34 *Guardian*, 23 May 1998.

35 *Guardian*, 25 May 1998.

36 Letter from Peter Mandelson to Alastair Campbell, 11 May 1998.

37 *The Sunday Times*, 24 May 1998.

38 *Guardian*, 31 July 1998.

39 Ibid.

40 Donald Macintyre, *Mandelson: the Biography*, HarperCollins, London 1999, p. 422.

41 *New Statesman* interview, 11 September 1998.

42 TUC, 17 September 1998. Excerpts on TUC website.

43 LPCR, 1998, p. 34.

44 *The Guardian*, 19 October 1998.

45 Macintyre, *Mandelson*, p. 422.

46 Lance Price, *The Spin Doctor's Diary: Inside No. 10 with New Labour*, Hodder & Stoughton, London, 2005, entry 13 December 1998, p. 161.

47 *Sunday Telegraph*, 22 November 2008.

48 Mark Hall (Industrial Relations Research Unit), Government Refinements to Fairness at Work proposals, European industrial relations observatory on-line, 28 January 1999.

49 *New Statesman*, 29 January 1999.

50 Sarah Veale, Senior Employment Rights Officer TUC, *Trade Union Group of Labour MPs Newsletter*, Winter 2002/3.

51 Tony Dubbins, *Tribune*, 27 January 2006.

52 *Financial Times*, 16 March 1999.

53 Ewing and Hock, *Next Step*, p. v.

54 Cridland CBI, interview with Edmonds, *Positioning Labour*, p. 14.

PART III
Crisis and control

15

The crisis of party management

Management successes

After over five years of leading the party, Blair and most of his advisers could consider their management activities, the culture and its code of behaviour with some satisfaction. The party officials had almost shed their civil service ethos and become Blair's personal machine. Clause IV had been triumphantly changed, as had various old policies and old images. The NEC, feared by the leadership as a potential rival centre of power, was now a shadow of its former self, virtually but not quite denuded of its policy-making role. The Partnership in Power arrangements provided insulation for the government, avoiding regular full frontal confrontations at the party conference. The conference operated under extended and heavy control. New parliamentary candidates appeared highly supportive. Although the government's performance did not live up to all expectations, nevertheless economic management underpinned the sense of impressive competence and optimism about the future. No votes had been lost in the House of Commons and, in the No. 10 Political Office, defeats looked unlikely.

Union votes at the party conference had been reduced, sponsorship of MPs had been changed, union representation on the NEC and at the NPF had been reformed. Yet the majority of unions remained regular supporters of the management. Important legislation covering the minimum wage and employment relations had been introduced without doing damage to the government's relationship with business, which grew ever closer. Tactical activities of the spin doctors and managers had succeeded in defusing or neutralising the worst potential media and electoral problems. The publicly off-putting ghosts and monsters of the past had been suppressed or inhibited.

Across the party, a complex of management devices and supportive self-control seemed to avoid all the worst outcomes that the Leader had worried about. It still appeared that the minority of dissenters in the party and dissatisfied ex-Labour supporters had effectively nowhere else to go. The discredited Conservatives were without effective public leadership, and continued to lag behind in the polls. The spin about the quality of 'New Labour' professionalism and the supremacy of the Leader reinforced managerial pride in their own record. Diminished accountability covered over mistakes and other flaws. There was, it seemed, a complete rationality as well as effectiveness to the 'New Labour' approach to party management – except that in the eyes of some leading managers there needed to be more of it.

Other voices

Awareness of the dangers of arousing distrust in the party had limited influence on the performance of the central managers. Their operation found manipulation necessary and permissible in various forms noted in this study. The extensive hidden managerial organisation was itself especially deceptive, and the role of manager included at times the fake and the misleading in communicating and informing, whilst the leadership, as indicated, had few qualms about bad faith in keeping the spirit of agreements. The rhetoric of democracy and partnership covered the reality of the rolling coup that expanded Blair's power, the repetitive fait accompli of the bounce, and a range of controlling procedural devices and communicational controls.

Against this, there were always some critical voices which were raised privately in discussions with managers about this form of leadership and management culture. Obsession with strong leadership could distort both partnership in power and the democratic process in a way which would provoke a defensive reaction in the party. Spin could be deemed manipulative and a poison in the body politic. 'Control' might become increasingly contentious and an adverse message drowning the impact of favourable substantive policy discussion. Trust within the party and in relations with unions could be undermined by the methods and attitudes of management. Regular manipulation did not create an atmosphere to encourage a sustained cooperative response to new proposals for internal change or the passing of the crucial message of trust from the party to the people. The warnings were given,[1] but supremely confident in their diagnosis of the major problems and prescriptions, and their understanding of public opinion, for the moment Blair and his orthodox managers ignored them, or soon lowered their attention.

Shocks to the consciousness

Philip Gould, in his preface to the paperback edition of *The Unfinished Revolution* in 1999, noted, or at least presented, little to disturb the glowing portrait of success and great difficulties overcome. Control and spin were judged to be misunderstood, trust received only a one-word mention. There was no reference to the difficulties produced by party management and manipulative politics, nor would there be in Gould's future public analysis of political problems under Blair. Then suddenly, seemingly out of the blue, in the summer of 2000, the Leader, his advisers, managers and loyal supporters had to come to terms with a series of shocks to their consciousness. A flurry of leaks of Gould's advisory memos gave an insight into the development of a dawning and deepening realisation that 'something has gone seriously wrong', which leading advisers, including Gould and Mandelson, could not understand.[2] That was primarily because the problem came not from the circumstances they might have expected but heavily involved the character of 'New Labour' politics, its party management and the unanticipated public responses to them.

The challenges to management

Media management and party management

In approaching that understanding and the complex series of developments which took place from 1999 to 2001 and produced major repercussions throughout the 'New Labour' years, it is useful to begin with media management and its relationship with party management. The assumption was that management and spin was unreservedly a good thing in dealing with media devilry. Few in the party would have doubted that. There was a constantly pressing concern that the Tories were easily able to mount and sustain attacks because of what Campbell and many in the party regarded as their corrupt and ruthless relationship with the press. The resulting pressures added to the imperatives of leadership command and control to adhere to and even pressurise along the media strategy and tactics.

Yet behind the scenes, media management also began to draw some discreet critical attention from amongst the party managers because not only was it not always as successful as reputation implied, it also created tensions and problems which at times made consensual party management more difficult. It focused on the media appeal of a proposal or solution with at times much less concern for the difficulties and costs involved in gaining party acceptance of the policy and putting it into practice.

The problem-causing record in the party was clear. From 1989 to 1993, the separationist spin from the modernising leaders had undermined unity on proposals for reform of the unions in candidate selection; that memory and its consequent distrust hung over all future union relations. In 1995 the spin against 'the unions' after the Clause IV result made public enemies of supportive unions and almost became the disaster of a party portrayed as acutely divided. A similar spin that year limited the reform of sponsorship. In 1996 the spin on the Road to Manifesto ballot almost destroyed the process before it started and public unity had to be rescued. In 1996, the spin representing Partnership in Power as a controlling response began a major division on the committee producing it. Similarly the pre-release spin on the PLP Review that year undermined the possibility of a consensual trustful initial PLP support for it.

There was also a big problem with what became recognised as 'a culture of humiliation' in the way that power was trumpeted in advance through the media against internal enemies. If the activists in the CLPs were to continue to be a regular target for media denigration, this raised the question of what that would do for their morale and level of activity. And if every story implied a split worth seeking suppression and then winning, what impression did it give about the claim to have achieved a unified party? In addition, constant reassurance to business and the media about control over the unions made union cooperation, even with the regularly friendly and also demeaned TUC, more difficult and grievance-ridden.

Then again, after 1997, the personalisation of media management fed a deep resentment when individual ministers, particularly David Clarke at the Cabinet Office, thought themselves under pressure from orchestrated briefings by the government spinners.[3] Two very independent-minded and at times truculent women did not easily fit into the new managed discipline. Clare Short and later, particularly, Mo Mowlem saw themselves at different times briefed against by what Short called 'the people who live in the dark'.[4] Though media managers consistently denied it, the women diagnosed that a mix of spin-doctor hubris and aggressive protection of the Leader had affected the way media managers behaved towards them.[5]

This linked to another problem which became more acute. Every senior Labour politician, and others less senior, had an alter ego of the disembodied spinning voice. It gave a sense of power to the presenters and was a seductive encouragement to irresponsible and competitive advantage-seeking behaviour. More than ever before, the age-old problem of inter-ministerial rivalry was played out by Blair and Brown, often by spinning proxy and sometimes in semi-public view, producing its own accentuation of personal distrust and embittered grievance. Even after the eviction of Mandelson and Whelan, the damaging spin war continued.

Spin, the public and the media

Spin produced other vulnerabilities, especially public distrust. Following the Labour media management success in attacking the Major government, and the acknowledgement of the skills of Labour's media management, a strong counter-attack from the anti-'New Labour' government media had already made its appearance shortly after Labour won the election, drawing attention to how the management was conducted. Mandelson and then especially Campbell provided high-profile targets. In the face of incessant attack, some of which was grossly exaggerated, prudence might have led ministers and media managers to take increased care not to give confirmatory evidence of devious and culpable behaviour to their critics. Yet the leadership and management became subject to an overconfident attitude about their skills and the experience of 'getting away with it' in various features of domineering party and media management.

The need to keep satisfying great public and party expectations about delivery drove them on. From putting a case most effectively in its best light, and repeating a message so frequently that it registered, media management slipped into a 'serious politics' dishonesty of constantly re-announcing policies as though they were new and double-counting the financial delivery. This applied particularly to Brown's treatment of health-service financial provision and the distrust it engendered. Some of that health-service spin generated particular distrust amongst public-sector workers. In doing so it undermined their potential role as positive ambas-sadors inside and outside the party about the condition of the heath service. The art that had begun as a means of handling media bias and mani-pulation could now be much more easily portrayed in the media as a government device to manipulate the people. Private polls for the party indicated that the public view that Blair was 'not delivering' and was 'all spin and presentation'.[6] Spinning became equated with deceit and that brought gifts of ammunition for those challenging Blair's claim to repre-sent the public interest.

Candidate selection and the generation of distrust

All this fed into a deeper growing public concern with the government's conduct of politics and the politicians' manipulation in British political life (more fully explored in Chapter 16, pp. 509–13). Noteworthy here is par-ticularly what had happened in reaction to the fixing of candidate selection in the highly controversial mayoral election in London following 'the rigged election' in Wales, examined in Chapter 12. The managerial activities had generated a distrustful reaction against what one respected commentator, Andrew Marr, had described as 'the baby-faced Machiavellis of New Labour'.[7] The experience was acknowledged by some party strategists to be damaging and undermining trust amongst Labour voters[8] although, in general, it was not taken as a challenge to the culture of party manage-ment, One exception came in an impressively pointed contribution of Blair's aide Peter Hyman, quoted in the private memo of Philip Gould which emerged in press hands. Hyman had captured accurately the way that the politics of the London mayoral-election process was a 'combination of spin, lack of conviction and apparently lack of integrity'.[9] The 'New Labour brand' had been 'badly contaminated'.[10]

A fundamental managerial assumption which had prevented an honest reappraisal had been that the vigilant and heavy control, including the serious politics of procedural fixing, was necessary to protect the people against the potential damage from 'Old Labour'. The axiom was also that the dangerous alignment would be that of party and unions versus the government and the people. The expectation was that 'for the government to stay in tune with the party, the party must stay in tune with the nation'.[11] Blair later claimed to have appreciated the danger of a developing alliance between the party and the people against the Leader.[12] That must be doubted. Certainly, none of that sense of danger came through to the managers of Party Into Power in 1996–7. There had been little conscious-ness in the way that the No. 10-influenced General Secretary led the discussions that the party might be at times the authentic voice of the people, whilst the government might be unresponsive to the party and failing to defend the public interest.

Over Livingstone in London it had proved to be easy, with few misgivings, to move to the early assumption that if the desired outcome of impeding 'Old Labour' was morally right then so were the procedural means, even if the movement in manipulating the party also manipulated the electorate. By 21 September 1999, focus groups were already showing that 'the commonest image' of Blair was 'Phony Tony'.[13] This was probably a mix of the charge of insincerity over promises made but not delivered and the suspicion of pervasive spin. Now the charge crucially broadened, taking in the image of the mayoral election procedural manoeuvres detailed in Chapter 12. The fact that only 15 per cent of Londoners accepted that the electoral college result was fair[14] could not be insulated from their changing view of Blair.

By early 2000 the focus by critics had broadened to the perception of Labour as 'the vote-fixing party'.[15] For significant numbers their judgement on this had an element of anger over the betrayal of his implied promise to be 'different to the others'.[16] Procedural fixing and communicational distortion had produced a situation by 2000 where Greenberg, an adviser from the US, noted that there had been 'a loss of trust that would never be regained'. It 'made lack of authenticity and manipulation an inescapable part of the Blairite world'.[17]

The limits of strong leadership

What happened in London, in daily national focus, highlighted something else. Blair had found himself so ideally suited to the role he admired of the strong bold leader that, in his view and that of most of his managers, it was bound to be found admirable by a public that yearned for it. A *Guardian* editorial in November 1998 had offered the view that it was 'part of the British character to favour strong leadership'.[18] One prominent political scientist, Ivor Crewe, judged that 'being too strong' only upset 'a small number of Labour supporters and Labour activists'.[19] But Dennis Healey had pointed out that the appeal of strong government depends a great deal on 'what the Leader does with his strength'.[20] And Martin Kettle had warned, in an early article full of insight into the potential degeneration of the party titled 'Please don't bother taking me to your strong leader', that Blair's leadership behaviour was 'causing him nothing but problems and will continue to do so'.[21] It was an overstatement but it conveyed a truth that Blair's fixation on strength could not accommodate. Even the direct role of Blair in winning elections was a contested position.[22] The highly regarded electoral analyst John Curtice argued, as did others, that Labour double-digit success under Blair was inherited from Smith.[23]

As for his methods, there were traditions within the British political culture born of historic struggle against autocracy and unjust political representation which fed into the British political bloodstream a more qualified view of people's evaluation of strong leadership. With the spirit of democracy came an obstinate potentially rebellious streak. Alastair Campbell would later point out to Blair the 'bloody-minded and anti-establishment' feature of the British character.[24] Virtually unnoticed by observers, a 1996 State of the Nation survey which included opinion on the voting responsibilities of MPs produced results far from compatible with a strict adherence to strong leadership. The primacy of MPs' loyalty to the interests of their constituents (65 per cent) and loyalty to the views of the local party (12 per cent) was far greater than loyalty to the national party leaders (4 per cent).[25]

True, electors did not like the idea that a Prime Minister was losing control over events and responsibilities, nor that they were unable to rise to the critical occasions, especially those where security – personal or national – was involved. In that focused sense they always wanted 'strong leaders'. There was generally admiration for leaders whose opinions and behaviour expressed a determined coherent integrity. But strength, boldness and determination were received and judged in the light of wisdom, values and competence. Gould, often excited by his own portrayal of the qualities of Blair the Leader, had been sure that Blair had 'a sense of the destiny of the nation and of the pulse of the people'.[26] In the light of Blair's party management of candidate selection that had now been shown to be over-blown, the growing reaction to 'New Labour' as government indicated that in respect of strong leadership and controlling party management Blair had a far from impeccable sense of the people's pulse.

During the London mayoral battle, when asked why they would not vote for Dobson, the strongest public response was that he was 'a puppet controlled by the government'. Spin doctor Lance Price noted in his diary a development about which both the Leader and managers had been at times remarkably blinkered in their views on party management. Although Blair had urged London audiences to concentrate on policy and not on process, Price noted that the campaign was 'getting bogged down by questions of process'.[27] It was a development that some private critics of control freakery had warned about. And the performance of the Leader was seen repeatedly now as arrogant. At this time Hugo Young captured a new mood: 'a not insubstantial section of the electorate has given up on the seductions of strong leadership of any kind'.[28] Another major axiom of party management was in trouble. It was the axiom that proved least susceptible to change in the years that followed.

Somewhere else to go

It had also been an axiom of party management that whatever the dissatisfactions about process and policy amongst a small number of Labour activists and supporters, Blair could ignore them because 'they have nowhere else to go'. If that judgement of 'nowhere else to go' was about alternative and electorally credible left-wing organisations operating within a first-past-the-post electoral system, then that was still the case. But now it had been shown in Falkirk and London that a dissenting left-wing candidate could stand against the party as a critic of its form of management and win. There was a potentially troublesome if small increase in independent socialist electoral support to approximately 5 per cent and, more significant, increasing signs of stay-at-home Labour identifiers withdrawing from their electoral role entirely.

Individual Labour members also found that they had somewhere else to go in the sense that they could just leave the party. A rising membership had been the proud symbol of 'New Labour' success. The membership in 1992 had been 279,530, then in a surge from December 1993 it rose to 305,000. By the end of 1996 it was 400,485. Whether that was accurate or spun is uncertain. But from 1997, immediately after the Conservatives were defeated, membership clearly began to decline. By 2001 it was down to officially 272,000 but even the extent of that decline was obscured by abuse of the reduced rate and by keeping lapsed members on the books. Internally there was also, as noted, a decline in participation for NEC elections, and for NPF elections a decline in the number of candidates willing to stand.

This decline in party membership and activity was such as to remind veterans of the modernising Wilson government which had lost office in 1970 amidst the lament that 'the grass comes away from the roots'.[29] The reversal of the membership rise in the modernised party became a public mark of failure and warning of the collateral damage of party management. An optimist about the party might see here another reason for the Blair management to adjust, especially as the work of Seyd and Whiteley had also shown that the influx of new members in the period 1994–7 did not live up to Blairite expectations about the scale of their policy differentiation from that of old members.[30] Members old and new found declining incentives to participate in Labour activity under Blair.[31]

Management and reappraisal

Re-evaluating management

Until the London mayoral debacle and in some measure long after it, it had been particularly difficult to get a hearing at senior levels of the party for the view that there were dangers in the degree of top-down controlling management and the politics that went with it. Around the Party into Power meetings in 1996–7, drawing attention to the potentially adverse consequences of manipulation was regarded by senior managers as unhelpful and, at times, placed the proponent 'offside'. Even when judged as not ill-intentioned, the proposal to shed any of the political armoury when facing the party's problems and enemies was regarded by the managers as naive, and ignored.

Yet in 2000 even if they did not understand it they could not ignore what was now happening amongst the electorate. One poll from a starting point in January 1998 of 56 per cent agreeing that the government had been 'honest and trustworthy' had by September 2000 fallen to 35.8 per cent.[32] Other polling, which in 1997 had 36 per cent judging Blair honest and trustworthy had only 12 per cent making that judgement in September 2000. That rose only to 17 per cent in the pre-election April of 2001.[33] The problem for No. 10 was that much of the 'New Labour' argument since 1994 had focused on what was regarded as the deep-rooted problems of Labour's culture and its inability to change. The emphatic historical work of Gould on Labour's conservatism had failed even to consider the important features which had facilitated Labour's change in the past. Blair, his allies and the managers found special difficulty in seeing that Blairism had its own cultural problems, its own pathologies and its own conservatism. At one point in November 2000, Blair privately expressed himself to Gould as mystified why 'a government that is doing well economically should not be popular', and blamed the press.[34]

A search for answers produced considerable bafflement in a busy 10 Downing Street not well attuned to fundamental post-mortems. For some of the managers, it was difficult to think of the adverse new developments other than in terms of temporary difficulties and cock-ups – each was 'a blip'. The instinct was to blame the Tory Press for the fact that the 'New Labour' professionalism of strong leadership, discipline and presentation were being turned into vices of arrogance, control freakery and style without substance. This was a half-truth more comfortable than facing the fact that all the virtues always had the potential to become vices and that the character of management was causing problems. Gould in 1998 had drawn attention to a focus-group response to the Tories when they were in government – 'People felt used and they felt manipulated'.[35] Yet what Hennessy called 'the great evangelist for a more commanding centre',[36] in spite of his own focus groups, did not appear to see the extent to which Labour's own managerial power structure was producing the same response. He was still arguing that 'we are not strong enough at the centre'.[37]

One deeply ingrained 'New Labour' managerial response to their problems was to find others in the party whose fault it was and make them the deflection. In November 1999 at a meeting of political advisers in No. 10 there was a rehearsal of the answers to be given to the charge of control freakery in selections in Scotland, Wales and London. The message was to be that it was 'a Scottish thing', it was a problem 'in Wales', it was 'London'. Basically, it was '*not us*'. Loyally reproduced in the PLP, this was reported back to No. 10 when they were seeking to find what the PLP was thinking and to an extent finding themselves misled by their own propaganda.

There was one other consistent deflective No. 10 theme which was to be raised in importance all the way through the London crisis to the

General Election and what followed. If critical attention focused on central management, the problem, it was said privately and emphatically, was 'Millbank'. For their part, officials in that building defended a deep resistance to changing behaviour on the grounds that change was what 'Tory tactics' intended. Their resistance was reinforced by a particular doubt as to whether Blair wanted to see any significant change in management control or had any reason to do it. However, a small but growing minority amongst the managers took a different view. Between 1999 and 2001 their acknowledgement of major problems brought repugnance and some in-house discreet non-cooperation with the crudest forms of the ethic of delivery. After 2001 there came an emphatic, if private, disassociation from it as some found their way out of party employment.

Adaptation and the new dilemmas

A minority of managers were also prepared to admit that there had been overkill in the earlier period and the less acceptable features of their own operation might no longer be justified. There had been no psephological analysis of this crisis focused specifically on manipulation but there was an illuminating contribution from Peter Kellner, a leading polling analyst who had been close to the modernising strategists. He found the electors detecting a lack of authenticity of the 'New Labour' voices arising out of the excess of zeal for enforcing a disciplined line. It was a salutary critique of something that had become fundamental to the character of 'New Labour' party management.[38]

From this and the discontent rising in the party over the controls, it was possible to envisage now a significant shift in management away from the manipulation and the undermining of partnership. However, it became clear only later that in No. 10 they had been discussing other solutions. They had to appear less preoccupied with getting their own way; could they 'loosen things a bit' without losing control? Could Blair's strong leadership be preserved whilst adjusting or hiding its most off-putting characteristics? Adaptability struggled against atavism. Pragmatic flexibility wrestled with habits of mind and character formed in the confident early days of 'New Labour'.

The message they put out of 'Tell them to remember the 1980s!' also played back into their own minds. Old instincts died hard and some did not die at all – as will be illustrated later. For Blair there was a particular problem. He, a man with supreme confidence in his own judgement, had to come to terms with the fact that his party management had been based on some major false assumptions and produced some unfortunate consequences. Seeing himself and not the party as the cause of major problems and the reason for pressing changes to deal with the damaging accusation of control freakery involved a very tricky contortion and produced an incomplete adjustment, especially as he now had other priorities.

New Tonyism

Frustration and party management

The challenge to managerial control freakery came at an especially in-opportune time for the Prime Minister. Mixing with the sense of success across his political project was a range of frustrations and dissatisfactions with government.[39] He was especially struggling with managing the coor-dination of governmental delivery of major elements of the domestic agenda in the face of a civil service regarded as a deeply conservative force. He was working also with the powerful, successful and at times aggressively non-cooperative Chancellor Gordon Brown who had tense relations with several colleagues and a deep feud with Mandelson.

And though it may not have appeared this way, his frustration was not simply over this governing experience. Not fully appreciated was the extent of his frustration over managing the party behind the projection of his supremacy. The leader of the most reformed, delivery-driven and extensive internal management process that Labour had yet known felt now in various ways held back, and had reasons for forebodings about future developments in the party. Achieving transformation of the Labour Party had, as we have seen, met various constraints that limited his efforts and caused him trouble in spite of the managerial successes. Some of this con-straint was rooted in the Smith-trade union settlement. Difficulties were reinforced by the reciprocity of relations with Prescott over the party. Blair was even skilfully held in check at times by the caution of Morgan and by the policy reservations of Cruddas – key Political Office aides.

Especially vexing was that in the party, local organisational change driven from above had come to an abrupt halt in the face of considerable distrust, and that there were limitations on management sanctions over the PLP. He had been astute enough to cautiously accept Partnership in Power, with the confidence that he was sheltered behind a series of covert man-agement controls which reinforced his autonomy and insulated him from accountability. It was the same with the role of PLP departmental com-mittees in policy-making. But in both areas expectations had been aroused about the obligations of leadership which potentially could lead to greater interference with his personal policy formulation and his radical aspirations. Tough management had succeeded in restricting that possibility so far but even at times when he was winning virtually across the board, he was not winning as he would have liked. Presidential plebiscitarianism over the party, his preferred style, had been discredited, even in the eyes of some of his own managers.

There was a special aggravation about Brown's constant pushing for his people to fill posts and what was suspected to be the build-up of his own parallel structures and platoons inside the party. And there was deep sus-picion that his ambitions might produce a second-term attack on Blair's position from a strengthened party position. General frustration also arose from the vitality of the party's traditions of pluralistic and democratic process now embedded in the participating role envisaged in Partnership in Power and the policy inclusion of the PLP departmental committees, both of which might produce problems for the core managerial culture he had encouraged.

Over several years the Political Office in No. 10 gave out the repeated reassurance that Tony 'feels better about the party now'. The fact of this repetition in itself cast suspicion on its veracity. Also, as one of Blair's spin doctors Lance Price pointed out later, at the time of the party's anniversary in 2000, Blair's body language at the centenary hardly expressed his deep love of the party and pride in its history.[40] The reality was that, as his more radical followers quietly bemoaned, the party had not been changed enough. It was a view that Blair shared. He never felt that he and his aides had enough power, either in the government or in the party, and in both cases he would have preferred to be leading a different kind of organisation in a different way. For his mission in the second term, he was not free enough and there were too many obstructions and the potential threat of more. Gaining more freedom and more control over the party was a priority.

Aspiration and ambiguity

Yet also, around the special man with a special mission there were increasing numbers wondering what that mission was exactly and where Blair might now want to lead. There were many complexities to the intellectual composition that was 'New Labour', and no consensual characterisation summed up the mix of continuities, differences and developments from the past. Espousing electoral triangulation and cross-dressing, lacking an ideology, practising rapid rebuttal and seeking the closure of vulnerabilities in response to right-wing press criticism produced a weakening of identity, and stimulated perplexity from around him. To Campbell their position looked too much like being all things to all men.[41] What had become Blair's 'Third Way' approach to the party's purpose,[42] taken forward also by Anthony Giddens,[43] was 'widely regarded as vacuous',[44] and even smiled at, when mentioned to the No. 10 Political Office.

Philip Gould had admitted in a leaked memo that 'there has been no shared agreement about what is the New Labour project for government'[45] and 'We don't know what we are'.[46] Derek Draper, once an insider in the Mandelsonian network of Blairites, diagnosed the 'congenital defects' of 'detachment from Labour's historic social democratic values' which involved 'short-term electoral gain bought at the expense of a meaningful identity'. His overall conclusion was that 'it might have been new, but it wasn't Labour and nobody understood it'.[47] Mandelson, looking rather pleased, found no problem in telling a fringe meeting at the 2000 party conference that Blairism was 'what a Labour government does'.[48] This gave the project a flexibility which was potentially an asset in managing some problems. But it gave also an elusive and at times an unconvincing purpose.

Back in 1996 Mandelson, with Liddle, had attributed to Blair the belief that 'clarity in the Party's goals and principles' was 'a precondition for success'.[49] Yet, much later, after his departure Blair described himself as having governed to this point in 2000 'with a clear political instinct but without the knowledge and experience of where the instinct should take us in specific policy terms'.[50] Even so, late in 2000 he sent out a confident-sounding message through party managers that in the second term 'I will be more radical'. For those on different wings of the party who thought that his policies had been too cautious, here was a new promise, but what would he be radical about?

Towards new purpose

The world stage

That was never fully revealed to the party and it only gradually became clear when Blair himself was sure that he had found out. His sense of himself as a special man on a special mission had been partially satisfied by the European proselytising over flexible labour markets, but found a new opportunity for his talents and horizons in 1999–2000. The role of war leader over Kosovo and then Sierra Leone and his response to ethnic cleansing gave him a mission and a world stage. Kosovo was seen as a moral challenge, taken up boldly and with conviction, despite the weakness of allies and international institutions. In the speech in Chicago in 1999, noted in Chapter 10 (see pp. 329–30), Blair's passionate appeal for international community action in an integrated world placed within a new doctrine of international cooperation and intervention invited a pressing and morally appealing discussion. Yet it was not integrated within his 1999 conference speech although it could have been fitted into the broad anti-conservative modernising perspective which was its central theme.

What dominated considerations of that theme was Blair's search for a new domestic dynamism focused on delivery of public-service reform in a way which would fit the triangulation tactical positioning. In August 2000, The NHS Plan proved to be a landmark on the road to radical second-year policy, with extensive organisational changes designed around the patient but also edging open the door for private sector involvement. Again, this was never systematically opened up to the party nor addressed directly in the Partnership in Power dialogue at the NPF. By this date the policy discussion there had been closed down.

This treatment of the party can be judged as a potent illustration of what at the time of the 2000 party conference Alastair Campbell was telling Hugo Young: 'Tony is not interested in having arguments, only winning them'.[51] Even so, at this very moment the special and unanticipated new headache was that he now had to shake off the control freak reputation at a time when he was looking to engineer more room for his bold leadership. A Leader who had to be seen by the public to be always in control now had also to be seen not to be obsessive about it. That had not been in the script of party management. How that script was rewritten began here, before the election, before the 9/11 terrorist attack and well before the Iraq invasion. There was no absolute consistency in this and no master plan but in a remarkable series of developments and interventions, misadventures and manoeuvres, most of which were covert in part or in whole and never fully noticed by observers, Blair's position began to be adroitly and extensively strengthened.

Pre-election management adjustment

Small shifts

The most subtle managerial judgement became that it was possible to change in limited ways some aspects of leadership and managerial behaviour, and to change some of the appearance of Blair's behaviour without doing much damage to his control. In this attempt, there was an important change of tone in 2000, notably in the public emphasis on 'we are listening'. There was eventually an apology over the treatment of the Wales leadership election. Within the Commons, the old system of discreet lobby briefings was reviewed by Campbell, and summaries put 'on the record', with his comments attributable to him. Before the party conference, the old practice of showing supremacy by publicly threatening what the leadership was going to do to the conference opposition was virtually abandoned.

Over candidate selection, the *21st Century Party* document had a new accommodating tone in its advocacy of selection procedures which were 'consistent transparent and fair'. OMOV was to be adopted in all selections with each section of an electoral-college system splitting votes according to the candidates' support. Although that was never fully put into operation and management intervention continued as will be shown, there was an acceptance of some new public restraint. Negotiation of peerages and parachuting candidates became less obvious. No. 10 Downing Street moved itself further away publicly from the mechanics of controversial selection, and with the notable exceptions of Sean Woodward at St Helens and David Miliband at South Shields, Blair put on no pressure for the placement of individuals. Reselection controversies over removing MPs were avoided. All these were influenced by the reluctant pragmatic admission that some of the past excessively controlling behaviour either 'didn't work anymore' or 'we can't get away with it all any more' (with, more sotto voce, the qualification 'not openly').

The turnings that never happened

Business as usual

There were more important changes that might have taken place at this point but did not. As has been noted, whilst problem issues relating to trade unions now barely registered in electoral terms, a poll in 1998 had found a majority agreeing that Blair paid too much attention to company bosses and not enough to ordinary working people.[52] The closeness of the government to the wealthy and their influence on government policy had become an issue of public as well as party concern. Open declaration of large donations had generated further public suspicion. State funding for political parties remained highly unpopular but in January 2001 a Gallup poll found 58 per cent believing parties' 'reliance on donations from a select number of wealthy individuals undesirable'.[53]

Countering party pressure for a reordering of relationships was the close relationship with the CBI, consolidated by the politics of the Employment Relations Act. Showing closeness to business was also still considered to be an asset in targeting ex-Tory voters, in spite of changes in broader public opinion. It continued to be the Treasury view that if not subject to too much interference, the booming City of London would remain a success story which could be associated with 'New Labour', and provide an important source of finance for increased public spending. There was no problem about the greed of such people; their desire to be more rich contributed to their motivation and innovation. Opposition to limiting taxation on the aspiring and the risk-takers became increasingly emphasised as a central feature of the 'Blairite' identity. The commitment in 1997 not to raise tax on higher earners was now renewed before the 2001 election.

Unions Today, firmly under No. 10 control, sought to put out the modernising message and strengthen the government's links to loyalists in the unions and, for the moment, the dominant view in the unions was that they could live with the settlement. Realism influenced the view that it was 'the best we can get' and loyalism that 'we have to give the government a bit of support' for what had been gained. Amongst union members, weaknesses in their ability to take action were not fully apparent until the exceptional situations where action was required. For the majority at the grass roots there was no great rebellious mood over conditions, nor, immediately in the atmosphere explained in Chapter 14 (see pp. 449–50), over the limitations of what had been gained. The ERA did have a beneficial effect on new recognition agreements by 2001.[54] Decline in union membership was arrested; but density continued to fall.[55]

The unions had been unable to organise new workers; the rise in 'nevermembers' accounted for nearly all this decline in union density.[56] Although Blair had no intention of unpicking the settlement, let alone agreeing to a major improvement, at the final Parliamentary Committee held before Christmas 2000, in a discussion of the limited consultation of British workers shown in the closure of the Vauxhall plant at Luton, he did appear to be hinting at future legislation to defend workers' interests but 'not at this time at least'. It was to prove a rhetorical deflection.

There continued to be a current in the unions strongest on the left, and amongst some sections of activists and the middle and lower representative ranks, that a Labour government should involve a more or less continuous gradual improvement in the conditions and rights of industrial labour. For them the new legislation ought to be the first phase of several which would be formulated in conjunction with the party. In the summer of 2000 a senior TUC official, going round the union conferences, was noting that the generally supportive mood had changed. Sections of speeches from the platform which congratulated the government on its various measures for people at work and their objectives, were beginning to be met with decreasing enthusiasm inside the unions.

Management personnel; continuity and changes

Epitomising the continuity of 'New Labour' and business as usual, Geoff Norris retained his role as a skilful and highly trusted manager liaising with business. He again produced the business manifesto consulting amongst ministerial insiders, but outside the new party-policy process and without any information being supplied about it. It focused on deregulation where possible and, where it was necessary to regulate, doing this with 'a light touch'. Another pre-election letter by Labour-inclined business supporters was produced, enthusiastically backing the government.

But Blair had grown dissatisfied with the union liaison from No. 10, and the evolution of Cruddas's semi-independent position had become uncomfortable for both of them. Recognising his limited room and the direction Blair was moving, Cruddas became a parliamentary candidate and was elected in 2001. With his impending departure, Blair took the opportunity in 2000 to bring in Nita Clarke from UNISON, initially on secondment until the General Election, after which she retained the post. A deep Blair loyalist, at times belligerently so, Nita Clarke's expectation was that there would be no major political shifts in the union leadership. Moderates, loyalists and those sympathetic to Blair's modernisation would be strengthened on the basis of moving away from past models of thought and behaviour. Developments in the CWU, RMT and ASLEF had produced more left-wing leaders, and Dave Prentis had replaced Rodney Bickerstaffe in UNISON, but this was not considered to involve a major reorientation of the unions.

An amalgamation envisaged for 2001 was about to produce a new union, Amicus, as the second-largest union, and the largest private sector union, out of the merger of MSF and the AEEU and, later, UNIFI and the GPMU. Although the addition of the GPMU added a new centre-left component to that union, the Amicus amalgamation was envisaged and welcomed in No. 10 as a strengthening of the traditional right loyalist current with a realistic view of the industrial-relations settlement. To assist the process of gathering support, it was planned that there would be an increasing attempt by the government to influence union policies and agendas, and bring various up-and-coming union officers in line with Blair's project.

Manifesto and relations with the party

The manifesto as partnership symbol

There might also have been a new relationship with the party built upon a shared involvement in forging the policies on which the manifesto for the next general election would be based. It had been a major argument in the Party into Power discussion that partnership would create a consensual second term for government and party. In the event, as will be explored later, the last thing which could be said about Blair's second term was that it was consensual. As for the manifesto-making process, it was a decidedly odd form of partnership. The Party into Power deliberations had produced no formal arrangements for the involvement of the National Policy Forum or other PIP institutions in the manifesto production. This gap might have been the opportunity to return to the first model of Blairite party management – the plebiscite. But now there was no question of excluding the unions, and a genuine plebiscite with choices would be too risky. A plebiscite which was restricted in choice, as on the previous occasion, would be embarrassingly 'false' as they acknowledged in No. 10. It could remind the party and the electorate of the damaging 'control freakery'.

It had been expected that the new institutions would be involved in some way in manifesto consultations, but in a memo to Blair from David Miliband in the Policy Unit on 11 December 1999 it was argued that, because of the need for protection against leaks, party working groups on the manifesto 'must be avoided at all costs'. The Policy Unit – Ed Richards in particular – would do the drafting. The policy commissions were closed down after September 2000, although the commitment to using them as a channel of 'ongoing dialogue' had been explicit in Partnership in Power. Even the JPC was closed down. As for the business manifesto, that, as before, had no party input. A special NPF meeting on 9 December 2000 appeared to give an opportunity for offering views on the content of the party's manifesto in line with NPF policy. But there was no invitation to discuss the future manifesto.

The unexpected

Composition of the Clause V meeting

However, alongside these new controls, there came an unexpected and curious development. None of the Party into Power officials or discussants in 1997 had noticed the effect on the composition of the Clause V manifesto meeting of the NEC and the Parliamentary Committee arising from a change of name of the government-PLP linking 'Liaison Committee' to the 'Parliamentary Committee'. This had happened back in 1980 at a time when there was pressure to give the PLP a bigger role in making future policy, a development confirmed by PLP Secretary Alan Howarth, supported by PLP Chairman Soley, and not disputed at the present Parliamentary Committee. It meant that now, for the first time in history, the government-PLP committee would be included in the Clause V meeting but the Cabinet as a body would be formally excluded from its normal place alongside the NEC in the manifesto-authorisation meeting.

The Cabinet members who were not members of the Parliamentary Committee included the Chancellor, Gordon Brown, and Home Secretary, Jack Straw. Ways were found of getting all the senior ministers into the meeting in 2001, but by edict of the Leader, not by right. It led later to a tennis match of manoeuvres between officials of the party and PLP seeking unsuccessfully to rectify the situation. And it later aroused unjustified suspicions of deliberate Blairite skulduggery from some in the Brown camp. Amazingly, this went on without anybody in the media noticing it for the next four years.

The new PLP input potentially most enhanced back-bench influence on the issue of hunting with hounds where Blair wanted a compromise, but the government had already been forced to give ground after Gordon Prentice's amendment to the Countryside and Rights of Way Bill had been backed by over 100 MPs, defying pressure from the whips. Officials of the PLP considered that in practice the renewed manifesto commitment to allow a free vote in the Commons and an early opportunity to express its view was an important step towards abolition.

Manifesto process

The NPF and the manifesto

Nita Clarke was given the job of ensuring that the NPF process and particularly the trade union input was taken account of in the preparation of the manifesto. Geoffrey Norris did the same for relations with the CBI. After all the talk of 'the members' party' and 'partnership' the CLPs do not appear to have registered much at all in this process. On the three radical issues said by Robin Cook, the NPF Chairman at Exeter, to have originated in the NPF process, two – on fuel poverty and free nursery places – were simply new timing commitments and included. The third, on loan sharks and predatory lending to the poor, was much more important – the kind of creativity in problem diagnosis that made the NPF's focus innovative and worthwhile. It could have been highlighted in the manifesto as part of the government's anti-poverty policies assisting the most vulnerable in deprived communities. But it raised fears of interfering in the market and disturbing the CBI and was omitted completely from the initial Nita Clarke appraisal of potential manifesto problem issues. After an internal protest, it was finally fitted discreetly into the manifesto under 'Supporting British Business' and at the end of a sentence after 'unfair terms in contracts'. It was easily missed.

The multiple problems involved in the campaign for an elected mayor in London, and the disappointing turnout, had the effect of reinforcing Labour Party internal criticism of the elected mayor policy and substantially raising public opposition. And yet it was at this time that support for elected mayors amongst its relatively small number of adherents around the Leader took on a further element of zealotry. Though the Local Government Act of 2000 had given directly elected mayors as an option, the manifesto became a blunt commitment: 'We support the introduction of elected mayors for our cities'. It was a position that neither the NPF nor the conference had ever agreed to and the electorate also proved unenthusiastic.

The union input and non-input into the manifesto

In contrast to the manifesto preparations in 1997, the TUC was heavily involved in consultations about the second term through David Miliband. There were also bilateral meetings with some of the union leaders. From the union side there was a strong element of sensitive pre-election restraint. On an anticipated information and consultation directive from the EEC, with pressure from European unions, the TUC side thought that they were heading the right way and agreed not to push a detailed position. The manifesto said that implementation needed to be 'appropriate to national traditions'. The possibility of a move towards a more explicit nationally organised social partnership was dangled by No. 10 with a flirtatious verbal reference to something labelled 'British Social Partnership'. But this was never given content and did not go in the manifesto. Another omission concerned 'fat cats' remuneration. Stephen Byers, Secretary of State for Trade and Industry, had announced new proposals designed to strengthen the link between directors' pay and their performance.[57] This had been heartily welcomed by the unions who had been campaigning against board-room greed and escalating salaries. Opposition from business led to a veto on the Byers proposal from Brown backed by Blair and the issue was buried. However, there was no reference to privatisation of the Post Office either – a union and party victory. And with the assistance of Nita Clarke the UNISON-pushed commitment, that the private finance initiative should not be delivered at the expense of the pay and conditions of the staff employed in these schemes, went in, as did the policy of statutory union learning representatives.

Manifesto meeting

As for the Clause V meeting itself, it had a larger than normal composition and was held on a very hot day in a room too small for the meeting and with no air-conditioning. There was a sense of acceptance and fatalism that 'this is what Tony wants' and even some of the more pluralistically inclined members of Cabinet accepted the line that 'We can't have an argument at the Clause V meeting'. As in 1997, loyalist members of the NEC were consulted in advance of the meeting and some helpful verbal changes made, but they were discouraged from regarding the formal meeting as an amending process. The agreement at Exeter, such as it was, and the bilateral discussions with the TUC were used to ensure that there was no sudden pressure from the unions. Only an amendment on miners' compensation was of any significance, consolidating various past representations from amongst others the PLP Parliamentary Committee: a ring-fenced £400 million to help ex-miners suffering industrial diseases.

One final development added to the generation of distrust and became a signal of extending the territory of 'serious politics'. With no warning, there was a change to the wording of the manifesto *after* the Clause V meeting. The document had committed the party to introduce anti-discrimination legislation covering age, sexuality, disability and religion. This reflected NPF decisions. But all this commitment had disappeared from the manifesto when it was published at a time when it was too late to do anything about it. A strong complaint was made later in a letter from the TGWU about 'a serious breach of the constitution of the party'.[58] That was not a consideration that counted much with Blair and his managers.

The personal penalisation of those involved in environmentally damaging business activities, supported at the NPF and at the conference, was ignored. In terms of the themes and issues which would dominate the second-term major discontents, the manifesto was far from a clear guide, with no mention of foundation hospitals but with a commitment *against* top-up fees. On the public services, there was a reference to giving patients more choice but no mention of markets and competition. There was nothing that would suggest intervention for liberation nor the need for further potential military preparation to deal with Iraq unless that was derived from the supremely ambiguous 'We need . . . to fight and keep the peace'.

Campaign spin and going private

Now there also came a pivotal development which affected party management and the mood of union-party relations for years to come. Even the day before the manifesto launch, it had been thought by experienced Labour Party watcher Patrick Wintour that the key message of the manifesto on the public services consistent with Labour's social-democratic credentials would be that salvation lies in extra funding.[59] A major problem had been that the government was spending less on core public services as a percentage of GDP than had the Major government.[60] In the middle of a hospital crisis in 2000, Blair had made a new commitment to raise the level of NHS spending to the level of that of the EU. That became embodied in increased expenditure plans for the next four years announced in the 2000 Comprehensive Spending Review. This investment would, it was thought, produce a clear line of disagreement with the Conservatives who emphasised tax cuts.

Yet with a close eye on the media reception, the manifesto also picked up from a policy document which had gone through the NPF, a reference to 'specially built surgical units, managed by the NHS or the private sector' which would 'guarantee shorter waiting times' and the use of 'spare capacity in private sector hospitals'. This had roots in the government's NHS Plan in 2000, but the NPF had expressed specific qualifications about private sector involvement in connection with clinical services, and a general turn to the private sector had not been part of the manifesto consultations.

However, once it came to the spin on the manifesto at the launch, an increasing private sector involvement in the public services was boldly and dramatically raised to centrality. Articles by prominent political correspondents Michael White: 'Blair goes private';[61] Andrew Grice: 'Like it or loathe it, Blair's "big idea" means more private sector involvement';[62] and Philip Webster: 'Blair orders the public services to ditch dogma and go private'.[63] This was linked to an IPPR report said to be favourable but later repudiated as distorted by Matthew Taylor, now the Director of IPPR.[64]

The spin was apparently Campbell's response to journalist criticism that there was little new in the manifesto.[65] The response was closely attuned to Blair's thoughts fitting into the attack on conservatism, helping an electoral strategy of pleasing the marginal Tory voter and soliciting approval from the business community. But in party terms it had a damaging effect which lasted as long as Blair did. Thus, far from the manifesto being a prelude to a new party consensus and more trust, this became a further provocation which undermined cooperation especially amongst public sector workers. It was noteworthy, however, that on the day of the second Blair election victory in 2001, in the markets 'Sterling was steady as a rock, gilts were unmoved'.[66]

New victory and new uncertainty

Blair's recovery

The closer the election approached, the more it became clear that the Conservatives had not recovered in public esteem. Blair, damaged by internal and public events in 2000, nevertheless gained now in contrast with the old discredited party enemy. The ballast of an element of renewed trust in Blair and 'New Labour' at this election was the government's manifesto implementation, its competence and especially its management of the economy. As the campaigning Brown told the PLP, 'nothing was more important than stability versus boom and bust'.[67] So it turned out, short- and long-term. That plus a passionate promise from Blair of more support for the delivery of public services had, Labour managers generally agreed, earned something like 'a second chance'. The second landslide produced a new Labour government with a majority which had dropped only from 179 to 167 and appeared as another major triumph for Blair and 'New Labour'.

(But see the further analysis in Chapter 16, p. 510 which gives a qualified picture.)

Landslide, social class and the unions

Remarkably, but well in tune with the 'New Labour' strategy, support amongst the AB and C1 social category of voters had actually risen by 3 per cent in each. But, in the C2 category it had dropped 5 per cent and in the DE category it had dropped 9 per cent.[68] Also, perhaps responding to the message of 'New Labour' independence, there was no sign of the party's links to the unions damaging electoral support. The polling indicated that it was simply not an issue. In another development, Sheffield University research led by Steve Ludlam showed that union campaigning (under the umbrella of TULO) did encourage union members to vote Labour, and the unions did target key seats effectively.[69] In recognition of that constructive contribution, and in dialogue with Ludlam after the election, TULO succeeded in having its existence acknowledged in the party constitution. It was also a sign of the changing times that Mandelson, once more out of government, now argued that the link to the unions must be retained or it would destroy Labour's character.[70]

Reaction to the manifesto

This was a time of chaotic post-election changes in organisation and personnel within No. 10 combined with an element of confusion of purpose and uncertainty about what exactly was going on over public sector policy. Campbell admitted in his diaries that he got into 'a bit of a muddle' afterwards on the private sector public services policy.[71] The immediate response of one key 10 Downing Street official to the sharp words coming from critical union leaders, and to the anxious enquiries of loyalist MPs, was an astonishing admission. 'We don't know what it means. There is no master plan for anything. That's bollocks. We did not intend that section to be the big theme. It was the spin. It may be all wind and piss.'

Both Brown and Prescott are said to have quietly and privately distanced themselves from the spin. A few ministers, particularly Milburn, endeavoured to give substance to it in terms of more local autonomy and enterprise.[72] Blunkett observed deep uncertainty at a dinner with Tony and Cherie Blair and the new public sector ministers Steve Byers, Alan Milburn and Estelle Morris where they 'went all round the houses'.[73] Yet this policy was to become the major domestic crusade for the second and third terms and the cause of much trouble for the management of the party.

Contrasts in polling

Early polling done for the unions suggested considerable opposition amongst voters about private sector involvement in public services. In June, 53 per cent of voters agreed that the Labour government was placing too much emphasis on using private companies to provide public services.[74] In July, only 11 per cent of those polled thought that bringing in private sector companies would be most likely to lead to significant improvement.[75] And in September, another poll indicated a likely shift of support of 8 per cent away from the Labour Party over private sector involvement in public services.[76] In contrast, in October, it was found that 68 per cent believed that private sector companies should be allowed to run public services 'if they can do so more effectively'.[77] This was said to highlight an overwhelming public pragmatism towards private sector involvement, and from this Blair moved ahead with the changes about which he was now a militant leader.

The 'end of control freakery' and the strengthening of the Leader

The reaction from affiliated public-sector unions to what was seen as spin-led policy-making and the adoption of unpopular private sector involvement was an intensification of distrust which fed into their party activity. It fused with other developments from which managers feared a possible future threat from within the party. That might arise from what was thought to be Brown's party network or from the party 'partners' using the procedures in the PLP and/or the wider party agreed in 1996–7.

It is generally believed that Blair's lack of action to move Brown at this time was the centrepiece of a failure to strengthen Blair's position after the election in the way that had been tentatively discussed in No. 10. It was also tempting to see the terrorist attack on the World Trade Centre on 11 September 2001 as the primary impulse to Blair's new turn to the practice of a stronger quasi-presidentialism and a new ascendancy over the party. Certainly alongside the domestic public-sector agenda it gave him another powerful cause to fight for. His impressive reaction to the attack boosted his electoral and party support.

Yet steps towards boosting his position had covertly already been taken. There was no master plan, just a close managerial attention to 'what Tony needs': a greater assured personal control over the party, a strengthening of his support, and the weakening of potential and actual obstacles from within the party. As will be shown below, the steps included the appointment by the Leader of a Party Chairman and with it the curtailment of the party role of other politicians, the attempt to rebuild a radical new No. 10 advisory team and the private assertion of the Leader's rights over party finance. Later came the new limitation of the potential PLP role in policy-formulation and then the evasion of a review of Partnership in Power.

The Leader's Party Chair

A new post of Party Chairman had been publicly suggested by Mandelson and Liddle in 1996,[78] and it was under consideration around the Leader for some time. Amongst the various reasons given for the post in 2001 was that he or she would be the voice of the government and the party to the people, putting over to the public the main campaigning and rebuttal messages – 'Minister for the Today Programme' was one description. He or she would also be a driving force for organisational renewal including financial recovery. But the crucial selling point to the party in 2001 was that the Party Chair, as known inconsistently until becoming the norm in 2006, would be the voice of the party in the Cabinet when policy was being discussed. The limitations of this scenario in terms of the Cabinet acting as a collectivity under Blair were not addressed. The NEC, and the party more generally, were encouraged to see the new post as part and parcel of a more receptive form of relations with the party.

Charles Clarke's appointment to the post was amongst Blair's first decisions at the commencement of the second term. Clarke immediately announced a commitment to 'the end of control freakery'.[79] The well-connected *Independent* political columnist Andrew Grice, feeding from Clarke, told readers that 'Mr Blair shares Mr Clarke's concern that the Labour Party could become moribund unless it is given more influence over government policies'.[80] It was now being put out privately by No. 10 that control freakery 'began when Tom allowed Margaret to do what she wanted'. Margaret and 'Millbank' now became a means of insulating Blair (and 10 Downing Street) from the odium of excessive control which had become an electoral as well as a party problem.

Advance discussion of the post had never been brought to the National Executive Committee. Since the party was founded, a Chairman and Vice Chairman of the NEC had been elected (in practice emerged by seniority) from its members. That was in the rulebook,[81] as also was that the person holding that office also became Chairman and Vice Chairman of the party[82] (increasingly referred to as Party Chair and Vice Chair). The rulebook remained unchanged for fear that any proposal to change it would be defeated or raise issues over an election. So now there were two 'Party Chairs'. By this stage, making rules by imposition was not an unusual event. Even so, this one was striking. As Anthony Howard pointed out, 'there could hardly have been a clearer or more blatant example of an *ultra vires* decision by a party leader'. Blair he thought had 'delusions of grandeur'.[83] But this was no delusion; he had much more instrumental purposes hidden away behind all the rhetoric.

There was a concerted managerial effort to create an acceptance of the Leader's appointment and, as with other elements of the rolling coup, ignore the rulebook. It helped receptivity to the new post that Clarke promised members' genuine policy-making.[84] What he did not say was that playing his major unidentified role as Party Chair he was, as senior party manager, expected to ensure delivery of the policy that the Leader wanted. This remained hidden behind the clever theme of 'the end of control freakery' and 'a voice in the Cabinet'.

Stopping 'the politicians'

There was also more to this extension of the managerial coup. It was controlling what was referred to in No. 10 as the 'the politicians' in their relations with the party. Blair had known before the election what Brown reaction would be when he found that Blair would not be going for another ten years: Brown would explode and Blair at that stage did not know how to handle it.[85] He continued to shy away from sacking Brown or taking governmental action to weaken him, seeing Brown's huge capability and the value of their governmental relationship when at its best.

He saw also that taking action directly against Brown risked putting on the back benches a resentful opponent who, it was thought, was already operating a shadow organisation in the party. Mandelson later suggested that the reason why Blair never felt strong enough in the party to take on Brown was that the Leader was a Labour outsider.[86] That seems unlikely given what Blair had already done as the outsider. More plausible is that Blair's reluctance was enhanced by the new need to distance himself from a media search for heavy-handed behaviour seen in Wales and in London. Acting directly against Brown risked provoking an internal crisis in the party by the now discredited practices of 'control freakery'; that could be a potent assault weapon by Brown who might even welcome aggressive action against him.

Hence the party managerial coup was an alternative to a frontal governmental battle. In 2001, it was said privately in No. 10 that because of 'the competing politicians' in party headquarters, 'Tony needed a clear political leader directly answerable to him'. Bringing in a Leader's Party Chair had the advantage of building a party defence of Blair's supremacy against Brown all the more effective as Clarke and Brown did not get on. That was probably why, when he heard of the post and the appointment, Brown in Powell's words, 'had a fit'.[87]

The post was also a way of dealing with Prescott, which also was no small matter to Blair's aides, although not accompanied by the venom that affected personal relations of Blair with Brown. Prescott in the summer of 2000 had been seeking to get back more into a deputy role with less time on the departmental work.[88] Now, with Clarke's appointment, Prescott's hitherto protective informal role as voice for the party was diminished by the presence of a new officer given responsibility for speaking on behalf of the party but under the overall supervision of the Leader. Prescott was given his own department and Office of the Deputy Prime Minister in May 2002. Over Iraq later he played an important supportive role, but as Blair's policy on the public sector became more controversial, Prescott privately articulated his doubts and his position was seen as moving nearer to that of Brown.[89] For the moment the main development in terms of party management was that until the final stage of this second term, Prescott was squeezed and taken out of the dissident wider party managerial role he had previously made his own.

Changing the Advisors

Meanwhile, new organisational changes were brought in which had the intention and effect of strengthening the centre of government and enhancing the freedom of action of the Prime Minister.[90] Circumscribed by fear of Blair being labelled arrogant, Blair's aides were less prone to flaunt the language of presidentialism to journalists and observers, whilst where necessary boosting its practice. There was a new Delivery Unit and a new Strategy Unit. In addition, Andrew Adonis, a believer in prime ministerial rather than cabinet government,[91] became head of an enlarged unit now the No. 10 Policy Directorate. He was in tune with Blair's radicalism although he created a bigger problem for Pat McFadden later when he became head of the Political Office, and found himself working to policies initiated or affected by a policy team hard-of-hearing in relation to the political concerns of the party.[92]

In these post-election moves after the appointment of Clarke came significant change in aides with the temporary sidelining of Sally Morgan to the House of Lords so that Blair's old friend and adviser Angie Hunter could be given Morgan's portfolio enhanced in title to Director of Government Relations as a means of persuading her to stay in No. 10. In an envisaged triumvirate, alongside her were the chief of staff Jonathan Powell, and Alastair Campbell whose formal position was enlarged by becoming Director of Strategy and Communication.

As Blair told Campbell, Hunter's appointment would bring an angle nobody else in No. 10 had, of attention to 'the upper end of the middle class' constituency.[93] She was, as Hyman protested, 'the least Labour person in the operation'.[94] It would mean, as Blunkett noted, a diminished liaison with the PLP and the wider party.[95] Since 1999, Morgan had moved in response to the discovery of the huge problems of party management and was not instinctively impressed by unremitting unvarying radicalism. Some of the political sensitivities missing in practice when she was pushed to one side quickly became obvious. Angie Hunter left after only a short spell in her new job. Morgan was brought back, and, as it happened played an increasingly important role without any break on Blair's trajectory.

The party's finance and the Leader's power

It was not just over the appointment of a Party Chair that the Leader made important party decisions by fiat. With Angie Hunter's new designation of post went a huge increase in salary which Blair declared would be paid for by the party. Margaret McDonagh, still General Secretary at this point but near the time of departure, fiercely challenged his right to make these financial decisions. As General Secretary she was responsible for party finance and said so. But Blair drove ahead and got what he wanted. It was another significant example of Blair's lack of respect for constitutional proprieties and of traditional demarcations of responsibility. It also revealed a man with a proprietorial attitude towards supervision of the party's finances.

Managing the forums

The multiple purposes of the new post of Party Chair required an acutely difficult balancing act from Clarke (with initially no staff and no government resources). How these new managerial arrangements and 'the end of control freakery' worked out in practice will be introduced briefly here, covering each forum in the immediate period after the 2001 election.

NEC

The Leader's appointment of the Party Chair provoked considerable resentment particularly as it appeared later that only Maggie Jones, the NEC's elected chair from October, was kept informed of what was happening. Why then was it accepted by the NEC? Part of the answer was that it was Blair's politics revisited. Bounce them, look to loyalists for hard-core support and in effect challenge others to repudiate you and damage the government. Jones, with Wall the Vice Chair and next-in-line, were as usual very cooperative. They even rang round to smooth down the situation. Reassurance was given that 'He won't be interfering in the NEC'. As for the title of Party Chairman or Chair, the NEC was urged by Blair and Clarke to focus on the beneficial role, not the title. It was said that he was to be given that title because they could not think of another more suitable. Of course they never did. In any case – and this was the most important factor – as he toured the party, Clarke came across as a breath of fresh air in terms of openness, free debate and his potent critique of control freakery. He did seem more like the party's voice.

He was also in various ways ideal for the job, having lived through the experience of being an outsider to the Blair regime and a critic of the 1994 party management, noted in Chapter 12 (see p. 371). He was aware of growing public and party disenchantment with the style of political leadership and management epitomised by Blair and Brown. London Region officials were particularly famous or notorious for their attempts at assiduous control of the party. When they were told by Clarke, in 2001, that there was to be more open debate it is said by those close to the event that jaws dropped. On the other hand, Clarke now in effect chose the new General Secretary, a trade union leader from the education sector, David Triesman. In the interview for this post the NEC was at first told they could not ask questions, then allowed to ask just one. It was one of several features that, as will be illustrated in Chapter 16, did not quite fit the new rhetoric.

On an NEC away-day on 9 October, held to examine party processes, there was a new mood of openness and liberality. There were also some private attempts by the more reform-minded party officials in headquarters to build greater party confidence in party selections – including proposals for more independent scrutiny. Some officials even talked about 'the end of the war room mentality'. Yet none of this happened, no concession was made by the officers to rebuilding the NEC's own policy role in Partnership in Power and there was no open discussion of the politics of party management, why it had arisen and what its limits might be in terms of control. In general this still remained the love that dared not speak its name. Charles Clarke did at one stage in 2002 half-attempt it. 'Political fixes will not work if they are seen to have been imposed; openness is the key'.[96] But that was all.

NPF

At the first NPF in July, there was a 'fresh start' theme to the contribution from the new Party Chair and a passionately impressive speech from David Triesman, the new General Secretary, which emphasised the involvement of party members and the importance of debate. It was followed by an amazing procedural session examining the experience of Partnership in Power, in ways that said much about the oppressive culture of Blair's party management in what had been under Smith a beacon of deliberative democracy. Only now was it clear at the NPF how many grievances had remained unaired over the party's involvement in policy-making under Partnership in Power, as representative after representative poured out heartfelt criticism of one feature after another.

Ian McCartney on the platform joined in, adding a knowledgeable summation of the problems. 'How wonderful it is to be able to say these things', exclaimed one forum member who had said her piece. All this had the happy effect of encouraging the acceptance of a new dawn which included the post of Party Chair. It also probably preserved, even inspired, the continued commitment of the representatives of both CLPs and unions to the principles of a partnership in power even though, as the General Secretary of the Fabian Society noted, it was 'almost universally regarded by the membership as a sham . . . hijacked by the party HQ at Millbank'.[97]

Another development helped overcome Clarke's lack of legitimacy. There did appear to be a new policy responsiveness by the Leader embodied in a small rash of u-turns and party-pleasing measures. Cannabis was to be downgraded to a class C drug, Railtrack was to be forced into administration, industrial tribunal fees were to be axed. All-women short lists were to be legalised. NPF members were even told by Blair that it had been their influence which had caused the leadership to rethink the whole issue of imposing student fees.[98] The immediate clear indication to the NPF was that, difficult though it was, there would be radical reform in tune with the party. Patrick Wintour's report in the *Guardian* was headed 'The Ministers are for turning'.[99] That proved to be optimistic or misleading. The turn to the party never came.

The PLP

Meanwhile, a new Chief Whip, Hilary Armstrong, replaced Ann Taylor. With the No. 10 Political Office and other managers, she was initially sanguine about the likelihood of large-scale dissidence in the PLP. Allowing individual MPs more time in their constituencies on local campaigning would still mean that there would be a reduced but regular government majority of around 50, rather than the formal majority of 161. But this anticipation had to be recast in the light of events in the PLP, reported by one of the whips to Cowley as 'they came back in the most foul mood'.[100]

This description could be taken to indicate a psychological condition, even an irrational spasm. That was how Blair saw it, as the Campbell diaries later revealed. It was 'unbelievable . . . what's there to complain about?'[101] It was very believable, built on the longer-term view that he and his aides did not listen and now by a heavy political reaction to the central campaign message of bringing in the private sector to reform public services, with total lack of advance consultation with the party. The post-election Parliamentary Committee as well as the PLP meeting with Blair on 27 June poured out this criticism of policy and called for more consultation and less imposition.

The new political mood was identified early by Clive Soley, a shrewd observer of the political realities, who had considered serving another term but now resigned on 4 July rather than facing defeat. Jean Corston, elected as the PLP Chair with 183 votes, was from the soft left and had contributed to various important dissenting discussions on the future of the party. Although politically close to Soley in terms of attitudes to party management, she was determined not to play the high-profile public role of defender of the Government. Nevertheless, she was considered 'safe' and consensual and was significantly backed by ministers and Blair loyalists. Tony Lloyd, who was again seen as the focus for outright back-bench dissent, got a substantial 167 votes – another indicator of mood. In PLP elections to the NEC, the MEP Michael Cashman defeated Soley but, through Dennis Skinner and Helen Jackson, the PLP representation continued to have a left-of-centre complexion.

There was an irony that Charles Clarke's appointment now temporarily added to the ingredients of the new dissent. In the PLP meeting on 4 July, his frank emphasis on past managerial failings found a receptive audience and encouraged a new assertiveness. Robin Cook, moved from the Foreign Office to be Leader of the House, in a change which avoided for Blair a potentially problematic wrestle over ethical foreign policy, also saw a new opportunity and wasted no time in signalling that his view of modernisation involved an emphasis on a more assertive Commons and better scrutiny of the government.

As before, much could be learned from the back-bench elections to the Parliamentary Committee, where the results, announced on 18 July, came as a shock for the Leader and the Whips. In spite of the fact that the electorate included around 35 PPSs who were not strictly speaking back-benchers, there was a clear swing towards more assertive independents and critics. Elected to the committee in July 2001 were Ann Clwyd, Helen Jackson, Tony Lloyd, Andrew MacKinlay, Chris Mullin and Gordon Prentice. Still, in spite of all these signs, Downing Street managers and the incoming whips were confident in seeing no great problems in the PLP over plans to remove from their post as chairs of the foreign affairs committee and the transport committee Donald Anderson and Gwyneth Dunwoody. This was not an arbitrary decision by the Chief Whip; several managers were consulted and all accepted it on the assumption that it would cause no trouble. Even though there were some complaints over this in the PLP meeting on 11 July the list was accepted with a vote of 88 votes to 39 – another indication that, in its private votes and limited attendance, the PLP tended to reaffirm its party loyalty.

But the managerial action was a public-relations disaster provoking the *Independent*, in an editorial, to reconstruct a government election promise of 1997 into 'We ran as control freaks and we will govern as control freaks'.[102] On 16 July in the House, in the free vote promised by Cook, there was a fierce reaction to the whips' recommendation on the committee chairs. The whips' proposals were rejected with 125 Labour members voting against the government on one vote and 118 on another.[103] These rebellions of what were labelled with some irony by Donald Anderson 'the revolting peasants'[104] allied with votes from other parties, defeated the proposals and led to the production of a revised list. It also led to new arguments about taking this process out of the sole control of the whips, bringing into sharp focus a tension between two different perspectives on reform.

One view emphasised parliamentary identity and the other emphasised party identity. The former accepted a new pluralism which involved, in some spheres, sharing power with other parties in order to advance the influence of the Commons. The latter was suspicious of this development, viewing it as a way by which Conservative and Liberals could potentially limit, even subvert, the Labour government; that view proved a useful loyalty asset to the managers in responding to and guiding the reformist current.

PLP players and the new mood
Blair had become sorely troubled by the mood in the PLP. It had revealed some worrying signs of a potential loss of control and a challenge to his supremacy in policy-formulation. Ignoring the difficulties created by his own style of leadership, he simply saw 'the old Labour Party at its worst'.[105] His tone, as conveyed by Campbell, was increasingly 'I'm always right'[106] and he now 'constantly defined himself against the left rather than against the right'.[107] In contrast, around this time Steve Richards reported that 'CBI leaders are amazed at the number of times they have gone into

Downing Street with a negotiating position only to find that Blair has given them everything before the negotiations begin'.[108]

Given his new position on public-sector policies, his reinforced relations with business and his worries over the PLP encouraging the unions, how was Blair to deal with a stroppy PLP whilst still talking of the end of control freakery? One response was very familiar. After a Parliamentary Committee, Mullins in his diary described him as giving 'a good impression of listening'.[109] But there was a contrary and more decisive move discreetly afoot. On 24 July a subcommittee of the Parliamentary Committee was set up to explore future relations between the PLP and the government during the summer recess. It included all the major new managerial players: the new Chief Whip, the new Party Chair and the new Leader of the House Robin Cook, the new Chair of the PLP Jean Corston, the two new deputy Chairs Ann Clwyd and Helen Jackson, the Prime Minister's new Political Secretary Robert Hill and the PLP Secretary. They began their discussions ready to report when the new parliamentary term began. What happened on this report was remarkable even by the normal standards of Blair's party management (see below, pp. 495–6).

The party conference 2001

Meanwhile, in September, the atmosphere at the party conference was influenced by the heavy pre-conference public and private discussions about declaring war on the Taliban, who had a congenial home in Afghanistan. The atmosphere (and the management) following the terrorist attack on 9/11, and the huge support for Blair's handling of it, added to his stature and produced a general understanding with the unions to limit public disagreement. There had been limited policy-making through the Partnership in Power process because the policy commission process had been slow to be resurrected after the general election. Lack of resources but also a habit of mind encouraged by the non-activity of new institutions after September 2000 meant that the documents taken through the NPF in 2001 had never in detail been through the commissions. It also turned out that, effectively, the rolling programme ceased to exist.

The spin around the manifesto had further undermined confidence in Partnership in Power and now gave an extra and unforeseen legitimacy to a much greater input of contemporary resolutions compared with that of previous years – a move not to the liking of the managers but irresistible under the circumstances. Exhibiting the weakening confidence in the whole 'partnership' process came the evidence from elections to the NPF at the party conference that with 26 places to be filled 14 candidates were elected unopposed and one position had to be left vacant.[110]

In 2001 the CAC had consulted with the NEC on the principles involved over contemporary resolutions, following the problems at the 2000 conference over pensions and following also the pressure for the CLPs to have separate but equal rights to vote four of their submissions onto the agenda.

This meeting was uncomfortable. There was general agreement that the contemporary resolutions were a legitimate part of the process and had proved their worth over pensions as a safety valve. But, in repudiation of the role declared by the CAC officials in 1999 that it was also a means of amending PIP documents, it was emphasised that this must not 'circumvent' the PIP process. There was resistance from the managers, including a majority of the CAC, to having separate 4:4 votes by the CLPs and the affiliated organisations, but there was now an agreement to a weighting of votes to give the CLPs more chance of determining the outcome. For the moment there was uncertainty over what the formula might be.

As it happened, other considerations intervened. The long dialogue at leadership level with the major unions over regarding this as 'a war conference' involved seeking extra cooperation in ensuring no defeats for the leadership. Over contemporary resolutions this did lead to something of a negotiating process between the union leaders and the two new party managers Clarke and Triesman. Clarke as, in effect, senior manager, chaired the final internal managers' meetings and became prominent in the negotiations with the unions. He ensured that there were no defeats for the platform. CLP proposals for adding two seats to the CLPs' representation on the NEC (for Scotland and Wales) which appeared to receive majority CLP support, was defeated by union votes in agreement with the managers.

Unions fall out

There was an important tactical argument between two unions, the GMB and UNISON, over cooperation and the tactics of challenging public-sector reform. Neither was convinced by the claim that the proposed Blair reforms would protect the public services from a future Conservative government. On the contrary, they saw this as potentially easing the Tory path. UNISON General Secretary Dave Prentis had a carefully worded resolution on public services which, in tune with the mood of the unity war conference, was composited into deep ambiguity. By contrast Edmonds from the GMB was determined to wage a fierce war against what he regarded as unauthorised and indefensible moves to privatisation. He let their much sharper resolution stand alone. That stimulated a new managerial determination that the GMB must gain nothing as punishment for its intransigence. UNISON, in contrast, was treated with more accommodation as (within limits) it had been since 1999. Building on the manifesto commitment of 2001, that union helped encourage Charles Clarke and Employment Secretary Steve Byers to a stronger commitment that 'where evidence of a two-tier work force is found to exist we will take action to end it'.[111] Inter-union tactical recriminations over tactics reverberated for some time.

Meanwhile, a new asylum-vouchers resolution from TGWU had not been pushed to a vote by the union, but Blunkett the new Home Secretary promised a genuine review and later delivered on abolition. In encouragement of the new order Clarke elaborated on the implications. It had been right for the government to do U-turns on vouchers for asylum seekers and tuition fees after an outcry from its own ranks.[112] There would be 'no fixed outcomes over discussion documents'. It gave him new kudos as the voice of the party.

The central focus of the conference, Blair's speech, was widely acclaimed as he emphasised the power of 'the international community' in dealing with the Al Qaeda terrorist threat harboured in Afghanistan. The speech was described by Mullins as 'a minor masterpiece' rather than 'the usual verbless New Labour claptrap'.[113] But indicative here was that in an action-directed speech there was no mention of the difficult or possible criteria for intervention noted in the Chicago speech, which might apply to future conflicts. There was no Leader's question-and-answer session either. That, it emerged later, had finally disappeared with 'the end of control freakery'.

PLP policy formulation and the quiet counter-revolution

The subcommittee of the Parliamentary Committee reported to the PLP on 14 November. 'Giving the PLP a Greater Stake in Government' included a proposal which came from the No. 10 Political Office for individual members of the PLP to be more closely involved in the government's work by acting as 'champions' (later changed to 'sponsors') of particular areas of special interest. That drew most attention and suspicion after a leak which suggested that it was a plot by the whips to extend collective responsibility within the PLP. Amidst some slight fuss the proposal was accepted by the PLP but never properly took off. Over the highly contentious question of Labour nominations to select committees, initially, in the draft the stipulation had been that the recommendations be from the whips (the old system), but after pressure from the Parliamentary Committee it was altered to read that the recommendation be made by the Parliamentary Committee after discussion with the Chief Whip. The PLP would have a further opportunity to propose and vote on amendments, deletions and alternative nominations to the proposed chairs.

Then came the big move. Blair had let it be known privately that he realised that the PLP wanted more involvement. There was a surge of confidence around the PLP office that 'this time Blair meant it'. After a discussion between Howarth and Robert Hill, who had led the discussion on party management at the No. 10 internal away day, it was accepted in the PLP office that, in the light of first-term experience, the government was not going to operate what were now described as the 'over-prescriptive' arrangements laid down in 1996. On the basis of this being a signal of a fresh start, in good faith, they settled for another proposal which No. 10 thought more practicable.

The original standing order K12 had stressed 'that the Government knows and takes into account the views of backbenchers when making key policy decisions', and the guiding principle was said to be that 'except in exceptional circumstances, backbenchers will be consulted before major policy decisions are taken'.[114] In its place, a new standing order K12 made reference to following 'aspects of best practice'. It was said that 'Ministers should brief officers of Departmental Committees on major announcements as a matter of course', but there was no longer a reference to ministerial obligations in relation to the preparation of legislation. The practice of 'giving an indication of policy areas or delivery issues they would be working on over the next year and inviting departmental committees to submit ideas or papers or holding special sessions on these issues' was simply noted, not made a recommendation.

The extraordinary procedural feature of this change was that though the PLP Secretary came under pressure for a debate on involving backbenchers in policy-making, not only would this not happen 'until the changes are bedded in', but the proposal for changing the standing orders was not mentioned in the executive summary of the report given to the PLP. That was why, in spite of the resentment over the manifesto bounce over policy towards the public sector, and the 'foul mood' at the summer meetings of the Parliamentary Committee and the PLP, the changes in government-party processes on policy formulation were not met by a loud bellow of negative response, and closely watching journalists and academics made no report of it. They just did not know about it.

Sometime afterwards, important members of the Parliamentary Committee thought (or at least, said) that it had never happened. Amongst those who definitely did not know about that 2001 change was the multi-representative Helen Jackson. To the observer, from a distance, it might be regarded as an adroit and perhaps the most important extension of the rolling managerial coup.[115] It released Blair and the ministers from procedural obligations which might cause him a problem as the controversies built up, and it was around this lack of early consultation and potential challenge that there would develop so much resentment in the second and third terms. As for Blair's indication of realising that the PLP wanted more involvement, he had that kind of tactical reassurance down to a fine art. It meant only that he knew what they wanted.

The new receptivity and its limitations

At the party conference, a 'debate' on Partnership in Power featured one speaker after another who failed to articulate any of the criticism heard by speaker after speaker at the NPF – and made no request for a review. The observer could be forgiven for thinking that behind the new rhetoric, 'control freakery' was alive and as vigorous as ever amongst the managing officials who had become expert in organising a misleading impression at the conference. Only the speaker replying for the NEC, Margaret Prosser, managed to get some balance in her contribution.

For Blair, the significance of the 'end of control freakery' had always been presentational. As headquarters managers saw it, whatever the intimations of potential change, he would soon lose any enthusiasm for adopting a new model of leadership and management. He was simply dealing with the significant public problems that the more overt and heavy forms of control had begun to cause him. In No. 10 it was conceded that he had in the past said 'yes' to the more open ways of dealing with party problems but then acted 'no' when the pressure was on – or appeared to be threatening. It would not be the last time. Stringing the party along had become his speciality.

This now fused with the sentiment of many of the unconverted managerial defenders, including Blairite 'conservatives' on the NEC. The perpetual underlying anxieties which had shaped the managerial culture in 1994 lived on most vividly amongst them in the view that 'We won in 1997 on a controlled agenda with all features interrelated, avoiding open division and avoiding giving the hostile media any opportunity'. It was also the case that for hard-line NEC loyalists, a new liberalisation was also a potential threat to their own role. Clarke's rhetoric was regarded as raising dangerous populistic expectations.

As Clarke rode the two horses, Leader's control and more party freedom, – albeit with an increasing tendency towards control – there was still from him a genuine argument. 'The end of control freakery' was sincerely meant as a contrast with what had gone before. To the loyalist doubters on the NEC his response was 'Yes it is a risk. But the bigger risk is leaving it as it is.' Privately, his caveat was that if it did not produce the right outcomes then, as politicians, they would have 'to find a way through it'.

But defenders of the old order became regular voices warning privately of the managerial problem that might emerge. From them, No. 10 heard messages that reinforced all the old fears of the reappearance of the ghosts and monsters of 'Old Labour'. In practice, once Blair was pursuing a mission made more focused and urgent after 9/11, the forceful word coming down to the senior staff in head office was that there should not be any new powers given to the party. There might be some further change to a more receptive style but there was to be no loss of control. As the older management style got its confidence back, some managers inclined towards reform began to leave.[116]

Vanishing review

The party at large was not privy to this retrenchment but a suspicion of it emerged in the vanishing review of Partnership in Power. This had been promised for 1998 and 1999.[117] There had been a reminder of it from Matthew Taylor before he left Millbank in 1999.[118] It was alluded to by NPF Vice Chair Margaret Wall, at the NPF in November 2000. After the critique mounted at the July NPF in 2001 there was a consultative process in the form of a questionnaire. At the NEC away-day discussion in

October there was a thorough exploration of what needed to be done to create a genuine partnership dialogue, involve the membership and make clear that the leadership was listening. It was reasonable to assume that this was the start of vigorous review and major reforms to be given a further stimulus at the second NPF meeting in November.

In No. 10, however, there was now a growing apprehension about where the new more liberal regime might lead in the wider party, especially as at the CBI conference in November Blair announced that 'support for business', was 'a founding principle of New Labour and it will not change'.[119] Notwithstanding that only recently had Hugo Young reported 'in the public mind business now seems more like an enemy than the unions',[120] 'Blair's love affair with big business'[121] became reflected in a deference to business in policy-making where even some in No. 10 bemoaned later that 'being wealthy' was 'taken as proxy for wisdom'.[122].

Around this time also it was candidly admitted in the Political Office that Partnership in Power was 'an effective control mechanism'. With stormy waters lying ahead over the new domestic radicalism agenda and the form of the 'war against terror', concerns over conceding more influence to the party affected the second NPF meeting of November 2001. In managing this regime, Clarke was elected unopposed as NPF Chair and two committed ultra-loyalists, Margaret Wall and Anne Snelgrove, were elected as Vice Chairs. In a move which covered a bitter behind-the-scenes personal battle over Clarke's push for supremacy, the retiring NPF Chair Robin Cook proposed Ian McCartney as an Honorary Vice Chair to keep him involved after an attempt was made to push him out.

As the NPF began its meeting, the procedural session, which might have followed up on the changes proposed in the previous Forum, was suddenly pre-empted. An announcement was made that there had been strong representations that the forum ought not to spend too much time on procedures but 'get on with policy-making'. This was met with a sudden startling Monte Cassino roar of loud clapping from the centre of the room (where a phalanx of managers and supportive loyalists had clustered). It did the trick. A majority of hands went up for discussing policy, not improvements to partnership procedure.

The NPF was generally very responsive to remonstrance about not being 'obsessed with process'. Close observation of management activity at the NPF suggests that in this culture the only people allowed to be 'obsessed by process' were the managers when it suited them. Without announcement, it slowly emerged that there was to be no detailed review of the PIP process. According to a very uncomfortable senior CLP loyalist-manager, speaking privately in 2002, 'The review just fell off the agenda'. The NPF in which many representatives continued to provide a responsible, pliable and at times deeply frustrated component moved on in the old routine within its old managerial constraints.

Notes

1 The other voices here include my own warning to Blair in a letter sent via Murray Elder, then the head of his office managers, on 10 October 1994 at Elder's suggestion after discussing with him the problem of trust; a special warning about public reactions to strong leadership given to Blair's emissaries at the final session of the Party into Power meetings in 1997 noted in Chapter 7 (see p. 219), a letter on the damaging electoral consequences of managerial control sent in 1998 to the General Secretary, a letter on the drowning of substantive issues by procedural rows, sent in 1999 to a senior minister who became a leading party manager.

2 Memo from Philip Gould, written in May 2000, reported in *Guardian*, 19 July 2000 and with full details, 20 July 2000.

3 Nicholas Jones, *The Control Freaks: How 'New Labour' Gets its Way*, Politico's, London, 2001.

4 Clare Short, *New Statesman*, 7 August 1996.

5 Private conversations with Mowlem and Short over several years.

6 Data leaked from a Philip Gould memo, *Sunday Times*, 11 June 2000.

7 *Observer*, 21 November 1999.

8 *The Times*, 24 February 2000.

9 *Guardian*, 19 July 2000.

10 Ibid.

11 *Partnership in Power*, p. 5.

12 Tony Blair, *A Journey*, Hutchinson, London, 2010, p. 201.

13 In Ion Trewin (ed.), *The Hugo Young Papers*, *Thirty Years of British Politics – Off the Record*, Allen Lane, 2008, entry 21 September 1999, p. 619.

14 ICM/*Evening Standard*, 21 February 2000.

15 *The Times*, Leader, 24 February 2000.

16 Derived from extensive conversations with London Labour supporters at this time.

17 Stanly B. Greenberg, *Dispatches from the War Room: In the Trenches with Five Extraordinary Leaders*, Thomas Dunne, New York, 2009, pp. 230–1.

18 *Guardian* editorial, 30 November 1998.

19 BBC Radio 4, *PM Programme*, 1 August 1996.

20 Ibid.

21 *Guardian*, 10 August 1996.

22 Michael Foley, *The British Presidency: Tony Blair and the Politics of Public Leadership*, Manchester University Press, Manchester, 2000, pp. 235–7.

23 *Independent*, 11 May 2007.

24 Alastair Campbell and Richard Stott (eds), Extracts from *Campbell diaries: The Blair Years*, Hutchinson, London, 2007, entry 26 June 2001, p. 553.

25 Patrick Dunleavy, Helen Margetts, Trevor Smith and Stuart Weir, Joseph Rowntree Trust/ICM, State of the Nation Survey, September 1996.

26 Philip Gould, *The Unfinished Revolution; How the Modernisers Saved the Labour Party*, Little, Brown, London, 1998, p. 193.

27 Lance Price, *The Spin Doctor's Diary: Inside No. 10 with New Labour*, Hodder & Stoughton, London, 2005, p. 158.

28 Hugo Young, *Guardian*, 21 September 2000.

29 Lena Jeger MP, *New Statesman*, 5 April 1968.

30 Patrick Seyd and Paul Whiteley, *Labour's Grassroots: The Politics of Party Membership*, Clarendon, Oxford, 1992, pp. 50–9 and pp. 68–9 and p. 71.

31 Ibid. p. 109.

32 Anthony King and Robert Wybrow, *British Political Opinion 1937–2000: The Gallop Polls*, Politicos, London, 2001, pp. 181–2.

33 Leader Image, MORI website, October 2006.

34 Trewin (ed.), *Hugo Young Papers*, interview with Philip Gould, entry 7 November 2000, p. 673.

35 Gould, *Unfinished Revolution*, p. 246.

36 Peter Hennessy, *The Prime Minister, The Office and its Holders since 1945*, Penguin, London, 2000, p. 485.

37 *Guardian*, 20 July 2000.

38 Peter Kellner, 'Mo Mowlem and the Campaign for Real Politics – the Kellner/Saunders Index', YouGov, September 2000.

39 Peter Riddell in Anthony Seldon (ed.), *The Blair Effect: The Blair Government 1997–2001*, Little, Brown and Company, London, 2001, pp. 21–40.

40 Price, *Spin Doctor's Diary*, entry 28 February 2000, p. 198.

41 Alistair Campbell and Bill Hagerty (eds), *Campbell Diaries*, Vol. 3: *Power and Responsibility*, Hutchinson, London, 2011, entry 13 April 2000, p. 288.

42 Tony Blair, 'The Third Way: New Politics of the New Society', Fabian Pamphlet 558, Fabian Society, London, 1998.

43 Anthony Giddens, *The Third Way*, Polity, Cambridge, 1998; Anthony Giddens, *The Third Way and its Critics*, Polity, Cambridge, 2000.

44 Steven Fielding, *The Labour Party: Continuity and Change in the Making of 'New Labour'*, Palgrave Macmillan, Basingstoke, 2003, p. 81.

45 *Guardian*, 20 July 2000.

46 Price, *Spin Doctor's Diary*, entry 10 October 1999, p. 152.

47 *The Times*, 20 July 2000.

48 *Independent* fringe meeting, 25 September 2000, my verbatim notes.

49 Peter Mandelson and Roger Liddle, *The Blair Revolution: Can New Labour Deliver?* Faber & Faber, London, 1996, p. 49.

50 Blair, *Journey*, p. 480.

51 Trewin (ed.), *Hugo Young Papers*, entry for 14 October 1999, p. 623.

52 *ICM/Observer*, 27 September 1998.

53 Gallop/*Daily Telegraph*, 19 January 2001.

54 Roger Undy, 'New Labour and New Unionism', *Employee Relations* 24(6), 2002, p. 649.

55 John McIlroy and Gary Daniels, 'An Anatomy of British Trade Unionism since 1997: Strategies for Revitalisation', in Gary Daniels and John McIlroy (eds), *Trade Unions in a Neoliberal World: British Trade Unions under New Labour*, Routledge, London, 2009, pp. 122–3.

56 Alex Bryson and Raphael Gomez, 'Marching On Together? Recent Trends in Union Membership', PSA paper 2003, p. 44 and p. 62.

57 BBC website, 8 March 2001.

58 Letter shown to me by an official of the TGWU.

59 *Guardian*, 16 May 2001.

60 Maurice Mullard, 'New Labour, New Public Expenditure', *Political Quarterly* 72(3), 2001, pp. 310–21.

61 *Guardian*, 17 May 2001.
62 *Independent*, 17 May 2001.
63 *The Times*, 17 May 2001.
64 *The Times*, 25 May 2001; *Independent*, 31 May 2001.
65 Campbell and Hagerty (eds), *Campbell Diaries*, Vol. 3, *Power and Responsibility*, entry 1 May 2001, p. 605.
66 *Guardian*, 9 May 2001.
67 Alastair Campbell and Bill Hagerty (eds), *Alastair Campbell Diaries*, Vol. 3, *Power and Responsibility*, Hutchinson, London, 2011, entry 9 May 2001 p. 595.
68 Populus drawing from MORI data, *Daily Telegraph*, 11 June 2008.
69 S. Ludlam, A.J. Taylor and P. Allender, ' Indispensible Officer Corps or Embarrassing Elderly Relatives', Paper presented to the Political Studies Association Conference, 2002. Steve Ludlam and Andrew Taylor, 'The Political Representation of the Labour Interest', *British Journal of Industrial Relations* 41(4), 2003, p. 734.
70 *Independent*, 18 June 2001.
71 Campbell and Hagerty (eds), *Campbell Diaries*, Vol. 3, *Power and Responsibility*, entry 16 May 2001, p. 605.
72 Fielding, *Labour Party: Continuity and Change*, p. 214.
73 Blunkett Tapes, entry 25 June 2001, p. 278.
74 IpsosMORI for UNISON, 11 June 2001.
75 IpsosMORI for GMB, 10 July 2001.
76 IpsosMORI for GMB, 18 September 2001.
77 IpsosMORI for New Local Government network, 17 October 2001.
78 Mandelson and Liddle, *Blair Revolution*, p. 223.
79 *Guardian*, 5 July 2001.
80 *Independent*, 5 July 2001.
81 Rulebook, 1999, Clause 3c6.1.
82 Rulebook,1999, clause VII para 2.
83 *The Times*, 24 July 2001.
84 *Guardian*, 5 July 2001.
85 Steve Richards, *Whatever It Takes: The Real Story of Gordon Brown and New Labour*, Fourth Estate, London, 2010, reporting a conversation with Blair's friend Barry Cox, p. 77.
86 *Independent*, 2 September 2010.
87 Jonathan Powell, *The New Machiavelli: How to Wield Power in the Modern World*, Bodley Head, London, 2010, p. 150.
88 Campbell and Hagerty, *Campbell Diaries*, Vol. 3, *Power and Responsibility*, entry 3 July, p. 361.
89 Blair, *Journey*, p. 327.
90 Hennessy, *Prime Minister*, p. 486.
91 According to Foster, the Poll Tax was used incorrectly by Adonis as an example of the case for prime ministerial government. Christopher Foster, *British Government in Crisis*, Hart, Oxford, 2005, pp. 105–6.
92 Robin Cook, *The Point of Departure: Diaries from the Front Bench*, Simon & Schuster, London, 2003, p. 249.
93 Campbell and Stott, Extracts from *Campbell Diaries: The Blair Years*, entry 11 April 2001, p. 519.

94 Campbell and Hagerty, *Campbell Diaries*, Vol. 3, *Power and Responsibility*, entry 12 March 2001, p. 549.
95 Blunkett Tapes, entry April/May/June 2001, p. 258.
96 Unions 21 'Talking Points', quoted in *Tribune*, 1 March 2002.
97 Michael Jacobs, 'Minding the Gap', *Fabian Review*, Autumn 2001.
98 My notes.
99 *Guardian*, 30 January 2001.
100 Philip Cowley, *The Rebels: How Blair Mislaid his Majority*, Politico's, London, 2005, p. 83.
101 Blair, *Journey*, p. 340.
102 *Independent*, 13 July 2001.
103 Philip Cowley and Mark Stuart, 'Parliament', in Anthony Seldon and Dennis Kavanagh (eds), *The Blair Effect*, Cambridge University Press, Cambridge, 2005, p. 21.
104 *The House Magazine*, 1 October 2001.
105 Campbell and Stott, Extracts from *Campbell Diaries, The Blair Years*, entry 13 July 2001, p. 557.
106 Ibid., entry 17 July, p. 557.
107 Ibid.
108 *Independent*, 29 July 2001.
109 Chris Mullin, *A View from the Foothills*, Profile Books, London, 2009, 24 September 2001, p. 226.
110 Ann Black, NEC Away day paper, 9 October 2001.
111 Mullins, *From the Foothills*, p. 227; Charles Clarke, LPCR 2001, p. 72.
112 *The Times*, 15 November 2001.
113 Mullins, *From the Foothills*, p. 227.
114 Report of the PLP Review Committee, 1996, p. 2.
115 I received a discreet indication of the change sometime in 2002 but only received full confirmation of my suspicions about how it had happened nine years later, in January and February 2011.
116 These included two senior national officers, David Evans who left in 2001 and Andrew Sharp who left in 2002.
117 *Partnership in Power*, p. 5.
118 GS3/11/98, Review of Partnership in Power report 1998.
119 *Daily Telegraph*, 16 November 2001.
120 *Guardian*, 11 September 2001.
121 Ibid.
122 Geoff Mulgan, ex-Head of the No. 10 Strategy Unit, giving evidence to the House of Common Public Administration Committee, Answer to Q 74, 16 October 2008.

16

Distrust, management and the long road to Iraq

Leadership and management success

The covert managerial changes which followed the second landslide election victory of 2001 were a major triumph for 'New Labour' internal leadership and management, at least in the short term. Within the party, Blair had moved to a new position of security, control and policy focus compared with the internally pressurised and puzzled period around 2000. The 9/11 attack on the United States and 'the war against terror' also changed what Blair called 'the political calculus' and led to a further tightening of the concentration of power. In relation to Afghanistan and then Iraq, he became a war leader-prime minister relying even more on his close advisers Campbell, David Manning the foreign-policy adviser, Morgan and Powell rather than the Cabinet.

Standing shoulder to shoulder in solidarity with the right-wing President of the USA George Bush, he was a world-stage figure, much bigger than those around him in the UK. The war aims shared with the US and the domestic reform policies on the public sector were driven with fervour and ever more certainty. 'There is now a clear agenda for this government' Blair told the BBC, in October 2002.[1] It was an agenda which was already creating an increasing gap between him and the party's centre of gravity. Nevertheless his unwavering convictions were conveyed with, at times, what appeared to be a serene confidence, in one impressive public and party performance after another.

Cooperative trade unionism

The TUC role

Despite a deep grievance and a new cause of distrust over the behaviour of No. 10 spin doctors around the election manifesto, there continued to be a strong cooperative pragmatism in much of the union activities in relation to party management. And the TUC continued to be a moderating realistic force on the response of the unions to the disappointments of 'New Labour'. As Keith Ewing, a leading and often critical academic, acknowledged later, the government had 'brought considerable benefits to the trade union movement which had been empowered politically, industrially and legally', although 'not as great as the trade unions would have wanted'.[2] Access worked well with most government departments, although some were less accommodating in their working methods and attitudes. Relations with the DTI improved considerably after heavy criticism of its failings from Monks and Bill Morris in 2002.

With Nita Clarke keeping close and cooperative relations, and Charles Clarke, who had long experience of fruitful backdoor relations to the TUC, doing the same in the role of Party Chair, the linkage from No. 10 worked better with Monks and his deputy Brendan Barber than that with many of the Labour-affiliated union leaders. There were regular quarterly meetings of senior TUC officers with the Labour leadership. The Political Office in No. 10 became a subtle discreet backdoor influence over the TUC's public positions. At one point there was the beginning of a new informal advance warning system from No. 10 about oncoming problems, and in January 2002 there was the first one-to-one unaccompanied discussion between Blair and Monks. Relations with the Chancellor also improved following the inauguration of tripartite talks on the knowledge economy and productivity, which for a short period after 2001 brought the TUC, the CBI and the government together.

Filters and review

In relation to what emerged through EEC initiatives, the filters continued to be influenced by the CBI and the British government's attitude to limited regulation. The British opt-out from the working time directive was heavily defended. The information and consultation directive of 2002 was introduced in stages to 2005 and applied only to firms employing 50 or more workers. Over the promised review of the Employment Relations Act, the government view was that the Act was working well and there was no case for making major changes. In the new Employment Act, in 2002, minor changes were treated with a now well-developed 'ping pong' of balancing concessions between employers and unions. There were some small union gains: a clarification of the right of union representatives to make a full contribution in disciplinary hearings, a legal right to access union services, and earlier access to workplaces in recognition cases.

To the carefully moderate *Times* journalist Peter Riddell, this had the appearance of 'stringing the unions along'.[3] General Secretary-elect Brendan Barber joined other union leaders in declaring that the review was too influenced by business.[4] But given the clear message from Blair and his managers that the basic settlement was untouchable, the realistic view was that a heavy TUC campaign pursued through the PLP might rebound. It might further strengthen the alliance of the government with the CBI, and opening up closed issues from the settlement might even result in losses to the unions.

PLP trade union group

The TUC's restraint contributed to the fact that the PLP trade union group became much less of a significant presence than in the first term. It was partially limited by the fact that no one dominant issue excited a large section of the PLP as it had in the original battle for union recognition. The new push to the left, beginning to happen in union leadership battles, also began to fracture some of the earlier unity.

More important, there was also a very different interaction with the managers compared with that in the first term. Frank Doran as secretary of the group still kept close links with McCartney, who was influential and in close contact with No. 10 before he became the Leader's appointed Party Chair in 2003. Their relationship, a pattern from 1998 of taking up cues about what it was useful to push, now involved receiving the heavy message from No. 10 that re-running major elements of the Employment Relations Act was a non-starter. It was a settlement and that was that. Here 'the end of control freakery' appeared to be accompanied by more managerial control. Meetings of the group were not enthusiastically organised and they became poorly attended. At an important meeting with ministers and advisers, only six MPs turned up in support of the officers.

Achievable gains

In March 2002, Monks announced his decision to move from the TUC to become secretary of the European Trade Union Confederation, and was replaced by Brendan Barber with the emphasis on continuity. TUC officials and Unions 21, a think-tank pressure group which worked closely with them, continued to focus on establishing processes that built better relations and a productive dialogue with government and employers' organisations and on seeking limited but achievable gains. They saw Monks's approach, and a cooperative relationship with the political leaders, paying off in a well discussed agreement on education and training and over raising the minimum wage. This increased roughly in line with earnings in October 2002 and thereafter outstripped both prices and average earning until 2005.[5] By 2002, a sense of gains was also affected by the major expansion of public-sector employment.

Dissentient and distrustful trade unionism

Intermingled with the cooperative and restrained behaviour of the TUC there was another response emerging from some party-affiliated trade union leaders. The increasing source of acute dissatisfaction was the policy of more private sector involvement in the public services, a policy never agreed through the partnership procedures and now with increasing emphasis on markets, competition and choice over which the party had not been consulted. Because of the tightly focused drive from Blair and his views on leadership, seeking alternatives involving the workforce or a combination of the unions together with the consumers was never tried. In line with the attraction of strong leadership, the view in No. 10 was simply and emphatically, 'we decide the policy'. Given their view of the attractions of private sector vitality and an increasing accommodation with business, what they decided went remorselessly in that direction.

Not giving the workforce and the unions a chance to participate in problem-solving and the form of the solutions imposed by the government left some of the unions even more distrustful of where they were being taken. In the Political Office in No. 10, there was later a private admission that because reform could only work with the support and involvement of the workforce, the management of party and government policy on public-sector reform from its inception had been badly handled. And in this crucial period of the second term with the beginning of a shift in union leadership, there was no 'keeper of the cloth cap' giving effective union representation at Cabinet level. Prescott had not played this role on policy issues and his relationship with the unions deteriorated when he became involved in new tensions with his own union the RMT and, later, in very fractious negotiations with the FBU.

Changing affinity and its effect on union members

In contrast, down below, union members were reacting against what was seen as a move away from the ratchet of progress in the conditions of labour and towards a one-sided emphasis on the flowering of relations with business. In a survey in July 2002, 37 per cent of all those polled took the view that Blair 'pays too much attention to the interests of business and not enough to the interests of trade unions'.[6] Only 14 per cent took the reverse view.[7] There was survey evidence also that at the grass roots, support for the Labour Government was 'plummeting' in union branches because of PFI and what was seen as a lack of commitment to public services.[8] In UNISON the uncertainty of government belief in public sector solutions was eating away at the position of its strong segment of loyalists. That union and others felt new pressures from members for a change in the priority of their funding of the party, especially when they wanted to finance independent campaigning. According to the ex-TUC economic adviser Coates, TUC research had shown that workers wanted unions to be both independent and cooperative.[9] But polling also found that trade unionists favoured 'standing up to the Government' by 60 to 21 per cent.[10]

The unions, finance and party management

Financial crisis and TULO policy coordination

Within the party the tensions between party managers and the unions became particularly intensified under the pressures of a post-election financial crisis. In 2001, the election had to be temporarily postponed because of the foot-and-mouth epidemic and this added to the election costs. Margaret McDonagh had set up plans for a rise in affiliation fees from 2002 and for financial stringency including a move of functions from headquarters. But McDonagh, as always, was focused on the priority of winning and delivering the resources that the politicians expected. Neither the NEC nor the Trustees were in a position to challenge the outlay.

Only later was it realised that the party was in debt not for the expected two million pounds but what was found to be nine million pounds by 2002.[11] There were conflicting views on the cause of the deficit depending on whether the interpretation focused on McDonagh's expenditure or on Triesman's delay in dealing with rebuilding the income. McDonagh and Triesman disagreed strongly over this. In the view of a closely involved senior party officer the truth was said to be 'Six of one, half a dozen of the other'.

This controversy also involved the aggravation to senior union leaders that TULO's own money in the party accounts had disappeared with the huge party debt, without TULO officials being consulted. At the same time, the No. 10 preference for the new TULO Liaison Officer was rejected by the unions who had the right to make the decision. This was followed by a cold war between the General Secretary and the TULO office under its new young Liaison Officer Byron Taylor, after Triesman complained over the cost of the TULO office in the building. Eventually, there was an agreement to write off the debt to the unions but allow TULO to continue to use facilities in the building.

The government's lack of consultation on the new public sector policies was provoking some in the unions into a search for ways to lever more influence in the policy arrangements. As explained earlier, with assent from No. 10 in 2000 TULO had been involved in some policy coordination over the Exeter NPF but that in practice provided a basis for tighter management control. Yet it had also left in the minds of union leaders, Edmonds and Morris particularly, a view that union political coordination should continue independent of No. 10. To the chagrin of the latter, that was what now happening, with TULO under Byron Taylor proposing to re-open some contentious policy issues.

Threats and counter-threats followed which included that Blair would not be attending TULO (which had not often happened anyway) and the TULO union leaders saying that when they were meeting on their own, as they intended, they did not want Nita Clarke from No. 10 sitting in with them. Backing up the union definition of its policy-making involvement, in TULO's own constitution, the formulation of 'matters of common concern' had developed a bullet-point expansion to mention 'policy' amongst other matters of common concern. It was in Edmonds's words 'simply a recognition of the reality' after Exeter, but it was very unwelcome to the managers in No. 10 and headquarters.

Financial sanctions

It had been noteworthy to the close observer that in spite of the difficulties and conflicts between Blair and the unions since 1994, the union leaders had abided by the prohibition on threats of financial sanctions in relation to policy. Similarly they avoided threats of sanctions in relating to the voting in the Commons by sponsored MPs. But in November 2001 that appeared to change dramatically following a GMB Executive Council decision to reduce the union's affiliation to the party from 650,000 to 400,000. With it came an announcement that the decision was in protest against the government public sector policy; the union would be using the money to campaign publicly against the policy as part of the TUC General Council plan to campaign for 'better public services run by public servants'.[12]

Edmonds's private explanation was full of foreboding. He saw 'something really dark happening to this government' in the paths they were prepared to tread and the means they now used to establish 'policy'. A new dimension of distrust built up over the consideration that the direction of government policy development was making it easier for a future Conservative government to move further and faster on 'New Labour' coat-tails. This was denied by the Leader and his aides. It was, they argued, the way to preserve the public sector's ethos and its delivery. The linking of union money with policy claims infuriated them, and was also widely regarded amongst affiliated union leaders as unhealthy and unhelpful. It would give an opportunity for some in the political wing to open an argument over the union link on the worst possible terrain for the unions. A later correcting interview with Derek Simpson, the Amicus (previously AEEU) General Secretary, was quite explicit: 'I think it's short-sighted and irrelevant . . . because it's raising the principle that you actually pay for policies'.[13]

There was also concern that this would further energise ultra-left forces in the unions who were attempting to organise ballots of members to decide where their money should go, thus – it was hoped – swinging finance away from Labour Party affiliation. In March 2002 an unofficial conference of trade union delegates organised by the anti-Labour left-wing Socialist Alliance agreed to campaign for this agenda. In the CWU where Billy Hayes the General Secretary continued to fight this year-by-year battle against cancelling or swinging the finance, he now announced the cutting of a third of its affiliation over the following three years.[14] In the RMT, led by Bob Crow who was, unusually, not a member of the Labour Party, the GMB move encouraged them to a more militant stance.

The union wrote to its list of MPs whose constituencies were reviving development-plan finance, asking the MPs to confirm their support for key union policies or be removed from the list of financially supported constituencies. Concern was expressed by Opposition MPs that this constituted a breach of privilege. The judgement of the Speaker was that the information provided to him did not justify a reference to the Standards and

Privileges Committee.[15] But again, the fact that this issue had been raised at all was regarded by most affiliated union leaders as unhelpful, even though some of them were increasingly struggling with their own distrust of and dissatisfaction with the party management.

Public distrust and the anti-manipulative ethos

Responses to 'New Labour'

The distrust and dissatisfaction growing in the party-affiliated unions following the manifesto spin was paralleled by a changing and adverse public context in which 'New Labour' politicians now had to operate. In his introduction to *The Blair Revolution Revisited* published in 2002, Mandelson, continuing the 'New Labour' diagnosis that the problem of distrust had been countered by a shift from Old to New Labour, explained that 'the government through its actions has largely rebuilt the relationship of trust between the Labour Party and the public that was destroyed in the 1970s and 1980s'.[16] In reality, in the conduct of politics there was a growing distrust between the public, the politicians and the government. The major forces at work were not unconnected with party management, and they have to be covered here within a canvas which takes us briefly backwards in time and outside the party.

Although there was a continuing strong commitment to democracy, a general disenchantment with politicians and government was a phenomenon of most advanced industrial democracies in the late 1990s, but with major variations in the timing and pace of decline[17] and with idiosyncratic national factors also in play.[18] In the context of this study it is useful to separate out here some of the distrustful national factors in the UK and the form that they took. Philip Gould had diagnosed it initially in 2000 as cynicism coupled with fickleness born of the Labour failure to make clear the project.[19] Yet it had a rational and an indignant ethical element about the way that politicians, particularly 'New Labour' politicians, behaved.

An important starting point in understanding how this developed is the hope raised by features of Blair's unusually intense honeymoon. No peacetime Prime Minister had achieved a higher satisfaction rate than Blair in September 1997, which was above 60 per cent for 20 consecutive months.[20] His verbal commitments had encouraged the expectation that he was a different kind of politician determined to nourish a new straight way of doing politics. Yet, for reasons given in Chapters 4 and 5 and uncovered throughout this study, 'New Labour' management politics under Blair had involved in practice a covert culture which eased, justified and at times lauded skilful manipulation in a way which shed some of the constraints of the past.

Its implications for and extension to wider practice in British political life gave the behaviour of 'New Labour' politics and politicians an especially disappointing and disillusioning character. The spinning practices of media management and the behaviour of Blair and the party machine during the 'vote-fixing' battle over the London Mayor had fallen far short of the hopes that Blair had raised, and they generated among the public another perception of him. At a time when there was accumulating evidence in Western Europe of the influential role played by character-based evaluations in the public's judgements of politicians, the winning of public trust in British politics, far from being a constantly replenished task of 'New Labour' protected by the party management, had become seriously undermined in part by that management.

An analysis of Blair's 2001 election victory suggests that it was not a cleansing away of the adverse reactions to him which had emerged strongly in 1999–2000. Although after the election Blair was judged to be more trustworthy than Hague – 46 per cent contrasted with 41 per cent[21] – both were judged equally untrustworthy.[22] That was in effect an expression of a very diminished expectation of Blair as a new straight politician. Further, Labour's support had declined in 2001 by over two and three-quarter million votes and there was a huge increase in non-voters, with more than five million fewer people voting in 2001 than in 1997. For most non-voters in 2001 this was a deliberate act of dissatisfaction.[23] In BBC polling the low turnout was ascribed by the electorate to the belief that voting would change nothing: 77 per cent, and a lack of trust in politicians: 65 per cent.[24] Amongst the concerns of the non-voters was found to be that politics was 'too stage-managed' and politicians were 'more interested in getting across what they say, rather than engaging in genuine dialogue'.[25] Overall, one important academic analysis judged that this election 'may have performed the traditional function of bolstering trust but it still left the electorate in predominantly cynical mood'.[26]

Social change and motivation

An analysis of the response to the changing perception of Blair and 'New Labour' reveals that in spite of what has been diagnosed as a decline in agreed moral or religious codes,[27] the public consistently and consensually regarded honesty as the highest virtue of people and organisations.[28] Although it would probably be accepted that there are limits on the obligation to be truthful, research on Britain's moral values showed that people rated honesty most as a personal quality.[29] It was also the most important quality sought in a public leader.[30] This assertion of the value of honesty was an underpinning for the growing reaction to what was regarded as political manipulation.

In delving further into this response, it can be conjectured that a long-term contributing factor was the change in child-rearing practices which encouraged autonomy and self-expression. These values had become pivotal to some of the dissatisfactions of the age expressed in a resentment at disempowering limitations. This spread amongst a now more educated electorate which had diminished deference and weakened loyalist party attachment. It was not necessarily accompanied by a claim to participate in all decision-making but certainly it stimulated an opposition to the pollution of influences which interfered with understanding and whatever decision-making was attempted.

This was integral to a broader response. David Boyle diagnosed that from all classes and ages, a growing minority described as the 'inner directed' (people who defend their autonomy and follow their own voice[31]) sought to recapture the real rather than the phoney, rejecting the fake, the virtual and the spun.[32] In the UK a little less than half the population was driving a demand for authenticity.[33]

Academics writing in the *Journal of Advertising Research* had earlier reported growing distrust by consumers,[34] viewing the majority of advertising as more manipulative than informative.[35] In 2001 it was authoritatively acknowledged within British marketing by its leading spokesman that 'everyone in the communications business' was now faced with 'a fundamental decline in trust'.[36]

In commerce, that had led to a dual development with potential political significance. First, independently amongst consumers there was a new assertiveness in challenging the communicator and self-proclaimed experts, with consumers choosing to adopt word-of-mouth trust from people they knew rather than being reliant on advertising;[37] it became the common sense of effective advertising that getting validation from the word-of-mouth network was 'no longer optional'.[38] Second, amongst producers in the advertising industry, there grew a greater acknowledgement of the importance of honesty and social responsibility in their conduct. As leading brand consultant Mary Portas put it ten years later, 'nothing buys customer loyalty quite like honesty'.[39]

In politics, that adjustment proved to be patchy as the covert code of 'New Labour' management produced what became a contradiction between 'New Labour' rhetoric and practices. This was embodied in the various political tricks involving a distortion of genuine choice, produced by the loaded spin of political communication and the procedural mechanisms exhibited in the London mayor election. A strong public reaction was fed by traditional British ingredients of adherence to fair play and antipathy to the abuse of power.

There is also an insight to be gained here from the path-breaking study of Lying, by Sissela Bok, first published in 1978.[40] Her work had arisen initially out of worry over declining standards of truth-telling in the USA. When the study was reissued in paperback in 1999,[41] it coincided both with the controversy over the management of opposition to Livingstone's mayoral campaign and with anecdotal but respectable evidence in the heavyweight British newspapers of an increasing UK trend towards dishonesty and deception in different spheres.[42] However, in an illuminating new preface, Bok now noted a dual and counteracting international pattern. Although, thanks to the media's global reach, the public was made aware of 'many more lies' with disproportionate attention on the newsworthy fraud, corruption, cheating and the practices of deceit; she now also detected public revulsion and a reaction even within some of the mass media, and some societal and political shifts towards supporting greater honesty and accountability.[43]

It was argued later by Blair that it was the media who were 'distorting, manipulating, lying, spinning control freaks'.[44] There was much to substantiate that description, and a strong case was also later made by the journalist John Lloyd that behaviour of sections of the media had a corrosive effect in promoting disengagement and distrust.[45] But the media had a dual effect, with a second facet acting as the regular and informed agency for the deconstruction of political behaviour. A general movement away from face-value reporting towards demonstration of the hidden reality was noted at the time of the general election campaign.[46] That practice increasingly exposed and detailed the political strategies, tactics and mechanics of influence. From the first, some of the critical exposure was heavily partisan politically, but some of it was also founded on a real public-spirited alarm over manipulation.

This media behaviour was all the more significant because a large majority of the public expected politicians to behave according to a higher standard of moral political behaviour and financial honesty than ordinary people.[47] Sir Nigel Wicks, Chairman of the Committee for Standards in Public Life, judged that people cared more about standards now than they did forty years ago.[48] The existence of the beneficial and moral activities of politicians began to become more submerged in public awareness, or discounted against the broader movement of hostile opinion. Reprehensible manipulative activities tended to be anticipated more easily and found out more quickly as empathy declined for the difficulties facing politicians in seeking delivery of their promises.

Blair 'form' and reaction to manipulation

Although the adverse movement of trust in Blair before 2001 had been partially obscured by the general election contest with a distrusted Conservative Leader, Blair's 'form' before that election campaign made him vulnerable to later reminders of his past manipulative behaviour. Every manipulation that made an appearance or could be presented as such was used by unsympathetic media to confirm the darker characterisation of his role. Early second-term failure in delivery, particularly on the NHS finances, quickly became a target for accusations of manipulative deceit over promises made. The explosion in use of the internet and later of political blogging added to sources of information and misinformation, at the press of a few keys, giving new opportunities to find out what others were thinking. It facilitated speedy sharing of deconstruction, sometimes challenging the mainstream media and calling politicians to account.

At the same time, and partially in response to this calling to account, public representatives presented a new target as supervision of party and government financial activity became more stringent. The government and individual MPs found themselves with new problems of any shortfall in their behaviour as judged by the Committee for Standards in Public Life set up in 1994, the new Register of Members' Interests set up in 1996, and the Electoral Commission responsible for supervising rules on party and electoral finance under the Political Parties, Elections Referendums Act of 2000. A Freedom of Information Act was introduced in 2000 and came into effect in January 2005. Although to advocates it was a disappointment in its provisions, it now added to the resources of evidence-gathering by the savvy, opening up more hidden information.

Reaction to manipulation was not the only root of the growing aggravation and dissatisfaction with politics and politicians.[49] In particular, the bickering and at times rancorous style of the crudest form of adversarial party politics seemed to feed an unnecessary sharpening and boring repetition of difference. In partial tension with this was another important resentment, about the lack of real electoral choice, and of inter-party consensus on the European relationship and on immigration which acted as a restraint on the people's national democratic participation. And although British politics was relatively clean by international standards, there was still a deep suspicion that many politicians looked after themselves, seeking various forms of personal and party – rather than public – gain. However, the now ingrained suspicion of what manipulative politicians said and did produced increasing scepticism about the reception of much of what politicians of all hues said and did.

That included reception of the case presented to the public in terms of the qualities of the politician, the claim to competence and, especially later, of the claim to have delivered. It also affected expectations of the fairness of procedural management and innovation. Although for only a minority of electors did these developments produce total distrust of politicians, they created a much wider circle of distrust.[50] This was in effect the development of what can reasonably be described as an anti-manipulative ethos, contemptuous of some age-old normalities of political trickery as well as especially antipathetic to some of the modern practices. 'New Labour' behaviour was still affected in part by a view of the continuing ruthless manipulative conduct of the media enemies that it faced, but where that and the new normality of party management practices had now taken Blair's politicians made themselves the primary focus of media attack and the most subject to public distrust and disapproval.

The further undermining of Blair's reputation

Contesting the reputation for manipulation

For Blair and his aides, attempting to counter that distrust of their political behaviour proved to be very difficult. In his introduction to *The Blair Revolution Revisited*, Mandelson emphasised the importance of the move to 'New Labour' and its competence as an underpinning of trust, but also frankly recognised that they had been hyping more than they were actually achieving[51] and that media spin had fallen into disrepute 'through overuse or misuse, when in inexperienced or over-zealous hands'.[52] Yet though he declared 'trustworthy character' to be one of three foundations of 'New Labour',[53] he failed to explore why that character had been so susceptible to this and other features of political degeneration.

There was no reference to the distrust problems engendered by the operation of covert and extensive party management and the behaviour that went with it, not even to give a gentle warning of allowing this kind of behaviour to become second nature in 'New Labour' politics. Special and unanticipated problems had been caused by activities in candidate selection which gained public prominence as a challenge to the people's right to choose. 'Control freakery' had become seen as a major fault. The damage done in the party had included reducing members' enthusiasm to act as a means of authentication, testifying on behalf of trustworthy policies and personnel. Within the party, countering distrust ran against the now-entrenched methods of management control. Amongst the electorate, countering distrust came into conflict with not only the 'New Labour' reputation for deceitful spin but also Blair's association with the 'vote-fixing party' events, which lingered in various depths of memory. That reputation and memory permanently contradicted Mandelson's view that there was a deeper public faith that 'the government's instincts' were 'in line with public opinion'.[54]

In general, the managers were unable to publicly accept or even to appreciate privately the full significance of the clash between the anti-manipulative culture and the 'New Labour' culture which insulated against accountability and permitted sustained manipulative practices. These were seen as the realistic ways of serious politics. From what found its way into public awareness and suspicion, Blair now carried with him a rooted public disappointment about the contrast with what had been promised about 'a new politics' in which things could 'only get better' and the reality which denied it. He and Campbell both had 'form' as presentational manipulators. Both of them announced a movement away from spin, but that met the cynical view from the media that this too was spin. Campbell's diaries confirm that Blair was not so keen to move away from the practice. Blair pressed Campbell for 'more communication'; Campbell commented that 'he meant more spin, which is what we were trying to cut out'.[55]

The later candid view from Lance Price, Campbell's ex-deputy as No. 10 spin doctor, bore out the private testimony of party managers about the influence of Blair's leadership on their conduct, covered in Chapter 5. And it confirmed the entrenched reputational problems produced by the managerial culture. Price's opinion was that none of the people who worked for Blair 'felt in any way inhibited by the sense that he might disapprove of what we were up to',[56] and Price accepted that 'by the time Downing Street signalled that it wanted to play straight with the media, most journalists doubted it would know how to do it if it tried'.[57]

Part of the psychological problem of dealing with the distrust was also that the 'New Labour' managers had been very good at much of what they did, judged within a short time-frame and over a narrow focus. They remained successful in some of their major combined party and media operations, especially maintaining Partnership in Power under leadership control. Recently they had helped dig Blair out of the unanticipated predicament of the pre-election period and implemented the covert controlling procedural measures following the general election campaign. Not only had the media management of 'the end of the control freakery' been markedly successful but the change of the standing orders of the PLP and the conflicts surrounding the composition of the Clause V meeting had been kept out of the awareness of the party and media to a remarkable degree. These reinforced the residual confidence that their skills could help get the politician out of even the most acute difficulties and urgent situations.

All that helps explain why there was little indication from managerial private comments and behaviour that they appreciated that there might be a serious problem for the party and the public in a cultural 'New Labour' managerial predisposition to embrace and at times privately extol the virtues of manipulation in managing a problem. The daily grind of party management, inter-party conflict and media struggle had involved for them, directly or indirectly, a repeated acculturation into some of the routine dark arts. The culture also reinforced and operated within a set of power relations which protected an absence of accountability. And within that culture there was a current of admiration for the creative ability to 'get away with it'.

As a result, as one semi-disenchanted party manager described it to me in 2001, 'they think that they can fix anything'. Later, Campbell's diaries told of a private Mandelson conversation with Campbell in 2001 in which Mandelson had expressed his 'love' of Blair's 'deviousness, his selfishness, the way he is able to turn everything to his own advantage'; his judgement was that Blair was 'different class as a politician'.[58] Just as interesting was that Campbell did not directly contest that view of Blair's character, nor Mandelson's political values; he focused instead on Blair's warning of the dangers to Labour governments of issues of ego and personality.[59]

What that, and the activities of the managers analysed here, highlighted was that trying to change to gain more trust was in permanent severe tension with this other mental framework, educated into a harsh culture of obligation about getting the internal and external jobs done, attempting always to neutralise problems anticipated or rising from ruthless external enemies, countering potential party obstacles standing in the way of major goals, feeling free to exercise and at times delight in the success of manipulative skills. Within that framework, sticking to the straight and narrow was often regarded as unrealistic and a distraction from the perpetual urgency of effective action.

A very good day for management

The emergence of new developments and issues fed media critics and increased public and party distrust. One highly publicised event in particular had reawakened an association of Blair and 'New Labour' with the worst example of insensitive underhand politics. It concerned Jo Moore, a Department of Trade and Industry Special Adviser to Secretary of State Stephen Byers. She came to public attention when it was publicly revealed in December 2001, by a critical colleague in her department, that she had used her media-management expertise to put out an email on 9/11 describing it as 'a very good day to get out anything we want to bury'.

The sheer scale of the horror of the 'very good day' (which she may not have fully known about at the time the email was sent) and the association with 'burying' became to many in the party and amongst the public the apotheosis of heartless manipulation. Blair was said to regard her behaviour as out of character.[60] Mandelson agreed,[61] and described it as 'a parody' of government behaviour.[62] Yet her response to the opportunity was attuned to years of socialisation into the normality of 'New Labour' professionalism engaged in the 'serious politics' grapple with its enemies.

More than that, before Mandelson and Campbell came on the national scene she had been a pioneer of attempts by people around Kinnock to find ways for the party to deal with an at times unscrupulously anti-Labour press. In the 1997 election campaign she was the party's chief press officer, an insider whose perceptions, skills and friendships overlapped with those of the headquarters and Downing Street staff. Her predicament after the email was revealed became a micro tragedy of 'New Labour' attitudes to politics.

Blair and Campbell assessed it initially as the misjudgement of a decent person, a professional who had given great service.[63] Moore would therefore be reprimanded and apologise. That meant that there would be no dramatic dismissal which would give a concrete sign to the party or the public of Blair's sharp disapproval of this level of unconstrained manipulation. The solidarity they showed with her came to be seen later as 'a mistake'.[64] However, it must also be noted that this was part of a pattern. A contribution to the difficulty of changing public perceptions of Blair over trust was that a public repudiation with sanctions did not happen to anybody found to be involved in any noxious management behaviour at any time during Blair's tenure as Leader.

There was a second development with party management implications involving Moore at Labour's spring conference on 3 February 2002. It was a strong reaction from the unions to a sudden Blair characterisation of the important policy arguments over the public sector in terms of 'reformers versus wreckers'. That was seen in the unions as yet another typical managerial assault on them, with a spin which they located as coming via Jo Moore. This focus was denied in No. 10, who stressed that the Conservatives were the target. Campbell in his diaries diagnosed that the unions were as unable to resist 'doing the victim thing'.[65] But Campbell's diaries also showed that there had been a parallel attempt by the minister Byers via Moore to label the unions as wreckers.[66] And as journalist and media commentator Nick Jones pointed out, Campbell did not seek to publicly challenge the extension of the target to the unions.[67]

From a senior ministerial source another view later emerged that this 'wreckers' accusation had been a deliberate attempt to isolate John Edmonds, the leading internal critic of the leadership from the unions.[68] If he was the target it achieved the wrong effect, producing an unusually strong reaction from Monks who had recently become more optimistic about new relations with Blair. Monks lambasted the attack on the unions as 'bizarre', 'juvenile' and 'destructive'.[69] His reaction was one of acute disappointment, but was also a product of the years of damage to trust in the unions from Blair's media spinners. The 'wreckers' charge had now also further enhanced a sense of mutual alienation which affected headquarters management-union relations (see p. 532 below) and it further tarnished Moore who was, it seems, simply doing as she was told. Evidence of another internal conflict in the Department of Trade and Industry, and a new internal accusation about an attempt to bury bad news, led to Moore's resignation, together with her principal internal combatant, on 14 February 2002.

Getting back to being straight

In April, Campbell told Hugo Young that the government had changed; there was no more double counting and over-claiming, and they were getting back 'to the straight and narrow', after the problem of Jo Moore.[70] In an effort to find new ways to overcome the problem of public distrust of Blair, and to build better relations with the media, there was an attempt to facilitate greater public scrutiny and what could be presented as the accountability of the Prime Minister. In June 2002, Blair instituted regular prime ministerial press conferences. He also accepted an invitation that he had previously turned down, to give evidence to the cross-party Liaison Committee of Select Committee chairs. These were an advance in procedure and accessibility and always handled by Blair with consummate ease and informative skill. He could change practice in this way, but he and his aides could do little to counter the equation of spin with deceit nor to redress Blair's now deep-rooted reputation for manipulation.

In a new dispute about presentation, highly publicised by media critics of the No. 10 spin doctors, Blair was damaged in June 2002 by allegations that through Campbell he had made a 'presidential' attempt to steal the limelight in the funeral arrangements for the Queen Mother. This was angrily contested by Campbell but, after a long series of arguments involving the senior parliamentary official Black Rod, a complaint from No. 10 to the Press Complaints Commission about this media presentation of No. 10 behaviour was withdrawn by the government without public explanation.[71] The episode had added new ammunition to critics of Blair and Campbell and their abuse of media opportunities.

Blair's public reputation as a manipulator was confirmed in a report by John Kampfner using a *New Statesman* focus group which found that the consensus came down to two phrases: 'he's always up to something' and 'he's not straight'.[72] At the same time, in a poll conducted by *YouGov* for the *New Statesman*, 67 per cent of respondents thought that Blair 'twists things according to what people want to hear'; well before the Iraq action only 28 per cent saw him as 'basically straight and honest'.[73] By the late summer of 2002 Blair was again, as adviser Greenberg put it, 'crashing' on trust and hitting a high on arrogance.[74]

Blair had another problem. Although most voters and most party members still preferred Blair to Brown as Prime Minister, judgement of the Chancellor's successful performance contrasted favourably in the public eye with that of Blair in his office.[75] Behind what was seen as his impressive economic record, Brown's role in the development of 'New Labour' first-term presentational manipulation in double counting had been obscured. The presidential Blair and his media grand strategist Alastair Campbell tended to take on major public responsibility for all the manipulative faults.

New media target: sleaze

From early 2002 the media criticism of Blair took on a discernibly more critical edge as it found new targets which had party management ramifications, notably accusations of Blair's willingness to deal with rich donors without a sense of propriety. In February 2002 Blair had been accused of assisting Indian billionaire Lakshmi Mittal to secure a Rumanian steel company, a month after he had given the Labour Party £125,000.[76] This added 'sleaze' to the other challenges being made to the Prime Minister's reputation. As Mandelson pointed out, the combination of funding diversification, which included business donations, and the new transparency was an invitation to sleaze-watching.[77] Accusations of impropriety were inherently difficult to substantiate and it could be argued, as Mandelson did, that in every case investigation revealed that the allegations 'added up to nothing'.[78] Public opinion took a different view. Those in 2002 now judging the government as more sleazy than the Major government had risen from 12 per cent in January 2001 to 18 per cent in February 2002, and those judging it as less sleazy had declined from 30 per cent to 22 per cent.[79] The effect of sleaze on voting behaviour at this point was uncertain, but the accusation added to the sense of an untrustworthy government with something to hide.

Within the party, there was an acutely adverse response when it confronted the moral standards of some of those providing the finance. This

had been the source of steady criticism by the Grassroots Alliance representatives on the NEC since 1998. Now, in May 2002, it became known
that the party had accepted a donation of £100,000 from Richard Desmond,
the owner of the *Daily Express* and various periodicals with pornographic
content. In an illuminating revelation of what seemed like a 'New Labour'
moral vacuum, John Reid, a senior Labour Minister with, at this time,
no particular responsibilities in this area, declared that 'Labour would not
be applying moral judgements to any donors',[80] presumably referring to
Desmond's occupation.

The Desmond donation and the response from Reid caused a furore,
led by angry women at national level in the party. Under pressure to manage the situation, Triesman responded by issuing a statement for donors
which usefully linked donations to support for the party's aims and values
and affirmed that they donated without seeking personal or commercial
advancement or advantage. A committee was also set up to advise the
General Secretary on the ethical basis of contributions. On the new committee was the Party Chair and a range of party notables of high repute,
together with the chief fundraiser, Lord Levy. The committee was first
referred to as 'The Ethics Committee' and then 'The Funding Committee'.
However, its limitations became apparent later, including the fact that its
responsibility was one step removed from the NEC's management role
(see Chapter 21, pp. 740–1).

Delivery in the public sector and the problem of reform

By May 2002 Labour had met nearly 80 per cent of its 1997 election
pledges, according to a major research project carried out by the BBC.[81]
Initially that had not stilled the critical media and public reaction to a
failure to deliver on the big issues of the NHS, education and, to a lesser
extent, public transport. However, in what appeared to be economic conditions of stability and continuous boom, there was a new confidence from
Brown arguing for an increase in National Insurance contributions by
employers to finance the expenditure. This was used to help pay for substantial extra public expenditure and, following past disappointments, was
received enthusiastically by the party. A proportion of 65 per cent of the
public also regarded the increase in contributions as 'good for Britain'. It
was the best finding for almost thirty years.[82] A few months later, in 2003
a new system of tax credits rewarded taking a job and staying in work by
boosting the incomes of low-paid families. These social democratic commitments were a potential basis for the managers to find an improved party
and union receptivity and continuing public support.

The major difficulty in the way of this was Blair's now rigidly adopted
preference for the form of public sector reform and the management of
what appeared to those in the NHS as perpetual change. Those plus the
strengthening union critique of the operation of PFI and, linked to these
issues, the growing union reaction to manipulative party management began

to drown the more unifying features of the new public expenditure. This moved Blair away from less dogmatic reformers, putting him in increasing conflict with a majority in the unions and substantial sections of his party. Instead of party management becoming easier through union appreciation of gains made in the public sector, there was an increasing concern over the direction that he was travelling, a feature which became characteristic of distrustful second-term intra-party politics.

Blair, Brown and new problems of party management

Inter-personal party management problems also now emerged acutely at leadership level. In spite of, and perhaps partly because of, all the planning to ensure more personal control by Blair, he found special new difficulties with Gordon Brown. A long-term clash over joining the euro, where Brown and Balls were thoughtfully and ultimately successfully resistant against Blair's pro-entry view, caused considerable aggravation throughout the second term, although it did not directly involve the party. But the new differences between them over public sector reform did. Blair defended his preferred public sector solutions as creating more and better delivery and a principled means of attuning them to the needs and choices of pupils and patients. Brown had reservations about the emphasis on choice with its potential dangers to equity. He also sought to demarcate the boundaries of the market in the public sector, seeing No. 10 as the source of ill-considered interventions on this with a dangerous absence of principled lines.

In the eyes of Blairite managers, the reservations and resistance which Brown encouraged evaded his full collective responsibilities, adding discreetly and, at times, semi-openly to the policy dissent in the PLP, on the NEC and through the unions at the conference. In effect it now fed an implied licence to rebel into the burdens of party management. Brown saw himself as in the principled policy position and saw Blair's attempts to strengthen his own position as moves towards breaching an agreement that there would be a second-term transfer of the Leader's post. Blair and his aides did not accept that any such agreement had been reached, and were furious at the Brownite dismissive treatment of the Leader.

The disagreements raised sudden flurries of suspicion and anger, with each regarding the other as the major problem. The accentuation of party management problems was believed by some in No. 10 and the whips' office to be part of a process of deliberately destabilising the Leader's position. On 19 December 2001 Blair had told Brown that he was easily the best person to be the next Leader, but Blair was not going to support him if he felt he was being forced out.[83] For his part Brown felt that his experience of Blair told him that he could not trust any agreement reached with him,[84] and he kept up the pressure to name a date.

All this affected the broader party management. The weakening of Brown's position in the party as a result of the appointment of a Party

Chair, and his awareness that Blair wanted to get rid of him,[85] added to the justification for him to send out semi-public signals which would have party appeal and to be more obviously friendly to others who shared criticism of Blair. A close Blair aide saw Brown still 'organising his own machine within the party', whereas 'Tony doesn't want us to organise. We'll just have to get on with it'. Yet something had already moved in the machine; the 'us' and 'them' character of 'New Labour' management vanguardism had become further split into a clearer Blairite-Brownite proto-factionalism, with the vast majority of party officials encouraged into a praetorian-guard stance more clearly assisting the defence of Blair against Brown. It was a role famously judged long ago by the academic analyst Robert McKenzie (see Chapter 1, n. 2) to be fundamental to the framework of supportive power for the Leader, but historically, primarily carried out by right-wing loyalist union leaders, not the party officials.

Cabinet disunity, Party Chair and party management

There was also an unexpected twist in the situation involving cabinet conflict caused by Clarke's interpretation of his role as Party Chair. The constitutional convention was that all ministers had to obey the doctrine of collective responsibility, publicly uniting behind government policies, or resigning. Yet, seeking to legitimise his role with the party, Clarke saw himself as licensed to comment in the name of the party on the areas of work of his colleagues, conceding for example that sections of the NHS now offered worse care than in 1997.[86] He even intervened in Brown's most specialised area, casting doubt on the economic tests for entry into the euro.[87] Criticism of the inadequacies of his colleagues became an occasional media story that 'Clarke warns Ministers to deliver or else', arguing that government should be more honest about the differences of opinion between Cabinet ministers.[88]

This did not fit easily into the heavily policed media strategy and the role that Blair had envisaged for his Party Chair. Arising from differences of tactics and priority as well as Clarke's personal dislike of the new job, his relationship with Blair and some of his aides became very strained. The reactions against Clarke eventually became semi-public, with Blair being urged, anonymously, to sack the 'disastrous' Party Chair because he was 'shooting his mouth off . . . without toeing the Government's line'.[89] This led to an even more acute problem, never envisaged by No. 10. Clarke was speaking in the name of 'the end of control freakery' and at a time when the party's private polling was showing the continuing danger of being seen by the public as too controlling and arrogant. Clarke therefore had special legitimacy in 'shooting his mouth off'.

In October 2002, following the surprise resignation of Estelle Morris, the Secretary of State for Education, Clarke was eventually moved from the job he now hated. He was replaced by the much more carefully loyal John Reid. But some internal divisions at Cabinet level continued to feed into the media. Clare Short, who had a long history of independent aggression towards the spin doctors and controllers, became increasingly alienated by Blair's attitude towards the party, his style of non-cabinet government and the way that he was pulling the country into war with Iraq. From 2002 she waged a semi-public and at times belligerent public campaign against Blair's policies. Yet she met no disciplinary response. Blair had created a situation where a highly publicised martyrdom of a dissenter, mounting an accusation of more 'control freakery', had to be avoided if a new party problem was not to be created and if a retoxification of this aspect of Blair's reputation was to be avoided.

New management of the PLP

The whips and management

Meanwhile, it helped initially in stabilising management relations in the PLP that Armstrong, the Chief Whip, had a close personal friendship with Blair and with Morgan. In spite of the change in the traditional whips' address in Downing Street that was thought by some to be a downgrading of the whips' office, it developed new status in what was envisaged as a staging post in the avenue of promotions. The office was enlarged to bring in extra MPs who were loyal, helpful and likely to progress as assistants to the whips. The Chief Whip became a more influential voice in reshuffles and promotions than either Brown or Taylor, although, given the controversies surrounding reshuffles, that did not necessarily improve her reputation. Her aggressive loyalty to Blair became at times off-putting and reduced the sense that the whips' office was involved in a genuine two-way process. Towards Brown and his aides her attitude was that their disloyalty and disruption was making Blair's job and the management task more difficult. Others in the PLP worried that Blairite anti-tribalism and his 'I know best' style were no encouragement to the collectivism that traditionally underpinned party unity.

There was now a growing accumulation of experienced ex-ministers often openly attached to areas of disagreement with the government. Some were offered the career carrot that by cooperation with the whips they might return to ministerial office, but many remained estranged. At the same time the huge 1997 intake of backbenchers were now more confident of their role, their policy specialism and their ability to handle their relationships in their constituency, without the same reliance on the reputation of the Leader.

The highly contentious second-term issues of Iraq, foundation hospitals and top-up fees had not been in the election manifesto and the lack of mandate reduced the legitimacy of the whips' role as 'the corner stone of democracy'. Following 'the peasants revolt', the managerial consensus shared by the Political Office, the whips and the new Parliamentary Committee became that they were now dealing with a new breed of MPs, who were, on the whole, more determined to make up their own minds. In agreement with Blair, the emphasis at this stage shifted in the whips' office towards a more proactive, 'political approach', said to be engaging with colleagues at an intellectual level in securing approval of legislation and defending the Labour Government. The whips had to be more clued-up about policy in order to be more persuasive. They would also place more emphasis on the personnel function.

There was an acceptance in the whips' office that there was little possibility of introducing a harsh disciplinary regime, particularly now that the Leader's appointed Party Chair was proclaiming, with No. 10 encouragement, 'the end of control freakery'. A few months later this was reinforced by the furore following a highly publicised verbatim report of the Chief Whip vigorously attempting the dressing down of the Labour MP Paul Marsden, a dissident over the bombing of Afghanistan. Her remonstrance that war could not be a matter of conscience (in terms of the PLP standing orders) rattled around the national letters columns. Marsden became an open critic of 'control freakery' and 'intolerance' to a degree which even alienated some on the party left. Left-wing MP Alice Mahon defended the tolerance of PLP managers about dissent, arguing that 'rebellion is alive and well'.[90]

At this point, ironically, defending the government's tolerance became the unifying position. It further reinforced the inhibition against using managerial sanctions on dissidents as the idiosyncratic Marsden went off to the Liberal Democrats. Meanwhile, management was quietly strengthened in other ways. Armstrong appointed as her special adviser Fiona Gordon, a strong-minded official who had, for a time, worked with Margaret McDonagh at Head Office but also had retained good working relations with some from Brown's inner circle. There was an increased covert whips' office role in wider party management including that taking place in relation to the party conference.

New arrangements for appointment to select committees also helped, by giving the PLP a sense of having improved its position. By the time that this procedure had got under way, appointments had already been made and the only decisions that remained concerned replacements. The replacements list was now produced at the beginning of each session by a meeting of the Chair of the PLP, the Chief Whip and the PLP Secretary. The arrangement worked on consensual criteria of representation by gender, region, age and so on. Some left-wing members of the PLP, including Kelvin Hopkins and Alan Simpson, got on committees where they might not have done before. Overall the system was agreed by PLP officials to be working well, sometimes beginning in a different place but moving towards agreement. It had yet to be tested at the beginning of a new term.

Blair and parliamentary management

Blair had still not become 'a House of Commons man' in traditional style. He saw no reason to waste his time in the chamber just listening to the debate. He was rarely there except for Prime Minister's questions and he was disdainful of the older symbolic gestures adopted by past Leaders, which included chatty visits to the tea-room. However, his record of attendance at votes improved from 6 per cent in 2002 to 9 per cent in 2003.[91] And as his new media adviser pointed out in 2004, his statements in the House were more numerous than had been those of Thatcher and Major in a comparable period.[92]

Blair and his aides also recognised what needed to be done in terms of his personal involvement in PLP relations. He made himself increasingly available for meetings with groups of Labour MPs, especially on the big problem issues. His attendance and contributions to the PLP meetings rose to an average of five per year and his performance in these meetings, without notes and with what appeared to be a major element of spontaneity, was widely rated as very impressive. He was 'a class act', as one critical MP admitted; 'extraordinarily resilient' was the view of another regular dissenter. At difficult times his utter confidence over the direction of travel, his easy command over policy and his informal style carried a great sense of command. It gave the loyalists heart even though it could not conceal 'the deep unease' that people like Chris Mullin discerned.[93] Blair continued to be adept at drawing out the sense of appreciation of what the party had achieved and, in effect, reminding them how important it was not to damage and certainly not to lose him.

PLP revolts

Yet the policy gap between the government and its backbenchers, exacerbated by the re-emergence of the Blair one-alone policy-formulating style, brought an increasing tendency to revolt. Cowley and Stuart showed that from the General Election of 2001 to November 2003 – the end of the second session – 197 Labour MPs voted against the whip, more than did so in the whole of the 1997 parliament.[94] Amongst even the 40 new recruits of 2001, 23 had voted against their whip by the end of the second session. Another feature of the new propensity to revolt was the changing behaviour of a significant section of those who would have been categorised previously as loyalists. There were 43 who had not rebelled in the past parliament but had done so in this one.[95]

At the same time, the whips continued to have a problem of dealing with the Lords after removal of the hereditary peers. The next phase of Lords reform produced no agreement. Blair was not in favour of reform and his attitude made it unofficially obligatory for the whips to covertly deliver for him in the 'free' vote; the result was that every option was defeated. Still, the 1999 reform of the Lords had the effect of strengthening the sense of legitimacy of the Lords in revolts, and the Labour Party in the Lords was less cohesive than the other parties in the period 1999–2002.[96] In a highly unusual move, in November 2001 Lord Stoddart had been expelled from the Labour Party for backing a candidate opposed to

Shaun Woodward at the 2001 election. But as was the custom in the Lords, the Labour disciplinary system in relation to voting remained liberal and became a frustration to government whips in both houses.

New party management outside the Commons

The Leader's Party Chair

Outside the Commons, from 2001, the major managerial changes were the performance of the new Party Chair and the sharper factional definition of the machine as protection for Blair against a challenge from Brown. Little detailed advance work had been done on what exactly would be involved in the post of Party Chair, and there was no clarity about the relationship with the General Secretary. Triesman had formally the same terms as had Whitty, Sawyer and McDonagh, and his view was that the relationship between him and Clarke was an equal one. In practice, over political management, with the possible exception of managing the politics over Iraq, the Party Chair drove the game.

He and his second-term successors in this role were front-bench 'big hitters', and in spite of the claim that this gave the party a new voice it was normally an authoritative voice speaking for Tony. Occupants of the Party Chair were politicians used to being abrasive in hand-to-hand political combat, but their demeanour was more sensitive and less consistently confrontational compared with that of McDonagh. In addition, all worked closely with the No. 10 Political Office staff, especially Clarke with the Political Secretary Robert Hill. Clarke also linked with the Chief Whip and Chair of the PLP without treading on territorial toes. At the NPF he became the Chair of that forum also, and its chief manager. Despite the promises that had been made on his behalf, Clarke continued to be involved in all significant policy decisions around the NEC, and he chaired the party management team at the party conference. His strong personality, clever tactics and disassociation from the past treatment of the party helped stabilise control over the NEC where, as shown, the simmering pre-election revolt over heavy-handed tactics and control freakery had earlier produced signs of repetitive revolt.

In spite of some developing tensions with No. 10, especially over some of Clarke's public comments and over his relations with the unions (dealt with below, see pp. 532–5) it was in the nature of Clarke's appointment that when the pressure was on about big government policies he, and his successors Reid and McCartney, tried to find ways to manage delivery against, at times, a rising tide of opposition. Some managerial defenders of the role thought the Party Chair was a useful communication channel from the party to government, if only in the limited sense that at least somebody might be reminding other ministers about the party. But early in 2002 Clarke was complaining privately to Blair that he did not have a real say in the politics.[97] There was no prospect of changing any of the major policy positions that Blair adopted and that was not the point of the chief party manager's job – as was to be shown emphatically over Iraq (see below, pp. 542–3).

'The end of control freakery' but the preservation of managerial control

Acceptance that the leadership meant what was being said about 'the end of control freakery' was fed by some strong initial polemical contributions from Triesman as well as Clarke. On internal party appointments, although Triesman asserted his right to control them he agreed to consult the NEC on them. For a period, information, including policy documents and a report of the NEC meetings, was more freely available through a more informative website. There was more encouragement of emails to members who had registered for them. The rulebook was now placed on the website although not regularly, and the website was often just as partisan in covering internal policy debates as it had been. As Russell noted, head-office briefings did not attempt to express the breadth of opinion.[98]

The general media acceptance of 'the end of control freakery' was an impressive management story. Control freakery was said to be 'in the past', and generally the media stopped looking for it. In reality there was no major change in the managers' own codes and no significant change in attitudes towards rules. They followed, as before, what was believed to be Blair's real instincts and signals from his aides. 'This is not laissez-faire. We have our electoral strategy' was the judgement of a senior No. 10 aide. Following this, it was even said by one headquarters manager that 'to make this work, we need more management'. The covert managerial organisation was still run from the General Secretary's office.

Perhaps the crucial expression of limitations of 'the end of control freakery' was the reappointment of Alicia Chater (later Kennedy) as head of the office of the General Secretary. She had played that role under McDonagh, shared her confident sense of legitimacy and was a similar bold risk-taker in party management. She was not Triesman's first preference but she was the preference of the Political Office in No. 10 and of influential voices in the party machine. Her appointment created new tensions with Triesman and also signalled the diminished importance of the role of General Secretary.

Close supervisory links to Downing Street over the management of the party in this 'end of control freakery' period was preserved through an institutionalised series of meetings. On the Monday morning after Blair had held a Downing Street strategy meeting which included the Chief Whip, there was a tripartite meeting of Party Chairman, General Secretary and Political Secretary. Then in October 2002, the same procedure followed after Charles Clarke was replaced by John Reid as Party Chair. These meetings were always followed by a regular meeting between the Political

Secretary and the important party manager Alicia Chater. The defensive view in the Political Office was that they would have liked to play less of this role in the party but were drawn in by the limited experience of the General Secretary. But also, Chater's experience as a knowledgeable, skilled and at times heavy fixer was regarded as an asset to them.

The criticism of intervention in the Brighton Kemptown CLP, organised from the General Secretary's office over the 2001 NEC elections, noted in Chapter 8 (see pp. 242–3), was never investigated by party headquarters even though privately the intervention was confirmed. Routine intervention in elections by the central party machine was brought to party attention with the leak of a set of directions to party officials in a series of emails from Chater, beginning in February 2002 and revealed by *Tribune* journalist Barclay Sumner.[99] Following complaints from members of the NEC including Ann Black, the General Secretary was reported to be 'looking into the matter'. But according to Sumner, he received no enquiries from the General Secretary.[100]

As the hands-on manager who had to do the party delivering, Chater saw no difference between the pre- and post-'end of control freakery' conditions under which headquarters worked. Nor was there any obvious evidence that this was out of line with Blair's own view of what the politics demanded. It was said in the Political Office in March 2002, with a 'busy-man' implication, that 'Tony does not bother about the detail, he just wants the job done'. There was another way of putting this, as a bold senior official in headquarters did later with an indicative edge to his voice: 'He doesn't give a shit about how you do it as long as it's done'. On a highly unusual occasion in 2002, when pressed, a senior manager did say that Tony was 'very angry with the illegitimate process' of electing representatives to the National Policy Forum, but it is hard to give much credibility to that, given initial Party into Power discussions on this procedure, and nothing came of his anger. Indeed as will be shown there was an increased covert managerial boldness in intervention which made an appearance later in 2002–3, with no constraint from No. 10.

NEC management

Management of the NEC followed the same pattern as the changes driven through after 1998, uncomplicated now by the antipathies aroused by McDonagh. Sawyer's closest allies, particularly Jones and Wall, became Triesman's closest allies, linked closely with Nita Clarke from No. 10. Membership continued to fall, affecting the finances. In July 2001, influenced by arguments over financial stringency, the NEC agreed a shift to biennial NEC elections in spite of a two to one majority for annual elections in the replies to a consultative document. Financial reasons were also used to justify the reduction in length of the party conference by one day. Again, it says much about the subordination of the NEC that most of its members did not know who had made that decision, and learned about it from the travel timetable. Financial reasons were now given to join the Women's Conference with that of conferences for Europe and Local Government although, as Diana Holland from the TGWU pointed out to the NEC, it had not in the past been loss-making. The NEC seating at the party conference continued to be a source of tension as changes were made which implied their marginality.

In the NEC elections in 2002, being on the official slate was still seen by three of the incumbents as a liability. Robinson, Malik and Turner now did their own thing although they also received covert official support. All six incumbents were re-elected. The turnout was again low at 23 per cent, but it was higher than in 2001 when it had been only 18 per cent. Given the problems that the government were facing and the scale of revolts in the PLP and the unions, this continuity of the incumbents could be seen as a victory for the leadership and the managers, but the GRA was pleased that their candidates' share of the vote had increased by 4.5 per cent, despite signs of the increasing organisational weakness of the left in the CLPs.

NEC: policy and organisation

In response to the adoption of 'the end of control freakery' there was some pressure on the NEC for a greater policy role, although no concerted effort to recover a separate party channel upwards into the partnership procedures. *Foresight*, an interesting exploration of future development and problems by Matt Carter, the new Policy Director, was met with some scepticism as another way of going round the NEC, but produced a good introductory offering to the 2002 NPF, although it was not organisationally sustained into policy development.

A resolution by Mark Seddon backed by the GMB had in 2001 tried to resuscitate the NEC process of discussing policy resolutions but failed, as did the managerial attempt to establish a tighter prohibition. The more independent-minded NEC Chair in 2002, Diana Holland, made the ruling that it was a matter for her whether a resolution was acceptable but agreed that her decision could be challenged. This compromise reflected the depth of disagreement on the policy role of the NEC and it did not please the managing officials and the NEC ultra-loyalists acting as representative managers. They saw 'a problem' arising for management in the future, as indeed it did, as will be shown below over Iraq.

Elections and appointments

The highly publicised emblem of control freakery in the public mind had been candidate selection, especially of the Leader in Wales and the Mayor in London. Some changes here were encouraged, which would help neutralise the adverse image. European selections now involved members deciding, by OMOV ballot, the ranking of candidates. The 21st Century Party document in 2000 had re-asserted the commitment to OMOV in selections, including electoral college arrangements for all major selections – Leader of the Labour Party, the Welsh First Secretary, Scottish First Minister and, where these were directly elected, mayors in England. This measure was introduced in 2001, although there was a long wrangle stretching into 2002 over the role of affiliated organisations (see p. 534 below).

The problem of how to accommodate party unity with national autonomy was dealt with by more background discretion and less offence. In Wales there was acceptance that the incumbent Rhodri Morgan was doing the job well. The selection after the death of Scottish Leader Donald Dewar was dealt with without interference. In London, for the moment Livingstone remained outside the party, and his public success produced a different kind of problem to be faced later. There were no new ambitious Conservative floor-crossers seeking urgently to find Labour seats. The Prime Minister could now keep clear of high-profile selection controversy where his publicised interventions had caused him particular trouble.

In selections for by-elections in 2001 some alterations were made to the panel at the request of the NEC but, as before, an inner circle of 'trusties' was well represented as ballast. Some insiders said privately that the Ipswich by-election selections involved all the old controls. An argument ensued after the Ogmore panel failed to put the *Tribune* Editor Mark Seddon on the shortlist. Others, including Clarke, saw Seddon's performance as undiplomatic in relation to Wales having revenue-raising powers. There was an important proposal from Andrew Sharp, Group Head of Party Services with responsibilities for party organisation and public policy issues, that to give some major sign of fairness an independent element should be introduced into adjudicating on particular selections. This was eventually dropped after discussions between senior officials, the Party Chair and No. 10.

One further revealing feature of the limits of the end of control freakery was the limited rehabilitation of OMOV. It did not stretch to the process whereby CLP representatives were elected to the NPF even though the conference was drawing in fewer delegates, and therefore warped the representation from there even before the managers got to work. The delivery of a good outcome remained the primary criterion for judgement of 'what worked' as a procedure. The hustings were not revived and arrangements remained a corrupted version of what had first been established in 1998. Nor was there any revival of OMOV for the National Constitutional Committee or, more justifiably, for the trigger in reselection.

Partnership in Power and policy-making

In December 2001, as a concession under the new regime, the NPF had secured reforms of their representation in the policy-making process. On each policy commission there had been one NPF representative; now there were three, one each from the PLP, CLPs and unions. But still managerial guidance continued on a high level through the loyalist-manager links. Vice

Chair Snelgrove, working with the managers, added to her patronage as the leading figure in the loyalist group of 16–18 people. Loyalists gained all places on the commissions. The NPF officers became a distinct managerial entity operating with freedom from the JPC and, as before, with no formal procedures of accountability to the NPF.

An expanded Joint Policy Committee of 32 now comprised the sixteen co-convenors of the commissions (eight from the NEC and eight ministers) plus the Leader, Deputy Leader of the Party, the (Leader's) Chairman of the Party, the President of the Party of European Socialists (a minister), the Leader of the Labour Group of the EPLP and the Leader of the Labour Group of the Local Government Association (who was also a member of the NEC). This made the non-ministerial NEC representation nine, the ministerial representation twelve. There were again three NPF members who were from the PLP, CLPs and unions. But as there was no significant change in the role of the JPC, its political dialogue remained limited and its NPF arrangements activity was managed by the Policy Director and the Political Office in No. 10, this expansion of the committee was not of great import.

There were some efforts to change the format of documents to make them more engaging and more stimulating but they remained variable in form, and often flat and timorous. Charles Clarke had said that there will be 'no fixed outcomes over discussion documents'[101] and there was to be more encouragement of new ideas in the first phase. But always, the routine central thrust of the government policy on issues was a given starting point, and avoiding a clash with government policy was a priority. Some attempts were also made to improve the performance of the policy commissions with an exchange of information on best practice but, as before, much depended on relations between the co-chairs. Commissions varied widely in the way they worked and the relationships within them but they continued to be dominated by ministers less enthusiastic than others about sharing with the party. And some from the NEC were less assertive than others in pushing a party view. The health commission covering some highly controversial areas of NHS reform had long periods when it did not meet at all.

There continued also to be unsatisfactory linkage from the policy commissions to the membership. Though there was a record number of local submissions, the mechanisms of feedback and information were still very limited. Submissions could be read by commission members in the headquarters but emailing them out was resisted on the grounds that it was inequitable. Also there was the usual fear of revealing material to the media and a nagging concern over being swamped with work. The better officers read them all and could pick up significant points but in terms of dialogue with those making submissions, none could cope with the volume and so the failure of feedback continued.

Limited improvement in feedback took place through *New Forum*, a quarterly newsletter covering the process. The Policy Director Carter did try, within the mechanisms of control, to find adjustments that would make the process more acceptable. NPF officers were authorised to speak to the media in order to keep the membership better informed. In a significant reversal of the controlling practices of the past, addresses and telephone numbers of all NPF members were now made available to each other. There was acceptance of personal reports on the NEC by Ann Black on her website, and she sent out a continuing series of sensitive and scrupulous emails covering the NEC, the conference and the NPF.

NPF and government policy

The problem of government deviation from party policy was raised in acute form in the second term. As the second term progressed so it became clear that there was an obvious range of issues enacted in government which ran counter to National Policy Forum decisions. Helen Jackson, convenor of the PLP group of the NPF and an elected member of both the NEC and the Parliamentary Committee, at one point called a meeting of the PLP representatives to the NPF to discuss the deviance of the Queen's speech from NPF policy discussions, but this was held to contravene the 'moving on' culture and had little impact.

The deviance involved the government dropping of the anti-ballistic missile treaty, the introduction of faith schools and the abolition of community health councils, each of which were reversals of the policy agreed in the NPF. Health Service private sector involvement ran counter to what the NPF had agreed in connection with clinical services. There had been no mention of foundation hospitals in the document agreed at the NPF. University top-up fees had not been agreed – just the opposite: it was specifically opposed in the election manifesto. Despite NPF and much party opposition, elected mayors had become government policy but could not gain a momentum of public support. The scheme achieved notoriety in Hartlepool in 2002 when a businessman Labour candidate, well respected by Peter Mandelson and by No. 10, was defeated by a monkey-dressed football mascot. It was now said by Prescott and supported by the Parliamentary Committee that the policy had been dropped.[102] But Blair was not happy with the change and some of the more fervent aides were simply waiting to return to it.

Partnership and management

Charles Clarke, who had said 'I want party members to play a central role in shaping policy',[103] resisted attempts to give more facility for NPF decisions on contemporary issues, and there continued to be strong scepticism about policy-making amongst activists in the party. A shortage of finance had led the NEC in 2002 to agree that two cycles of documents through the PIP process be made into one. It meant that there would be no NPF votes on documents in 2002 and none at the party conference until they were all done together in 2004. Black and Snelgrove ran an impressive extra meeting at the Newcastle NPF in November 2002 (the first two-day meeting since 2000) at which it was said that the NPF was 'on trial with the members . . . given a last chance'. The network of CLP loyalists was not getting enough out of the process, especially the policy commissions, and they did not know how to express their independence without being disloyal. The normal way of expressing independence, it was said, was 'to shout or to write critical articles in *Tribune*'. But that was 'not the NPF way'.

Unions and the managerial counter-attack

In the summer of 2002, deeply hostile to the idea that policy should be swayed by financial considerations, and under the pressures of funding problems, also possibly influenced by what looked like a guiding spin about unions being 'wreckers', Clarke and Triesman prepared to go over to the attack. Around the two of them there was talk of a decisive change in government-union relations. Clarke had always been in favour of the government building better links to the TUC rather than the affiliated unions; his relations with Monks now became closer. There was also a consideration of various alternative party rules changing the union method of funding with any gap filled by state funding. Others who favoured even more radical reform also intervened. Matt Cain with Matthew Taylor advocated a £5,000 cap on donations that would include affiliation fees. It was a proposal that floated unhelpfully above the party reality; there was little exploration from them of the practical problem of getting a conference agreement for the change nor of the dangerous wider political consequences.[104]

The possibility of the sacking of Labour staff union members was now quietly being blamed by managerial critics of the unions on their lack of financial support. There was even a discussion within the national party machine of the GMB being blacklisted as a union for party officials. One party official deeply opposed to these moves saw this as a managerial attempt not only to drive a wedge between the GMB and UNISON over their members in the machine but also to extend this divide more deeply to public sector policy issues. Everything began to point towards a major and unprecedented crisis, financial and political, coming to the boil at a party conference where the unions, particularly the GMB, would come under fire, perhaps even from its own party staff members.

Ten days that did not shake the Labour Party

Contrasting perception

To the close observer, the conflict over party finance proved to be hugely illuminating about the unions and party management, beginning with what had really happened in the GMB. Following decline in union membership and political funds in recent years there had already been a general pattern of decline in annual union affiliation. To assist the party, the GMB had resisted automatically reducing its affiliation as its levy-paying membership declined. It turned out much later that the GMB Executive at its meeting on 17 July 2001 had not taken the decision to reduce affiliation on political grounds. It was advocated as reasonable financial prudence bringing the union into line with the TGWU. There was a separate decision to allocate £100,000 to campaign on the private-public issue. In the use of spin by his press officer Dan Hodges to give another meaning to the union financial decisions, Edmonds saw the union as simply responding to the methods of the senior politicians, as a means of 'giving them pain' in the attempt to make it appear less worthwhile for them to go down this policy road.

Clarke and Triesman, on the other hand, now saw developments in the GMB and more generally 'the unions' as destructive obduracy. They developed a total pessimism about the unions helping the party, even if it was on the point of crashing. Consequently, these two leading managerial figures appeared to cease looking for a constructive way to find financial agreement. Yet the historical evidence was that neither Edmonds nor the other union leaders were immune to a crisis appeal regardless of other differences. The GMB historical record was of responding quietly to the urgent appeals of different General Secretaries.

It was significant that whilst Clarke was getting bolder in this area a divide was opening up in No. 10 about the impending battle with the unions. Whilst some voices returned to the old battle cries, Tony Blair and some of his other political aides were not only becoming concerned at the worsening of the financial crisis but also anxious to avoid a fundamental political confrontation with the unions. The most influential voices around Blair took the view that such a battle would reach an unbreakable impasse at the party conference, thereby probably splitting both the government and the party. There was another well-hidden factor at work which only emerged years later. Blair was hardening his position on Iraq and not looking to cause an internal civil war with the unions whilst looking for support over military action.

At the TUC on 15 July 2002 the word was that the affiliated unions had dug themselves into a complete refusal to assist the party in its financial difficulties. That was the understanding also in No. 10. From my conversation with Byron Taylor on 16 July 2000 came an understanding of the unions' historic behaviour together with information on contemporary attitudes, both of which indicated that the union leaders could be persuaded unconditionally to come to the aid of the party if the financial crisis was so acute that it threatened the party's viability. It also became clear that the union leaders had not fully appreciated the scale of the financial problems. Made more aware of the finances, and also reassured that Blair himself was not using this conflict to push towards an engineered crisis, the union leaders, meeting informally at a TUC party that evening, became convinced that the crisis was being manipulated by the two senior managers Clarke and Triesman, in a way which was aimed at setting the unions up as the cause of all the party's financial problems.

Tensions with the two new senior officers were further exacerbated over differences in the implementation of the 21st Century Party commitments on electoral-college voting for choosing the Labour candidate for the London Mayoral election. With five options in front of them, there was an attempt by Clarke and Triesman to support individual member OMOV and keep the affiliated organisations out of these selections. On 23 July 2002, in effect, the senior managers Clarke and Triesman were overruled by the NEC voting for a college of individual and affiliated members and without a commitment to split voting.

Edmonds now replayed his old 'chair of the trustees' persona as union leaders began to plan their support package in avoidance of what appeared to them now to be a huge political trap. One notable upshot of all this was to firmly unite the public sector unions' leaders, including the partially estranged Edmonds and Prentis. Inadvertently, Clarke and Triesman became the agency of the unity which later solidified a new union counter-managerial organisation (see Chapter 17, pp. 563–6). On 24 July, at a hurriedly convened meeting of all TULO leaders, ten days after the crisis was seen as irresolvable, Morris led off by an appeal for them to play their historic solidarity role and save the party. One after another, the leaders spoke out in support, even representatives of the RMT and the CWU. So the unions enthusiastically agreed, without conditions, to supply an immediate grant of £100,000 and, in principle, to produce a larger package based initially on a proposal from Taylor to Triesman, involving increased affiliation fees with no reduction of affiliation. There was a repeated suggestion from the party side that there should now be a five-year package but this was beyond the possibility of union financial or political delivery. Otherwise the General Secretary was left to consult and then formalise the proposal for financial assistance.

So nervous were No. 10 and managing officials that in spite of its propriety the rescue might be misrepresented by the media that, at their suggestion, and with some reluctance on the union side, the whole rescue episode was deliberately not publicised. There were also some on the party side who feared the union generosity might result in an extension of their influence. This may explain why, in an extreme case, in an interview with Jonathan Glancey in the *Guardian*, Mandelson said that he remembered Jack Jones in the 1970s taking exception to Labour's transport policy and at one point saying in a meeting at Transport House 'We're the landlords here; we want it off the agenda'. 'This was', said Mandelson, 'a defining moment in my politics'.[105] Yet that incident was not recalled by any union representative questioned about the use of union finance for political purposes during the Jones era.[106] Nor did any word about Jack Jones or this 'defining moment' appear in the impressive biography of Mandelson by

Macintyre.[107] Though the now elderly Jones did not want a public battle, he privately repudiated vehemently the Mandelson account,[108] in line with his previous outrage at any question of landlord pressure.[109]

It did seem that, misunderstandings aside, this financial cooperation might be a potentially fruitful opportunity for a new period of unity and perhaps new 'rules' and protocols which would put the relationship on a firmer basis. But in Downing Street, the prospect of a change of that kind disturbed years of routine media strategy messages about union subordination, years of deeply embedded managerial attitudes towards control and years of development of an often contemptuous mindset about the unions. Again it was shown that mutual rules and an internal settlement were not on the 'New Labour' agenda for the union-party relationship. So there was little follow-up from No. 10 or headquarters officials. Everybody went on holiday. When they returned there was still poor liaison with the union leaders.

Impasse on major delivery: more boldness in management

As a result, on the eve of the party conference, a meeting of TULO that was thought would be fairly straightforward turned out not to be. Triesman's three-year plan presented to the meeting was rejected, not as a snub nor as leverage, although it was spun that the unions were 'playing hardball' with the General Secretary.[110] In fact the proposal as it was presented was regarded as over-complex. Worse, there was limited advance discussion of the detail with friendly union leaders. It was not surprising therefore that in the meeting rejection was led by exasperated loyalist union leaders, particularly Bill Connor from USDAW.

However, as a helpful final proposal from Morris, it was agreed to restart discussion through the party trustees and increase the affiliation fees immediately by 2.25 per cent per annum from January 2003. In a speech to the conference, Triesman stated: 'We need income and we need a stable arrangement with the unions, and I pay tribute to those union leaders I met earlier in the week who are working hard to make sure that we do get back to stability.' He made no reference at all to their agreement on the raising of affiliation fees.[111] This was in line with managerial reticence already conveyed to the unions.

However, there was also no formal rule-change conference decision on the affiliation rate. Later it was said privately by a senior party official to TULO representatives that it had been overlooked. Nevertheless, the rule-book that became operative on 1 January 2003 included the change that increased the affiliation rates, and it was duly reported to the Electoral Commission. In that connection it must also be noted that around this time a further bold development in attitude towards rule-making and the party conference had begun to emerge amongst senior headquarters officials, in discussions with TULO representatives. It was that constitutional reform, including varying affiliation rates, could legitimately take place outside the formal conference process. It was held that the existing rules gave the NEC, and in practice the officials through NEC authorisation, the right to take such decisions. Changing the rulebook on finance without conference authorisation may have been 'a mistake', as was claimed, or a continuation of the political reticence, but it also fitted this new managerial view and the precept that managerial skills were reflected in testing the limits of how far individual rules could be taken. The following year, as will be shown, a similar 'mistake' occurred.

Further moves on finance

That important issue will be returned to in Chapter 17, but at this point the big surprise was that, for reasons that were obscure even to Blair's very irritated aides in No. 10, there was no speedy follow-up from the General Secretary to initiate new discussions with an adjusted package to secure further union financial support. A short informal meeting in January 2003 which was, in union eyes, faced with similar proposals from the General Secretary, had led nowhere.

In another significant twist to the story, the general union response to the GMB and RMT behaviour in 2001–2, the party's submission to the Electoral Commission which defended the affiliated relationship, and the emotions behind 'saving the party', all had the effect of reinforcing the prohibition against financial pressure by leaders in relation to policy outcomes. The more amazing feature, given what happened in 2001 and early 2002, was that as will be shown later the unions through TULO did come up with a further package of two years of increased affiliation fees, and they did so in the middle of the acute policy battles of 2003 – again with no strings attached.

Managing the conference

Finance aside, the conference of 2002 had some very uncomfortable and distrustful undertones and some heavy managerial defensive operations as well as some intense policy conflicts. There was a continuing improvement in making publications available earlier, a CAC newsletter with more useful information on the mechanics and new attempts to reduce the time of ministerial speeches. That apart, the politics of this conference confirmed that, whatever was being said about 'the end of control freakery', the conference headquarters' management felt it right to keep a very tight hold.

The push to manage the CLPs was if anything strengthened. Regional political liaison work by organising staff, which had once been to some extent a matter of personal choice, now became regarded as integral to the job for all of them. The changes in party organisation after 2001, which had increased the regional staffing for electoral purposes, provided an enhanced resource in liaison work for the conference. The developing culture of delegates not sitting through conference debates was now further encouraged by the announcement of other party activities whilst regional liaison teams chased up only loyal delegates, when needed for votes. The practice of regional officials sitting in the delegation consolidated the process of socio-political pressure – what one regional official privately called the 'hassle', but critics of some officials saw as bullying.

Contemporary resolutions and PFI

With a change in the cycle of policy-making involving no policy votes at the 2002 or 2003 NPF, that left a gap in policy authorisation opening up more justification for the use of contemporary resolutions at the party conferences of 2002 and 2003. In the procedural conflict which had been taking place on and off the CAC and NEC over contemporary resolutions, a small but significant change had taken place. On the Conference Arrangements Committee, CLP representatives Cooper and Twigg joined Aitken in arguing for giving CLPs a stronger voice on contemporary issues, although there was no agreement on the 4:4 split proposed by CLPD. But it led to an important concession by the CAC in 2002 that if more than 50 per cent of the the CLPs voted for a subject other than one of the four chosen by the unions it would be timetabled for debate. There continued to be an attempt to produce managerially favoured subjects by officials giving unofficial encouragement for CLP delegates to vote for particular issues to be debated in order to avoid others.

A GMB rule amendment which would have precluded peers from standing in the CLP section was the first union initiative on constitutional issues under Blair. But other than this, the managers were generally relieved that the unions concentrated their priority attention on domestic issues rather than the looming problem of Iraq. Nevertheless ministers and managers were unhappy with a contemporary resolution moved by UNISON and supported by other public sector unions, calling for an independent review of PFI. For years, over PFI, No. 10 and party officials had carefully and selectively accommodated to the conditions of labour agenda and directed interest and debate away from the public-interest impact of PFI. Now the unions clearly shifted the argument on to public value fundamentals, over which they were unable to secure change through the NPF. And failure of attempts at ministerial intervention over the content of the UNISON resolution made it clear that union resolutions were now an inter-union arrangement, with the managers having little influence over topics or content.

One huge and unusual managerial misjudgement soured the atmosphere further. Pre-conference spin to the media included some unusually provocative boasting, which publicly drew attention to their instigation of supportive resolutions on PFI for the conference.[112] Nine almost identical motions on PFI were submitted supporting the government, and accusations followed from CLPD that in some cases no formal meeting of the submitting CLP had authorised it.[113] The official managerial view as usual was that that was up to the CLP; they had no time to police such things.

The UNISON resolution was carried by 67.19 per cent to 32.81 per cent. The NEC statement which simply noted the concern was lost by 53.62 per cent to 45.38 per cent. Amongst CLP delegates, the managerial argument for not 'putting off projects' or deterring investors and focusing on what was needed now in terms of hospitals and schools had more influence than the 'lack of competence in PFI' and 'burden of debt' arguments from UNISON; only 41.5 per cent of the CLPs voted for the union resolution; 57.5 per cent voted against.

Once again, the managerial spin focused on the CLP representatives' support for the government as an indication of strong support by party members. Spontaneously, and also primed by the managers, there was continuing criticism of the collective union voting by some in the CLPs. The heavier than expected defeat for the government stimulated private managerial mutterings about 'doing something about the block vote'. As for the response to the resolution on PFI, no review took place and it was simply sent to the economic policy commission dominated by ministers, and ignored. UNISON saw it as having the backing of the authority of the conference. Managers argued that it had no special status and should never have gone to the conference. It was a view that did not fit easily with the 1999 CAC judgement that such resolutions could amend second-year documents, but by managerial edict that judgement had now become null and void.

Party distrust and controlling the controllers

Meanwhile as indicated, in spite of the formal commitment to 'openness, transparency and fairness',[114] the managers' real code of conduct varied little from the early heavy managerial phase. The idea that the party officials might be regarded as civil servants rather than political organisers was still described privately as 'bizarre'. There were regular complaints of staff partisan involvement at the conference and over internal party selections and other decision-making.

In recognition of the complaints, the distrust and the proliferation in number and diversity of internal party elections, a series of discussions led to the Organisation Committee, chaired by Mike Griffiths, attempting to establish some firmer procedural positions that would underpin all future elections.[115] A new code of conduct laid down that, 'Party staff will not use or abuse their position, party resources or time in the process of an internal selection or election so as to further the interests of themselves or their personal preferred candidate(s)'.[116] Nonetheless, in a move which transformed the thrust of the document, under pressure from the in-house unions which once again under 'New Labour' had become the protective voice of the management, it recognised that party staff had various rights as party members. They were declared to be 'entitled to have a political life as party members' and 'to have an opinion and to express it'.[117] They also had the right to stand for public office and to be elected to local party office. The party staff were even entitled to attend the conference 'as delegates from their CLP, Trade Union or other affiliated body'.[118]

In an equally unprecedented development, it was agreed that party staff were entitled to stand for election to national committees. This presumably included the NEC. If so it was an agreement that past generations of Labour politicians and senior staff would have regarded as a deeply repugnant replication of Communist Party traditions, leading to the apparatus substituting itself for the party. The document's reference to unacceptable staff behaviour was couched entirely in terms of the individual employee. It made no reference to the fact that acting as a party manager on behalf of the leadership might well involve a regular partisanship and devious practices which could be viewed by others as an abuse of power. Party management was, yet again, a love that dare not speak its name, let alone place limitations on its function. In the event, although there were some potentially hugely controversial elements here, minutes of the Organisation Committee for 17 March 2003, but not the background documents, were circulated for the NEC meeting on 25 March 2003, and according to the NEC minutes were 'noted' without special attention being drawn.

Complaints about staff behaviour continued in 2003–4. NEC member Ann Black wrote 'sadly, the manipulation of party elections continues'.[119] But her calls to action were continually ignored by senior staff. In formal mode at the most senior level, they were still saying that the partisan intervention of officers 'doesn't exist. It's just a criticism from the left'. An official code of conduct which prohibited party staff from using their position, party resources and time furthering the interests of any candidate in an internal election was regularly reissued. But infringements continued, legitimised by the managers' own discreet codes of conduct.

Accord and the two-tier workforce

Not all was imposition and manipulation and not all moves in policy moves were away from union preferences. There was some improvement in managerial links with the unions after Charles Clarke moved to the Education department post in October 2002 and John Reid was made Party Chair. Gerry Sutcliffe moved to the DTI from the whips' office and became more free to play his past linking role with the unions. Ian McCartney was also brought in unofficially by Reid to help relationships with the unions. Pat McFadden replaced Robert Hill and became Director of Political Operations. He made an effort to strengthen liaison between No. 10, the unions and the party, although relations with the PLP was not given much emphasis. Working with Nita Clarke, there was a renewed focus, building on developments in policy since 1999, towards eradicating the two-tier workforce in line with the promises made in 2001.

This faced strong opposition from business and some resistant government departments. Nevertheless, in February 2003, they got backing from Blair and a major advance on what was on offer. New recruits to the private sector in the health service were to get the unions' preferred formula of 'no less favourable' terms and conditions. To this agreement covering the NHS was added a retention of employment clause by which workers employed under NHS PFI agreements were given the status of NHS employees. Polly Toynbee reported that it was 'the boldest the government has ever been in facing down business pressures'.[120]

The pressures diagnosed

In response, in the media once again, there were voices which said that financial pressure was the explanation. It was even declared that the deal would result in unions signing 'a 40 million donation'.[121] But, as we have seen, there were other complexities to party financial negotiations, and the two-tier discussions did not enter into it. It was also argued later that the threat of serious industrial action was a factor.[122] Perhaps so, but as shown, the issue had a long pedigree through party channels and for management purposes. Nearer the heart of it was that the issue had to be settled; otherwise it was going to overshadow every conference. It was also hoped that it would pull UNISON away from the GMB into a new ballast managerial role at the conference. But the NHS agreement still left the non-delivery of what the unions regarded as a commitment to an across-the-range prohibition of two-tier working. In any case, the search for new management-supporting alliance was now too late, given the build-up of antipathy to the ways of management, the dissatisfaction being shown in union elections, and the misgivings in the unions about the coming war with Iraq.

The road to Iraq

Managing and the value of success

Blair was almost invariably an impressive communicator, and that facility developed further after 9/11 as a new passion entered his contributions. That being said, it remained the case that the assumptions and predispositions of party tactical management and its code of behaviour were essential elements of the repertoire of important political skills taken by Blair and his managers into the management of winning party support for his Iraq policy. Once committed to staying close to the US President in tackling Saddam Hussein, it had become essential for Blair to find means of producing room for manoeuvre and a degree of insulation in relation to the war policy.

Over and above the international policy cause on which Blair felt passionately, there was much to be gained simply in terms of Blair's future premiership and party leadership. As war with Iraq came close, some of

Blair's closest advisers and friends could fantasise about what would be achieved by him and for him, through success in the war. Victory would be followed by a public reception reminiscent of the welcome given to the fleet returning from the Falklands. Blair's emulation of Thatcher as war leader would have stolen a policy march on the Conservatives' political territory. His international reputation would be enhanced and his role as closest ally and hero of the US would be secure. The more hawkish of his office politicians and back-bench allies could share privately, with rising voice and particular relish, the thought of how a strengthened Tony with huge party backing would settle accounts with those around him who had not given full cooperation and loyalty. The Leader would then be in a truly supreme position. It would be Blair's liberation from party frustrations as well as Iraq's liberation from Saddam.

In winning over the party, a willingness to use force against Saddam Hussein could draw strength from its traditional hostility to tyranny and its respect for the UN whose decisions Saddam had failed to follow. The special Blair emphasis was on the capacity of the Iraq leader to use weapons of mass destruction and/or pass on that capacity to international terrorists. It also focused on the benefits to the people of Iraq from disarming a tyrannical leader. Blair drew authority from his personal diplomatic success over Northern Ireland and his lead in the military success over Kosovo. But public opposition to a war was intense and increasing, as was the opposition in the party. That came from suspicion of the aims of a US-led war and also not so much from the pacifist tradition but from the same values which had driven the party during the Suez Crisis of 1956 – law not war; if forces proved necessary it must be multilateral, acting against a clear threat and carried out after specific authorisation through the UN. These party views were generally shared by a majority of members and public opinion. Holding the party voice in check was therefore not only a managerial priority in restricting its influence over its parliamentary representatives but also in curbing the alternative party voice to members and particularly the electorate.

Management of the party involved the attempt to control information and discussion and the use of agenda mechanisms in each authoritative forum of the wider party: the NPF, the NEC and the party conference. The forums interacted with each other and influenced the wider party membership. The tactics of managerial operation were, as usual, not to be regarded as a challenge to integrity but as a serious pursuit of moral ends. And the striking feature here epitomised two general patterns already covered in other activities. As illustrated, the party officials as self-defined 'political organisers' performed their managerial role according to a code which gave them room for the exercise of more power, even a liberation from control in securing the Leader's objectives. In contrast the so-called trade union 'bosses' and their supporters generally performed their role in relation to political policies and party regime change, according to a role definition which was heavy with inhibitions and constraints and varied in its priorities forum by forum.

The NEC and Iraq

In 2002 the managers of the extra-parliamentary party were still sticking closely to its initial tactical response of keeping things quiet in the party over Iraq. Charles Clarke was still proclaimed to be the voice of the party to government, and he bravely admitted at one point that in practice the Partnership in Power policy-making process 'had created an atmosphere of cynicism and scepticism among Labour members'.[123] Yet by the summer, over Iraq there were complaints about the failure to hold any party 'Britain in the World' policy commission meetings since January. Not until July, after Mark Seddon demanded an emergency meeting of the NEC for a discussion of Iraq, did a telephone conference take place between the Foreign Secretary Jack Straw and the commission. It discussed, amongst other things, the reply being sent out to pressing representations from the party over Iraq and the Middle East.

Meanwhile, although there was strong feeling in the unions against an Iraq invasion, as evidenced by their contribution to the TUC discussions, the unions' four priorities for the party conference resolutions had, as before, followed domestic priorities. But in the new procedure where topics were accepted for debate if supported by more than 50 per cent of the CLPs, overwhelming support was given by CLP representatives to debating Iraq. The managers had been involved with instigating 'helpful' resolutions into the party conference. These together became composite resolution No. 5. It recognised that the Iraq situation could 'in the last resort . . . involve military action . . . taken within the context of international law and with the authority of the UN'. Commitment to the UN gave it consensual appeal, but it did not have an unambiguous commitment to an explicit UN decision before action was taken. That could be taken to give the freedom of action that Blair needed.

The policy commission met again on 18 September, during the week before the conference. Its role, including drafting the reply to party submissions, was taken over by the NEC on 29 September with ministerial backing – an irony given the attempt to kill off NEC policy-making. In practice, it is now known from Campbell's diaries that the draft was done by Blair himself.[124] Blair's message to the NEC as in the PLP was that 'nothing has been decided'. What became clear much later was that a quickening of party policy on Iraq in September followed Blair's further meeting with Bush, at which it later emerged that a promise was given of British military support if the UN route failed.[125] With the world's press on the doorstep of the NEC meeting, pressure from Blair's managers urging public unity was especially heavy. An attempt by Grassroots Alliance members on the NEC to amend the Blair draft, requiring that any military action be explicitly endorsed by the UN, was rejected with only four votes in favour.

However, a further amendment from trade union representatives would have brought into the resolution a section of the TUC General Council Statement passed at the September Congress. That had affirmed that seeking regime change in another member state was not consistent with the requirements of the UN charter and opposed any military action on a unilateral basis. This was more narrowly defeated on the NEC by 18 votes to 13. Following this vote the TGWU, GMB and UNISON representatives all warned that without a paragraph on the lines agreed by the TUC there would be difficulty in their conference delegations. That being ignored, when it came to the lunchtime before the debate, in both the TGWU and GMB delegations, led by the main candidate for the impending election of the two union General Secretaries, criticised the NEC statement, and the delegations decided to oppose the statement. Observant delegates coming back into the hall after lunch noted a speedy shocked run-round by Clarke and Triesman which secured no change. That was followed by an unannounced recall of members of the NEC behind the platform. To avoid defeat, for the first time in party history the agreed NEC statement was suddenly withdrawn – without a formal committee vote.

This left on the agenda just the contemporary resolutions, another irony given the sustained managerial attempts to kill off this procedure. Ultra-loyalist Margaret Wall chaired the session, working as usual to a prepared list of speakers. The normal speakers' manager Greg Cook was replaced to make room on the platform for Triesman, the General Secretary. Speakers were then selected in such a way as to enrage critics of government policy. Pro-government voices in the debate supporting composite 5 outnumbered the critics by 13 to 4. The blatant scale of it even aroused concern among Political Office staff that it might ignite a public reaction of a 'return to control freakery' given the public sentiment over Iraq, compromising the victory already arranged on the resolutions taken. But in a further unusual development, Blair's senior aide Morgan was unable to get her cautionary message heeded on the platform managed by Triesman and Wall.

On a card vote 40.22 per cent of the conference voted to support composite resolution 4, an unqualified anti-war position, with 59.78 per cent against. There was a majority of 67.51 per cent against it in the CLPs with 32.49 in favour; from the affiliated organisations it was 52.04 per cent against and 47.96 per cent in favour. But the crucial managerial feature was that conference was never allowed the choice of a wording prohibiting force without a second specific UN resolution. As the well-informed Patrick Wintour from the *Guardian* reported, 'Conference managers were eager to avoid such a choice'.[126] The leadership-supported composite resolution No. 5 was declared carried by Wall on a show of hands but no card vote was allowed in spite of calls, even from the delegate moving the resolution. Campbell's diary description that 'the Iraq row never really took off'[127] was economical with the managerial reality.

On 29 November, at the NPF held in Newcastle, there was concern expressed across the Forum over failure at the centre to respond to the record number of party submissions on various issues. There was a recognition by John Reid, the Leader's new appointment as Party Chair, of the limitations in the Partnership in Power process, particularly in the dialogue over 'blue skies thinking and over immediate policy issues'. But he took no observable action over the latter. United Nations Security Council Resolution 1441 on 8 November 2002 had offered the Iraq leader a final opportunity to comply with its disarmament obligations. What that meant in terms of giving specific authority for action was and remains contentious. If ever there was an issue which needed a separate session of small workshop group dialogue at the NPF, with an expression of overall opinion in a plenary session, it was this and now. But the forum was organised to plough on through the timetable of seven policy papers on domestic issues.

Not only that, but in the National Policy Forum Newsletter (created to improve feedback to the party in this era of 'the end of control freakery') the withdrawn NEC statement on Iraq was initially reported as having been 'overwhelmingly endorsed'.[128] Later, after vigorous complaints by NEC members and NPF representatives, an edition was published which carried a correction. Reid as Party Chair became a key manager giving strong principled reasons for the party to be supportive of the government. He assured the Cabinet that people were not leaving the party over Iraq.[129] The general message put out from the party machine at this time was also that there had been 'no recent rise in resignations'. In reality, membership continued to fall, some of it unquestionably due to Iraq as a senior manager later privately confirmed by reporting (inaccurately) that, 'we've got them all back now'. As Kampfner tells us also, Reid was active with the Chief Whip Armstrong in checking the number of dissidents.[130] This was from the post accepted by the NEC in 2001 as the new voice of the party in the cabinet.

On 28 January 2003, as the momentum to war mounted, a motion submitted to the NEC by Seddon and Black on Iraq said that 'war at the current time is not justified'. What happened to this motion raised major procedural and managerial issues. The managers in headquarters and in No. 10 wanted it to go just to the policy commission and not to the NEC. But there was a quiet determination from the NEC majority that after the policy commission met there must be an NEC debate. There were two ingredients to this mood. There were those on the NEC who had never accepted the manipulated abolition of the NEC independent policy role. But also the NEC was receiving a large number of resolutions from CLPs on Iraq that gave little support for unilateral or bilateral attack. The NEC was now confronted with the question: if the NEC was not to discuss this huge issue now, what could it discuss and when?

The Chair of the NEC this year, Diana Holland, who still had the rule-book status of being 'the Party Chairman', insisted on taking both a draft NEC statement and the resolution and allowing a full debate on them at the February NEC. The NEC statement drew heavily from the carefully managed Composite 5 supporting, 'in the last resort . . . military action . . . taken within the context of international law and with the authority of the UN', but again with no commitment to a specific second UN author-isation. However, it included a recognition of 'the widespread concern within the party and the country at large'. That acknowledgement troubled the leadership but helped get it through the NEC by 22 votes to 4. The motion from Seddon and Black then fell. Still, the reluctance by headquarters management to give a wider circulation of the ' widespread concern' led to the statement not being circulated at the party's spring conference on the grounds that the media would find division. After that the statement disappeared.

Union management of the anti-war position

The development of the union voice and its management was potentially highly important in party decision-making. Debates on the General Coun-cil of the TUC were impassioned. Some who normally were regarded as moderates and loyalists were fiercely opposed to a war without a specific UN authorisation. Statements that emerged were not voted on (in order to keep unity) but on 26 February 2003 one stated very clearly its concern at increasing indications that 'the United States administration backed by the British Government . . . is intent on military action within weeks, and that action might be taken without the explicit authorisation of the UN Security Council'. It affirmed that 'this is not supported by working people and their families' and expressed the view that 'moral repugnance towards any regime cannot on its own be sufficient justification for war'. However, as often with the unions on political issues, action was constrained over judgements of priorities and differences over wider political considerations. To help Blair, statements of TUC policy were spun by the TUC staff in a way that was judged least damaging to the government and their relations with it.

When the decisive vote in the House approached, the incoming TUC General Secretary Brendan Barber did not accept any invitations to speak at anti-war demonstrations and other public activities. There were reinforc-ing reasons for his stance. He was very aware of the old symbolism of 'moving back into Trafalgar Square' and the damage that that might do to the years of changing the TUC's respectable insider image. Increasingly also, the anti-war movement was seen by some of the TUC officials as led by people they regarded as left-wing sectarians.

The PLP and Iraq

The movement towards war had generated both an alarmed body of PLP opinion and a passionately determined support for Blair's position. Both fed into the PLP meetings and into the Parliamentary Committee. The PLP Foreign Affairs committee also met regularly with the Foreign Secretary and facilitated meetings between backbenchers and the government. In response to the considerable disquiet, Blair gave repeated assurances that no decisions had been taken and that he was attempting to influence the US and exhaust diplomatic processes. He also challenged them regularly to face the acute problem of weapons of mass destruction in the light of strong intelligence warnings about Saddam's activities.

The PLP Secretary Howarth became a convinced supporter of the government policy and the attempt to preserve unity behind it. PLP Chairman Jean Corston moved the same way after early doubts. Clwyd, previously a regular and effective critic of past government policy, became a passionate and influential defender of the Iraq policy to deal with tyranny and protect human rights. In a small but significant change in composition, the determined maverick McKinlay had been replaced on the committee by the loyalist Bridget Prentice in the elections of October 2002, but McKinlay became convinced by Blair, spoke in support at the party conference and also voted for the war in the House. MPs Jackson, Lloyd, Gordon Prentice and Mullin remained consistent sceptics but with differences over the tactics of handling the issue through the PLP. At the Parliamentary Committee meeting on 8 January Blair was still saying that there was no immediate threat of war.[131] In February 2003 a second document which became known later as 'the dodgy dossier' was issued. Like the first dossier in September 2002 it gave in considerable detail what was presented as a well-sourced cause for concern over Saddam's armoury and objectives.

A critical motion on Iraq was introduced at the Parliamentary Committee on 5 February 2003 by Gordon Prentice and Tony Lloyd. The long argument went over predictable grounds including the dangers of public disunity if a resolution was put to a PLP vote. Prentice made continued attempts to push the resolution but was defeated on the committee. It was agreed that a full discussion of Iraq would take place at the next PLP meeting and it was also suggested that as the NEC had reached a settled position, the NEC statement would be available. Later, it was argued amongst the managers that the PLP could not be seen as subordinate to the NEC, and the NEC statement was not circulated to the PLP members with the weekly whip documents.

The scale of the opposition to the war on Labour's benches was clear on 20 February 2003 when for the first time there was a full debate in the Commons. There were 121 Labour MPs voting against the government – many more than Downing Street expected – and there were a large number of abstentions. As the time for decision approached, pressure mounted on the Labour benches to ensure that there would be a vote as well as a substantive debate. With the Leader of the House Robin Cook arguing the parallel procedures of the US Congress, and the Foreign Secretary Jack Straw under pressure from backbenchers and defending the right of MPs to decide,[132] after initial reservations from Blair, he became convinced that it had to happen.

Deselection and management of pressure from the CLPs against the war

It was later suggested by Russell,[133] citing Cowling, and taking a line which Short recorded the Party Chair and Chief Whip had taken to the Cabinet in February 2003,[134] that the procedure for mandatory reselection by CLPs was a pressuring feature of the situation, pushing PLP rebels. Certainly deselection could reasonably be described as a back-of-the-mind concern of MPs in some CLPs during the period of the peak of the selection cycle. But back-of-the-mind was not necessarily determinant, especially as the most striking feature here, given the emotions involved, was how very few efforts were made to put the procedure in motion. When it arose in three cases it was for personal rather than political factional reasons, and only in two of these, Reading and Tooting, did the eviction succeed. In this sense it was the lack of this procedural pressure here that was the more significant feature. MPs were relatively free to dissent from CLP opinion, providing that they handled it with sensitivity and were vigorous in their own local welfare and political campaigning role.

It was also a feature that, as already noted, since 1998 the affiliated union branches had under Blair a strengthened influence on reselections. They had become accustomed to the conservative role at this level. Over Iraq also, in the major unions they were not encouraged from above by their leaders to get involved in high-profile 'political' moves on deselection which might be portrayed as a backdoor attempt at regime change in the party and thus complicate both the Iraq issue and domestic agendas. The union stability role went universally unregistered in any analysis of Labour's internal politics over Iraq policy. Part of the explanation for this is that in the regular private commentary by party whips and officials it was not the 'New Labour' line on the unions to stress their importance, especially if they were doing something praiseworthy – as we have seen over finance.

Over Iraq, it was also a significant constraint that in March 2003, following reports that deselection was being encouraged by emails from the Labour Against the War Group, the Parliamentary Committee was told that a warning had been given by the Chief Whip to leading officials of the group who were Labour MPs that, by convention, MPs did not interfere in the territory of their colleagues. This was strongly supported by the committee. As for the role of union groups in parliament, the majority of anti-war union leaders including Edmonds, who with his Deputy General Secretary Steve Pickering had carried the union banner on the Glasgow march in the spring of 2003, took the same view of their parliamentary group as they did of instigating political action from the CLPs against MPs. It could be counterproductive in the way opponents could use it as 'not their business'; it would be divisive in the union and damage other activities. That applied also to the trade union group of the PLP. Although officials of the group individually voted against the war they also made no attempt to engage the group collectively. Yet once more the managers found the situation less of a constraint and more of an opportunity. Pro-war NEC union loyalists, discreetly working to the No. 10 Political Office, used the phones to selected union group members to help build up the supporting vote for war.

War management in the Commons and outside influences

Although there were signs from MPs comments that a majority of the PLP favoured a delay in military action, Blair was being pulled behind the US timetable. He in turn drove the PLP by a hugely impressive speech in the House on 18 March which came across as both a candid diagnosis and a powerfully persuasive prescription. It carried the message of a real and present danger to be expected from a tyrant who had failed to comply with UN Resolution 1441. A French 'veto' was said to have prevented a second resolution 'whatever the circumstances'. Saddam had now had his final opportunity to get rid of his weapons of mass destruction. A claim to have destroyed them was, Blair said, 'palpably absurd'.

He reiterated his warning of a potential threat from the link between weapons of mass destruction and terrorism, which had to be dealt with. And that the 'only true hope of liberation' for the people of Iraq, who were subject to 'pitiless terror', lay in the removal of Saddam. Overall, the impression was heavily conveyed that this was a man who understood better than anyone in the House or the country precisely and accurately what was being faced and the responsibility of taking action. The situation facing Britain was he suggested, akin to that facing the country over the Munich agreement in 1938 and the failure to act over Czechoslovakia. In effect, he gave Labour MPs the sharp choice 'to stand British troops down and turn back' or 'to stand firm to the course we have set'. If action was not taken, 'who will celebrate and who will weep?' So magisterial and committed was this speech that it made personal the unstated choice being offered. It was Blair or Saddam; a defeat would see the Prime Minister's departure.

Cowley, in his study of dissent in the PLP in Blair's second term, gives an incisive account of some of the organised influences brought to bear by leading ministers and whips in moving PLP support behind the invasion; their operation was systematically targeted on the basis of information about the recipients.[135] More noticeable, in heavy symbolism as well as pragmatism Blair broke with his past behaviour and decamped into a highly visible tearoom persuasive role. Important also but much less obvious was that a crucial background loyalist role was played by Prescott in mobilising support, even though he remained a private critic of some of Blair's governing arrangements. But the extra-parliamentary battles explored in this chapter also fed into parliamentary influence in ways favourable to the government. Crucial battles had been won in managing every forum and in circumscribing the repercussions. The potentially hostile pressures from the wider party on the PLP, in what was seen as a knife-edge decision, had been alleviated by this management intervention and by a union restraint, which left more room for the whips, ministers and government supporters to make their appeals.

Opposition weaknesses and management

At the same time, there were important weaknesses of the war opposition at the highest level, affected by personal differences, the tactics of party management and a divisive association of the anti-war leadership with regime change in the party. Gordon Brown had not taken a prominent public or party role over Iraq. What was regarded as his weak support in this battle infuriated some Blairite managers and provoked speculation about what damage he might, in the end, cause over the invasion. Nevertheless, encouraged by Prescott, acting as a bridge to Blair on this, Brown became heavily involved in securing support for the crucial vote in the House, as were his primary supporters. In a follow-up, discreetly organised by PLP managers to see what the reactions to him had been, Brown was seen as effective with those he targeted.

There had been little attempt by the two leading cabinet opposition figures, Cook and Short, to work together within the party. This was influenced by differences of temperament, past territorial tensions fed by media stories which set them in competition, a tactical judgement to avoid the charge of factionalism and, crucially, different attitudes towards the Leader. In the absence of a second legitimating resolution from the UN, Cook resigned before the vote. His resignation speech was as brilliant as that of Blair and later read as much the wiser course. But Cook was unwilling to push the challenge of his speech in a way which might damage Blair and bring in Brown. In the choreography of his resignation Cook worked cooperatively with Campbell. The resignation speech was made before, not during, the Iraq debate, which had been his original intention, limiting its potential effectiveness in influencing the outcome.

Despite what was reported privately as major misgivings amongst ministers there were only two other ministerial resignations: John Denham, Minister of State at the Home Office and Lord Hunt, Health Minister, both on the eve of war. Clare Short, by far the fiercest of Blair's public critics, favoured the Leader's replacement by Brown and was utterly uninhibited in making challenges, but nevertheless did not resign immediately at the onset of the invasion. At that time, after booking her resignation speech slot, she came under a barrage of private supplication, some of it managed by the No. 10 Political Office, to avoid a double Cabinet resignation. Blair sought repeatedly to persuade her to stay; eventually successfully. She did not make the speech of opposition to the war that she had partially prepared but accepted a continuation of her international role when given assurances over the Middle East roadmap and the guarantee of support for the leading role of the UN in post-war planning. Later, after angrily judging that she was being 'conned', Short resigned from the Cabinet on 12 May 2003 with the war in progress. Her appeal to history then came in the resignation speech with a fierce and weighty attack on Blair's method of governing.

On 18 March the Government with Conservative support won the Commons vote by 396 votes to 217. There were 139 Labour MPs who voted against their whip, said to be more than half of the 264 non-payroll vote,[136] although less than half of the PLP. But Conservative support over Iraq guaranteed a Blair victory. Also, at the time, as the Worcester, Mortimer and Bains team from IpsosMORI put it, only 26 per cent of the public approved of British involvement without a 'smoking gun and a second UN vote' but 'the British people got neither'.[137] Then, inevitably, some opinion began to move in solidarity behind 'our troops' as the day of invasion approached.

Following a swift military victory, the initial light loss of British lives and reports of joy in Iraq as the tyrant Saddam Hussein was driven from office were presented as vindication of Blair and spun with gusto. His public popularity immediately soared. It was assumed that careful plans for the occupation had been made. His party management seemed on the verge of a new supremacy built on the permanence of strong and bold war leadership and the controlling mechanism strengthened after 2001.

New union leaders and reactions in No. 10

Meanwhile, the conflict over Iraq, as already indicated, coincided with developing changes in the union leadership. In elections carried out by OMOV ballots, at the grassroots there was receptiveness to critical union assertiveness against the political leadership. Candidates for union positions quietly or obviously supported by No. 10 tended to get defeated. Leftish leaders with independent voices emerged. The earlier change in leadership of UNISON in 2001 had replaced one moderate left leader by another, but Dave Prentis was more involved in internal Labour Party politics than Bickerstaffe had been and within the year was working with new and assertive colleagues in major unions.

True, a moderate from the traditional right, Kevin Curran won in the GMB but on a platform much more attuned to the traditional union industrial positions and highly critical of the government. In the TGWU, the left had been split, with Morris backing a weaker candidate. It led to the emergence of Tony Woodley, a complicated figure with strong industrial trade union experience and old connections to the Militant left. The biggest shock was in the AEEU-Amicus where a knighted union leader, Ken Jackson, close to No. 10 and standing again at 65, proved to be out of touch with his members. He was replaced by an unknown left-winger and ex-Communist Derek Simpson who (at that time) saw Tony Benn as an inspirational figure.

These union leaders were highly critical of 'New Labour' and distrustful of Blair's management of the party. They were also distrustful of the TUC, its political style and accommodations with government, indeed suspicious also of London influences, especially the involvement of No. 10 managers trying to determine union internal matters. In the AEEU particularly, accusations were made of interference from the Transport Minister Spellar during the elections, but Spellar had always been active in this, his own union. Nevertheless it sharpened the sense of 'us against them' trying to subvert the unions and they were not taking any more of it.

In June 2002 *Unions Today*, the bimonthly created from No. 10 to forge new understanding with union loyalists, had folded after it failed to reach its target circulation. There were new worries in No. 10 that the carefully built-up image of a party and unions under control and the Leader's supremacy could be threatened in the right-wing press, disturb the CBI and cause electoral damage in the marginals. There were deeper fears also that the changes might threaten the new political landscape of the party and bring in political shifts of the kind that the Jones-Scanlon generation had initially helped to bring in train. This was the 'New Labour' nightmare – the title of a book by an experienced left-wing union adviser.[138] The initiating actions of the two aspiring union leaders in their delegations over Iraq had been a particularly worrying development.

Nevertheless it was doubtful if these militant union leaders represented a fundamental political change in shop-floor attitudes amongst the majority of members, a point made by the limited later studies noted in Daniels and McIllroy.[139] In No. 10 from some there was a sophisticated awareness that these men were inexperienced in national political life, and that the Jones-Scanlon generation had within a few years made its accommodation with the political leaders in pursuit of joint priorities. With the exception of a scornful attack by the ex-union leader and now minister, Alan Johnson, referring to union leaders 'from Planet Zog',[140] the response from the government was in the main, publicly, very restrained.

But that accommodation with Jones and Scanlon had been firmly made only in the context of a TUC-Labour Party Liaison Committee which forged greater trust and mutual commitment. Such an institution and its priorities was anathema to Blair and Brown. At their most worried, in No. 10 the immediate problem ahead remained that it appeared to be possible that Blair's managers were about to lose control over the party conference and maybe the NEC, as the domestic grievances of the unions became more forcefully expressed and more potently focused. However, more hopeful was the thought that such a development might well be countered in the party by the mood expected to be engendered by Blair's triumph over Iraq.

Notes

1 BBC *Today* programme, 2 October 2002.
2 Keith Ewing, 'Rethinking the Law of Work: The Continuing Role of Trade Unions in Labour Law', unpublished appraisal, circa 2003, privately supplied to me.

3 *The Times*, 1 October 2002.

4 *Independent*, 28 February 2003.

5 Information supplied by the TUC.

6 ICM/*Guardian*, 30 July 2002.

7 Ibid.

8 *Labour Research*, October 2002, pp 10–12, cited in J. Waddington, *Annual Review* article, 'Heightening Tensions in Relations between Trade Unions and the Labour Government in 2002', *British Journal of Industrial Relations* 41(2), 2003, p. 339.

9 David Coates, pamphlet *Raising Lazarus*, Fabian Society, 2005, p. 3.

10 ICM/*Guardian*, 18 September 2002.

11 Labour Party (NEC) Report 2003, p. 27.

12 *Guardian*, 18 July 2001; *Morning Star*, 18 July 2001.

13 Kevin Maguire, interview with Derek Simpson, General Secretary-elect of Amicus, *Fabian Review*, Autumn, 2002.

14 *The Times*, 29 March 2002.

15 Speaker's Statement, *Hansard*, Column 885, 10 July 2002.

16 Peter Mandelson, introduction to *The Blair Revolution Revisited*, Politico's, London, 2002, p. xv.

17 Pippa Norris (ed.), *Critical Citizens: Global Support for Democratic Governance*, Oxford University Press, Oxford, 1999, in which particularly Russel J. Dalton, 'Political Support in Advanced Industrial Democracies', pp. 63–5. Russel J. Dalton, *Democratic Challenges, Democratic Choices: The Erosion of Political Support in Advanced Industrial Democracies*, Oxford University Press, Oxford, 2004, pp. 29–30. Gerry Stoker, 'Explaining Political Disenchantment: Finding Pathways to Democratic Renewal', *Political Quarterly* 77(2), April to June 2006, pp. 184–5.

18 Dalton in Norris, *Critical Citizens*, p. 62.

19 Ion Trewin (ed.), *The Hugo Young Papers, Thirty Years of British Politics – Off the Record*, Allen Lane, 2008 entry for 7 November 2000, p. 676.

20 IpsosMORI, *Blair's Britain: the Political Legacy*, 2007, p. 29.

21 MORI website, 15 October 2000.

22 Ibid.

23 MORI/Hansard Society, 'None of the Above: Non Voters and the 2001 Election', 2001, p. 1 and p. 3.

24 Robert Bennett, *The British General Election of 2001 at a Glance*, Parliamentary Library of Australia. Research Note 35, 2000–1, p. 3.

25 Ibid.

26 Catherine Bromley and John Curtice, 'Where Have all the Voters gone?' in Alison Park et al., *British Social Attitudes*, Report 19, Edition 2002–3, Sage, London, 2002, p. 141.

27 Anthony Seldon, *Trust: How we Lost it and How to Get it Back*, Biteback, London, 2009, pp. 32–3.

28 Gallop/Saga, 20 July 1999, Future Foundation/Consumers Association – research into corporate citizenship and freedom of information, February 1999. Helen Haste, 'Mapping Britain's Moral Values', study with MORI for *Nestlé Family Monitor*, 30 March 2000.

29 MORI, 30 March 2000.

30 Ibid. p. 43.

31 Derived from David Riesman, Nathan Glazer and Reuel Denney, *The Lonely Crowd: a Study in the Changing American Character*, Yale University Press, New Haven, CT, 1950.

32 David Boyle, *Authenticity: Brands, Fakes, Spin and the Lust for Real Life*, Flamingo, London, 2003, p. 4.

33 Ibid. p. 43.

34 Sharon Shavitt, Pamela Lowrey and James Haefner, 'Public Attitudes Towards Advertising', *Journal of Advertising Research* 38(4), October–December, 1998, pp. 7–22.

35 Abhilashe Mehta, 'Advertising Attitudes and Advertising Effectiveness', *Journal of Advertising Research* 40(3), May/June 2000, pp. 67–72.

36 Neil Fitzgerald, Chairman of Unilever, Address to the Advertising Association, May 2001.

37 *Trust in Advertising: a Global Nielson Consumer Report*, October 2007. See also the present volume, Chapter 20, n. 63 and Chapter 21, n. 89.

38 GFK Roper Consulting, *On the Horizon*, July 2009.

39 *Sunday Telegraph*, 18 April 2010.

40 Sissela Bok, *Lying: Moral Choice in Public and Private Life*, Pantheon Books, New York, 1978.

41 Sissela Bok, *Lying: Moral Choice in Public and Private Life*, Random House, New York, 1999.

42 There were extensive articles on this in the *Sunday Times*, 2 May 1999; *Guardian*, 14 July 1999; and *Observer*, 12 March 2000.

43 Bok, Preface, p. xviii.

44 Alastair Campbell and Richard Stott (eds), Extracts from *The Alastair Campbell Diaries: The Blair Years*, Hutchinson, London, 2007, entry 24 July 2003, p. 729.

45 John Lloyd, *What the Media are Doing to our Politics*, Constable, London, 2004.

46 Kim Fletcher, *Daily Telegraph*, 17 May 2001.

47 70 per cent, IpsosMORI, 'Trusting the politicians', Roger Mortimer website. 27 September 2002.

48 Notes of a speech given at Leeds University, 28 November 2001.

49 A range of these dissatisfactions were later explored by, amongst others, Meg Russell, *Must Politics Disappoint?* Fabian Society, London, 2005, Gerry Stoker, *Why Politics Matters, Making Democracy Work*, Palgrave Macmillan, London, 2006 and Colin Hay, *Why We Hate Politics*, Polity Press, London, 2007. Peter Riddell, *A Defence of Politicians (In Spite of Themselves)*, Biteback, London, 2011.

50 On this see particularly Chapter 17, p. 559 for the first audit of political engagement carried out by IpsosMORI for the Hansard Society in 2004, and also the reasons for distrust uncovered in IpsosMORI/BBC polling 22 January 2008, details of which are in Chapter 21, pp. 741–2.

51 Mandelson, *Blair Revolution Revisited*, Introduction, pp. xiv–xv.

52 Ibid. p. xliv.

53 Ibid. p. xxvii.

54 Ibid. p. xiii.

55 Alastair Campbell and Bill Hagerty (eds), *Alastair Campbell Diaries*, Vol. 3, *Power and Responsibility*, Hutchinson, London, 2011, entry 23 July 2001, p. 676.

56 Lance Price, *Where Power Lies: Prime Ministers v the Media*, Simon & Schuster, London, 2010, p. 392.
57 Ibid.
58 Campbell and Stott, Extracts from *Campbell Diaries, The Blair Years*, entry 20 Dec 2001, p. 594.
59 Ibid.
60 Price, *Where Power Lies*, p. 359.
61 *Guardian*, 17 May 2002.
62 Mandelson, *Blair Revolution Revisited*, Introduction, p. xliv.
63 Campbell and Stott, Extracts from *Campbell Diaries, The Blair Years*, entry 9 October 2001, p. 578.
64 Ibid. 11 March, p. 609. Also Mandelson, *Guardian*, May 17 2002.
65 Alastair Campbell and Bill Hagerty (eds), *The Campbell Diaries*, Vol. 4, *The Burden of Power: Countdown to Iraq*, Hutchinson, London, 2012, entry 3 February 2002, p. 157.
66 Ibid. p. 156.
67 Nicholas Jones, *Control Freaks: How New Labour Gets its Own Way*, Politico's, London, 2001, p. 308.
68 Chris Mullin, *A View from the Foothills*, Profile Books, London, 2009, entry 4 February 2002, p. 254, quoting a conversation with Secretary of State for Health Alan Milburn.
69 *Westminster Hour*, BBC Radio 4, 3 February 2002.
70 Trewin, *Young Papers*, discussion with Campbell, entry 14 April 2002, p. 784.
71 Price, *Where Power Lies*, p. 360. Also cited there was that on 14 June 2009 on the BBC *Politics Show*, the parliamentary official Black Rod had said that he had 'refused to lie' on behalf of No. 10.
72 John Kampfner, *New Statesman*, 1 July 2002.
73 YouGov/*New Statesman*, 1 July 2002.
74 Greenberg memo to the PM, 1 August 2002, cited in Stanley B. Greenberg, *Dispatches from the War Room: In the Trenches with Five Extraordinary Leaders*, Thomas Dunne, New York, 2009, p. 248.
75 Anthony King, drawing from You Gov/*Daily Telegraph*, 29 September 2002.
76 *Daily Telegraph*, 2 February 2002.
77 Mandelson, *Blair Revolution Revisited*, Introduction, p. xlv.
78 Ibid. p. xlvi.
79 Robert Worcester, Roger Mortimer and Paul Bains, *Explaining Labour's Landslip: the 2005 General Election*, Politico's, London, 2005, p. 98.
80 *Guardian*, 13 May 2002.
81 BBC research project and website, 3 May 2002.
82 IpsosMORI, Social Research Institute, Delivery Index and commentary, September 2002.
83 Campbell and Stott, Extracts from *Campbell Diaries: The Blair Years*, entry 19 December 2001, p. 592.
84 Brown discussion with Short, revealed to me in detail by Short in 2003.
85 Tony Blair, *A Journey*, Hutchinson, London, 2010, p. 340.
86 Clarke, interviewed on BBC Radio 4, 28 November 2001.
87 *Sunday Times*, 6 January 2002.
88 Ibid.
89 *The Times*, 25 August 2002.

90 *Tribune*, 4 January 2002.
91 *The Times*, 2 January 2004, cited in Christopher Foster, *British Government in Crisis*, Hart, Oxford, 2005, p. 131.
92 David Hill, Letter to *The Times*, 27 December 2004.
93 Mullin, *From the Foothills*, entry 16 January 2002, p. 250.
94 Philip Cowley and Mark Stuart, 'Parliament: More Bleak House than Great Expectations'. Paper presented at the University of Nottingham, April 2004, p. 3.
95 Ibid.
96 Covering 1999–2002, Philip Norton, 'Cohesion without Discipline: Party Voting in the House of Lords', *Journal of Legislative Studies* 9(4), 2003, p. 66.
97 Campbell and Hagerty, *Campbell Diaries*, Vol. 4, *The Burden of Power*, entry for 14 January 2002, p. 140.
98 Meg Russell, *Building New Labour*, Palgrave Macmillan, Basingstoke, 2005, p. 231.
99 *Tribune*, 27 February 2002.
100 Telephone discussion with Sumner, March 2004.
101 *Inside Labour*, June 2002, p. 8.
102 Robin Cook, *The Point of Departure: Diaries from the Front Bench*, Simon & Schuster, London, 2003, p. 230, entry for 23 October 2002.
103 *Inside Labour*, June 2002, p. 8.
104 Matt Cain with Matthew Taylor, *Keeping it Clean: the Way Forward for State Funding of Political Parties*, IPPR, London, 2002.
105 *Guardian*, 23 August 2002.
106 In forty years' research I found no evidence from the unions or the politicians to sustain this accusation of threats relating policy to the TGWU role as landlord.
107 Donald Macintyre, *Mandelson: the Biography*, HarperCollins, London 1999.
108 In a telephone interview with Jack Jones, 27 August 2002, he used very strong language in his denial, expressed contempt for the accuser and agreed that his response could be used when appropriate.
109 Minkin, *Contentious Alliance*, pp. 512–14.
110 *Guardian* editorial, 30 September 2002.
111 LPCR 2002, p. 113.
112 *Guardian*, 26 September 2002.
113 *CLPD Briefing*, Sunday 29 September 2002.
114 *21st Century Party*, p. 39.
115 Conduct of Internal Party elections – organisational principles, NEC Organisation Committee, 21 January 2003.
116 Ibid.
117 Ibid.
118 Ibid.
119 Ann Black, *Tribune*, 21 May 2004.
120 *Guardian*, 14 February 2003.
121 *Observer*, 14 February 2003.
122 Shaw, *Labour Soul*, p. 127.
123 *The Times*, 14 March 2002.
124 Campbell and Hagerty, *Campbell Diaries*, Vol. 4, *The Burden of Power*, entry 24 September 2001, p. 640.

125 John Kampfner, *Blair's Wars*, Simon & Shuster, London, 2003, pp. 196–8.
126 *Guardian*, 1 October 2002.
127 Campbell and Stott, Extracts from *Campbell Diaries, The Burden of Power: Countdown to Iraq*, entry 3 October 2002, p. 319.
128 Ann Black, National Policy Forum Report, 29/30 November 2002, dated 12 December 2002.
129 Excerpt from Clare Short's diaries contained in Clare Short, *An Honourable Deception? New Labour, Iraq and the Misuse of Power*, Simon & Schuster, London, 2004, p. 182.
130 Kampfner, *Blair's Wars*, p. 292.
131 Mullin, *From the Foothills*, p. 344.
132 Cook, *Point of Departure*, pp. 189–90.
133 Russell, *Building New Labour*, p. 279.
134 Short, *An Honourable Deception*, p. 169.
135 Philip Cowley, *The Rebels: How Blair Mislaid his Majority*, Politico's, London, 2005, Chapter 5, pp. 106–28.
136 Kampfner, *Blair's Wars*, p. 309.
137 Worcester, Mortimer and Baines, *Explaining Labour's Landslide*, p. 83.
138 Andrew Murray, *A New Labour Nightmare: The Return of the Awkward Squad*, Verso, London, 2003.
139 Gary Daniels and John McIlroy, *Trade Unions in a Neo-Liberal World: British Trade Unions under New Labour*, Routledge, London, 2009, pp. 147–9.
140 *Guardian*, 18 April 2003.

17

New challenges and management on the road to Warwick

Leadership and management

Blair under attack

But the politics of Iraq had very different consequences. The Iraq insurgency and counter-insurgency became a protracted and bloody affair, exposing the lack of appropriate preparation by the occupiers and bringing to Iraq the forecastable linkage between organised and violent resistance against an occupation and 'international' terrorism. The suicide of the government scientist Dr David Kelly, whose body was found on 18 July 2003, brought to a shuddering halt the celebration by the Prime Minister's entourage of his triumphant American reception.

The Hutton enquiry into the death of Kelly was watched, monitored, blogged and replayed to a gripped national audience. What was learned from there fed a growing public and party view that the country had been misled into the war. Hutton's report on 28 January 2004, which in effect formally cleared Blair of every charge against him, appeared so manifestly in conflict with the evidence presented to Hutton that it surprised even some in No. 10.[1] It created a strong sense shared by a substantial minority – 31 per cent of the party membership – that its conclusions were a whitewash.[2] From this point on, new evidence accumulated over the years that what had been presented to be a true and accurate account of the Saddam situation in April had in fact fallen far short of it.

Amongst these discoveries, contrasting with what the party was told in his PLP meetings and what he claimed publicly, was that Blair had reached important hidden early understandings about joining an invasion with the US government. His interpretation of the French 'whatever the circumstances' UN veto was discovered later to have been a misinterpretation. He had also declared 'beyond doubt' what was much more uncertain in the intelligence about weapons of mass destruction, and had overstated the 'growing' problem from Saddam. The claim in the September dossier of an Iraq capacity to deploy weapons of mass destruction within 45 minutes of the order being given, and a press story of his ability to launch a missile attack which would hit those serving in British Cyprus bases, were never repudiated by the government, but were later found to be false.

No. 10 and the intelligence organisations appear to have encouraged each other in the task of effectively warning and clarifying for the party and people what they believed to be the urgency of impending danger from Saddam. Yet his weapons of mass destruction were never found, to the surprise of more than Blair but especially damaging for him, given their centrality in his arguments.

The self-serving form of Blair's prime ministerial governance over Iraq was confirmed by the evidence gathered of his 'sofa government' contained in the Butler enquiry into *Intelligence on Weapons of Mass Destruction* which reported on 14 July 2004. It raised the major criticism that 'The informality and circumscribed nature of the Government's procedures' including the absence of proper Cabinet papers, the lack of a formal agenda, the failure to take minutes of all meetings, risked 'reducing the scope for informed collective political judgment'. As Kampfner pointed out, at no point did he produce a formal government paper setting out the options; the Defence and Overseas Policy Committee did not meet in a way which would have been the normality in the past.[3] What also became at issue was the Prime Minister's restriction of a full balanced report by the Attorney General on the legality of the war from open discussion in the Cabinet. All this practice emanated from Blair's view of effective government in organisations. And if his policy on Iraq was as Clare Short questioned, Blair's version of 'honourable deception',[4] then as she recognised in her own frequent past criticisms, it was a version regularly in play in party management.

Amongst the public, Blair's personal support fell far more sharply than public support for the war.[5] Public trust in Blair which had been at plus 15 per cent in April 2001 had already sunk to minus 23 per cent in October/November 2003 and it had dropped to minus 29 by April 2005.[6] In September 2003 a poll of the now further depleted party membership found 57 per cent thought that it had been 'wrong to go to war'.[7] By 3 May 2005 only 19 per cent of the public saw Blair as having always told the truth about Iraq.[8] Consequently the view of spin as deceit had received a further boost. As Mattinson put it, her focus-group evidence showed that 'The ability to manipulate the news agenda regardless of the facts came to symbolise the gap between politicians and people perhaps more than anything else for the disillusioned electorate.'[9] What was found out about how Britain was led into that war replenished and heightened the image of Blair as a practitioner of manipulative politics, boosting an already critical opinion anxious to expose and punish errant politicians. A substantial section of the 'New Labour' coalition moved away from Labour support, alienated by Blair's policy and process.

Spin, mistrust and departure

Even so, from IpsosMORI, Bob Worcester's informed conjecture was that the increased level of public opprobrium was deflected somewhat from

Blair and fell on Campbell.[10] The media manager had developed a strong sense of the damage that the media-government war was doing to his role and the reputation of politics, as by now had Gould, but the battle with the media raged on. Campbell was by nature a warrior, who increasingly took the view that the media enemies were poisonous. He was ever ready to fight from the government corner even if he had doubts about Blair's policy and positioning in relation to the party. Handling those tensions had become a massive burden on Campbell and he had been thinking about resignation for some time. On 29 August 2003 he went, and at his suggestion was replaced by the experienced but much more low-key media manager David Hill.

Meanwhile, confidence in government communication and the use of government statistics had markedly diminished. Findings from a survey of public confidence in 2004 found 60 per cent believing that official statistics were changed to support particular arguments, 59 per cent denying that the government used official figures honestly and 58 per cent disagreeing that official figures were produced without political interference.[11] Spin and the use of statistics were not the only features that drew caustic criticism. In 2004, an experiment in compulsory postal voting was argued by John Rentoul, who was by no means a regular critic of the government, to be 'a shameful exercise in electoral manipulation'.[12]

Mistrust and the audit of political engagement

In 2004, the first audit of political engagement carried out for the Hansard Society found 51 per cent of the public with 'not very much trust in politicians and 19 per cent who trusted politicians 'not at all'. Only 27 per cent of the public trusted politicians 'a great deal' or 'a fair amount'. That this distrust was related to the character and behaviour of politicians was captured in the public's images of rats, weasels, snakes, foxes and vultures – emphasising, as the report said, 'the sly, greedy and deceitful'.[13] That deeply negative characterisation also expressed the common cultural representation of politics described in 2005 by Ben Page of the MORI Social Research Institute as highlighting not only a craft but 'a set of tricks and a dark art, to be used in the service of gaining advantage for personal and party gain'.[14]

Leadership, governance and party management

Blair denied that he had undermined cabinet government, but what became revealed about the Iraq policy process appeared to confirm the earlier conceptual encapsulation contained in Graham Allen's analysis that, 'we are for all intents and purposes, ruled by a hidden Presidency'.[15] Clare Short's important resignation assessment was that 'we have the powers of a presidential type system with the automatic majority of a parliamentary system', in spite of the fact that, as Short lamented, his large majority in the House was based on the support of only a quarter of the electorate.[16] Tony Wright, Chairman of the Public Administration Committee, agreed that 'The absolutely penetratingly true line out of what she said was not so much the tyranny of the centre, which is well known – it was the fact that we had this particular combination of presidential government and a parliamentary system'.[17] A fundamental underpinning of this combination was Blair's party management, both in the House and outside it.

Party management and government controversy

The managerial efforts to limit pressure over Iraq from the party outside the Commons, and to curb the public expression of the party's authentic voice, flowed into the managerial avoidance of party accountability inside and outside the House. With the aid of Blair's managers there was no post-mortem on the Iraq policy in the PLP or on the Parliamentary Committee or the NEC. In line with the practice of Blair's party management there was also no calling to account of managers about the unsatisfactory elements of their use of the party's policy process. Meanwhile, the lead-from-the-front-and-pull-them philosophy in policy formulation took on an even harder edge in managing the radical domestic policy drive. It became a routine priority for the managers to seek to avoid any specific advance commitments from the party outside the House and then to seek to 'move on' after policies were introduced and implemented, avoiding inquests and accountability.

Increasingly party members were a declining entity and those who remained became a more disheartened audience as much of the policy-formulating process continued to exclude them. In July 2003 Blair saw the people's mistrust problem best addressed by reconnecting with people on the issues they really felt strongly about.[18] At one stage he was challenged by Straw that distrust was not just policy-based; part of the problem was the Blair practice of defining the government against the party; as a result we 'alienated our own people' and sometimes win the vote without being clear about winning the argument.[19] Blair made very clear that he disapproved of that contribution.[20] Over the two most controversial domestic policies, foundation hospitals and education top-up fees (see below, pp. 573–6), the initial policy announcement or leak was made without any preliminary consultations with the PLP, let alone advanced sharing in the policy process. They both moved away from the party's understood position.

On 12 June 2003 came a reshuffle which reinforced Blairite ministerial support and, in a press release, the abolition of the post of Lord Chancellor and the setting up of a new US-style supreme court in place of the law lords was announced. There was no consultation with the party or the Opposition before the changes were announced and some confusion afterwards about both the reshuffle and the details of the major constitutional changes. That fitted closely into an image of governance seen by some as both arbitrary and dysfunctional, and in that sense, a government in crisis.[21]

Party managers go and come

No. 10 and new management liaison

Meanwhile, in April 2003 John Reid had replaced Alan Milburn at Health after the latter had resigned to spend more time with his family. With a new awareness of the desperate state of the party organisation and the need for it to be rebuilt, McCartney was first encouraged by Reid to get involved and then was brought back by Blair as Party Chair from 4 April 2003 to 4 May 2006. As it happened, he was from October 2004 to October 2005 also Chairman of the NEC, and in this conjunction the argument over the legitimacy of the Leader's appointment virtually disappeared. He also became chair of the NPF and gave proactive attention to relations with the party and the unions – although, in practice, what happened to management was still heavily determined by Blair's style of leadership and positioning.

Evicting the General Secretary

The McCartney appointment produced an immediate new problem. As so often with 'New Labour' proposals, the post of Party Chair had never been thought through in terms of its potential problems as well as its advantages. Not the least of these was the query of what happens if relations between a new Party Chair and the General Secretary deteriorated, as they did. Relations between them were always very prickly, part of the bitter residue of the attempt to push McCartney out of the chair of the NPF in 2001. Since then, Triesman had done two big jobs that No. 10 needed, disassociating the image of party management from McDonagh and reducing the deficit, reported as dropping from nine million pounds to £924,000.[22] As part of the financial rectification, the headquarters was moved out of Millbank to Old Queen Street in March 2002, a shift that also embodied a symbolism of image distancing from 'control freakery'. Only later did it become clear that the new headquarters, chosen by Triesman, was physically inadequate for the purpose of fighting elections. He had not come well out of the handling of financial negotiations with the unions, and in No. 10 they grew concerned at what appeared to be a lack of focus on the needs of campaigning, a criticism emanating also from inside party headquarters after Labour's first by-election loss since 1998 at Brent East on 19 September 2003. His unexpected departure was conveyed publicly on 3 November 2003,[23] without consultation of the NEC and just prior to the committee's planned two-day November meeting.

Matt Carter, chosen as replacement, effectively by No. 10, was young but more experienced and knowledgeable on party organisational issues, and well-schooled in the ways of the machine. However, the position of General Secretary was now clearly more diminished. McCartney as the Party Chair became a more significant political managerial figure. His links to the unions had the advantage of getting union cooperation, but that record also meant that he had to work harder for the Leader to keep his job. In terms of the reality of power relations it is important to note also the development of the history of the Ethics (Funding) Committee. After Triesman's eviction, the committee was run down and eventually ceased to meet after its members had raised complaints about not being kept properly informed. No report of this was made to the NEC until a crisis over funding and honours forced it on everybody's attention (see Chapter 18, pp. 631–2).

Trade unions and neo-liberal immovability

Neo-liberal hegemony and myth

A permanent atmospheric problem affecting union-managerial relations in the party continued to be that Blair, Brown and the Treasury were helping to drive the European agenda more strongly in the anti-regulatory neo-liberal direction and in that project working with the CBI. In response, the TUC kept up its critique of the major premise and assumptions behind the whole policy. In February 2003 a Congress House document argued that, 'the alleged burden on business from new rights in the work place is grossly exaggerated'. International evidence suggested that there was no systematic link between employment regulation and either job generation or unemployment and, as concluded in the Labour Market trends review, 'it appears more important that the range of and type of legislation adopted in a particular country is appropriate and works well with other labour market institutions'.[24] In November 2004 in the face of government determination but a paucity of evidence against the adverse effects of regulation, the TUC produced a comprehensive attack on 'labour market myths'.[25]

But the government's economic diagnosis and its political underpinning was unwavering and, as there was only a limited union push for a new economic framework, the TUC settled mainly for finding the scope for change indicated by the government and then after constructing arguments around it, pushing a bit further in ensuring gains. Within the government-imposed limitations, education and training had become a fertile common ground. But this left still a range of industrial and social grievances. The Employment Relations Act 1999 had given the government power to introduce regulations to outlaw the blacklisting of trade unionists, but not until 2003 did the government consult on draft regulations. Nothing was done as there was said to be an absence of hard enough evidence. There was a growing problem also that an increase in new employment came in part-time and temporary low-paid employment with limited legislative protection. Over this insecure and under-protected employment there was a continuing reluctance to legislate. Exploitative employment practices became an emotive public and party issue after the deaths of 23 cockle pickers in Morecambe on 5 February 2004. Under public pressure mediated through back-bench MPs and the TGWU, ministers gave support to The

Gangmasters (Licensing) Act 2004, but it was restricted to agriculture and food processing. All this fed the mood towards more aggressive union action through the party and an attempt to build a counter to the heavy party management on issues of major concern.

New union leaders in action

Awkward squad attitudes and rhetoric

The party management and the Leader now faced union leaders new and old who were an especially difficult squad to relate to, let alone to manage. Simpson of Amicus and Woodley of the TGWU were alienated and heavily critical. Edmonds had always been an independent and creative figure. Linking with Prentis, who had played a more mainstream role although he too was deeply critical of 'New Labour' policies and management, they formed a powerful 'big four'. Billy Hayes of the CWU, the sixth-biggest union, who had been the first elected into office, fitted easily into this left-wing trade unionism but uneasily into the 'big four' operation. The fifth-biggest union USDAW, led after 2004 by the General Secretary John Hannett, was outside this development, still solidly associated with the trade union right.

Like previous generations, 'the big four' were bound-in by the union mandates unless, as in the past, the agenda choices gave them more space. Simpson and Woodley had been elected with a strong push from union activists with grievances that 'the great majority of restrictive legislation passed between 1979 and 1997' remained on the statute book.[26] Though the greatest alarm to the party's leaders and managers was caused by what appeared to be a hard-line political rhetoric which emphasised traditional socialism, opposition to the war in Iraq and an intra-party project specified sometimes as 'reclaiming the party', there was, as friendly critic Gregor Gail noted, little sign of an alternative political vision.[27] In the resolutions the unions submitted there was a focus on domestic policy issues. No attempt was made to push constitutional changes which might have strengthened the unions or limited the leadership. There was no move to make easier and clearer the process of evicting the Leader.

New union developments inside the party

But there was a move against traditional intra-party cooperation and this was to generate further developments. Distrust of party management was such that at the 2003 party conference, for the first time since Blair became Leader, there was no pre-conference collective meeting of major union leaders called by Blair to influence their managerial support role. There was plenty of evidence that the new union leaders were not prepared to play the managerial game. This was one major, if hidden, feature which made the conference of 2003 a departure point in party management. There was a second reinforcing development. In 2003 was the last conference fringe meeting held by the traditional union right from USDAW, Community (ex-ISTC), TSSA and the MSF section of Amicus. Two union leaders, Rosser of TSSA and Lyons of MSF-Amicus, were on the point of retirement. The only subsequently significant victory in the unions for Blair's supporters was support for Shaun Brady against Mick Rix as ASLEF General Secretary for reasons mainly peculiar to that union. Brady took up the post in October 2003, was suspended in May 2004 and sacked in December 2004 after bitter internal infighting. In 2005 he won his industrial tribune case but never regained his position.

Managerial responses

The uncooperative mood from the new union leaders led to or was further precipitated by new preparations from the managers. Before the conference assembled there was a renewed emphasis on the Blairite 'great and good' of the PLP, meeting privately to discuss giving assistance to the conference management. Their discussions focused on the failings of the unions and the pivotal importance of the CLPs. And there was also a new managerial assertiveness in protection of the Leader and avoidance of accountability. Although the NEC had asked in 2002 for more question-and-answer sessions with ministers, at the 2003 conference they were drastically reduced. The most important change here was the ending of the session on foreign affairs which would have covered Iraq.

As an alternative, extra official policy seminars were added on international affairs and public services. They were to meet on the Sunday morning at around the time when for a century the trade union delegations had held their meetings. The managers later argued that this was an unfortunate outcome of timetabling difficulties. To unions, not even informally consulted, it evoked the suspicion that the managers, developing a reputation for small acts of systematic subversion of the unions – even creating problems for them with documentation, as a senior official later privately confirmed – were finding additional ways for one-way influence over constituency delegates. It was patronising but not too surprising that the move was seen by the unions as 'leaving innocent constituency representatives to be brainwashed'.[28]

The senior officials in the unions became more aware of the means by which the CLP representatives were being managed in other ways. In the middle of debates, sections of delegates were now systematically asked to leave the hall to meet ministers or the Party Chair for what was said to be a 'feedback session'. In practice, it was to be persuaded of voting for foundation hospitals and against the constitutional change being proposed on contemporary resolutions. A few short questions were allowed but no discussion. As a result of this, and various other worthy distractions, CLP delegates were not encouraged to sit in the hall throughout the debates unless the liaison officers were targeting delegates for a vote. Managers now asserted (as if it was an unfortunate independent phenomenon) that 'there isn't a culture of sitting through the debates'. There was also much moving around of seats, encouraged by the managers to ensure that the front of the hall looked full. Various delegates complained at what they saw as visitors voting, but no attempt was made from the platform to warn visitors that they should not vote. 'We had too few votes for it to be an issue' was the unconvincing explanation offered privately by a platform official later.

New union leaders' tactical activity

As they came into increasing conflict with the managers, the priority tactical aim of the new union leaders became to further consolidate their own coordination. Aware of the leadership's past tactics of dividing the unions, they now evolved an agreement that, on domestic priority issues, the union delegations would vote for each other's positions. Unlike in 2001, the affiliated unions would focus on TULO and the party process in determining the next term's union claims on government, and not initially prioritise the TUC with its direct channel to Government. The TUC-Government phase would follow on after the commitment had been made. The growing reaction against the past and present tactics of party management was such that Prentis of UNISON even privately apologised to other union leaders for some of the past divisive role of his own union representatives. All were aware that a key ex-UNISON official, Nita Clarke, was now working from No. 10.

At the 2003 Conference, Iraq was not prioritised for debate by the majority of CLP delegates or the unions. Although there was some resentment about the war and the way that Britain was taken into it, the appeal to 'finish the job' after occupation and to 'move on' was regarded as realistic, and it fused with union domestic priorities. Still, there was a critical emergency resolution on the issue from the RMT. It was ruled out by the CAC, discussed behind the scenes for three days and ruled out again. Debate was confined to an innocuous Britain in the World report.

The big four union leaders – Curran over pensions, Woodley over Labour law, Prentis on health service marketisation and Simpson over manufacturing, led on the contemporary resolutions, which were focused on the most highly contentious group of issues since the procedure had been initiated. With Billy Hayes of CWU, the big four also organised their own fringe meeting 'Putting Labour back into the Party' – a title changed under pressure from No. 10 to 'Towards a radical strategy for the Third Term'. For their part the Downing Street managers, particularly McFadden, were aggrieved that over the NHS, despite a clear advance in avoiding the two-tier workforce, there wasn't more accommodation from the unions, particularly UNISON, in strengthening management.

The tensions here revealed some deep-rooted differences in perspectives on managerial relations between union leaders and party managers. Managerial behaviour by Clarke and Triesman over the party's financial problems had consolidated distrust of party management amongst union leaders, and this was strengthening over their manipulation of the party's policy-making process. In any case, there was an increasingly acute problem of reconciling the unions' historic solidarity role in sharing party management, with their industrial obligations as representatives of a workforce whose interests and concerns they considered were not adequately embodied in government policies. So UNISON, taking Blair's promise in 2001 at his word, now attempted to roll out the prohibition of the two-tier workforce from the NHS across the public sector with the same 'no less favourable' terms and conditions. The public–private battle shifted also to foundation hospitals, another policy foisted on the party and the unions without prior discussion.

Simmering conflict over what was legitimate and what was not in union use of the party policy process in this way became sharper, particularly the ministerial criticism that the unions were raising industrial-relations issues through the party and organising a block vote against the Leader. In the unions this critique of the block vote was met with some derision; the Leader's managers had been attempting to organise a block vote like that for years, whenever 'it worked for Tony' in defending the leadership from the CLP membership. There was another tactical aspect to this which further soured the atmosphere. The managers were pressing quietly that 'We won't deliver on two-tier workforce unless they concede on foundation hospitals' and, more openly, that 'We didn't say [of ending the two-tier workforce] that we would deliver it now'. With half a mind, they were probably already thinking about the content of limited concessions which would form part of the pre-election unity.

For the moment their anger at the new assertive and cohesive role of the unions was uppermost. It was made worse when, in a policy area which managers had thought closed off, what had come to be a routine pro-government NEC vote responding to resolutions on the conference agenda, the one supporting foundation hospitals was carried by only 16 votes to 15, with 10 of 12 trade union representatives voting against it. Also irritating to No. 10 was that a TGWU-led composite resolution on employment law, which included changing the legal rights of companies to dismiss workers after eight weeks of lawful industrial action, was accepted by the NEC and later the conference. They met it privately with the view that 'We'll ignore it', although it did not work out like that (see below, p. 596).

The tactics of the GMB union then played into the hands of critics. The GMB composite on pensions was late in being agreed in the conference because the GMB got the compositing meeting recalled after its new leader Kevin Curran had had second thoughts about it. The NEC for the first time in memory decided not to take a view of it because it was too late. Although the action by the GMB leader greatly irritated some of the CLP representatives, the resolution was carried in the conference on a hand vote. But it had left a precedent and managers were eagle-eyed in spotting new opportunities (as will be seen, Chapter 18, pp. 619–20).

There was no conference debate on top-up fees but there was a controversial series of managerial defeats over foundation hospitals. First, on the Conference Arrangements Committee, the attempt by officials to prevent a debate was defeated. In the hall on a card vote the pro-government policy resolution from Shrewsbury and Atcham CLP supported by the NEC was lost 55.99 per cent to 44.01 per cent with 75.82 per cent of trade unions voting against, although only 36.15 per cent of CLPs against. That could be claimed as 'support by the party'. However, a hand vote on a more critical resolution on foundation hospitals resulted in a defeat for the government policy. The failure to hold a card vote on this led to much recrimination against the chair, Mike Griffiths, a trade union NEC representative. Some managers argued that he had been guided to hold a card vote by the platform official Greg Cook and should have taken the advice – a revealing managerial perspective. But Griffiths thought it was clearly carried and as no call for a card vote came from the conference (which was not disputed) he declared it like that. The managers were convinced that the card vote would have shown a majority in the CLPs in favour of foundation hospitals.

There was also an unusual development concerning constitutional reform over the allocation of contemporary resolutions. That had emerged from some CLPs and the CWU. It proposed to formalise eight contemporary resolutions to be debated at each conference with the CLPs guaranteed four of them. This appeared to deal with a long-standing CLP grievance over 'perceived union domination of the agenda'.[29] The whole NEC CLP section had supported it when it came to the NEC. In the conference the amendment was passed by 54.72 per cent to 45.28 per cent with the affiliated organisations voting for it by 33.49 per cent to 16.51 per cent. But, to some amazement, a majority of the CLPs rejected it by 28.77 per cent to 21.23 per cent. Perhaps it was that the managerial arguments that the reform would damage Partnership in Power were found convincing, as managers said. But the result appeared as something of a mystery to the unions and added to suspicions of managerial methods.

CLPs and moral victory

What the managers portrayed as 'a moral victory' amongst CLP delegates over foundation hospitals, and over the constitutional change, enabled the managers to downplay the significance of resolutions which were passed by union majorities. Once again, the word was put out to the media that the CLP members had now become the source of loyalty and stability. There is, however, good reason to question this portrait of the CLP membership as opposed to their delegates. One poll in the *Observer* in September showed a majority of party members opposed to foundation hospitals and higher tuition fees (and favouring higher top rate of tax).[30] Another poll in the *Guardian* in February 2004 found that members were 'old Labour'; 66 per cent favoured increasing the top rate of tax. They did not approve of key government policies on public sector reform and only 5 per cent favoured increased user charges.[31] Later, in 2007, polling of members showed only 23 per cent favoured a reform of schools and hospitals to give parents and patients more choice.[32] And a poll found that 82 per cent of members favoured funding for local councils to build low-cost council housing on the same basis as housing associations.[33]

Unions, continuity and again the myth of financial pressure

The role of union representatives still involved some strong continuities. On policy issues, union attitude towards industrial priorities dominated over their attitude towards wider political objectives. The remaining traditional right representatives in the unions were still more instinctively loyalist in party terms. Party obligations often weighed against union obligations on the NEC and CAC, influenced by the ethos of those committees. Individuals with official party positions generally retained their greater sense of the primacy of party obligations. By the middle of 2003, in the midst of growing tensions over policy and management, a crude view of the way unions used their financial muscle within the Labour Party would judge that if there was ever a time to put on the financial pressure it was now.

The internal battle in several unions was growing as some left-wing separationists focused on redirecting union resources to other organisations and campaigns. In spite of that, it was at this point, following two meetings of TULO on 23 July and 16 September, that the unions delivered without conditions the further financial rescue plan agreed in principle in the summer of 2002. Why should this happen?

Several developments led to their decision. In January 2003 the Leader, through McCartney, improved the atmosphere by reconfirming the movement towards a limited public funding of parties which would not be at the expense of traditional party structures. The party submission to the Electoral Commission (agreed with TULO) defended the link to the unions and accepted the maintenance of a broad balance of party income. The Electoral Commission refrained from proposals which would interfere with Labour internal arrangements. In July 2003 Blair, accepting the new importance of TULO, delegated to McCartney his joint chairmanship of TULO, which was accepted with the proviso that it 'would not prevent unilateral meetings of trade unions taking place under TULO auspices'.[34] In a further boost to the status of TULO, McCartney brought onto the JPC three of their representatives, although with no discernible improvement in their policy influence.

Most important was that some strategists in the unions were now beginning to be acutely aware that the issue of the non-delivery of the money was constantly being raised in relation to the unions – as was the accusation that financially they had the party over a barrel. In TULO meetings, it now became the pressing wisdom that until the issue of finance was out of the way, the unions could not use their new cohesion in practice to press effectively on the industrial policy issues, and opponents of the unions were using financial accusations against them.

So, the remarkable end result of the series of developments on party finance, which had started in 2001 with the GMB attempt to exert influence, was to reinforce 'the rules' prohibiting financial pressure by leaders in relation to policy outcomes. It was embodied in the delivery of additional finance as an act of good faith. Building on the agreement already in preparation whereby trade union affiliation fees would increase for 2003 from £2.25 to £2.50 per member, the unions agreed a further two-year package of increased fees. They would raise affiliation fees in 2004 by 25p and in 2005 by a further 25p with a guarantee of no change in affiliation levels. That amounted to an increase of approximately £2 million as at December 2005. All of this was given without policy strings.

Management and rulebook authorisation

It was formally ratified by a meeting of all the TULO unions on the eve of the party conference. However, as with the original commitment the year before, there was no public welcome from the party for the support, in fear of what the media might make of it as 'bribery', even though it was taking the money out of the political conflict. The new finance went through the normal accounts and was duly reported to the Electoral Commission. But here again the verbatim report[35] indicates that it was not presented for the approval of the party conference. And in a new development, there was no immediate alteration of the rulebook. Meanwhile, it should be noted again that since 2002 it had become very difficult for observers to get hold of the verbatim conference report, even after many requests. The officials were always 'too busy' to get it ready.

This was significant also in that around this time there had arisen at senior level in headquarters an interpretation of the rulebook which gave the officials acting for the NEC the right to change the constitution without going through the conference. This view was not put directly to the NEC, and TULO officials were very unhappy with it. Much later, under continuing pressure from Byron Taylor and TULO, and after Gordon Brown became Leader, the failure to get authorisation by the conference was eventually understood to have been 'a mistake', and after a decision of the NEC Officers' meeting, a rectification of fees was made in the rulebook in 2007 covering affiliation fees from 2003.[36] It was retrospectively and discreetly reported to the party conference in the NEC's annual report, and the rulebook was then amended accordingly. This whole performance reinforced the view in TULO circles that the party management must be reformed but, under Blair, how could it be done?

The Leader's conference speech

After the Iraq invasion and the emergence of controversial issues of domestic policy, and with his public rating as more honest than most politicians having dropped from 25 per cent in November after the 2001 election to just 8 per cent in September 2003,[37] the 2003 party conference was seen by some of those around him as an especially tough task. He rose to the occasion, handling Iraq with delicacy, carefully making a plea to understand his intentions in taking the decision, and taking the audience through the exercise of putting them in his place. 'Imagine you are the Prime Minister . . . there was no easy choice', and concluding that 'whatever the disagreement, Iraq is a better country without Saddam'.

Confirming his role as a conviction politician, he referred to the passage in Clause IV, 'by the strength of our collective endeavour we achieve more than we achieve alone', and now gave this the status of 'a fundamental restatement of ideology', ignoring its hidden history but more surprisingly, going against years of denying an ideology. In a passage focused on the fight against the Tories, there was no acknowledgement of the huge loss of electoral support taking place to the Liberal Democrats and to abstention, affected by both policy and a distrust of being misled. His basic message on conviction politics was that he did not have a reverse gear. This was interpreted as a reinforcement of his determination on public sector reform and a replay of Thatcher's past theme, 'the lady is not for turning'. It was an indication that whether relating to party or people Blair was still addicted to the appeal of a form of bold leadership that Peter Hyman, his ex-aide in No. 10, later labelled as 'the shit or bust' style, to which 'listening' was subordinate.[38]

Nevertheless, talking directly to the party, at one point he now seemed also to announce a shift in leadership style. In stark contrast to his response to Straw's private criticism in July (see above, p. 560), he told the conference 'I know the old top-down approach won't work anymore. I know I can't simply say "I'm the leader, follow me"'.[39] This apparent shift then led into his announcement of 'the biggest policy consultation we have ever taken': The Big Conversation, a reasonable proposal in itself, operating as a sign of receptivity and reaching out. It might have even been heard as a new involvement of party members. However, it had not been discussed with the NPF or the NEC nor with the party officials who would have to operate it. Indeed, Prescott had to weigh in to ensure the party was involved at all. Later, an exasperated Helen Jackson, lamenting the exclusion of the partnership policy commissions from the processes of The Big Conversation, wondered whether the partnership 'was always a bit of a fraud'.[40]

Talking with the public in small groups rather than talking at them was, on the face of it, more useful that previous practice. But it was also subject to managerial intervention to vet some of those involved, to avoid findings which could have fed further internal revolt and to interpret what the managers wanted to report (or not). In a way that was very 'New Labour'; an idealistic aspect of mutual education became buried under the culture of control. In this it was a continuation of what Labour Minister Chris Mullins diagnosed in 2000 as 'a classic New Labour wheeze designed to create the illusion of consultation'.[41] In practice its effect on Blair's policy was minimal and the 500 Big Conversation meetings held from the launch in November to February 2004 did little discernible to boost Blair's public support.

The reception for that Blair speech at the conference was seen as an indication of the party's continued acceptance of his authority after Iraq. Yet some of the fears in No. 10 of problems from the delegates were misconceived. Though sections of party opinion had become more distrusting and more hostile to Blair, his reception amongst delegates did draw from a mixture of party moods sometimes within the same individual. There was a continuing party mood of not wanting to damage the government and appreciating the difficulties of the job. The speech was increasingly a theatrical event and a thoroughly organised celebration of the party and the government as much as of the Leader. Urged on in advance by the managers and the liaison teams, loyalty was called upon to defend the Leader against 'them' in the media. And in 2003, more than ever before, the party managers left nothing to chance, in preparation to ensure success. There was a tight script of organised vocal responses and an in-the-round setting, which Blair liked; the platform behind him was packed with specially selected politically verified, visually representative young people, being discreetly signalled when to clap. To the close observer of continuing 'New Labour' managerial behaviour against this background, it was unsurprising that a proposal to restore the question-and-answer session for the Leader was not entertained. All this reinforced an atmosphere of veneration which was not congenial to critical responses.

The continuing managerial control over the conference alerted some in the press to the activities of the apparatchiki-clap organisers during Blair's speech. The press comments were in turn reported to the delegates the next day by the Chair, Mike Griffiths. The beginning of his protest against the inaccuracy of the media portrait was drowned in the chorus of derision directed towards the press by delegates and managers. It was one of the great moments in the history of managerial ascendancy. Years later, ex-General Secretary Peter Watt described the conference as having been an 'annual torture-the-leader session by the sea'.[42] But, it had been part of Watt's job, and the successful managerial project to avoid any torture and to ensure that the speech met annual acclamation.

Over the intensification of managerial politics, the bitter arguments that followed this conference produced, on the NEC, an agreement to a demand for there to be more NEC involvement in the preparation of the agenda, as there had been for years past before Partnership in Power.[43] In practice, it was never fully complied with. There were always managers like the

Chief Whip to express disapproval of the legitimacy of 'interfering' with the CAC, as usual ignoring the role of the party officials in that process. Private reports to the union leaders through TULO conveyed that at the end of the 2003 Conference, Blair, at his discreet meeting to thank the conference managers, was talking further in terms of 'dealing with the block vote'. Managers began to spin that the unions were 'playing with fire'.[44] This was once again couched in terms of the unions 'riding roughshod over constituency activists'.[45] Judging by other managerial comment, hovering behind all this appeared to be the usual anxiety to reassure business that the unions and the party were not in charge. On 17 November 2003 on BBC *Newsnight*, Murdoch's voice was heard in his first BBC interview for many years indicating a possible change in support to the Howard-led Tories.

PLP management and dissent

In the PLP, the managers had been given an increasingly difficult task. Over the whole period 2001–5 there was a higher rate of rebellion than in any other post-war period.[46] In discussions on the Parliamentary Committee, the Chief Whip was in no way critical of the practices of an exclusively leader-centred policy formulation, although she had reminded Blair in a Political Cabinet that to avoid division the PLP had to be listened to.[47] On the committee she was candid about the problems she now encountered, not only over voting dissent but also with unauthorised individual absences by MPs. These absences were increasingly explicable in terms of the evidence that incumbents nursing their constituency could be rewarded in electoral terms. That added to a shift of focus by MPs to their local surgery work which proliferated as local councils became increasingly administrative agencies of the centre.

The confidence of MPs about their local role gave them an increasing sense that they and their local parties were generally closer to and more understanding of Labour voters than those advising the Leader in No. 10. Some of that mood even affected some of the Labour Lords who could also take a principled stance regardless of public opinion and the Leader's wishes. With no party holding a majority the Lords defeated the government on 245 separate occasions 2001–5 across a wide field of legislation, inducing a range of concessions.[48] By strengthening the position of Commons dissidents, Lords rebellions added to the work of the ministers and the Labour whips in the Commons. The absence of major public disapproval of serial Lords rebellions was probably an indication that Blair's government was judged to be too strong.

Facing regular revolts, the promotion from back bench to front bench grew through a further increase in ministers including unpaid ministers attached to the whips' office, and an increase in the number of individual PPSs. This led to a situation by August 2003 where the total number of

MPs involved in government, which had been 129 in 1999, had become 146.[49] Blair's aides also attempted to engage PLP loyalist backbenchers more directly including regular meetings with ministers and more small group visits to No. 10 to see the Prime Minister. Blair found it necessary to raise his attendance at the PLP meeting to five times in 2002 and six times in 2003 but then kept it at five in 2004. In these appearances Blair showed an extraordinary public resilience which evoked awe even from major critics. He remained consistently at his impressive best. In assistance, in meetings where the pressure was on, vocal loyalists acted as a protective and at times intimidating shield; some loyalists, including the militant chief whip, gave regular loud robust commentary whilst critics were speaking.

Officials emphasised that, in spite of criticism to the contrary, anybody who wanted to speak at the PLP meeting could generally do so and no organised effort was made to give dissenters a rough time. One defensive nostalgic from the whips' office implied that they were 'not that good at organising the PLP anyway'. Yet it was part of the job that they routinely worked with allies in building morale, as they saw it. Organised or spontaneous loyalist shouting sent a message of government support to the dissidents present and to the media outside.

Policy, party management and the intensifying battle with Brown

Brown, party management and contentious issues

Brown's push as Blair's replacement became a more open running sore and all policy differences were judged by No. 10 and the whips' office in terms of his attempt to stir further party problems for Blair. Over foundation hospitals Alan Milburn produced the policy in accordance with the Blairite quasi-market model, but there was a hefty and leaked opposition from the Chancellor at an early formulative stage, resulting in change to the policy over the issue of borrowing powers. There was also a critique shared by Brown and a variety of critics that it would create a two-tier NHS with increasing disparities. More discreetly, around Brown they let it be known that the framework could make it easier to move towards privatisation. Their positioning, rhetoric and personal influence was seen by Blair's managers, including the Chief Whip, as exacerbating the management problem in the PLP, even giving the rebels assistance on the financial calculations involved in the legislation.

Brown's hands were seen (and exaggerated) also in influencing the trade union vote on the NEC which came close to defeating the Leader on foundation hospitals. More indicative was a decision of the Conference Arrangements Committee, of which Yvette Cooper, a close Brown ally, was a member. Her vote in the face of some severe backbiting from No. 10 helped secure a debate on foundation hospitals at the 2003 party conference. That led to a defeat for the platform, only a few weeks before the vote in the House of Commons. At this time, a poll found 84 per cent of the electorate opposed to foundation hospitals.[50] The government took no notice of the conference decision or the poll and won the vote in the House of Commons on 19 November, yet with a majority reduced to only 17. One important concession with the potential to be an important general precedent was induced by the weight of revolt. The back-bench party suspicion that foundation hospitals would open the door to privatisation had led to a limit being placed on the number of private patients in foundation trust hospitals with a formula which made that a very small element.

Brown, the NEC and policy-making

The growing division with Brown opened up another contentious flank of party management. Brown had voluntarily announced that he was standing down from NEC in 1997 and under the unanticipated changes of 2001 had lost his right to automatic membership of the Clause V meeting as a member of the Cabinet. On 6 November 2003 in a television interview he complained that Blair was excluding him. This was not a flaunting of his invulnerability as suggested by Peston.[51] It was almost the opposite. The behaviour of the NEC at the 2003 Conference over foundation hospitals had indicated that the apparently dormant NEC still had a potentially significant policy role. And the NEC had also become potentially an important player in the Clause V election-manifesto meeting which Brown wanted to attend, as of right. In excluding him as one of the three government representatives on the NEC, there was an element of punishment but there was also worry in the Political Office that there could develop a difficult fight over the public sector policies at the manifesto meeting. Things were now so bad that they were not certain how Brown might vote. Not until 2005 was the composition of the Clause V meeting reformed to the satisfaction of both Blair and Brown (see p. 600 below).

Top-up fees and the near thing

The personalisation of conflict within the leadership of the party also became part of the politics of policy-making over higher-education finance. Top-up fees for students had been specifically rejected in the 2001 manifesto, and following the campaign where charging fees was acknowledged to be a doorstep problem, Blair had promised to undertake a review of state funding and student contributions. But he faced an intensifying dilemma after new representation from the universities on the seriousness of their financial situation. A review which appeared in January 2003 accepted the need for a supplementary funding mechanism in the proposal that universities would be able to charge students a variable top-up fee.

In the PLP, opinion was influenced by conflicting considerations. These included a view of the realities of the financial position but the injustice of asking taxpayers who had not been in higher education paying more for those who were. On the other side, Brown's background opposition was mainly to the inequity of the proposed policy; he favoured a graduate tax. There was also strong PLP opposition to the marketisation of universities and the danger of discouraging students from poorer and more risk-averse backgrounds. In the wider party the new proposal went into a Partnership in Power policy-commission discussion and because of this, contemporary resolutions on it were prohibited from the 2003 Conference. Huge support built up in the PLP behind Ian Gibson's broadly drawn EDM 7, 'Alternatives to Variable Top-up Fees'. In the three weeks between the Queen's Speech and the Christmas recess it attracted 159 Labour signatories. Opposition to upfront top-up fees had support in public opinion polls. It became clear that Blair could not deliver it.

Finding an acceptable alternative was left in the hands of the ministers, Charles Clarke and Alan Johnson. They were widely judged to be very skilful in handling party concerns whilst retaining focus on the central problem of raising finance. Chipping away at the opposition came through numerous meetings including departmental committee meetings but also the introduction of ad hoc seminars run by Clarke. Their work began to pay off in terms of the changing mood. Detailed polling by Populus for the *Times* on 7 December indicated that the emerging package did have public and Labour supporters' acceptance as a fair way to raise extra funding. The Labour students organisation, which at leadership level was heavily Blairite, also quietly moved into line.

Yet by the turn of 2004 there was still confidence amongst the dissenters, led by two ex-managers who were close to Gordon Brown, Nick Brown and George Mudie, that they were about to inflict the first defeat on the government and the management under Armstrong. That clash of two sets of managers seen as the instruments of the two leaders made the politics before the coming vote exceptionally fierce and significant. A PLP meeting held on 14 January 2004 to discuss the issue was said by the whips to have involved a movement of 'the silent majority'. Clarke, leading off, and defenders of the new proposals emphasised the abolition of upfront fees, safeguards for poorer families, a maximum level of fee, and a system of repayment of loans which would begin only when students were earning £15,000. Some detailed qualifications were expressed over particular items but a large majority of speakers made generally supportive comments. The first of only three outright opponents chosen to speak at the meeting, Harold Best, defended the manifesto mandate and argued that policies were driving away members. He had to be protected from the severe barracking by an appeal by the PLP Chair to be 'given a fair chance'.[52]

On Monday 19 January, with still the strong possibility of defeat but with the gap in support expected to close as it normally did approaching the vote, a second PLP meeting was held, addressed this time by Blair. He made a comprehensive case for the new proposals and again there were just three outright opponents chosen to speak. However, Blair was also questioned about the policy process and the point was made that more should be learned about pre-legislative scrutiny. Blair's answer was that it was possible to learn from how they had arrived at this point and that was the reason for the Big Conversation. That view was countered gently by a supporter of the policy with the request to consider extending the Big Conversation to the PLP and inside the Labour Party.[53]

A decisive move towards a government victory came on the day following when Gordon Brown announced his support. He had earlier privately told Blair that he would not vote against him on this.[54] But it appears that he was not believed – a growing feature of the relationship on both sides. In the discussions that followed Gordon Brown's public stance, Nick Brown, but not Mudie, also decided to vote with the government creating a new momentum towards a government victory. It was said by Brown supporters that in the end he helped deliver the victory because the damage to the party and the government would have been too immense if Blair had been defeated. It would also have saddled Brown with a reputation of seeking to be a destructive usurper, a fear that was a constant constraint upon him. He gained no kudos for his action in No. 10 or the whips' office. They were still angry at his aides' encouragement for the original revolt and now saw him seeking not to help the management so much as not moving too far from Rupert Murdoch who was in favour of reform. The second-reading vote giving the government a majority which was only five votes – the narrowest result yet – was a further psychological undermining of Blair's position, but it also reflected the limitations of both Brown and Blair in influencing rebels on an issue where the PLP felt very strongly. There were signs here of a sustained problem of party management under either Leader unless the behaviour of the Leader changed.

Leadership style

In February 2004 Blair told the Parliamentary Committee that he was not anxious to have majorities of five.[55] Optimists on the committee again took this as a sign of encouraging a possible change in the policy-making process. Indeed it might have opened up a thorough discussion of Blair governance including that an unhealthy fatalism-realism was developing about influencing policy formulation. In February 2004, Helen Jackson, a member of the Parliamentary Committee and also a PLP representative on the NEC and on the NPF, circulated privately a document which drew attention to Blair's 'drive to consolidate control over government in himself and the No. 10 machine (and that) cumulatively the process is driven along without thought for the implications'.[56] Chris Mullin had noted in his diary in March 2003 that 'we shall have to have a serious conversation with The Man about his style of government'.[57] But inhibition about being portrayed as oppositionists or being seen as working to Brown's ambitions, together with the loyalty of the party officials to Blair, led to a situation that discussion of the problem of Blair's method of leadership, and constructive change in it, never happened on the Parliamentary Committee nor, as far as can be discovered, in any other party forum. Here Brown's aggression had become an asset.

Departmental committees and policy formulation: problems revisited

Back in January 2003, a report to the Parliamentary Committee on the operation of Departmental Committees, given by the Senior Committee Officer Catherine Jackson, had noted that although there was a structure to maintain dialogue it was not as successful as had been hoped. Now, after the top-up fees result, dissatisfaction with the way that backbenchers were uninvolved in initial policy formulation moved into the centre of attention. This suggested the possibility of reopening a discussion of the understanding reached in 2001 on relations between the government and the Departmental Committees. That might in turn have led to an attempt to re-inject the obligation for an early element of joint consultation with the party. But again no discussion took place on the changes in obligations in 2001 which were known to only a few, nor on other proposals for a higher level of advance policy consultation as envisaged in 1996. The possibility of changing back to the proposals of 1996 was not raised by the PLP officials themselves because the fatalistic-realistic view of Howarth and Jackson was that there was no point: it was 'not going to happen', even though Blair told the Parliamentary Committee that a change in process was no problem for him.[58]

At this time, Wintour reported that Blair was 'wary that consultation will become an excuse for indecision'.[59] Yet, more importantly, he would not have been happy with others making decisions which were in tension with his role as authoritative culture carrier of the future; as he had ensured over Partnership in Power and over the responsibilities of ministers in relation to the departmental committees. His role had to be untrammelled regardless of what was said or hinted at to the party. There was also a strategic consideration that, although consultations on individual pieces of legislation were carried out in the latter stages much more in terms of Labour's traditional values and party perspectives, and controversial measures became in the end significantly different to the original version, each retained a movement forward in the direction that Blair had initially chosen. They could, at some future date, be expanded and in spirit and goals extend the Blair project into other areas and possibly under another government. In that sense he could feel that Blairism was winning.

Yet there was no way of escaping from the criticism that it was far from being a satisfactory way of making policy; indeed it was seen, even by Byers, a senior Blairite ex-Minister, as an example of 'how not to go about developing policy'.[60] Its critics considered that the policy formulation had produced faulty bills and added a dangerous edge to stored-up distrust, made cooperation more difficult and lowered morale in the PLP, indeed in the party as a whole.

There was a further problem facing MPs. In informal discussions around the decline in attendances at the departmental committees, some MPs thought that the Cook reforms – modernised family-friendly hours of work after January 2003 – whilst welcome in principle were becoming a detrimental influence. They filled in more morning times of the two working days, Tuesday and Wednesday already being taken up with more select-committee meetings. It meant that PLP members had to ration their party meeting times more than ever. The extra pressure of time was also a reinforcement of the problem of absenteeism from the House, with now about 40 MPs, both left and right, who felt that they had better things to do in their constituencies than attend weak committees.

Given poor attendances at the departmental committees, there was even a discussion amongst some of the least enthusiastic party officials in 2004–5 about abandoning the committees altogether and possibly instituting just ad hoc seminars. But here again what happened in the PLP was affected by its wider integration in the party. At the Warwick NPF of July 2004 PLP representatives linked with the departmental committee Chairs in their prior discussions and afterwards sought to build more systematic links to the committees. It was also re-recognised, with little enthusiasm, that if the departmental structure was abandoned there would have to be another structure put in its place.

Reasserting PLP discipline

Loss of sanctions revisited

Alongside private discussion of the problems of Blair's leadership there was also a hardened loyalist current in the PLP which was growing increasingly frustrated at the public criticism of him by Labour members and the incessant revolts. What was to be done about this indiscipline? It was argued by some of them that a liberal policy which aimed to build good relationships as credit in the bank 'did not work' in halting rebellions. So discussion turned once again to the fact that behind the scenes in the PLP and on the NEC, proposals involving sanctions had been constrained. A sense had grown that precedents had been established and it was time for these to be questioned. Support for more disciplinary action by the whips against 'disloyalty' was picked up by the well-informed Andrew Rawnsley. The more tough-minded of the Prime Minister's circle, he said, 'want to hear some firmer slapping'.[61]

Yet having in 2001 successfully undermined the image of his control freakery, Blair still found himself constrained by it. An important feature here was that a sudden move to the authoritarian could hand a propaganda weapon to the dissentients and carry with it some dangers of a new public reaction. Since rebels still voted overwhelmingly with their party[62], there could be even more trouble if as an independent separate group they developed, after sanctions, their own esprit de corps. It said something about the anxieties of the PLP managers about Labour Members' attitude towards disciplinary action that it was the party procedures outside the House which were used in relation to accusations against the openly dissenting MP George Galloway. He was charged with, amongst other things, inciting attacks on British troops and urging British troops to defy orders. Galloway was not suspended by the PLP till these NEC proceedings began and did not have the whip withdrawn before the ultimate sanction of expulsion by the National Constitutional Committee took place in October 2003.[63]

The two edged sword of this exclusion was that in 2005, fighting an unrestrained campaign, Galloway retained the seat. If sanctions were to be imposed in the PLP, that kind of consequence had to be borne in mind. It also had to be done in a way which did not set the 'control freakery' accusations flying again in the media, did not open up an internal war and could not point to the man in No. 10. That was especially difficult given the closeness of Armstrong and Blair. The hope of the Leader and the whips was that local loyalism, wanting action against disunity, could be quietly encouraged to constrain MPs against indulgent public gestures, thereby changing the climate of opinion. Blair was reported as telling the PLP after the top-up fees revolt that the Labour Party's call centre had been inundated with complaints from members about MPs who seemed to want to damage the party.[64] How representative that was must be uncertain given the managers' skills in instigation.

The immediate target became Clare Short who kept up regular pointed public criticism of Blair after her resignation. But Blair, Armstrong and Morgan were all wary of the special dangers of making her a martyr, especially as her criticism of his style of policy-making had a public credibility as well as party resonance. Opinion in the very limited Parliamentary Committee discussions on any of this was generally dominated by the view that attempts at disciplinary action through the PLP would simply split the party and draw more media attention. Eventually there was an uneasy accord between Armstrong and Short and some restraint on both sides. In leaving decisions on action against MPs to their CLPs, there was also some hope from mainstream critics of Short that she might be vulnerable to deselection. In practice, the unions, still playing the stabilising role encouraged under Blair, were reluctant to take part.

Privately, discussions amongst the managers moved on to how they might at least set the scene for more management control in the third term when there might not be such a huge government majority. In March 2004 some of that discussion was leaked in a very unhelpful way. Armstrong, it was reported, wanted the NEC to use the Chief Whip's report on MPs to organise 'show trials to axe MPs disloyal to Blair'.[65] That suggestion did evoke some serious private support amongst disciplinarians but there were some angry responses to the rumours and it was reported as being 'dismissed by the party machine' which would attempt 'to shame serial rebels into line'.[66] That was not surprising at all. There was no reason to believe that the NEC acting as a party managerial body would be more amenable to disciplinary sanctions than it had been in 1999. The attempt could easily rebound putting the Chief Whip in an embarrassingly weaker position. So, in the end, in an amazing and revealing turnabout, the Chief Whip's Report never even appeared at the NEC, although this had been considered an obligation under the rules. The revolts continued and the managers and the hard disciplinarian minority seethed with frustration.

Reactions to management

Breaking collective responsibility

In the post-Iraq-invasion period Blair's troubles were a signal to some that a leadership election and probably a deputy leadership election were not far away. Hain, a supporter of the war, played a role he had adopted before of working to the approval of the soft left in the party whilst keeping close in to the Leader. He had had some licence for this form of dissent accepted by the Political Office. But seeking to build party support he broke loose and twice went further than his licence in making his appeal to and for the party. On 21 June 2003, Hain called for the rich to pay higher taxes. Angry but frustrated, a campaign against PLP and Cabinet dissenters via the managers and loyalists in the party was now a favoured option of No. 10. There was an orchestrated series of messages to Downing Street calling for more discipline from Cabinet Ministers. After a period of quiet, Hain counter-attacked in a pamphlet focusing on 'censored' policy-making but also now extending the challenge to party management and efforts to manipulate internal elections.[67] It was an open rejection of the controlling system and received hefty support from a *Guardian* editorial, 'Hain is right . . . the over-centralised undemocratic and closed approach of the past has to change'.[68] That met an angry response from No. 10 though there was little that could be done without apparently confirming that Hain was right.

Weakening leadership and the limits of presidentialism

Here was the point at which, integral to the kind of supremacy over his party to which Blair had aspired, he might have engaged more directly with the electorate, speaking over the heads of the party to reinforce his position. But from the summer of 2003 he was in a weakening position to do so. The method of getting approval for invading Iraq had undermined public trust, and some of the contentious policies he brought forward had limited public enthusiasm. Unions had begun to consolidate a counter-organisation against the way that the party conference was managed (see pp. 590–1 below). If provoked by any attempt to go presidential, they and opponents in the party could have made their own public call and caused him and the government even greater trouble. Further to this Blair could see that unless he was careful he could create much ammunition for the party's media opponents about a publicly divided Labour party, adding to the damage done already by the Blair-Brown conflicts.

Changing Tony and new relations with the party

In the various responses in No. 10 to Blair's predicament, one major viewpoint, which continued right up to the 2005 election, returned to the pre-Iraq agenda seeking ways of freeing the Leader from his party and collegiate encumbrances. That would give the natural abilities and tendencies of the real Blair more room, deal with the Brown problem and gather strength to assert his radicalism. However, Blair also came under periodic advice with a different perspective, particularly from Sally Morgan, attempting to strengthen Blair by moving him closer to the party and gaining more support by being more consultative and collegiate. From an influential sympathiser outside, on 11 May 2004, there was also concern for a change in the attitude and behaviour of the Leader towards the wider party. Martin Kettle lamented that Blair had fallen 'increasingly prey to the belief that when in doubt . . . he will always gain electorally . . . by confronting or ignoring his party rather than by listening to it'. Labour could soon be in opposition again unless he was prepared 'to adapt and change. The dreadful mood of the party and the country gives him little choice'.[69]

Back to old Tony

It was reasonable advice but it ran against the past form of a man who had an ingrained bloody-mindedness in relation to the party. The local and European elections produced bad results but not as bad as Blair had feared. In the light of the election results, it was argued plausibly again by Martin Kettle that 'the people want a different kind of Blair'.[70] But this Blair was now bouncing back on the high of his own resilience. He had also received a motivating push once again in what seemed to be a new threat from Brown. Following joint discussions at the Treasury, Matthew Taylor had given Blair a private report that the Brown camp 'were considering significant alterations to the tuition fees reforms'.[71] Few things could have been more likely to wind Blair up than news of a threat to turn back one of his advances.

The emphasis from Blair's Political Office was now on 'Tony is a gut politician', which was another way of saying that there was to be no change in his political style. As for trust in him from the party, as a headquarters electoral adviser noted at this time, 'We are limited in how much you can make people trust him. It is conveyed organically from his positioning, message, achievements, keeping promises'. This was acute observation but there was nothing conveyed of what there was in his past behaviour Blair might seek to avoid. Again, change was for the party and the unions, not for him. A vivid sign of Blair's comfort in distance from his party came on a free vote on 15 September 2004. After years of PLP pressure the Hunting Act went through its third reading, with Blair grinning broadly as he was seen to vote against it.

Party regime change

There was another view of leadership and dissent that now gained publicity. In July 2004 an important article by the respected Labour historian Ross McKibbin, entitled 'How to dislodge a leader who doesn't want to go', bemoaned the passivity of the PLP as 'surprising and depressing' and urged Blair's removal.[72] That summer also the CLPD began calling for resolutions to the party conference seeking a new election for the Leader. In defending the Leader against such calls the managers had a cultural asset. As Heffernan had pointed out in a centenary appraisal, Labour Leaders had had a major security of tenure compared with their Conservative counterparts.[73] There was no history of the party getting rid of its Leader since Lansbury in 1935, and that was not through a procedural move but precipitated by withering public criticism from union leader Ernest Bevin.

But it was not just the culture and the precedents that affected the security of Blair. Nor was it just passivity. There was an element of sober calculation. For all the strength of the rebellions within the House and the animosity and distrust which Blair aroused amongst an increasing number in the PLP and the party at large, the loyalist current was still a powerful force carrying a deep sense that the party owed much of its success to Blair in reaching people that the party normally could not. And it could be reasonably questioned whether the seventy Labour MPs in marginal seats could be sure in moving from Blair to Brown that the English electorate would go for a Scottish redistributionist.[74] It could also be argued that forcing a leadership election would lead to a deeply split PLP.

Blair's position was also reinforced by a deep ambivalence about Brown, shared to varying degrees in anti-Blair sections of the PLP. True, Brown was widely regarded as a very clever man and a very successful Chancellor with a commitment to worthy social democratic causes, more respectful than Blair of the party's values and instincts, and more likely to revive the party. But he had become a convinced neoliberal in economic policy, close to the City of London, excited by the enterprise economy and at ease with the privatisation shift. More important, for many the search was not just for some adjustment of policy, but for a new style of leadership. Here, the problem was that Brown was also at ease with the 'New Labour' management, and its view of 'serious politics'. He was comfortable with short-term tactical manoeuvres, and his forcefulness and determination could verge on the bullying and insensitive. Those who worked with him often saw him as an unyielding and an uncooperative non-team player. This, and a reputation for being a cautious, cards-close-to-the-chest control freak, did not make him an attractive Leader of a revived and participatory party.

And 'Team Brown', as he and his aides became known to insiders, carried with them also an unusual level of group loyalty, coupled in some instances with the sulky manners of cheated and grievance-ridden family rivals. At this time in 2004, although the team around Blair were very circumspect in their open comments about Brown, from close to No. 10 and the whips' office there were dark and semi-discreet allusions to what would happen if Brown became Leader followed by: 'You'll find out'. These features produced concern rather than unrestrained enthusiasm for Brown amongst some anxious members of the PLP. For their part, Brown and his group carried a mix of repetitive robust covert attack together with inhibitions on the scope of their actions, limiting their capacity to produce Blair's downfall. Brown and especially his long-serving aide Sue Nye saw clearly the possibility of a poisonous heritage left by driving Blair out, especially that it might further liberate the PLP into an oppositionist mode, making party management a nightmare.

Adjustments and new pressures outside parliament

NEC elections

It was a revealing sign of the times that Tony Robinson, alienated by the behaviour of the machine and voting against the managers on foundation hospitals and on representation of MPs, MEPs and Peers on the NEC, did not stand for election to the CLP section in the now biennial elections held in 2004. He had reacted against the methods of controlling the Youth Section which by 2004 represented a virtually moribund youth organisation. Here, as before, the managers relied in elections on Amicus and UNISON for support against 'oppositionists'. The managerial methods around the NEC taught Robinson the way that power corrupted the relationship between a politician and the members 'who are manipulated and are treated with disdain if not contempt'.[75]

In the NEC elections of 2004, in a now customary low poll, only 22 per cent of members voted. This in itself did not disturb the attitude of the managers, but there was more concern at the result. Once again there were two partially overlapping slates from Labour First and from No. 10. Peter Wheeler, an independent figure from the traditional right, organised on his own but was then taken on to the official slate and gained a seat. In spite of the grassroots decline of the left, but in tune with the various revolts taking place, the Grassroots Alliance won the same three positions and came close in two others. Top of those who failed to gain a seat was Louise Baldock, an independent Blairite and ex-party organiser.

It was beginning to be noticeable also that changes in the unions were beginning to feed through into a slow shift of their NEC political representation. Important also was the sharpening of resentment at the arbitrary way that the NEC was at times treated by the managing officials. Helen Jackson put it like this: 'The NEC of the Party feels belittled, and somewhat resentful of a perceived assumption that it is simply a biddable "endorsing" body, as described in the media. It has a core of independent voices – all driven by a party loyalty rather than a career opportunity – who actually do deserve the trust of the Labour movement'.[76] The NEC, however, was still too inhibited and integrated within the governing management culture for the tensions within the party to be fully expressed.

Nevertheless, one significant shift did take place in the position of parliamentary representatives who after election to the Commons had been allowed to continue to sit on the NEC CLP section until new elections for the NEC. As a result of movement from below led by regular pressure from the GRA, especially Ann Black, backed also by the GMB, a constitutional amendment from the Oxford East party was supported by the NEC with all six CLP representatives voting together for the change. It went further than the issue of continuation of NEC membership. No elected member of the Commons, European Parliament, Scottish Parliament or Welsh Assembly or House of Lords would in future be allowed to stand in sections I–IV of the NEC and must cease to be a member if elected to them. The Lord Tom Sawyer anomaly – that a peer represented the grassroots – was ended.

Building supportive candidates

The anticipated composition of the PLP after the coming election was a major managerial concern. It was estimated that the larger the swing against the government the more loyalists with small majorities would be caught in it. Selections in safe seats became all the more important. Influencing candidate selection now involved an improved system of networking between the party centre and the regions to locate seats for suitable candidates and to give assistance to their campaigns, including the earlier provision of membership lists to the favoured. This was a discreet turn to what was described privately as being 'more canny'.

The leading academic expert in this field, Byron Criddle, described the party as now seeking to use 'a centralised system of candidate selection to transfer reliable favoured policy advisers and party staffers from state or party bureaucracies to parliamentary and ministerial careers'.[77] In practice, that was more a career push than a management pull, but it was welcomed in headquarters as a means of strengthening 'New Labour' in the PLP. There was nothing automatic about the selections involved. The task had the increasing problem in 2005 of the often adverse reactions in CLPs to an association with No. 10, although in some cases this could be countered by the attraction of a potential to add to the reputation of the constituency. What the candidate did could be crucial. This was increasingly a matter of 'running for office' and much depended on the energy of the candidate.

Two Blair advisers, Liz Lloyd and Razi Rachman, failed to be selected in Bishop Auckland and Brent South.[78] They were judged by other managers as to have not worked hard enough for it. On the other hand, in Wolverhampton South East there was a clear win for Pat McFadden, a man with huge managerial connections but also a very hard worker with all-round political competence. A trio of very prominent Brown aides emerged as candidates, Ian Austin in Dudley North, Ed Balls in Normanton and Ed Miliband in Doncaster North. There was, at one point of high tension between Blair and Brown, some Blairite managerial discussion about who of these might be stopped, although in the end this came to nothing. Each had good relations with the relevant regional managers and each evoked strong CLP support.

No new cause célèbre drew down the kind of media fire on Blair's head that had been seen over Wales and London. But there was an illuminating example of Blair's pragmatism and attitude to rules in dealing with the popular and successful Livingstone. In 2003 an attempt to bring him back into the party was defeated on the NEC under the party's rules about re-entry, with the PLP leaders united against him. But, on 6 January 2004 at the Leader's initiative, under the same rules he was allowed back into the party by the NEC on a vote of 22 to 2 because he was now seen as un-defeatable at a time of declining confidence in Blair and the government. The public reconciliation over Livingstone also helped to bury deeper the control freak experience from 2000. In spite of some opposition to this 'bad precedent' from within the party machine, in November 2004 the Labour mayoral candidate Nicky Gavron agreed to stand down to allow Livingstone to stand. In a ballot of party members, the old rebel was over-whelmingly endorsed as the Labour candidate and again swept to victory.

In selections at this time there were attractions to be seen as an independent-minded but non-oppositionist candidate who was capable of speaking up for the locality, but it was rare now for an outright left-wing critic to be newly selected. Katy Clark, the legal officer of UNISON, was one rarity, winning the selection in North Ayrshire and Arran. But the most unusual case was at Halifax where left-wing candidate Linda Reardon, backed by the existing MP Alice Mahon with union and Cooperative Party support, won the selection. That result was challenged at the NEC by ministers acting on behalf of the managers who were convinced that Reardon would lose the seat. In a situation almost unprecedented since the NEC composition change in 1998 the government block was not united on the committee (The only previous occasion being when Prescott split over the time of the party conference ending). But the NEC, with strong support from members of the union group, voted 12–8 to allow it to stand. Reardon did not lose the seat in 2005. Indeed, against the national tide she was still there even after the 2010 election.

Another indication of an increase in countervailing power in some circum-stances came with the Leicester South by-election. By-election shortlisting had been invariably dominated by the leadership's preferences since the mid-1980s. But in 2004 against the wishes of Downing Street and the Chief Whip the panel, influenced by Mike Griffiths, aware of the local situation, did not vote to keep off the strong local candidate Peter Soulsby, who was easily selected, avoiding a big local conflict. He was, however, defeated by a Liberal Democrat in the election apparently justifying No. 10's position, but then he recaptured the seat in 2005 and held it in 2010 with swing towards him.

In 2002, legislation had been introduced which restored the power to have selection through all-women shortlists. The NEC responded by setting the long-term target of 50:50 representation and set an immediate target of 35 per cent representation in areas with particularly low women's representation. Late retirements were to be automatically made all-women shortlists, but the NEC also retained a power 'to authorise exemptions in special circumstances'.[79] This loophole was an opportunity for politics around last-minute retirements, of which there was an extraordinary number continuing till late in the day. There were 58 MPs who retired early, nearly twice as many as in 2001. An NEC Late Retirement Panel was constructed, which was by no means a patsy group for the Leader or the managerial officials. John Prescott also got involved in defending the independence and propriety of the process.

There was a digging-in-of-heels by members of the panel against proposals from various sources which were seen as attuning the occurrence of all-women short lists to the advantage of particular favoured sons or daughters. The most contentious seat was Copeland which was not an all-women shortlist, but non-partisan insiders judged that it probably should have been. Devonport went the opposite way, changed to an all-women shortlist. The outcome of all this was described by one independent senior NEC member defending the neutral criteria as 'We won some, we lost some.' It was a further advance for women. As Criddle pointed out, 23 of the new MPs were from all-women shortlists.[80]

Because of the past problems over women's representation in Wales, there was extra determination centrally to ensure that the candidature for the safest seat in Wales, Blaenau Gwent had an all-women short list. Crucially, the view in headquarters was that the Welsh reaction over the London treatment of Rhodri Morgan had left no significant legacy. Maggie Jones was a very capable candidate with strong local family associations. However, there was a local challenger, Peter Law, forty years a member, who had nursed the seat for some time. It was a seat with strong left-wing traditions where some of its members, including the retiring MP Llew Smith, harboured additional resentment against a Blairite 'puppet' from London, known to be a prominent and long-standing NEC loyalist. Defeated in the party ballot, Law fought the seat as an independent Labour candidate with his focus on the treatment of the London connection. The result was a parliamentary election result unparalleled in Labour Party history

– a swing against of 49 per cent. The senior managers, keeping an eye on the changing power relations around the Leader, were nevertheless confident that in spite of the signs of disenchantment below, overall the outcome of the selections was satisfactory in terms of the composition of the next PLP. And on the NEC there were few revolts against the leadership, for the reasons which had become dominant since 1998.

The grass still comes away from the roots

At the same time, the decline in membership continued and, as far as limited information allows it to be judged, after Iraq at an increased rate. It could be argued that the decline of party membership was a common international feature but, as Cruddas and Harris pointed out later, there were 'clear and addressable reasons for much of Labour's decline from the voice denied to ordinary members to the policies pursued'.[81] Rising membership had been an emblem of the vitality and distinctiveness of 'New Labour', and each Party Chair on appointment was urged by Blair to build up the membership.

Yet in 2003 the energetic and committed Chair, Reid became lost in seeking a way to build on the unpopular policies. At one stage, he and the other party managers had to fall back on attempts to obscure the extent of politically motivated resignations over Iraq by defining resignations only as those who had written to give that reason. It was also said by an official that the membership problem was often a case of them not being asked to renew. But, if true, that was also saying something about the low morale amongst constituency activists. Overall, try as they did, it was difficult to hide the politics of the loss of membership. Their own internally declared figures were that from 272,000 in 2001 it had dropped to 240,000 in April 2004. Of these, 30,000 were up to six months in arrears and 16,000 were over six months.

National Policy Forum and the road to Warwick

Loyalism and the problem of management

By 2003 a record number of constituency parties and affiliated organisations had made submissions to the policy process. The dialogue at the NPF continued to give its regular members a sense of it being a worthwhile experience. But at all levels there was scepticism about members' influence. Some in the NPF loyalist network had developed their own private doubts and frustrations. It had led to some divisions and defections amongst the loyalists, especially at the NPF in November 2003 at Newport when Anne Snelgrove was thought not to be standing again as vice chairman. Tony Robinson decided to stand but then Snelgrove did stand and defeated Robinson. Robinson was infuriated by the intervention of No. 10 and party officials in this election and the effrontery of their denial that it had happened. It reinforced his reaction to Blairite party management. Another leading loyalist, Daniel Zeichner voted with Robinson and was excluded thereafter from the loyalist group. Zeichner was then removed from the place on the policy commissions for a couple of years.

The loyalist group continued to emphasise that many important issues got discussed at NPF without a power struggle or a vote. Mental health was one example. 'A whole range of soft improvements were achieved in the documents adding to their quality' was their view. Working persistently with ministers was central to the loyalist focus of partnership. The managers, particularly some of the NEC trade union representatives, were acknowledged to be a big problem, always fearful of losing control. But if the CLP representatives tried to work round them, experience suggested that the managers would panic and behave in a worse way. It was important to build up the trust of the leadership so that you could say that they were wrong and be listened to. It was also believed by some of them that the managers thought that under new critical pressure they could not get away with the kind of tactics employed in 1998–2000. In that sense it was said that the managers had to have loyalist assent. But the loyalists had an immovable bottom line that they would not vote against the leadership, and that undermined their potential influence over the control-conscious management.

The managerial fear of losing control even made it difficult for anyone to pursue independent activity to reform the process. The PLP representative on the NPF Helen Jackson consulted MPs on their local experience of policy-making and the PIP arrangements[82] but copies of her findings were not open to discussion at the NPF because they did not have the agreement of the Party Chair McCartney and, behind him, a very resistant No. 10. Those still seeking a review of PIP were fobbed off on the grounds that a review had 'already been going on'. Unhappy at this lack of movement, the National Political Forum of UNISON called for a review and this was pushed successfully at the NEC in September 2003 by UNISON representatives, including Maggie Jones. It was slow going but the review was eventually undertaken by three NEC working groups examining engagement with the party, the government and the country. The composition of the groups was carefully chosen by McCartney and the relations with government working group was chaired by McCartney himself. An interim report did not appear until September 2004. It went to the JPC and then to the 2005 conference after the election.

The unions and changing party management

New Leadership and TULO

In October 2003, Bill Morris of the TGWU (who had sometimes played what was seen as an uncertain political role leading TULO) retired. The Chairmanship of TULO now passed to Tony Dubbins, the GPMU General

Secretary closely linked to Mike Griffiths as Chair of the Organisation Committee (from 2001) and John O'Regan as political adviser. The GPMU in 2004 amalgamated into Amicus and its senior political figures became in effect the political team of that union working with Derek Simpson. There was now a very easy and consistent relationship between this lead union and the efficient TULO officials working in Party headquarters, the TULO Liaison Officer Byron Taylor and his deputy (until 2006) Andy Bagnall.

Dubbins and the team around him saw their role as keeping the TUC and the affiliated unions working together but preserving their different responsibilities. This was a new coalition unionism seeking to keep the new union leaders within the broader representation of TULO and the TUC. It would be working to keep up a constructive dialogue with the Labour leadership whilst pursuing the united use of Labour Party procedures by its affiliates to ensure that the coordinated union voice circumvented management control and that the conference was fed by the NPF in ways which, in the practice expected under Partnership in Power, gave the conference a final say. From this, they aimed to take some firm commitments into a new manifesto.

The tactical divide and the battle in the party

This view was challenged by another strategy more focused on TUC-Government relations and advocated by the Unions 21 organisation as its think-tank of knowledgeable trade union participants and advisers. A pamphlet it published in 2003, *What Next for the Unions?*, criticised the Government's lack of an agenda which had a social place for trade unionism and the limitations of the Government objectives. But it also criticised the limitations of the new union agenda, and the failure of the unions to fully embrace the opportunities of what it asserted was a favourable public policy climate. It clashed with the new left union leaders and TULO in suggesting that the way forward was a way of managing relationships 'rather than a list of programmatic demands'.

Success, it suggested, should not be judged by the number of items from the TUC shopping list which went into the next election manifesto, nor should increasing the number of statutory rights be seen as bringing closer the elusive European social model. It was said to be a misunderstanding of that model which was as much about the way that the parties did business as it was about achievement of substantive legal rights. The unions needed to move on from the employment-law agenda and push for Labour market institutions that put unions at the heart of national as well as firms' decision-making.

For some of the new union leaders this was interpreted as a frustrating preoccupation with process that both expressed and reinforced the weakness of the TUC. The new leaders were deeply suspicious of what they saw as the integration of the TUC into the Blair government's objectives – subverted and demeaned by the government and the Downing Street managers. With that critique the new union leaders were also contemptuous of the paraphernalia of governmental rewards – peerages and knighthoods – and were constantly looking to establish other factors in the London set-up that caused past union leaders to be less assertive than they should be. The obvious signs that the Unions 21 pamphlet was being pushed by party managers made both Unions 21 and the TUC that much more suspect.

The unions' counter-management and the road to Warwick

Internal party action by the affiliated unions was also pressurised from outside. Bob Crow, the non-Labour General Secretary of RMT, argued 'How do you (fight from within) when you see that the Conference is rigged?'.[83] In 2004, Crow sought to build a broader political strategy including affiliation to the Scottish Socialist Party. After an agonised NEC debate the view taken was 21 votes to 3 that the RMT (the forerunner of which had initiated what became the formation of the Labour Party) was expelled as being in contravention of the rulebook. Privately, the argument was that if this had been allowed, it would risk further piecemeal disaffiliation. A long dispute between the government and the firefighters over a pay claim damaged relations – particularly with John Prescott after the government forced withdrawal of an offer brokered by the TUC. A settlement was reached but on 17 June 2004 after long recriminations the FBU conference voted to disaffiliate. No other unions followed the RMT's 33,000 affiliated members and the FBU's 20,000, and they made little or no attempt to form another party.[84] Disaffiliation remained a minority current in the affiliated unions but it did further provoke the unions staying in the party to organise for an advance that would show the value of their affiliation.

Examining party management
In the tense distrustful atmosphere following the 2003 conference, TULO unions held urgent discussions amongst themselves as to how the party management system worked and how party managers might be countered. What they learned seemed to give an understanding of the way in which unions failed to achieve what their members wanted through the party. A broadly shared union perspective on party managerial activities which had historically underpinned stable support for the leadership now began to underpin an institutionalised counter-management organisation.

The plan for the final NPF meetings
Coming up in March and July 2004 were the two very important forums which would agree the policy reports to be made to the party conference

and also had the power to register minority positions as had happened at the Exeter NPF. The NPF votes which were to be taken at the 2004 Conference that followed would give the unions their maximum leverage and the danger to the leadership that initiatives from the unions could create a well-publicised pre-election series of splits. Byron Taylor from the TULO office produced a strategic plan with Dubbins to focus preparation on the final NPF meetings. It would organise to keep maximum unity and avoid the seductions coming from the divide-and-rule tacticians in No. 10. This offered a counter to the new ginger group Labour Representation Committee, set up in 2004 by MPs from the Socialist Campaign group with four national union affiliates – RMT, FBU, CWU and BFAWU – with left policies and a focus on the failure of unions to be properly represented within the Labour Party.

But as in 2000, before the Exeter NPF, tactical movements within the unions were noted and paralleled by various managerial initiatives seeking to forestall or take the edge off what the unions were proposing. A major alternative possibility for No. 10 was to replicate the Morgan-Norris tactics of Exeter in 2000, turning these NPF meetings into a firmer base for pre-election unity which would avoid a major confrontation at the party conference. It would offer initiatives and concessions, of which many were not even part of the union agenda. This would cement agreement without crossing major lines of unacceptability and/or stirring up antipathy from the CBI. Ian McCartney as Party Chair with his special adviser Martin O'Donovan linking to Dubbins and Taylor in TULO became the major broker taking the principle to Blair for his assent. For No. 10, avoiding a potential conference 'disaster' was their central preoccupation, integrated with defending the settlement with the CBI.

National Policy Forum

The Warwick meetings

At this time, the Partnership in Power process was looking increasingly unhealthy and the informational feed-in from the grassroots was more restricted compared with that of the last cycle. At Exeter in accordance with previous understandings, the regional policy forum submissions had been circulated to representatives at the NPF to give guidance. These policy forums had become fewer, with lower attendances, and there was no such circulation at the two Warwick meetings. Also not circulated were national submissions from party organisations although they could be read at party headquarters if the journey was made.

The management of the March meeting, although it did not cover the range of issues dealt with in July, further reinforced the growing union suspicion of management behaviour. This began with problems caused by the party's numbering of policy documents in such a way as to complicate the unions' attempt at policy coordination throughout the Forum. More significant was a clumsy last-minute attempt by a combination of headquarters officials and No. 10 to revise the rules for the sequence of voting in a way that would, it was argued, avoid the possibility of incompatible positions being supported. That was a reasonable concern, although the verbally presented solution appeared to make the acceptance of minority positions more difficult. Perhaps the busy managers were simply misunderstood. But crucially, there had been no notification, let alone consultation, over the change; it had not been taken to the JPC which formally supervised the procedures.

This experience confirmed to union representatives of the need for maximum union watchfulness, organisation and unity and for more reassurance that any agreement would be kept. In the meantime, so great was the pressure against what appeared as an attempt to bounce through procedural change, that under McCartney's guidance, and after a new consultation, the old procedure was brought back. There was an understanding that Forum members could vote for which alternatives they wanted even if they were said to be incompatible. In addition and, in a step forward, the movers of amendments as well as the leadership were to be allowed to make short contributions before the vote was taken.

The March NPF also received a detailed report on the Big Conversation given by Matthew Taylor, who had replaced Adonis as head of the policy unit in No. 10. The Big Conversation website in the year of its operation made no comment on Iraq,[85] and Taylor's report was revealing in one key respect that it also made no mention of Iraq. Unusually, this was openly challenged at the forum, by the party's Policy Director, Luke Bruce. His view was that Iraq was an important background influence on everything.[86] This semi-public exchange raised an issue which had always been there in the conduct of the Big Conversation and similar mechanisms. How far was this genuine and how far was it yet another mode of presenting an image of receptivity by the government and spinning the most sensitive outcomes? For Blair's staff the problem of dealing with Iraq was all the more acute because, as Mattinson revealed later, Blair's star pollster Stan Greenberg was declared 'sacked for passing on the electorate's fury and urging Blair to apologise',[87] although 'somehow nobody ever did it'.[88]

As for policy development in this March NPF, much of the two documents examined were uncontroversial. Over public funding of political parties there was an important prohibition on donation caps and on proposals which would undermine the trade union link. The policy process over a Single Equalities Act was based on a renewed campaign launched by Angela Eagle MP but initially opposed by Government ministers as too difficult. Now it had the backing of the Secretary of State at the DTI Patricia Hewitt, and Deborah Lincoln, her special adviser. The consensus wording involved an agreement that committed the party to a review with the aim of drafting legislation.

An agreement was reached after the furore over the procedures which allowed an amendment, that the composition of the House of Lords be 'as democratic as possible', to get through as the alternative position only in the loose form that the leadership wanted. However, an amendment to delete the reference to NHS Foundation Trust Boards as an example of extending empowerment also got enough support to go through as a minority position. But the weak status of the NPF as an authoritative body on contemporary policy issues was further revealed first over a Palestine policy accepted at the NPF but publicly repudiated in the next few weeks, then over a European Charter of Rights also approved by the NPF but then repudiated by Jack Straw and made a red-line issue.

The Warwick agreement

Build-up

The second Warwick meeting from 25 to 27 July had the unpromising build-up of a series of critical speeches and articles by union leaders. Some of the preliminary meetings with ministers were described as sluggish. There was a lift to the process when a two-year-old commitment to end the two-tier workforce reached a final stage after McCartney took it to the Domestic Policy Committee of the Cabinet with the backing of the Prime Minister. That announcement, before the Forum started, pleased UNISON and the GMB in particular. It was part of a discreet agenda of offers. But Ministers also brought with them a note of heavy red-line issues covered by union submissions which were not negotiable. These included the reopening of labour law and its 'settlement'.

The TULO unions agreed their policies based on their own internal union mandates and a careful submission of agreed amendments. To the fury of the headquarters managers there was also an agreement, eventually secured by McCartney, that allowed the unions to work from an office on-site and from which they developed their own floor operation. Memories of how in the last round they had been damaged by the No. 10 divide-and-rule managerial tactics became a source of union-unifying strength. Although there were tensions, particularly between the big four and the next two largest unions USDAW and the CWU, who were not always brought into the huddles, they stayed together.

Pluralism and the politics of negotiation

Together with their new cohesion, new more open behaviour from the unions had knock-on effects to other groups. Unions kept closer links with the Grassroots Alliance and also responded to loyalist demands for private meetings. The PLP group made efforts to hold meetings with the trade unions, as did the Local Government Labour group. The healthy range of multiple informal meetings and extensive networking pulled in advocates for various lobbies including those covering the environment and housing which fed into and from the union concerns. So a stronger new form of pluralism emerged which gave participants the sense that an advance in the quality of the process was happening.

CLPs and managers

The union collective push had an effect on the assertiveness of the CLP loyalists and influenced their 'work with us, negotiate with us on policy' argument to the managers. Pat McFadden, Nita Clarke and John McTiernan from No. 10 were made aware of the need for the loyalists to come away with something in order to help produce a good story about the NPF. A relaxation of managerial activity took place which involved them being more prepared to live with what went into the documents. The loyalists who also worked at times with the Grassroots Alliance where they were in agreement were, in the end, very happy with what was achieved. Anne Snelgrove produced a huge list of items which together the CLP loyalists and the Grassroots Alliance had been, it was said, secured in the document. None of this was dramatic in content or immediately influential but was useful in laying down markers of opinion and legitimating the role of the CLP representatives.

PLP at NPF

The nine PLP representatives from the NPF elected in 2003 for the next two years – Vera Baird, Anne Begg, Anne Campbell, Parmjit Dhanda, Mike Gapes, Linda Gilroy, Jim Knight, Dari Taylor and Lawrie Quinn – were politically balanced, but again excluding the Socialist Campaign Group left whose members did not stand. PLP representatives had in the past operated as a group only to cover particular issues and decide who reported back. Now, prompted by the development in the unions, the PLP representatives also attempted to operate overall as a group supporting each other's positions. These positions in the form of a priority list were arrived at following discussions with PLP departmental committee chairs, back-bench members of the Parliamentary Committee and the trade union group and women's group of the PLP.

In this process, some significant tensions emerged between the PLP managers and headquarters managers when the PLP Chair supported sending a member of the PLP staff to assist the group but opposed an intervention by a representative of headquarters managers. In the final vote some of the members resisted sitting and voting together and on some votes, including housing, where there was not a pre-agreed position, they went their separate ways. But PLP representatives also came away with a strong feeling that in this pluralistic form the partnership in power was working. Issues thought to have involved gains included equality over women's pensions, opposition to two-tier education, support for policies to assist in congestion charges, assurances in relation to future development aid, and seeking agreement on the international finance facility.

Leadership tactics and the battle with the unions

As in the last round at Warwick, Norris, covering the business relationship, was the key figure representing the Prime Minister. The long-drawn-out series of negotiations involved the big four union leaders and Dubbins on one side, and a wide range of ministers, advisers and officials, including Charles Clarke and Alan Johnson with DTI special advisers Ian Stewart and Deborah Lincoln on the other. But Hewitt, McCartney and Sutcliffe did most of the negotiating work and in the complex and protracted discussions there was room for some ministerial discretion.

The union side began as deeply distrustful pessimists about the possibility of a major agreement and uncertain for some time about their priorities. That made their initial contribution unsatisfactory and awkward to the government side who privately criticised its intellectual incoherence. But the government side added to the problems by changes of personnel and sometimes a failure to express their position early lest the unions asked for more. At one point, the government came up with 15 pages of text obliterating existing amendments – a complete break with past practice not to mention the Taylor 'no parachuting' dictum. Discussions took many hours, with the first sign of agreement being a section on manufacturing which brought Brown and Simpson closer together. The final section was not agreed until 2 am on the morning the forum ended. As at Exeter, the TULO meetings with ministers were not attended by other NPF members including relevant policy-commission members. Although attempts were made to keep the NPF working groups informed about progress in the TULO talks, this independent sideshow again caused irritation amongst some CLP loyalist representatives, but this was against the background of other more satisfying relations. The vote on what became 'the Warwick Agreement' was supported by all the CLP representatives as well as all the unions.

The agreement covered between 56 and 110 items, depending on how they were grouped or separated. Results included final elimination of the two-tier workforce for the public services, a new 'women at work' commission, additional family-friendly rights including a review of the right to request flexible hours for parents and carers, maternity, paternity, adoptive and parental leave and extending respite care. Rights for migrant workers were included, stopping employers holding their passports. Once more it was registered that the Royal Mail would stay in public hands and legislation on corporate manslaughter (a 1997 manifesto commitment) would be in this parliamentary term. On pensions there was to be a move to make pensions a bargaining issue for recognition purposes and new measures on women's pensions. There would be training for pension trustees and a move to 50 per cent member trustees. In an agenda that went wider than work issues it affirmed that 'Labour is committed to narrowing inequalities in society, tackling the gap between rich and poor and abolishing child and pensioner poverty'. It also returned to the 'loan sharks' agenda with a broad call for legal limits to stop rip-off interest rates for credit. There was confirmation of support for the public funding of parties and there was what turned out to be a highly problematic policy of seeking to determine the precise role and boundaries of the private sector in the NHS.

Not obvious, but central to management of the agreement, was that according to union sources, no more than 40 of the 110 came from union claims; the rest were offered as government initiatives. These included change in the working-time directive. The UK had been the only EEC member where the directive of four weeks' annual holiday entitlement had been reduced to take account of eight days of public holidays. This was now set aside, with the government side claiming credit and some managers saying privately that they had always been opposed to the provision. The proposal for extra finance for the union modernisation fund, which was to become a particular target of criticism from the Conservatives, also came from the government side.

There was no commitment to International Labour Organisation standards and the leadership had retained its red lines on labour law apart from one issue which was of great concern to the TGWU. Protection from dismissal for strikers was raised from 8 weeks to 12 weeks, in line with the 2003 conference decision and in spite of Norris's discontent. Other than that all the other major labour-law issues which unions had brought to Warwick were rejected. A reconsideration of the 21 employees criteria for employment rights supported by research was said very quietly by the union side to have been verbally a final promise of an experimental change agreed through the minister, Sutcliffe. If so, following changes on the ministerial side it disappeared.

After Warwick

Reactions

Overall the agreement gained more than union pessimists had anticipated. As for the ministers and managers, they had avoided a crisis at the party conference with some private satisfaction that they had not been pushed further. Even the CBI, it was said, was reasonably happy, nourished by Norris after at one stage fearing worse. It helped that much of the agreement prepared on the government side was sellable as a modernisation package. There was no heavy hostile media reaction against 'the power of the unions'. Various explanations can be offered for this which are not exclusive. The claim of No. 10 insiders was that it showed that they had neutralised the union question. But it was also helped that there was no immediate public anti-union steer from around the Leader. Impressionistic evidence also suggests that by this time, some union assertiveness was seen by more people as a healthy counterweight to an over-mighty business influence and a government under Blair's one-alone style.

Warwick, finance and the myth of the piper

Within the relatively uncontroversial press reception was the *Sunday Times* description that 'Labour renewed its financial alliance with the trade unions through the Warwick agreement'.[89] That evidence-free account apart, there was a notable absence of immediate accusations of union financial power, or party dependence either in the media or from the party's opponents. Further, in the aftermath of Warwick, there was an intense post-mortem by individuals in No. 10 and in the unions over why and how it had come about, and what lessons might be learned. In those discussions nobody on either side reported any mention of financial pressure, anticipated or experienced.[90]

Yet later, out of the blue, this diagnosis suddenly took on a new authority after an academic study in 2005 by Butler and Kavanagh alleged that the agreement was 'prompted in large part by the need for union financial support for the general election'.[91] It was a mistaken focus given the cemented affinity with the wealthy, and what Peter Watt described later as the casual No. 10 assumption that the money would somehow be found.[92] And it missed the fundamental points about the new agreement.

One was the growth of counter-managerial organisation on the union side making more acute the growing managerial concern with pre-election unity at the party conference and in the manifesto meeting. That concern involved seeking to encourage the unions to play their old managerial auxiliary role at those venues. It has also been argued that this Warwick meeting was 'far more significant than any recent party conference'.[93] But this comparison does not take account of the interplay of the two institutions, what had happened to union organisation following the conferences of 2002 and 2003 and the problems for the management of the conference of 2004 if agreement had not been reached at the NPF.

The party managers did not get fully what they wanted in the Warwick discussions; a commitment from the unions to unite with the managers in opposing all amendments from the Grassroots Alliance. But the Grassroots Alliance itself did now agree to remit their amendments. TULO did go some way towards promising to regard the party conference as a pre-election rally but with reservations about what they were prepared to do. The leadership could not prevent rail renationalisation becoming an alternative position to the party conference and similarly with the housing 'fourth' option favouring a level playing field on social housing by which local authorities would be able to invest in existing housing.

Warwick: sanctification and grievance

In the weeks after Warwick and before the party conference, there were constant references from the leadership to implementing 'Warwick' and even a remarkable new emphasis on 'partnership' with the unions. Blair made the requested speech at the TUC advocating trade union membership, albeit carefully worded and offered with no great enthusiasm. Some of the sticky working difficulties within party headquarters in relating to coop-eration with the TULO unit disappeared. In October 2004, it was explained privately by a clever senior official that 'We are trying to be more straight. I hope that you think we are'. Nevertheless, the fact remained that no attempt was made to renovate the old 'rules' and protocols of the relation-ship, and the Warwick agreement had many uncertainties of specificity and commitment.

It was a conglomeration of proposals with varying wording and no detailed codification. One of the proposals, for sector working parties, fell to pieces very quickly immediately after opposition from UNISON. On the government side, 'Warwick' was interpreted as not reopenable by the unions but openable by the government which had the responsibility to govern. Later it became clear that the party management view of the *Warwick Agreement* had become what was in the final report of Labour's National Policy Forum, subsequently endorsed by the party conference. That included some important decisions not discussed with the unions which remained contested on the union side. This was most immediately relevant to an argument over ID cards, support for which was held by the managers to have been covered at Warwick.[94] As a procedure, this was challenged in some unions, notably UNISON, and also challenged in terms of the sub-stance of the Warwick decisions by NEC member Ann Black, 'It is the government which is breaking the bargain'.[95]

Conference management and Iraq

At the party conference in September 2004 CLP attendance showed a continuing decline. Of 641 constituencies only 500 sent representatives.[96] But the managers were heavily represented. It was estimated by one ex-manager that with normally five staff per region – some 50 people were involved full-time in the activity of gaining the intelligence, making the contacts, putting out the message and getting out the votes. The potential post-mortem on the deteriorating situation in Iraq was a managerial con-cern so it was an advantage that the NEC Report didn't go out in time for the CLPs to examine it before the conference. But Iraq did get on the agenda, topping the issues voted for under contemporary resolutions. Blair as well as the managers became actively involved in some hard pressure on Prentice, Simpson and Woodley to gain union support for an NEC statement which took a unifying future-focused position and not a backwards-looking criticism.

The TGWU had special problems here. It had been and remained strongly opposed to the invasion and wanted that registered, but it was also con-cerned over the defence of free trade unionism in Iraq. A representative of the Iraq trade unions addressed their delegation which met on more than one occasion before it made up its mind to respond to his call not to support a timetable of withdrawal.[97] In the conference debate, that representative also made a powerful speech which added to the influences pulling delegates behind the platform position. In the end, the TGWU joined a huge hand vote in favour of the unifying NEC statement and rejected a constituency composite resolution asking for an early date to be set for troop withdrawal. It was voted down by 85.8 per cent to 14.2 per cent, with the unions voting 90 to 10 in opposition. It was a significant unifying moment but leaving some unsatisfied with what they were voting for.

Partnership in Power: the final votes

In the ballot for contemporary resolutions as had now become routine, officials advised CLP delegates to vote for the union priorities because there was no time for other resolutions. As for the five alternative positions which had been produced by the NPF, two – one on NHS Foundation Hospitals Trust Boards and one on voting at 16 – were avoided by a delegate remitting, a problematic procedure as already noted over the 2000 conference. Of the remaining three, one on House of Lords reform calling for a more democratic and representative second chamber was now accepted by Lord Falconer, attempting to create new consensus around indirect elections and hoping to make this amendment the basis for legislative agreement. Defeats for the leadership came on rail renationalisation carried by 63.7 per cent against 36.3 per cent. Over 99 per cent of union votes supported this but remarkably 72 per cent of CLP delegates were declared to have voted against even though all the evidence from the membership suggested majority support.[98] They were also defeated over increasing the supply of affordable housing and creating a level playing field for local authorities to invest in existing housing. This was carried overwhelmingly across the conference on a show of hands. The unions helped the managers by regarding these as 'outside the Warwick Agreement' and a matter for individual unions. The managers later found other means to use Warwick as a block vote control mechanism in the manifesto discussions (see p. 600 below).

Blair, Brown and the departure date

Blair's surprise announcement on 30 September 2004, immediately following the conference, that he would serve a full third term but not seek a fourth term, added new political complications and provoked new calculations about what it meant for power and party management. In practice, although the wording of the commitment was to have an undermining impact on his position over time, for the moment he gained some security and a new opportunity to plan for more freedom to improve his position in the subterranean and occasionally open war with Brown. That reached a new damaging pre-election point where on 9 January 2005 in an advance

Sunday Telegraph extract from a book by Robert Peston, Brown was quoted as having said to Blair, 'There is nothing that you could ever say to me now that I could ever believe'.[99] Blair denied that it had been said to him.[100] Furious Blair allies regarded this as another stab in the back and it led to an acute intensification of the battle between the two camps. A PLP meeting on 10 January was heavily critical of the squabbling, although some centre-ground MPs at the meetings saw it as more a remonstrance to Brown than to Blair.

The manifestos and management

Meanwhile, the union-government relationship was moving more smoothly. Agreement was finally reached now over the composition of the manifesto meeting bringing the Cabinet formally back into it whilst also leaving in the Parliamentary Committee and, introduced for the first time in history, there was direct representation of the unions, through TULO. Three representatives of the CLP section of the NPF were also brought on, chosen by the NPF but in effect appointed by the managers in agreement with the loyalist group leaders.

A series of consultative meetings on the manifesto included advance meetings between the Party Chair, No. 10 aides and a TULO-TUC Contact Group, and also a meeting of the managers with NEC representatives and a separate one with the NEC trade union members. The meetings continued with the Parliamentary Committee officers and separately the three CLP representatives of the NPF. In the light of the manifesto draft commitment to deliver the Warwick policies 'in full', and a fulsome assertion of the importance of modern trade unionism, there was an especially cooperative atmosphere in relations with union representatives. And the repeated party rejection of privatisation of the Post Office was taken as represented by the commitment that 'we have no plans to privatise'.

In assisting the government, union leaders were prepared to avoid supporting renationalisation of railways in the manifesto because it was 'outside Warwick', although as individuals and as leaders of individual unions with union policy on the issue some would have thought themselves bound to do so if it came to a vote. There was an unprecedented request by the Party Chair that not only should there not be amendments in the Clause V meeting but 'in order to solidify the Warwick agreement' there would only be votes for or against the manifesto as a whole, taken at the end of the meeting. Only Helen Jackson with a compassionate amendment, which said 'we mourn the loss of life of innocent civilians and coalition forces in the war in Iraq', pushed in advance and then during the meeting, managed to break through the prohibition with an agreed insertion.

One tricky problem was that the draft prepared in No. 10 by Matthew Taylor included a commitment to using new providers in the NHS where they 'added capacity or promoted innovation'. That unqualified proposal had not been agreed by the NPF which had said that the ultimate intended share of the private sector 'needs to be determined'.[101] As expressed here it potentially left room for a virtually unbounded radical Blairite agenda, although in this more friendly union-government atmosphere it was understood that interpretation would be guided by an unpublicised agreement between UNISON General Secretary Prentis and the health minister Reid; the private sector would only be involved on the margins. If Brown had any policy reservations he did not open them up. The receptive atmosphere was also helpful to the Leader and his aides attempting to recommit to directly elected mayors for local government. Though it had not been rediscussed in recent NPF meetings nor in the policy documents, now suddenly it was in the draft manifesto and said to be 'no change from past policy'.

The draft did take account of the strong party feeling over the extension of social housing and promised to 'give local authorities the ability to start building homes again'. A radical proposal from Milburn to extend the right to buy to housing association tenants was stopped by Prescott. The CLP representatives were happy at it being 'a good manifesto' in terms of what they thought CLPs wanted and in tune with their own long-term contributions. But, as in the past, it remained hard to locate any significant item which would not otherwise have been there but for the CLP contribution to Partnership in Power.

From another part of the political world, the implementation of the Warwick Agreement was becoming subject to the cross-pressure between the parties seeking business support. MORI for the *New Economist* asked 200 directors of UK companies which party they thought was best for business. The Conservatives were named by 49 per cent of respondents, compared with only 23 per cent support for the Labour Party.[102] On 28 April 2005, Labour's business manifesto was launched. It made new promises to curb regulation in 'tackling red tape'. Blair again pledged not to raise the top personal-income-tax rate of 40 per cent. The usual letter from Labour business supporters was sent out. The *Sun* newspaper again endorsed the Government.

Party management and policy-making

Another new Tony?

Blair continued to be criticised for his attitude towards policy-making. The mix of inadequate intra-party process and concentration on presentation for maximum public impact was seen as a fundamental problem for trust and for government competence. There was a persistent complaint that the public sector workforce resented policies driven from above on the basis of prior positions rather than being consultative and evidence-based. Looking back later, Geoff Mulgan, head of the No. 10 Strategy Unit, noted that communication had been almost entirely one-way, rather than the kind of dialogue needed to take the public sector through a major process of change.[103] The workforce became subject to untested experimentation by a government which had almost no centre of expertise in methods of 'doing really good innovation'.[104]

As for the party members, in the autumn of 2004 a severe alert had come from the unlikely source of the Blairite minister Steve Byers. He noted regretfully that there was 'an attitude in some quarters that party members are really a bit of a pain'. 'They could be critical of the leadership at the most inconvenient of times, they wanted to hold ministers and MPs to account and they wanted to be involved in determining the overall direction of the party.' His strong advice was 'Give them back a say'.[105] That did not bring a receptive response from No. 10.

However, in February 2005, at Labour's spring conference, Blair suddenly began to articulate to the party what he described as his change in attitude to leadership. 'If you're not careful', he said, "doing the right thing" becomes "I know best". So, starting with the Big Conversation, I went back out, and rather than talking at, talked with people. This journey has gone from "all things to all people" to "I know best" to "we can only do it together". And we all know which is best of those three.'[106] Yet in the light of what happened subsequently, there must remain some doubts whether his views on 'doing it together' leadership had changed at all.

Campaigning and managing the unions

TULO coordination which had built up union unity was now an asset in securing their common approach to election policy. This facilitated a new emphasis shared with the minister, Douglas Alexander, on the importance of word-of-mouth communication, and the US union experience of acting as independent sources of recommendation based on surveys of union members' preferences and then using their trust of the union rather than the party.

Energised by the commitment in the election manifesto to the full implementation of the Warwick Agreement, the TULO role in the general election involved some improvements on previous union efforts in elections. There was a consistent union message, emphasising particularly industrial gains such as the adjustment of holiday pay, longer protection for strikers, maternity leave and a Women at Work Commission. There was also a new system of direct mail to individuals in the key marginals, a national network of key seat coordinators and, emulating the new political activities of US unions, a special website encouraging union members' participation in the process of taking the message to others.

But initiatives in the election period had to operate within longer-term trends and behaviour. Various features of the political strategy, tactics policy and party management of 'New Labour' continued to weaken its appeal to sections of its traditional support (see Chapter 18, p. 609). As the polls had indicated, there was some deep- rooted public sector workers' resistance to government policy and the constant change, some of it without any consultation, and there was a grievance-ridden movement away from Labour support. The union election effort strived in an uphill battle and though in that context it was judged successful in TULO and the closely linked Amicus union, in No. 10 they disputed the evidence about it and the value of it.

Behind all this also, although the Warwick Agreement was projected as a new basis for unity and trust, there was still a school of thought anticipating and radically interpreting Blair's thought, for whom 'Warwick' had left a residue of deep resentment about what they termed 'the process'. That was a reference to the union counter-management organisation at the NPF and the negotiations which accompanied it. It contravened a panoply of 'New Labour' party management control maxims developed since 1994. It was seen as threatening the culture carriers of the future. They had developed new tactical means of dealing with Warwick Mark I, but what might be the follow up in the third term? What might they be under pressure to concede? These considerations led to a search for a new way out towards more management – a perspective which united Blair and Brown.

Reforming union representation

One thought that re-emerged was to develop relations with the TUC as an alternative to TULO. It was a return to an old arrangement and also potentially a return to divide and rule. There was also a new prospect emerging which began to look like a silver lining. The concentration of union votes in a small number of large entities had been a major managerial asset to the leadership. It now looked to be offering a very useful target. A slow but consistent build-up of amalgamations over the years had in the early 1990s suggested that at some point there would be the major incongruity of three or four large unions dominating the politics of the conference. On the NEC trade union review group in 1993, Blair had focused on this. Subsequently that issue had changed complexion when there was the new 50:50 arrangement between affiliated organisations and CLPs which left the unions, which had previously had around 90 per cent of the votes, now permanently on marginally over 49 per cent of the conference vote.

Within the trade unions, the concentration continued as amalgamations reduced affiliated unions from the 27 in 1994 to 17 in 2005. In 2004 it was confirmed that two of the four largest unions, Amicus (631,000 affiliated) and TGWU (400,000 affiliated), would seek a merger the following year, then possibly unite with the GMB (400,000 affiliated), although that third element did not happen. On the anticipated figures the big two together would have around one million out of two and three-quarter million union votes, This was looked forward to in No. 10 as a necessary and useful focus for pressing a broader reform involving a reduced union

voting weight at the conference, and giving the CLPs more votes, a change
which it was hoped would ease the management.

Unions and membership failure

The fact that there had been a long-term decline in union membership
and affiliation, and no surge of union membership amongst unorganised
workers, also fed into arguments over reforming the position of the unions
in the party. One influential contribution to the discussion by the ex-TUC
official David Coates blamed union recruitment failure on the lack of appeal
of the union brand, product and marketing strategy.[107] That focus on union
responsibility was well received by those around the political leadership
who saw trade unionism as in permanent decline, of decreasing electoral
significance and yet casting votes in the party on a scale which was judged
to be an anachronism. In contrast, various academic specialists on industrial
relations blamed the failure on the limits and constraints of the legislation;
the ERA recognition processes were judged complex and cumbersome,
imposing too many hurdles and onerous obligations on the unions. Smith
and Morton diagnosed that employment rights 'are diluted by the limited
scope, difficulties in access and weak sanctions'.[108] That view dominated
union responses, albeit with varying degrees of concern.

Union scepticism

In the unions later, when news reached them of the No. 10 discussions
about reform which was followed by some not well informed, spasmodic
pushing of the reform agenda in the press, apparently coming from
No. 10, the reaction was derisive. At its most temperate it was regarded
as 'a bit rich' to use union amalgamations as an argument for giving the
CLPs more votes. The amalgamation of the two unions, which in 2005
created Unite-the-Union with 1,031,000 votes out of 2,720,000 union
votes, had no effect whatsoever on the distribution of votes between the
unions and the CLPs. In the unions they noted the consistent pressure from
the managers for the unions to support their managerial control over the
party members. From a minority on the union side who were prepared
reluctantly to think about a further reform which might overcome the
potential for misrepresentation of union power, it was pointed out to
No. 10 that in any adjustment, more trust, including signs of good faith
on the government side in the implementation of the Warwick agreement,
could help the discussion.

Managing Gordon

The failure of the No. 10 push to engender wider party interest in reform
of the union votes added to the feeling around No. 10 of being on the
defensive in different locations. Once again, proposals to weaken Brown's

position in government were held back and the same inhibitive considerations applied as in 2001. Still, various schemes of strengthening party management were played with which could come into effect after another Blair election victory. In March 2005, it became known that there would be a new move 'to rein in the Treasury' in the attempt to 'drive through radical reform'.[109] There was talk again that Brown would be shifted from his job.[110] Milburn was returned to the Cabinet and given the role of election-campaign coordinator, in effect doing much of what Brown had done in the two previous elections.

But once again the plan for supremacy went awry. Continuing party and public reaction to the disunity at the top did not involve a significant call for more powers for Blair from either of them. One revealing poll analysis by Bob Worcester was that Labour was seen as having 'a good team of leaders' but was 'too dominated by its leader'.[111] With Blair low on electoral trust and performance satisfaction, six election pledges of an unimpressive generality, the election-campaign advance preparations going badly, and Brown's public reputation high, it was judged that economic success and trust in economic competence had to be the major emphasis.

Following pressure from the PLP there was now intervention by veteran 'New Labour' forces, including Campbell and Gould, to arrange an accommodation. Polling by Gould showed the value to party support if the two leaders were working together.[112] Of all voters, 67 per cent considered that Brown would deserve as much credit as Blair, if the election was won.[113] Brown was now brought back into his old central position in the election organisation even though, according to Powell, Mandelson was very critical of this development.[114] There was a Brown duet with Blair on the basis of the tried and tested attack on Tory cuts and in defence of Labour investment. Three of Brown's lieutenants were brought into party headquarters from which Milburn was banished. For the moment, there was a publicly effective, ice-cream-sharing unity.

Notes

1 Conversation with No. 10 aide the following day.
2 ICM/*Guardian*, 24 February 2004.
3 John Kampfner, *Blair's Wars*, Simon & Shuster, London, 2003, p. 295.
4 Clare Short, *An Honourable Deception? New Labour, Iraq and the Misuse of Power*, Simon & Schuster, London, 2004.
5 Robert Worcester, Roger Mortimer and Paul Bains, *Explaining Labour's Landslip: the 2005 General Election*, Politico's, London, 2005, p. 91.
6 IpsosMORI, Trustworthiness of Politicians–Trends, IpsosMORI website, 12 October 2007.
7 YouGov/*Observer*, 28 September 2003.
8 IpsosMORI/*Financial Times*, 3 May 2005.
9 Deborah Mattinson, *Talking to a Brick Wall*, Backbite, London, 2010, p. 123.

10 Worcester, Mortimer and Bains, *Explaining Labour's Landslip*, pp. 93–4.
11 Francis Jones and Maryanne Kelly, *Omnibus Survey: Initial Findings on Public Confidence in Official Statistics*, ONS, London, 2004.
12 *Independent*, 3 June 2004.
13 Survey data and analysis by IpsosMORI for Hansard Society, *First Audit of Political Engagement*, 2004, p. 37.
14 'The Future of Political Parties', *Progress Magazine*, September 2005.
15 Graham Allen MP, *The Last Prime Minister: Being Honest about the UK Presidency*, Graham Allen, House of Commons, 2001, p. 4.
16 Short, *An Honourable Deception?*, p. 207.
17 *Independent*, 14 May 2003.
18 Alastair Campbell and Bill Hagerty (eds), *The Campbell Diaries*, Vol. 4, *The Burden of Power*, Hutchinson, London, 2012, entry July 10, 2003, p. 636.
19 Ibid.
20 Ibid.
21 Christopher Foster, *British Government in Crisis*, Hart Publishing, Oxford, 2005.
22 Labour Party Annual (NEC) Report, 2003, p. 27. One senior ex-party official contested these figures but they were generally accepted.
23 *Guardian*, 3 November 2003.
24 TUC document, 'Unraveling the Red Tape Myths', 14 February 2003.
25 TUC document, 'Labour Market Flexibility: Building a Modern Labour Market', 3 November 2004.
26 Andrew Murray, *A New Labour Nightmare: The Return of the Awkward Squad*, Verso, London, 2003, p. 56.
27 *Morning Star*, 14 October 2005.
28 Ann Black, email personal report, 23 September 2003.
29 Ann Black, email personal report, 9 October 2003.
30 YouGov/*Observer*, 28 September 2003.
31 ICM/*Guardian*, 24 February 2004.
32 YouGov/*New Statesman*, 14 March 2007.
33 You Gov for Cruddas, *Guardian*, 9 May 2007.
34 Minutes of the National Committee of TULO, 23 July 2003.
35 Surreptitiously made available to me in late 2004.
36 Minutes of NEC Officers meeting, 16 April 2007.
37 MORI poll of Labour leader image, fieldwork 1981 to 2006, MORI website 2006.
38 BBC *Newsnight*, 2 May 2008.
39 LPCR 2003 p. 98.
40 Helen Jackson, privately circulated memo, *Loyalty and the Labour Party*, February, 2004.
41 Chris Mullin, *A View from the Foothills*, Profile Books, London, 2009, entry 17 May 2000, p. 103.
42 Peter Watt, *Inside Out: My Story of Betrayal and Cowardice at the Heart of New Labour*, Biteback, London, 2010, p. 123.
43 NEC Minutes. GS02/11/03.
44 *The Times*, 2 October 2003.
45 *Guardian*, 2 October 2003.

46 Philip Cowley, *The Rebels: How Blair Mislaid his Majority*, Politico's, London, 2005, p. 231.

47 Campbell and Hagerty (eds), *Campbell Diaries, Burden of Power*, entry 10 July 2003, p. 637.

48 Philip Cowley and Mark Stuart, 'Parliament', in Anthony Seldon and Dennis Kavanagh, *The Blair Effect, 2001–5*, Cambridge University Press, Cambridge, 2005, pp. 38–9.

49 *Guardian*, 4 August 2003, Michael White, drawing from the work of Philip Cowley.

50 NOP for UNISON, *Morning Star*, 19 November 2003.

51 Robert Peston, *Brown's Britain*, Short Books, London, 2006, p. 335.

52 Minutes of PLP meeting 14 January 2004.

53 Minutes of PLP meeting 19 January 2004.

54 Peter Mandelson, *The Third Man: Life at the Heart of New Labour*, Harper, London, 2010, p. 375.

55 Minutes of the Parliamentary Committee, 11 February 2004.

56 Helen Jackson MP, *Loyalty and the Labour Party*, 8 February 2004.

57 Mullin, *From the Foothills*, entry 13 March 2003, p. 379.

58 Minutes of Parliamentary Committee, 11 February 2004.

59 *Guardian*, 5 February 2004.

60 *Guardian*, 7 May 2005.

61 *Observer*, 25 January 2004.

62 Cowley, *Rebels*, p. 51.

63 Noted in Ann Black's email 10 June 2003.

64 *The Times*, 5 February 2004.

65 *Daily Telegraph*, 2 March 2004.

66 *The Times*, 3 March 2004.

67 Peter Hain, *The Future Party*, Catalyst, London, 2004.

68 *Guardian*, 11 March 2004.

69 *Guardian*, 11 May 2004.

70 *Guardian*, 15 June 2004.

71 Tony Blair, *A Journey*, Hutchinson, London, 2010, p. 506.

72 London Review of Books, 8 July 2004.

73 Richard Heffernan, 'Leaders and Followers, The Politics of the Parliamentary Labour Party', in Brian Brivati and Richard Heffernan, *The Labour Party: a Centenary History*, Macmillan, London, 2000, p. 249.

74 Tom Bower, *Gordon Brown, Prime Minister*, Harper Perennial, London, 2007, p. 455.

75 *Red Pepper*, November 2005.

76 Helen Jackson, privately circulated paper, November 2004.

77 Byron Criddle, 'MPs and Candidates', in Dennis Kavanagh and David Butler, *The General Election of 2005*, Palgrave Macmillan, Basingstoke, 2005, p. 154.

78 *Tribune*, 11 March 2005 and 1 April 2005.

79 Criddle, in Kavanagh and Butler, *General Election of 2005*, p. 152.

80 Ibid. p. 153.

81 Jon Cruddas and John Harris, *Fit for Purpose: a Programme for Labour Party Renewal*, Compass, London 2007, p. 8.

82 Helen Jackson, *Policymaking and the PLP*, privately circulated paper, July 2003.
83 Murray, *New Labour Nightmare*, p. 101.
84 John McIlroy, 'Under Stress but Still Enduring: The Contentious Alliance in the Age of Tony Blair and Gordon Brown', in Gary Daniels and John McIlroy (eds), *Trade Unions in a Neoliberal World: British Trade Unions under New Labour*, Routledge, London, 2009, p. 182.
85 *Guardian*, 18 February 2006.
86 My notes, and confirmatory interview with Luke Bruce.
87 Mattinson, *Brick Wall*, p. 125.
88 Stanley B. Greenberg, *Dispatches from the War Room: In the Trenches with Five Extraordinary Leaders*, Thomas Dunne, New York, 2009, pp. 261–2.
89 *Sunday Times* editorial, 2 December 2004.
90 My notes monitoring this at the NPF and in the many private discussions afterwards.
91 Dennis Kavanagh and David Butler, *The General Election of 2005*, Palgrave Macmillan, Basingstoke, 2005, p. 25.
92 Watt, *Inside Out*, p. 86.
93 Lewis Baston and Simon Henig 'The Labour Party', in Anthony Seldon and Dennis Kavanagh, *The Blair Effect 2001–5*, Cambridge University Press, Cambridge, 2005, p. 115.
94 *Guardian*, 27 June 2004.
95 Ann Black, *Guardian*, letters, 28 June 2004.
96 Meg Russell, *Building New Labour*, Palgrave Macmillan, Basingstoke, 2005, p. 204.
97 *Morning Star*, 26 October 2004.
98 You Gov/*Observer*, 28 September 2003.
99 Peston, *Brown's Britain*, p. 349.
100 Prime Minister's Questions, Wednesday 12 January 2005.
101 NPF Report to Conference, 2004, p. 132.
102 *New Economist*, 28 April 2005.
103 House of Commons Public Administration Committee, 16 October 2008, MQ 84.
104 Ibid.
105 *Guardian*, 7 September 2004.
106 Labour Party press release, Blair's Spring Conference speech, 14 February 2005.
107 Coates, *Raising Lazarus*, p. 3.
108 Paul Smith and Garry Morton, 'Nine Years New Labour: Neo-liberalism and Workers Rights', *British Journal of Industrial Relations* 44(3), September 2006, p. 414.
109 *Guardian*, 13 March 2005.
110 Peston, *Brown's Britain*, p. 359.
111 Worcester's Weblog – the Blair Factor, MORI website, 29 April 2005.
112 Lance Price, *Where Power Lies*, Simon & Schuster, London, 2010, p. 378.
113 Populus, poll archives, April 2005.
114 Jonathan Powell, *The New Machiavelli: How to Wield Power in the Modern World*, Bodley Head, London, 2010, p. 126.

18

Managing for legacy

Into the third term[1]

In 2005 Labour under Blair achieved a historic third victory in a row, but its 35.2 per cent vote share was a drop of 5.5 per cent since 2001, making it the most unpopular party to form a government since the beginning of universal adult suffrage. There was a loss of 56 seats with the major feature being the swing to the Liberals from Labour. Whilst Labour's lead amongst AB category voters had risen since 1997, amongst the lowest social groups D and E Labour's lead over the Conservatives had fallen from 58 per cent in 1997 to 42 per cent.[2] In 'Labour's natural constituency', people in the working class and those living in council houses were most likely to have lost trust in Blair.[3]

In a PLP increasingly comprising professional politicians, the ex-manual working class was greatly underrepresented with only two new MPs from that class.[4] In a party created by manual workers, by 2005 there were only 38 in the PLP. In the declining manual working-class electorate there was a view growing since the days of Opposition that 'they are not interested in us'. For all that the government's policies in terms of countering poverty included an increase in the minimum wage which ran ahead of both prices and average earnings, in the three years from 2002 to 2005, as Larry Elliot and Polly Toynbee pointed out, the poorest 20 per cent saw their real incomes fall by 2.6 per cent.[5] Interwoven with this was resentment about the scale of immigration which was cultural and also heavily fed by problems over housing, jobs and wage pressures. It also involved a reasonable democratic lament that 'nobody asked us'.

It was difficult to see the election win as purely a victory for Blair. Brown's credit was expressed in Labour's significant lead of 26 per cent on the general management of the economy.[6] The invasion of Iraq and how the people were taken by Blair into that war was a major issue. Compared with what pertained in previous elections, there was a drop in trust in him.[7] A significant feature also had been the party dog that did not bark back; from top to bottom the party did not create a furore in Blair's defence over trust. That created a great Catch 22 of manipulation for the managers. Why did they not organise a response to assist Blair? The private answer was along the lines of 'We couldn't organise that defence because if we had been found out it would have added to electoral distrust of manipulation'.

The fact that the supportive party voice could not be heard raised some questions about how far Blair would now change his relationship with his party. Blair's message to Labour's spring conference in February 2005 had seemed to indicate he was on his way to that with a new level of self-criticism. And, at first sight, that appeared to have been reinforced by his electoral experience.

Leadership and party management

The new Tony: listening and learning

'I have listened and I have learned', he said as he stood outside No. 10. But, as in the past, Blair was not a changed man for long. Though the tactics of the election had been not to fight it as a referendum on Blair, his aides now stuck with the formalities; Blair 'had won it' and he would legitimately serve a full term with his programme of radical legislation. The Worcester poll analysis showing that Labour was 'too dominated by its leader' was ignored. Blair never did fully come to terms with the qualified public view of the strong leader. He was happier with seeking to emulate Thatcher's third-term radical push. Mandelson's view may have played a part here. He was convinced that some in the inner circle of No. 10 were 'sucking energy out of him by constantly telling him that he was politically weak, trusted less by the public and badly isolated in the party'.[8] To an observer this inner-circle perspective seemed simply a realistic and honest appraisal.

Indications of how Blair intended to proceed came in the No. 10 staffing where overall the changes strengthened assertive advocates of third-term Blairism. Jonathan Powell and David Hill remained in position as did the business anchorman Geoff Norris. Matthew Taylor took on the enhanced role of Chief Adviser on Political Strategy to the Prime Minister. John McTiernan was made Director of Political Operations including responsibility for party liaison. Ruth Turner became Director of Government Relations, Jo Gibbons worked as Deputy Director of Government relations and then Director of Events, Visits and Scheduling. There was a new head of the Strategic Communications Unit, Benjamin Wegg-Prosser, a new more technocratic head of the enlarged Policy Directorate, David Bennett; and a new speechwriter, Philip Collins. Nita Clarke, responsible for union liaison, stayed in the post of Assistant Political Secretary despite, or even because of her tense relations with the affiliated union leaders but continuing her more straightforward links to the TUC. Ex-union political officer, ex-minister and ex-Deputy Chief Whip Keith Hill, now very critical of the unions, became a PPS to the PM.

All this produced a management generally working enthusiastically with the flow of his most radical aspirations focused on delivery of the legacy.

He encouraged the team to think in these terms and the team facilitated the true 'organic' Tony, a bold man in a new hurry. In relations with the Labour Party and the unions the new personnel overall gave Blair a noticeably sharper edge. It was not just in No. 10 that the managerial composition had been replenished. Alan Howarth, long the PLP Secretary, had retired and moved into the Lords just before the election. His replacement had been declared by a party committee heavily dominated by central officials, with only the PLP Chair Jean Corston as the PLP representative. The committee had appointed the Chief Whip's special adviser Fiona Gordon, who was not the preferred choice of the outgoing Secretary nor of the PLP Chair. She was a highly experienced organiser, big on delivery, who emphasised being proactive in party management as in other activities and favoured the kind of radical PLP reorganisation that the party headquarters had been pushing for some time.

In her view, the PLP office 'had not been keeping up with the times', so she sought to link the staff more closely with MPs in integrating what MPs were doing in the Commons with the needs of electoral campaigning. The task was broadened to more personal engagement in linking to new members and improving their understanding of the government. The fear of some of the existing PLP Office members was that this was an attempt to transform the role from 'civil servants' to 'political organisers', building an auxilliary operation to the whips' office, moving closer to the central party machine and losing the jealously gaurded delicate line between the PLP and the wider party. By the summer of 2006 the PLP Office staff, forced to reapply for their jobs, had been completely changed. The PLP Office title was now PLP Political Services Staff.

The changing base of support

The strengthening of PLP management after 2005 was expected to bolster the support crucial to Blair's radical ambitions. True, there were yet more disappointed ex-ministers and never-to-be ministers, some of whom added to the body of discontent. Yet the Campaign Group had risen by only two members and the organised left in the party continued to weaken. A Labour majority of 66 would in the past have been considered easily workable in avoiding deep trouble. Although the reshuffle of ministers on 9 May 2005 was, like its 2001 equivalent, seen as unimpressive and bungled, at the first meeting of the PLP, on 11 May 2005, Blair was welcomed as a three-term victor. Once again he was in impressive and sensitive form, making clear that he understood the need for 'a stable and orderly transition' in the change of Leader but he wanted to go in his own time.[9] A few of the usual suspects, calling for Blair to step aside, were jeered whilst the Leader elicited his normal organised as well as spontaneous wave of loyalist enthusiasm.

In the immediate aftermath of the election, Brown did get agreement to recover his seat on the NEC and all plans for moving him to another post and/or reorganising the Treasury were opposed by him and sidelined, yet again. But the chance of sustained unity at this level was lost because, in the Blairite view, Brown immediately relaunched his demand on Blair to set a date of departure.[10] The Brownite view, confirmed generally by Seldon, was that Blair's promises to Brown on an element of jointness and consultation in governing did not materialise; he was 'the Prime Minister'.[11] Discussion between the two leaders about the future produced no solution and aroused a new aggressive resentment from around Brown. Yet Brown himself was still held back by a fear of the odium of regicide and the creation of an embittered opposition to his future leadership.

Turbulence, revolt and their sources

In the face of criticism No. 10 focused heavily, as did much of the media, on the dissenters from past conflicts, orchestrated or reinforced by 'Brown's people'. But underneath their role bubbled up a deeper and broader turbulence. Blair's main weakness, and the cause of the slowly growing support for a change in the Leader, was an accumulating reaction against his ideological 'line of travel', his governing-alone style of policy formulation, and the behaviour of his highly partisan party management. A concern amongst a circle of the PLP wider than the Brownites was that there should be a consensual timetable for Blair's departure. 'About 18 months' seemed to be a commonly held centre-ground view in the summer. Blair's aides met that message with a degree of truculent irritation and dismissal.

PLP elections

Significantly, over time in this more integrated party, before the final confrontation of September 2006, revolts of different kinds took place in each major national forum and within the party management itself, linking to and from what was happening in the PLP. Moving in and out, investigating these developments is essential in understanding what led to the final confrontations. The PLP election to the Parliamentary Committee results revealed an important starting point for the fragmentation and weakening of Blair's base of managerial support. As signs emerged that Blair and his new staff were becoming more assertive and more unified in their legacy-seeking radicalism, a new pluralism began to emerge amongst the managers in the PLP. The election of PLP Chair Ann Clwyd by an electorate which, as normal, included all ministers, was much closer than expected. She beat Tony Lloyd by only 167 votes to 156. In the elections for back-bench representation, it was no surprise that managers could not control a shift to more critical composition – the same had happened in 2001. Yet the scale of the shift was very significant. There was a complete rejection of the whips' slate, bringing in new faces from a broad-based centre left. Angela Eagle topped the poll and became Deputy PLP Chair, the others were Ann Cryer, Kevan Jones, Tony Lloyd, Joan Ruddock and Martin Salter.

None of them was a serial 'oppositionist', although Cryer remained a member of the Campaign Group. The variation in some of their attitudes to key policy issues showed in votes in the House but crucially, unlike the 2001 committee intake, in this committee role they worked closely together. They had a clear focus on reasserting the rights of the PLP but also sought to avoid the head-on policy collisions of the second term. Although individually in various shades they now prefered Brown, they were particularly focused on Blair's constant drift away from the maintream of the party, and later the refusal to name a date for his departure.

The most significant event was in and around an election for the PLP representative on the NEC to replace the retired Helen Jackson. The head office proposal to count the votes at the end of each day whilst the ballot was going on was said to be the normal procedure but was strongly challenged by Eagle.[12] Amongst some of the elected members on the Parliamentary Committee there was deep concern that if the ballot was not secure that could make it easier for the managing officials to refine their campaigning focus. After strong representations from the three candidates to the General Secretary, the proposal was dropped. In an electorate which included all those on the government payroll, the NEC position was won by Eagle by 125 votes to 124 against Janet Anderson, who was seen as the candidate backed by the whips' office. This was despite the Campaign Group candidate Lynn Jones taking 40 votes.

It has been a central theme of this study that in a more integrated party it is not possible to understand fully the behaviour of the PLP in relation to the leadership and management without seeing the linkage of represenation through the parliamentary committee to the wider management and counter-managerial politics. That connectedness was particularly important now because the growing irritation over Blair's leadership linked the backbench representatives on the Parliamentary Committee with elements on the NEC, and with growing support for more party accountability and a curbing of manipulation. Eagle, an ex-minister, could hope to regain a post if Brown became Leader but she was also a passionate critic of managerial behaviour and developed into a skilful Deputy Chair keeping regular communication to the PLP.

There were signs also that old behaviour patterns amongst the elected PLP managers were beginning to break down, with the development of a period of regular and highly unusual tensions between the back-bench group and the PLP Secretary. Later, in the selection of chairs of select committees on 22 July, some inter-party horse trading of the whips' office was recognised, but this was now partly superseded by an assertion of supremacy of the elected representatives over the whips' office preference for recently dropped ministers. This was neither factional nor follower behaviour, just a process of seeking now to speak with more clarity and strength for the PLP. The mood of this activity was captured in an extraordinary moment when the three governmental representatives Geoff Hoon the

Leader of the House, McCartney the Party Chair and Hilary Armstrong the Chief Whip, were asked to leave the meeting so that the elected PLP representatives could confer. After this, there was even talk of the creation of a 1922 Committee of Labour backbenchers, although that faded. The group also sought closer links with the women's committee and kept contact with the trade union group of the PLP.

The management of PLP meetings remained contentious. Managers acknowledged the general importance of allowing ministers to get the feel of real party opinion and the meetings were more open than often acknowledged. But the organisation of the meetings was also influenced by the importance of the issue and whether the Prime Minister was present. Ministers and the PPSs were expected to be there and most loyalists did not need reminding. For those that did, word went out from the whips' office to 'give Tony some backing' and the PLP office was always heavily involved in producing lists of speakers. How this operated in practice then depended also on who was in the Chair. Eagle was seen as more pluralistic than the now strongly loyalist Ann Clwyd.

Strong leadership reasserted

Meanwhile, on 29 May 2005 a French rejection of new European constitutional arrangements had got Blair off the hook of the British referendum promise foisted on him in April 2004. And any sense of Blair having his back to the wall was dissipated in early July by a string of well-received performances – a speech to the European Parliament, a successful G8 Summit covering aid and climate change, and active support in securing the 2012 Olympic Games for London. He was boosted most by his impressive immediate response to the terrorist bombs planted in London by a group of young British Muslim citizens on 7 July.

It might not have been a plus for him. There had been repeated warnings from critics of the Iraq venture and from intelligence chiefs that Britain would become an increasing target for al-Qaeda and that British Muslims could be radicalised. The terrorists' own videos later confirmed that Blair's foreign policy including the war against Iraq was a contributing factor in motivating them. Two-thirds of the electorate agreed that there was this link.[13] Yet Blair refused to accept it and in the strength of his conviction and his defence of the nation he initially drew support even from some regular critics. 'I salute you Blair' was the message of civil liberties critic Henry Porter.[14] Polls now found the highest rating of its premiership apart from after the fall of Baghdad.[15]

Here, then, was a Leader who now rested on potentially two of the strongest planks of sustained public and party support: economic success and defence of the public against suicidal terrorism. There was also record public sector investment and a public sector labour force 'growing at pretty much the same rate as in the private sector'.[16] This was a base which should easily have taken him into near completion of his third term. Yet, as will be shown, Blair's political management eventually undermined his own longer-term position and it began in a press conference of 5 August when he took the counter-terrorism agenda out of the hands of the new Home Secretary Charles Clarke, who was on holiday, with a twelve-point plan signposted with a headline-grabbing 'The rules of the game have changed'. Spokesmen for the two opposition parties later alleged that they had been given the advance impression by junior minister Hazel Blears that the announcement would be of very little significance.[17] It actually signalled major new hard-line measures against terrorism that further encroached on civil liberties, and came to be seen later by some critics as the cynical manipulation of fear and security.[18]

Once again, high in pursuit of his purposes, carrying a sense of his own rectitude and using his impressive communicational skills, he found the energy and commitment to drive ahead with his domestic policy reforms regardless of the balance of party opinion. In particular, over public-service reform, he pressed forward with the agenda of private sector involvement, and made no attempt to specify the ultimate share of its role. On another front, controversial city academies backed by private capital or religious groups or the voluntary sector were given enhanced freedom of operation and rapid expansion, even though it was judged by a House committee to be 'at the expense of rigorous evaluation.'[19]

NEC and new managerial division

On the NEC initially there seemed to be a new turn to hard Blairite control. Where over London, under McDonagh, harsh retribution for Livingstone workers was avoided, here it was supported. On 24 May, there was confirmation of the expulsion of 20 members of Blaenau Gwent CLP who had worked for the MP Peter Laws. But alongside this action, reinforced by anger from women seeking a fairer representation in the Commons, there were now important differences opening up within party management which rolled back and forth between different venues.

The managerial internal pluralism, which had shown itself in a new differentiation of the attitudes of representatives and officials in the PLP, now spread to the NEC. With the loss from the NEC of the ultra-loyalist duet of Jones and Wall, and some other shifts in union representation, the distinction between appointed officials as managers and elected NEC representatives as managers became much more of a political differentiation, and the representative managers became a more critical component. The regular meetings of party officers had in the past been mainly a status affair, although on occasions it had played an important role – as over the Clause IV consultation. Now they became increasingly important events. By the autumn of 2005 there was growing concern at the lack of attention Blair was giving to the party processes and decisions rather than his own personal objectives. His record of Year Zero distance from Labour history, his anti-tribalism and absence of sentimentality about the party came back now to produce a new note of anxiety about the old query. Where is he trying to take us? Under these new circumstances and with some further changes in party officers it led the NEC officers meeting to become more consciously assertive in defence of 'the party' and of the union-party relationship. This was further affected by what was happening over the Warwick Agreement.

Management, Warwick and union reform

In search of implementation

In terms of cooperative party management, it made clear tactical sense for Blair to continue to build up trust with the unions based on implementation of the Warwick Agreement. Yet just the opposite happened. Parts of the Warwick Agreement (and also a possible future Warwick Agreement) were regarded as potentially in tension with the Brown-Blair economic diagnosis being pushed heavily in Europe. Blair and Brown were politicially comfortable and increasingly integrated within relations with the City, and even more concerned that no new party arrangement must cause damage to it, especially if it was seen to expand the unions' influence.

Brown's speech to the CBI dinner in May 2005 had emphasised the aim 'to build a new trust between business and government'.[20] The deregulatory theme was confirmed in the Queen's Speech on 17 May which spoke of lifting 'the burden' of red tape. That was accompanied in No. 10 by a new evangelism against over-regulation and risk aversion. On 26 May, Blair took this up in a speech which included a passage heavily critical of the Financial Services Authority for its constraint on enterprising business; in reply the chairman of the FSA accused Tony Blair of undermining the role of the City watchdog.[21] This would eventually in 2008, after the Bank crisis, become a classic exemplification of the idelogically constrained limitations of 'New Labour' regulatory control. At the time it appeared in No. 10 as splendidly radical and legacy-making. But in the unions concern grew at the dangers, including to health-and-safety legislation, from the growing anti-regulation sentiment in the Blair government.

Changing the union vote

In the midst of this, the issue of reform of union votes at the party conference suddenly and clumsily emerged on the government side in discussions with TULO representatives, signalling an attempt from No. 10 to reduce the party influence of the unions in the new review of Partnership in Power. Now it appeared to the unions that, far from being a basis of new trust, the full implementation of Warwick was to be used as a bargaining lever over changing the unions' position in the party. It was a tactical move which No. 10 had been warned against by those who focused on the implementation of agreements as a means of creating a climate for con-sensual change. But, pleasing Blair, the governmental representatives were making an effort to deliver a new agenda.

On 6 June, a TULO *Briefing Paper: The NPF Review*, written by Byron Taylor after discussion with TULO chairman Tony Dubbins, was circulated privately to affiliated unions. It voiced concern that in a number of areas the Government was not fulfilling the commitments made at Warwick. Also, it now noted that 'there is a determination to rewrite the Smith settlement' on voting parity at the Conference 'in order to prevent a future Warwick Agreement'. Barrie Clements, the labour correspondent of the *Independent*, got hold of the story and it was given the heading that 'Labour chiefs attempt to cut unions' hold on the party'.[22] There was a short ghastly silence and then a hasty retreat from ministers and No. 10 as they distanced themselves, leaving behind nothing gained and more trust lost.

In an attempt at reassurance, the government proposed a process for the delivery and communication of the Warwick Agreement. There would be a sub-Cabinet political committee meeting convened by McCartney and Sutcliffe on a bi-monthly basis. There would be regular meetings of the convenors and No. 10 representatives with the TULO-TUC Contact Group at General Secretary level. After each sub-cabinet meeting there would also be a meeting of political officers and special advisers to develop a narrative of delivery and an effective communication strategy. This was welcomed at the TULO AGM in October. Yet the feed-in of the sub-cabinet political committee to a labour-market strategy document from the DTI, which would outline the timetable for the delivery, was long delayed.

Leader's Party Chair and management

McCartney's role as Party Chair became much harder during this attempt to deliver the big legacy. He was, as before, a major force seeking to influ-ence progressive party developments in ways which did not cause problems for the Leader. The long-delayed review of Partnership in Power, 'A Stronger Voice for Members', finally neared completion. In the process, attempts to replace contemporary resolutions by 'consensus resolutions' agreed with ministers were fended off by the unions. There were promises of support for NPF CLP representatives in attempting to liaise with their constituen-cies, with better feedback and a better focus on topical issues by the policy commissions which now received greater emphasis. The handling of Iraq by the Britain in the World policy commission in 2002–3 was now said to be the model for the future. Yet, it has been noted how contested this was at the time and the range of managerial devices used around it. As usual, the experience of managerial interference in subverting the spirit of Part-nership in Power was not one which was open to review. Privately, when this was brought up, it met the answer 'You can't keep the politics out of it'. It meant that the managers would fight any impediment to their operations.

But McCartney and Luke Bruce the Policy Director did adjust to the new research evidence that there was 'a common ground of agreement' between the policies of party members, activists and party voters.[23] There was little evidence to support the view that party activists were extreme in relation to the voters.[24] The key proposal which went to the NPF in July was that CLPs be allowed to amend the document directly at the final NPF stage. This important initiative was taken only as the last item of the NPF consultative weekend when people were ready to go. It met little enthusiasm from the majority of CLP loyalists, as potentially it reduced their own role in continuous deliberative procedures. Later, however, a new accommodation was initiated by Ann Black and agreed by the JPC. The CLPs' input would be processed through their existing representatives moving amendments.

Meanwhile, a new industrial conflict exacerbated existing problems between the unions and the government. The TUC drew ministerial attention to the evidence that indicated that low-paid Asian women workers at Gate Gourmet had been deliberately provoked into a strike in order to replace them with workers on lower pay and worse conditions.[25] That company's behaviour drew new calls for changes in labour law which would allow legal supporting action. The calls were resisted as a breach of the 1999 settlement and they also provided a new incentive for Blairite outrider Alan Milburn to express fear that Labour would 'revert to type' and swing back to the left after Blair departed.[26] Once again some Blairites saw themselves as the culture carriers now protecting their revolution from the unions, the party and the deviant brother from the 'New Labour' family. In effect, they gave signals to the media and particularly the business community that there was something to be feared from the election of Brown. That made Blairite-Brownite relations worse.

The word from Blair's aides in the summer of 2005 had been that 'Tony is going to try one last effort at party renewal but taking the party with him'. Yet there were few signs that any lessons had been learned about taking the party with him and curbing his trust-destroying management. Again we have to look at this management elsewhere to see the beginning of a wider undermining of his parliamentary position. The crucial source of change was the mood of the party conference, his method of seeking party renewal and the new reaction of the NEC majority.

NEC, party renewal and the conference

The 2005 party conference as it assembled gave signs of further party alienation. It was attended by only 491 CLPs.[27] Experienced attenders judged this a significant decline, although the General Secretary Matt Carter at the NEC meeting on 8 November judged it 'comparable to previous conferences'.[28] MPs commented privately that 'more than half of the PLP did not turn up'; others came and went after a short stay. All of it was educated guesswork because the officials, protecting Blair's success, would not give regular accurate updates. Votes at the conference indicated either a huge drop in CLP representation or massive abstentions.[29] Concerns expressed over loyalist resolutions submitted to the conference but not going through the CLPs' formal decision-taking procedures, and the fact that delegates were taken out of the debates for meetings with ministers, had been a consistent criticism of recent conferences; but allegation from NEC member Pete Willsman that, for CLPs with no delegates, voting papers were given to their MPs was new.[30] As usual, there was no reply from party officials to the accusations. In a rule change, councillors were now given the right to attend the conference in an ex officio capacity, an unremarkable innovation in itself but a future opportunity to fill empty CLP chairs with supporters.

The NEC, whose task force had worked on a new version of the *21st Century Party* document, was presented at its pre-conference meeting with an introduction to that document written by the Prime Minister and Party Chair McCartney. The introduction focused on making all-member CLP General Committees obligatory, in spite of this proposal being regularly rejected by the CLPs in consultation. On the NEC, the reaction was very significant. Under a barrage of criticisms, McCartney was forced to withdraw the introduction and replace it by another. This was a significant landmark. An attempt at an extension of Blair's influence over the party had been forced into retreat.

Aggressive management control was further revealed later. Throughout the whole of Labour Party history, the NEC had met prior to the conference debates to decide its reply to the resolutions on the agenda. There were four contemporary resolutions from the unions. Yet the Monday morning NEC meeting was suspended before a vote was taken, to seek an agreement after it appeared that in a vote the NEC would probably be supporting the TGWU resolution on workers' rights following the dispute at Gate Gourmet.

There was an additional development involving the NEC's rights. Within the unions there was a disgreement over the pensions composite. The GMB, led at his first conference by Paul Kenny, who had replaced Curran after his resignation, had agreed a resolution on the pensions' link to earnings which, though a long-established union position, had not been part of the Warwick Agreement. The resolution was changed after protracted discussions between union leaders Dubbins, Woodley and Simpson and McCartney. Out of their complex discussions also came an unexpected agreement that the NEC would not take a view on the acceptability of this resolution. It was a coup for the management controllers but a manoeuvre that left many NEC members seething about the imposition. It also caused new tensions within what was to become the new union Unite, between the TGWU NEC representative Jack Dromey who opposed the manoeuvre and from Amicus representative Griffiths who supported it. It did not help the mood of the NEC that the prepared managerial machine was still operating throughout, putting out the line against the GMB resolution through the regional liaison teams, in spite of the absence of any decision by what was historically regarded as 'Labour's ruling NEC'.

Resolutions and decisions

On some procedural issues where they had major concerns, the weight of the unions went in defence of the status quo. A constitutional amendment to give the party conference the right to make its own amendments to the final Partnership in Power documents was defeated; most unions favoured the form of a final Warwick-style comprehensive deal. With the review still under discussion and the politics of the NPF after Warwick potentially much more important, there was a successful intensification of the managerial organisation of NPF elections to increase loyalist representatives. Four sitting GRA candidates were rejected.

Once again the unions' votes and those of the CLPs went in different ways on some key policy resolutions. A resolution seen as a threat to the Post Office remaining in the public sector was defeated by 34.6 per cent to 65.4 per cent with the affiliates having voted 98 per cent against, but surprisingly, given past indications, the CLPs voted only 33 per cent against with 67 per cent in favour. A Gate Gourmet resolution from the TGWU 'permitting lawful supportive action at least where there is a close connection between those involved in line with ILO conventions' was supported by 69.4 per cent to 30.6 per cent. Again, the affiliates were the core of support, voting 99.6 per cent in favour but the CLPs only 39.2 per cent in favour but 60.8 per cent against. This difference again became the basis on which critics of the unions portrayed them as imposing their will on the CLPs.

On the health service, tempers became frayed in a policy clash that was to reverberate through the third term. In May, the Secretary of State for Health Patricia Hewitt had announced extra funding for a second wave of independent-sector treatment centres, increasing the private sector providers. She regarded it as electorally and substantively essential and claimed it to be 'very similar' to what the manifesto referred to as 'a plurality of providers to expand capacity'. But the new policy had not indicated limitations in harmony with the Prentis-Reid discussions. In an unprecedented intervention, the ministerial view was heavily contested as party policy by the normally restrained Jeremy Beecham, speaking as the chair of the conference.[31] On the role of the private sector in the Health Service, in a published letter, Beecham also challenged: 'The questions remain as to how much, for how long and on what terms such contracting should be part of the system'. On this 'there has yet to be a debate within the Labour Party'.[32]

The UNISON contemporary resolution calling for suspension of the proposed NHS changes on primary care trusts, a review of the use of markets and opposition to further expansion of the private provision was passed on a card vote with 71.1 per cent in favour to 28.9 per cent against.

Here the vote of affiliates was 99.9 per cent in support but the CLPs representatives gave a vote of only 42.5% in favour. These results were unsurprising in the light of past card votes but also noteworthy managerial victories given what was thought to be hugely adverse CLP opinion.

On housing, the debate returned to the Partnership in Power decision of 2004 which had not been fully implemented. A composite reaffirming the commitment to a 'fourth option' of 'direct investment' in council housing 'as a matter of urgency' was carried on an overwhelming show of hands with huge majorities in both the affiliates and CLP sections. There was no card vote. The now amended pensions-earning submission from the GMB also went through on an overwhelming hand vote but without contestation from the platform.

Many people remembered this conference for the Walter Wolfgang affair rather than these decisions. Police counter-terrorism controls were easily accommodated alongside heavy management controls over the conference audience. The year before, prominent dissent during the Leader's speech had been, in effect, prohibited. But a PR disaster of monumental proportion took place within the conference this year when, in the full sight of a TV camera team, Wolfgang – a venerable Labour Party dissident and a refugee from Nazi Germany – was manhandled out of the conference for heckling and subsequently arrested under the provisions of counter-terrorism laws. Played over before an appalled nation, it led eventually to repetitive groveling apology from the party officials and the Leader and a promise later that the CAC would examine further how to combine security with the needs of delegates.

In an email circular of 4 October, Ann Black lamented 'yet again' the reports of harassment of constituency delegates by party officials. The policy procedure remained frustrating. Conference resolutions were now the property of the policy commissions, and union leaders were told that they did not discuss party conference resolutions on the commissions. On the final day of the conference, David Miliband speaking on local government had said 'The product of powerlessness is anger'.[33] Had he focused on Blair, the party management, the harassment and the power relations experienced by the grassroots of the Labour Party, he might have seen the events and mood behind the scenes of this party conference as an important warning of what was to happen to the Leader. The rising in the party temper against Blair was by no means all about Brown. And it was also against a background where there was a rising net public dissatisfaction with Blair and a rising net satisfaction with Brown.[34]

Reactions to management and the Blair supremacy

Reaction to the conference and the NEC revolt

The No. 10 managerial interventions since 2003 had included strong attempts to divide the unions USDAW and Community, which were traditionally loyal to the leadership, from the rest of the TULO union alliance.

The GMB had decided not to join the big amalgamation, and its new Leader Kenny was encouraged to work alone. Amongst the noises-off during and after the conference were some which exacerbated Amicus and TGWU tensions and pushed the agenda of reforming the union role. They included Anne Snelgrove in the November 2005 edition of the journal *Progress*, writing on 'Rebalancing the Conference'. But, for the moment, the most significant reaction at and after the conference was over the managerial treatment of the NEC.

The annual NEC away day was held on 7 November, a session with the main focus being 'making the NEC work better'. It was a constructive discussion but it also became the setting for a powerful reaction to the management of the past eight years. One impeccably moderate and esteemed NEC figure from the tradional right had earlier said of this developing mood 'we are not trying to seize power – we just want them to behave'. The mood now was described by one aggravated centre-ground representative as 'fed up with being bounced, manipulated, treated like crap'. Here was another indicator of what would turn out to be a growing crisis in Blair's party management.

A new General Secretary

Meanwhile, in September Matt Carter the General Secretary had unexpectedly resigned without public explanation. Ray Collins from the TGWU, a man with a left-wing past but now close to Nita Clarke in the No. 10 Political Office where they were looking for a weakening of the TULO role, became spoken of as the favourite. But, at a late hour, the favourite was challenged by an internal candidate, Peter Watt, the party's Director of Finance and Compliance. The No. 10 staff became split but the Leader's preference remained for Collins. Yet, Blair did not attempt to force Watt to stand down, and in remarkably quick time, Watt built an unusual and multifaceted alliance, performed the best in the interview and won the vote on 7 November 16–10.

One factor involved here was undoubtedly a reaction on the NEC to what was seen as another imposition by No. 10. Brown's supporters specially liked him for that. Watt also appealed to some loyalist sentiment unhappy with the TGWU nominee and looking for practical administrative and electoral expertise; Amicus representatives split away from the TGWU. But possibly the most important factor was that Watt built up an accommodation with various forces, some of whom gained the strong impression from him that they were about to see a return to the role of the party officials as civil servants of the party. This also pulled in the GRA representatives.

In practice, little in his earlier history as a protégé of Margaret McDonagh indicated that Watt would find the change to acting as a civil servant as his preference. He was a bold and skilled organisational risk-taker especially in his view of the malleability of party rules. The ambiguity of his position was underlined with the continued rise to prominence of Alicia Chater (now Kennedy) who became Deputy General Secretary. She was married to another major fixer, Roy Kennedy, the party's Finance and Compliance Director who was also Secretary of the Conference Arrangements Committee. In No. 10, Blair had been consoled by a secret if unrealistic proposal from Watt to make sweeping changes in the power of 'the union barons'.[35] Watt also kept contact with Brown's emissaries, who became more confident that he was a man they also could do business with.

In addition to that, with some friendly silky presentational skills, he also sought to keep good links with the NEC unions and the now more active NEC officers meeting. In spite of this, the capacity of the officials to continue the old politics by steering without NEC consent kept re-emerging. Managerial interference in internal selections and elections continued. The private word to critics was that he was doing his best to control it. It was not clear who or what should be believed. In this period Watt had a close working ally in Mike Griffiths, Chairman of the Organisation Committee and a classic exponent of the skills of working both ways to reconcile different forces.

Indications of the continuing mores of the managers were contained in the new composition of the NPF on 24 January 2006. The new elected PLP representation was politically mixed apart from the voluntary absence of the Socialist Campaign Group, but some familiar managerial faces re-appeared. Margaret Wall, now a new peer, became a representative of the Lords. New MP Anne Snelgrove became first NPF then JPC representative from the PLP. McCartney was re-elected Chair of the NPF for another two years. A new post of Vice Chairman from the PLP arrived in the person of Anne Begg, without, it appeared, prior NPF discussion.

PLP

It was, as has been shown, a feature of management politics that the form of management in one area could affect the politics in others. The management of the NEC, the party conference and the NPF together generated a mood increasingly frustrated and resentful of the management practices. That in turn fed into the developing politics of the PLP. The Hewitt proposal for the devolution of primary care trust powers to GPs with power to commission from the private sector was seen both as an imperious measure on the basis of a contentious manifesto mandate and as carrying yet another threat of health workers being pushed out of the NHS. With Eagle in the Chair allowing free debate, Patricia Hewitt and the NHS policy were savaged at an early PLP meeting. There was a temporary retreat on these proposals but then the movement towards private sector involvement and marketisation continued.

Relations between the PLP, the Prime Minister and ministers responsible for particular legislation reflected Blair's ascendancy and his driving style, although in matters linked to financial and economic plans much depended still on Blair's relationship with Brown. A new crisis on the major issue of state-pensions policy was met by their joint involvement in a government commission on pensions. Blair favoured pensions increasing in line with earnings – a policy close to that pushed by the party conference in 2000 and 2006. Brown was unhappy with its financial implications and insisted on a long lead-in time. The continuing policy tensions with Brown added to the managerial problems Blair himself produced for the whips by his policies and the myself-alone processes of policy-formulation on other issues.

The Schools White Paper

The big divide that changed the scale and upped the tempo of revolt within the PLP came in October 2005 with the new schools white paper, *Higher Standards, Better Schools for All* (which became in February 2006 the Education and Inspections Bill). As was the Blair leadership style, there was no attempt to involve the PLP in the first stage of policy-formulation and the Cabinet was informed about the White Paper too late to change it. When the dialogue with the PLP did start, it was undermined by the Blair spin aiming to show its appeal to swing voters and its distance from the past – thus accentuating PLP distrust over his line of travel once again. Even the very careful Geoff Hoon publicly criticised the failure to consult the PLP on policy 'until the last minute'.[36] So much for the genuflexions from the Leader in 2001 and the change in leadership behaviour announced just before the 2005 election.

Months of argument spread across the party over proposals for 'trust schools' which now appeared to spread the loss of shared objectives into an area of party consensus. The emphasis was now on greater parental choice, giving schools and academies the power to operate outside local government control, running their own entrance criteria and receiving direct funding from government. It offered new opportunties for greater outside involvement on the school boards including the bringing in of business and religious organisations.

The shift away from party traditions and long-thought-through issues of principle was considerable and badly received. As one loyalist Cabinet Minister joked discreetly and grimly, 'The party is united on this policy – against it'. At an early stage when pressed at the Parliamentary Committee, it appeared that Blair did not know the extent of the opposition within the party which favoured fair access well ahead of choice. When informed, he also appeared dismissive of them, telling the committee 'our folks will have to come into line'.

The new members

He had considerable confidence in the newly elected MPs. It had been anticipated that as those in safe seats retired the new intake would be less rebellious. Managerial influence in the regions was seen as successful in avoiding almost all 'oppositionists' aided by the organisational decline of the CLP left. Interviews with the new recruits revealed 'a cohort' where the sentiment was 'don't rock the boat'.[37] Organised by the whips and by the PLP office there were also some new managerial influences encouraging cooperation, including a mentoring of new entrants to a greater degree than before, although some insiders saw this as 'unsophisticated'. There was a briefing of MPs' staff every Monday with hand-picked groups going to No. 10.

This new PLP had an unusual number of ex-special advisers, some with experience at the forefront of party management. Austin, Balls and Ed Milliband were and remained very close to Brown but shied away from urging systematic policy opposition; careful to avoid the accusation of subversion and also aware of the dangers of new MPs getting the habit of open rebellions. Pat MacFadden remained loyally close to Blair. All these factors may well have influenced the initial restrained mood of the new entrants. But then again, government support from a smaller majority made their role more important and their reponsibilities more inhibiting. What was happening under the surface and where opinion would eventually settle in terms of rebelliousness was uncertain. Some who sounded them out before the so-called 'September coup' (see below, p. 646) saw little difference in attitudes between them and those of the 2001 intake.

But in any case, PLP opposition was growing from a variety of motives and over diverse issues as Blair's line of travel and priorities undermined support. Cowley reported that the 28 revolts of this parliament were already higher than the 21 of the previous parliament which was 'itself the highest rate in the postwar era'.[38] Blair's attempt to put the responsibility for unity on the PLP whilst shedding it for himself in the name of strong leadership, fed increased aggravation. It particularly enraged those in the mainstream who had elements of their own agenda of progressive reform. Martin Linton, a thoughtful modernising MP, announced that 'discipline does not work if it's a one way street'. This had to be 'the end for top-down policymaking'.[39]

The education white paper provoked a constructive alternative white paper drafted by the four senior ex-Ministers John Denham, Angela Eagle, Estelle Morris (in the Lords), and Nick Raynsford backed, it was said, by 90 supporters. They sought 'to build a consensus' around their position. The government position brought outright criticism from amongst others the normally publicly reticent Neil Kinnock. Up to this point also, Prescott's mainly discreet interventions, wearing his party hat, had affected policy only on procedural issues including elected mayors, regional government and reform of electoral law. He had shied away from anything that could be presented by the media as a major policy split. Now, in a public attack on the education policy, Prescott broke with past form by, in effect, directly challenging the Leader.

Leadership, management and defeat

It was not surprising that the Chief Whip found her job increasingly difficult with one policy collision following another. Whilst the new education policy was churning up widespread opposition across the party, the big test for Blair came on other grounds of his own making, national security and strong leadership. Over the Terrorism Bill, Blair advocated an increase in detention of terrorist suspects from 14 to 90 days, regarding this as essential to protect the public and also convinced that it would secure overwhelming public support. Blair also saw no disadvantage in portraying the Conservatives, who (with the Liberal democrats) were opposing this shift, as compromising national security. If ever a policy was the flagship of a Leader building on his stance in 2001 and 2005 and potentially the means of strengthening his tenure, this was it.

His defeat on this issue – the first as Prime Minister – was due in part to scepticism over the evidence-base of the case for the 90 days, especially given its adverse implications for civil liberty. There were also doubts over its value as a defence of security. Much later the Director of Public Prosecutions disputed that he or the police had been the source of the pressure for the ninety days.[40] Warned by the whips and by the backbenchers on the Parliamentary Committee that he was likely to lose, Blair pressed ahead, encouraged by the thunderous enthusiasm shown in a PLP meeting which had been carefully choreographed in an attempt to help project his support. George Mudie, who voted againt the 90 days, had a pointed view of this. Blair was 'out of touch with the backbenchers' and PLP meetings were 'run like Nuremberg rallies'.[41] This management became an encouragement for Blair to see at the PLP meeting what he wanted to see.

Sent out from the PLP office to party members, who it was hoped would put pressure on MPs, was a cringe-making email questionnaire which quickly became notorious.[42] Its three questions were: Do you think that our laws shuld be updated to cope with the current security threat? Do you think that the police should have the time and opportunity to complete their investigations into suspected terrorists? Do you think that government should make sure there are new safeguards to protect innocent people? The attempted manipulation was so crude that it generated anger and rebounded from the CLPs. Blair and the Home Secretary Clarke both denied responsibility for the document. Clarke later apologised about it. A source in the management later said it had been a piece of managerial private enterprise.

On the central issue, Clarke was thought to have been privately seeking a compromise which would have moved past the 28 days but was not absolutely committed to the 90 days. Blair, however, was adamant, saying, 'Sometimes it is better to fight and lose than to win and do the wrong thing'.[43] That was presumably an example of what was admiringly viewed later by one of his advisers as the 'shit or bust' style of leadership.[44] Here it turned into a step towards the 'bust' of his political demise. On

9 November 2005 the Government was twice defeated on the Terrorism Bill with majorities against of 31 and 33. Brown, at this time, had been supportive, returning from abroad for the vote and getting his allies to try to organise to defend the Leader.

Aftermath

In terms of Blair's base of support in the PLP the significant feature was that his judgement here was questioned even by some very close allies. One view was that it was a ridiculous way of approaching what must be an uncertain judgement of the time period and a damaging failure to maximise support for the strongest position available. The *Guardian* made the point that doing the right thing and losing had never been a 'New Labour' governing principle.[45] Others worried that it was an encouragement to PLP dissidents on other issues to keep their actions in line with absolutist beliefs.

On the terrorism vote, from the 2005 intake there were two who were highly rebellious, Katy Clark and Linda Riordan, but now also for the first time there were four others.[46] They too heeded the no-compromise message. Not only had Blair not pulled the party behind him; strikingly, he had not pulled the country either. In a particular blow to his strong leadership, only 20 per cent of all voters and 21 per cent of Labour voters supported the decision to push on with the 90-day proposal when it faced defeat.[47] A finding of 63 per cent agreed that Blair's authority had been damaged by the defeat. Blair's behaviour was regarded as so over-the-top that, as Peston reported, concern grew that he wanted 'to bequeath maximum mayhem',[48] or at least did not care enough if it happened. That fear later deepened to Blair's cost.

Conservative revival

On 6 December 2005 the Conservatives elected a new young Leader, David Cameron. As he made clear, he was attempting to change public perception of the Conservative Party, losing its 'nasty party' image, copying the Blair style, and in effect moving on to some of the 'New Labour' political ground. For the first time since 1994, in the face of a reviving Conservative Party the government looked like being in serious electoral difficulties as Blair was judged to have 'lost his magic'.[49] But polling also indicated that with Gordon Brown as Labour Leader, the Tories would move even further ahead.[50] That finding strengthened Blair's personal position as did the decline of Brown's lead over the Conservatives on his economic performance. Later, in the Dunfermline and West Fife by-election on 11 February there was a huge swing to the then leaderless Liberals after a campaign in Brown's national territory in which the Chancellor himself had played a prominent part.

Meanwhile, as the battle over the Schools Bill wore on, in January 2006 the government suffered its third and fourth defeats on votes on two Lords amendments to the Racial and Religious Hatred Bill. One was defeated by ten votes, the other by just one vote and in the surprising absence of Blair. Brown again supported the government. The main explanation given for these defeats was that they were due to MPs filling in for the shortage of activists at the Dunfermline and West Fife by-election campaign. Armstrong had allowed around 20 MPs to assist there but then met a Conservative ambush bringing in members thought to be absent. In addition, it was said by some that 21 Labour rebels who voted against were the usual suspects and that they had been cooperating with the Conservatives in a planned move.

An alternative view was that there were only around ten or so MPs at the by-elections yet over 40 absent or abstained. This was diagnosed by some as reflecting a sinking morale and a managerial failure to keep contact with the rebels and party opinion more generally. At this time, various forms of non-cooperation with the whips, including hiding voting intentions, were also noted. That began to be seen by some MPs as part of a more or less permanent estrangement between the whips' office and a growing section of the PLP. Blair's absence in the one-vote defeat was in line with his low attendance record for votes, but it set a very bad example and seemed to signal management incompetence.

Discipline, management and the Parliamentary Committee

Following the defeats there was a new concern amongst some of the more assertive loyalists to change the atmosphere and curb revolts in the PLP. What was highlighted yet again was the degree to which Blair had lost control over sanctions. Just as after the first defeat, when the Chief Whip was said to be ready to punish dissenters,[51] so now she was said to be being urged to move against high-profile figures, particularly the 'oppositionists' in the Campaign Group and more especially against Robert Marshall-Andrews accused of colluding with the Conservatives.[52] To the disciplinarians, action seemed all the more urgent when the Conservatives moved into a 9 per cent poll lead.

Yet nothing happened about it. The whips' office, where Bob Ainsworth the Deputy was said to be less confrontational and less abrasive than Armstrong, was quietly divided and Armstrong could not guarantee support in the PLP for heavily imposed discipline. There was always the possibility that overreaction might produce a huge internal convulsion opening up a new front of disunity. Marshall-Andrews received the usual caution. On the Parliamentary Committee, where Blair's leadership was seen by back-bench representatives as an increasing problem, the report of the Chief Whip now usually took the form of 'nothing to report'. The only method available appeared to be keeping up peer pressure on the dissidents, whilst also encouraging pressure from below. The Party Chair played his part in this. He reported to the NEC on 4 February that what upset members most was Labour MPs voting against the Government.[53] Later

McCartney even called on party members to write in protest to those MPs who defied a three-line whip.[54]

Back to Schools Bill

Some compromise by the Leader became essential over the long-running battle on the Schools Bill, especially after a heavily critical report from the Labour-dominated education select committee, although even that did not go as far as many of the Labour Party opponents wanted. The proposals on admissions policy were strengthened in a way which seemed to preclude selection. Polling of Labour Party members between 2 and 8 March still showed significant differnces between their views and the bill.[55] Only a quarter supported the view that most schools should be run by outside organisations.

Neverthless, the concessions did prove enough to split its critics and Prescott came in behind the agreement. The Education and Inspections Bill was carried on second reading on 15 March, but there were still 52 Labour opponents and 25 non-voters,[56] and the measure went through because of Conservative support. By the time it came to votes on the third reading on 24 May, the Labour revolt was petering out as MPs became increasingly concerned over the electorate responses to constant party divisions. On 12 May a Populus poll for BBC 2 found 67 per cent agreeing that Labour was 'more interested in its own internal squabbles than in dealing with the problems that affect my life'. The legacy-seeking Blair did not take the hint.

Warwick Agreement, unions and disunity

Implementation in practice

At this time relations with the unions over the implementation of the Warwick Agreement were under new strain. The unions had been told that when the DTI published its labour-market strategy document, which would outline the timetable for the delivery of the Warwick agreement in full, there would be consultations with the TULO Contact Group on it. But after a long delay, when the document eventually appeared on 24 April 2006 as *Success at Work*, the TULO unions were given less than 24 hours to respond to it.

The document made no direct reference to the existence of a Warwick Agreement with its detailed provisions, although it did make reference to a number of issues which were also referred to at Warwick. Blair continued to publicly affirm that the Warwick Agreement would be implemented, and the general government reply to complaints was that a number of items from Warwick had already been delivered and that most other issues were in progress.[57] Privately, the government side talked in terms of about half of the agreement having 'been done'. On the TULO side it was seen as falling short of the spirit and text of Warwick in that some pledges had been reinterpreted and others passed over. The unions had become increasingly aware that the government found it more possible to implement elements which the government itself had newly introduced at Warwick than those proposed by the unions and agreed.

Old union divisions and old management politics also now came into operation. The unions through TULO were not geared up for the process of detailed follow-up, whilst at the TUC non-party-affiliated unions had felt some exclusion from the action taking place within the party. It was also argued at the TUC that working to government through the TUC was in line with past experience pre-TULO. In TULO the view was that it was through TULO that the agreement had been organised and established. This became an ideal situation for divide and rule tactics to be pursued from No. 10 playing to the tensions. The invitation to TULO to respond to *Success at Work* had been extended not directly but via the TUC. Following this, arguments about process and territory led to the TUC's withdrawal from the Contact Group.

Frustration over the procedures and and the delivery did not curtail the further build-up of TULO as an auxiliary campaigning organisation. There were 600,000 trade unionists targeted in the 100 most marginal seats and they received 1.8 million direct mails. Later, in local government elections TULO was privately acknowledged by managers to have given significant assistance in London, although no detailed follow-up polling took place.

Reforming the unions

Deteriorating relations over Warwick were compounded by Downing Street tactics over union voting reform. There was a spasmodic dribble of proposals which appeared to have been encouraged from No. 10. In November, Alan Johnson proposed a drop in the unions vote from 50 per cent to 15 per cent.[58] In December a Fabian pamphlet by ex-TUC official David Coates conjectured reducing the unions' conference vote to that of the NPF vote, exactly the same prescription.[59]

A meeting of TULO General Secretaries on 26 January 2006 agreed that they would not support change in the voting arrangements, although quietly efforts were being made to explore some changes in representation and other processes at the conference that might accommodate representation of the new Unite amalgamation, without threatening the Smith settlement. In a further intervention, David Coates and Alan Milburn warned that after amalgamation there would be 'irresistable pressure for a new constitutional settlement'.[60] Similar calls came from Steve Byers[61] and ex-union leader Bill Morris, now in the Lords.[62] But what was striking about this series of interventions was the utter inability of the No. 10 Political Office to provoke a sustained media correspondence or debate anywhere in the party around the issue which they were trying to highlight – changing the union vote. There was little support for it and not much stomach for the argument. Part of the problem for them was the clear recognition that – as Tony Robinson, a past critic of the union leaders, noted – it was 'Only when the trade unions vote against government policy that their collective voice becomes a matter of concern'.[63]

Sleaze and a new dimension

Loans for peerages and the government of the party

Regardless of legality it was a covert understanding of elite British political life that financial provision was an asset in seeking a peerage, but it was not something that many Labour Party members approved of. On 13 March 2006 it was reported that Labour leaders were facing a backlash from their own MPs after admitting they received loans from millionaire supporters who were then recommended for peerages.[64] In April, according to the General Secretary Peter Watt, he was informed that the party, like the Tories, had been taking loans from its supporters.[65] The NEC knew nothing about the practice and even the two most senior elected officials of the party, the Chair Jeremy Beecham and the Treasurer Jack Dromey, knew nothing about it. After a series of meetings when it was agreed to make only one statement through the NEC,[66] on Wednesday 15 March Dromey suddenly went public with an angry statement and series of media interviews.

In his memoirs, Blair gave an account of the sequence of events just prior to Dromey's public statements, and accuses Brown of threatening to open up an NEC enquiry on this unless Blair came into line with him on pensions policy, which Blair refused.[67] Powell partially confirms this but only in terms of Brown wanting to publicly circulate a critical paper.[68] Whatever the truth of any of that, the basic problem that the loans issue and Dromey criticism exposed was that there had been a continuous weakness of financial accountability at national level in the party. Members of the Finance Board, Jeremy Beecham and Dianne Hayter in particular, had often complained of lacking information. Beecham had complained as recently as at the 2 February meeting of the NEC. There was no indication whatsoever that managers were covering up self-seeking sleaze; rather, they were working to prevent leaks and working to the Leader's managerial agenda which had deliberately reduced the NEC's role and status. Blair had been uninterested in the past when informed of the inadequaces of the NEC control over finance.

It was therefore no surprise that there was no sign of concern in the later Blair or Powell memoirs that NEC supervision had failed. Nor was there an adequate contestation of Dromey's accusation that 'No. 10 must have known about the loans'. Dromey had also widened the diagnosis: 'I think it is a symbol of a wider problem in the culture of the Labour Party'. And he clarified his purpose. The party, its institutions and its democracy needed to be respected, including by No. 10. 'What I want to do is to assert the democratic integrity of the Labour Party'. In effect, Blair and his aides faced from Dromey what sounded like the charge of acting like a party within a party. This was, as copiously illustrated here, not far from the truth in terms of their general managerial behaviour. As for Blair's personal responsibility, his biographer John Rentoul had come to suspect that he was 'a man who takes a macho pride in his man of the world realism' and was then 'caught bang to rights' over loans for peerages.[69]

Another revealing feature of New Labour managerial realism which required investigation was the reaction of the Ethics (later Funding) Committee set up in 2002 to examine the ethical basis of party funding. After the removal of Triesman from his post there were complaints from members of the committee that they were not being kept informed of all the party's income. This was smoothed over for a time but the committee was then allowed to pass away without any reference to the NEC. Certainly, by the time of the crisis over loans and funding the NEC's Chair, the chair of the Organisation Committee, the Treasurer, and other senior NEC members had lost sight of its existence. An officers' meeting now formally declared its demise and the NEC agreed to take over its old responsibilities and propose new structures. On 21 March 2006, following an NEC discussion on the loans controversy, there was a telling recommendation 'that the NEC resume its rightful reponsibility for oversight of all matters of party funding and financing'. There would be a review of the lessons to be learned and revised processes and protocols would be put in place to preserve NEC accountability and the Labour Party's internal democracy.[70] At least, that was the intention (but see 'Donorgate'in Chapter 21, pp. 740–1).

Blair's immediate public vulnerability was that in the use of loans the party had evaded the rules on British political finance that he himself had initiated. Urged on by the Scottish Nationalists, a police investigation began and went on for over a year. There were continuing arguments over the scope and wisdom of this police activity. What appeared to be the leaking of police views together with the media suggestion of a No. 10 cover-up put constant pressure on Blair and also undermined the reputation of the police. The final decision was not to proceed with a prosecution but the whole episode had exposed Blair to yet another look at his political character, adding a sharper edge to the discomfort felt in the party about the sense of a degenerating government.

The debt, funding and the unions

Following this episode the party moved into a desperate financial position as high-value donors dried up, leaving a debt of something in the region of £27 million and with a major shortfall in income to pay for the £4 million annual running costs. Major financial cuts took place at the centre and in the regions. The unsuitable Queen Street premises, which the party had left to move into Victoria Street prior to the 2005 election, were sold with some questioning of the wisdom of buying it in the first place.[71] This now made the unions' fianancial support all the more important as an open transparent regular contribution which by August was now around three-quarters of the party's annual income. That was said to have heightened business fears of the unions' influence over the government.[72]

According to the crude myth of 'who pays the piper', this ought to have resulted in union financial threats. Also, given the growing union criticism of the behaviour of party managers, it might have been expected that there would be financial pressure for them to change or be changed. Some unions, individually, did increasingly support the new unofficial Commission on Party Accountability, but the unions remained very restrained in their direct behaviour. In the next months, the arguments over what the unions regarded as the unfulfilled elements of Warwick (calculated by the unions at about 50 per cent and with the majority of fulfilled pledges coming from the government's own input) dragged on, but still there came no financial threats from TULO. Since 2001, union leaders had faced growing pressure, pushed from the anti-Labour left in their unions, for withdrawal or reallocation of funds to other political organisations. All that had been fought off across the board, year by year. Nevertheless, in 2006–7 there were two exceptional cases in content and form which indicated trouble ahead.

In March 2006, there was an unprecedented move by UNISON following huge internal pressure over the government's alteration of the retirement date under the local authority workers' occupational pensions scheme. The action did not involve changing affiliation but temporarily withdrawing completely all its election support in all forms from the Labour Party during the local election period. The government still did not back down. It was not party finance but industrial action and the threat of other strikes which influenced negotiations and eventually produced a compromise which protected present but not future pensions. Nevertheless, it was an unprecedented move showing a relationship under deep stress.

In May 2006 in a move not led from its leadership, the UCW conference voted to withdraw finance from the party if the government went ahead with offering shares in the Post Office. This they considered would be a breach of both the Warwick Agreement and the election manifesto. But no sanctions threats were taken into TULO post-Warwick discussions, and the union policy was not followed up by UCW General Secretary Billy Hayes. Derek Simpson made the point about TULO explicit: 'we will not use our finance as a lever inside the party'.[73] Later, under pressure to completely withdraw funds at the 2007 UCW conference, Hayes was reported as responding by telling them that the union would 'consider' suspending its funds if ministers refused to heed the campaign against privatisation.[74] Nothing came of it, but it indicated a special case with special tensions and pressures.

Hayden Phillips

To some around Blair, the political-financial crisis provided a welcome opportunity to sort out the financing of political parties. The appointment of senior retired civil servant Sir Hayden Phillips to seek agreement between the political parties on reform of party finance also offered the moderniser radicals a big, perhaps *the* big, element in Blair's legacy, although it was not helped by failing to tell anybody in the Labour Party machine or the NEC before dashing off the press release.[75] 'Doomed from the start' was Watts's judgement.[76]

That was not quite true. For the Conservatives, it offered an opportunity of drawing on the writings of Blair's strategist Matthew Taylor in returning to their own long-standing attempt to break the collective affiliated structure of the Labour Party which Andrew Tyrie the Conservative MP saw as 'in hock to the unions'.[77] As his colleague McTernan revealed later to NEC representatives, Taylor drew up the terms of reference for Hayden Phillips. So, whilst the unions had had nothing to do with the way that the loans for peerages scandal had developed, nor of the use of party funds without NEC approval, they quickly became the target of internal and external forces who used each other as leverage for radical legal measures against the unions. It was believed in No. 10 and around the General Secretary that the union view was shortsighted in not responding to the party's interest, but that was not the party's view as it emerged from its institutions.

As the argument progressed at senior levels of the party, a leading academic authority, Keith Ewing, became influential on TULO in reinforcing their refusal to accept a cap on donations that would constrain union affiliation. He focused on the lack of symmetry between the political parties in their internal forms and funding. A legal uniform cap would be partisan and partial in the damage it would cause. It would threaten the rights of self-determination of the Labour Party. Funding arrangements in relation to the unions were already the most heavily regulated of British parties. And the radical critique of 'the problem' of the relationship from its opponents contrasted with the 1998 report of the Committee on Standards in Public Life which had found the legislation working satisfactorily and requiring no change in the law.

Although the public wanted reform, their view was also not as supportive of more radical proposals as had been implied by Hayden Phillips and the managers. IpsosMORI, on the basis of workshop discussions with representatives of the general public, had found that, as the participants gained more information, they took the view that the aims of bringing about 'greater control over the influence from the affluent few' and 'the invigoration of local politics' could be achieved 'with relatively little change to the current party funding system'.[78] The party and union emphasis remained on tighter control of what the parties spent so that there was nearer an 'equality of arms', full transparency, and a diminished attraction to secure other finance. There should, it was argued, be a modest extension of state funding, constrained as it was by the still intense public antipathy to financing the parties.

On the NEC and in the conference the party-union position on funding went through with no opposition (showing) and an avalanche of support for the relationship seen as under legal threat. In the light of the battles since 1992 this unity was an extraordinary historical twist but not the last. As the party discussion continued, McCartney, on behalf of the Leader, gave a guarantee that the party not the government would decide its policy on party financing in relation to the Hayden Phillips deliberations and conclusions. In confidential bilateral discussions with the Conservatives he became very sticky, much to the chagrin of No. 10.[79] That may well have sealed his personal fate (see below, p. 636).

Blows to Blair

In the meantime, the police investigations added to the factors affecting Blair's political standing. On BBC *Newsnight* on 20 April 2006, a nationally representative focus group of floating voters produced a hugely negative response to Blair, with a particularly pointed hostility to him over trust. On 25 April, the Government received an additional blow with adverse repercussions for Blair and changing consequences for the party. The NHS had received a huge input of finance and a substantial increase in staff, but suddenly there was a series of localised financial crises with new threats of hospital closures and job losses. Hewitt met an exeptionally bad reception at the RCN conference. It became a public-relations disaster on what had been Labour's strongest policy ground, driving forward the momentum of union and party criticism. Later, it was noted by academic specialists on voting behaviour that 'more than 40 per cent of British adults either work in or have partners who work in the public sector'. 'They talk about their enormous disillusionment. This spreads to the wider population.'[80]

Blair had intended to make law and security, and his own assertion of strong leadership, the central theme of the local government elections but in another setback on 26 April it turned out that 1,023 foreign criminals from British jails who were to have gone through a process of examination for deportation had been released without consideration. The government's reputation for competence and that of Home Secretary Charles Clarke were badly damaged.

Little publicised at the time, a survey of public attitudes between December 2005 and April 2006, which included attitudes towards Commons voting behaviour, added to the observation of a growing public reaction agains Blair's governing style. It confirmed that how the party leadership thought their MPs should vote ranked lower in public approval (36 per cent) than what the MPs' local party members wanted (58 per cent). Since 2004, a further shift had taken place in answer to a question with tougher phrasing about leadership action, whereby a third fewer of the public now thought that an MP 'should base his or her decision on party leadership orders' had dropped from 21 per cent to 14 per cent.[81] The weakening public legitimacy of strong personal leadership combined with the traditional managerial system had no noticeable effect on Blair's behaviour.

Leadership reassertion again

In the English local elections held on 4 May, Labour came third in the overall share of the vote, losing control of 18 local authorities. Anticipating the public and party reaction to poor results, Blair attempted to manage a relaunch. On 5 May, in a Night of the Long Knives reshuffle, Jack Straw, understood to have some differences with Blair over the Middle East, was replaced by Margaret Beckett as Foreign Secretary. Charles Clarke was sacked after refusing a move to another department. John Reid went to the Home Office where he appeared to rubbish his predecessors Blunkett and Clarke in a critique of a department which was 'not fit for purpose'. A month later, Clarke attacked Reid in reply. Their rivalry and the argument over competence virtually took out of contention for the Leader's post the two biggest anti-Brown players who might have built enough party support to seriously constrain and challenge him.

Hilary Armstrong, the Chief Whip, had been damaged by the defeats on counter-terrorism. She was seen at this time as increasingly short-tempered. In meetings, her incessant loud militant muttering whilst others were speaking did nothing healthy for the atmosphere and had become a useful target for Cameron in the House in questions to the Prime Minister. In the reshuffle she was replaced by a firm but less confrontational Blair loyalist Jacqui Smith, who would still have to manage the Blair defence operation. Gerry Sutcliffe was moved away from the DTI position which linked him to the trade unions and replaced there by consistently loyalist Jim Fitzpatrick. Ian McCartney was also now finally moved from the Party Chair role. There was a muted response from the unions because his role as their champion was now regarded as more surface than effective, and there was little response either from his past protector Prescott, who had developed reservations about the accommodating way that McCartney was playing the role. Hazel Blears, famed for her devoted loyalism, was moved into the post which was from this point more consistently referred to with the gender-neutral title of Party Chair.

In an attempt to reassert the authority of the Leader, the tasks of ministers were laid down in published letters. To Blears on party reorganisation he detailed what he expected – a ten year plan to be announced by June and then implemented quickly.[82] In an atmosphere increasingly concerned over his direction of travel and increasingly at odds with the failure to involve the party in consultation on policy-formulation, it aroused aggravated NEC protectiveness of their responsibilities. It also aroused Prescott to an extraordinary intervention which indicated a change in relations with Blair. In an unreported comment, he told the NEC that organisational matters 'were the NEC's responsibility and . . . it was not proper to write such a letter'. Nothing emerged of the ten-year plan. Blears did seek to get the Warwick discussions moving as a means of giving her some credibility with the unions. On 24 July 2006 in a memo showing movement on 25 items she argued that, 'given the substantial progress on most isues there are no grounds to make the argument that the Government is not committed to the Warwick Agreement . . . over the course of this Parliament'.[83] The unions saw it as taking relations and the discussion on unimplemented items no further forward.

The reshuffle and its aftermath were widely seen not as an expression of invigorated authority but as the act of a desperate man. Up to this point, Blair had refused to move away from his previous 'full term' commitment as Prime Minister, but now the commitment which had assisted Blair became a usable issue by critics. They pressed that it was producing an uncertainty which was badly affecting government and the party because it was not known exactly when the Prime Minister was planning to stand down. It could also produce problems for a coherent transfer of power and time for the new Leader to bed in.

Heavily questioned about this on 8 May, at a press conference before the PLP meeting, Blair now made a promise to allow his successor 'ample time' to establish himself. He also made what appeared to be his first personal endorsement of Brown as the successor he would prefer. But, as for an agreed timetable for transfer of the post, Blair would not give one: that, he argued, would 'paralyse' the government.[84] If there had been enough trust in Blair, that could have been regarded as a reasonable position. But around three-quarters of MPs contacted in a survey wanted him to set out a timetable,[85] and the acute problem was, as Nick Robinson the BBC Political Editor put it, 'If he says trust me the problem for many Labour MPs is that they don't'.[86] At the PLP meeting that day, chaired by Angela Eagle, those present were warned off the aggressive heckling which often particularly expressed loyalist disapproval at these meetings. The choice of speakers came from a broad spectrum of party opinion – other than from the Campaign Group members who did not turn up. The 'ample time' formula was repeated there by Blair and the commitment made to 'a stable and orderly transition'.[87]

The distrustful mood of this meeting marked a major shift. Blair felt it necessary to reassure MPs that he had the interests of the Labour Party at heart. Mullin questioned himself, 'Should we believe him?' and gave the answer 'On balance yes'.[88] But the doubts and distrust had grown, even amongst habitual loyalists. The sense was that because of the uncertainty about Blair and the damage of the Blair–Brown war, the party was in danger of falling apart. In the centre ground of the PLP there was beginning to be a move which saw Blair as the bigger problem. In that respect it was a contrast to the PLP meeting held in January 2005 when both had been warned about their behaviour; the subtext was that it was Brown who was the main difficulty. In line with the new mood, behind the scenes, there were even suggestions of bringing in eminent Labour figures as brokers and guarantors that Blair would deliver what he promised. It was hardly surprising that, couched in these demeaning terms, the attempt – if it was real – failed.

Two days later, a poll delivered more bad news for Blair. It found that he had become the most unpopular Labour Prime Minister of modern times. In May 1997 his satisfaction rating had reached 83 per cent. Now it was 26 per cent. On top of this deficit in leadership appeal, there was a growing sense of this being a fractious government. Only 6 per cent saw the Labour Party as united.[89]

Imposing discipline?

Given the disciplinary intentions of Blair's party management in 1997, it was not surprising that at this point dealing with the problem of this rebellious PLP was seen again by some loyalists and managers as having procedural solutions. But few raised their voices. At the NEC meeting of 23 May 2006, Louise Baldock, a loyalist now filling a vacant place on the NEC after Ruth Turner had moved into government, in a bold contribution directed at the Prime Minister and the new Chief Whip, complained about the lack of discipline amongst MPs. She dated that back to the failure to act over deselection in the wake of the vote on lone parent benefit.[90] But Blair himself, from a wiser position he had strongly developed since 2001, now warned that 'people would claim they were being martyred for their principles' and he argued again as an alternative that 'some colleagues need pressure from the party to stop them being so utterly destructive'.[91] The new Chief Whip did get agreement from the Parliamentary Committee for a new measure of disciplinary sanctions but of a very limited kind. Temporary suspension was allowed though only on condition it was not to be used against parliamentary dissent.

The tensions were further reflected in arguments over the conduct of the ballot for division V (PLP/EPLP) of the NEC in June. The row taken to the Parliamentary Committee focused on the whips' office, which was said to be seeking to mobilise ministers to vote for 'our candidate' Anderson against the incumbent Eagle. The Chief Whip repudiated the claim. But the main argument also focused on the proposal that votes would not be counted until the following day, a move which again evoked suspicions from deeply distrustful voices on the Parliamentary Committee. Eventually, it was agreed that the count would take place as soon as the ballot closed. Once again Eagle was elected. The ballot for the Parliamentary Committee was postponed until the next session of Parliament and then postponed further till December.

Meanwhile, on 30 June, in a by-election, Blaenau Gwent was lost again, this time to Dai Davies – the agent of the late Peter Laws – fighting on a financial shoe-string against the Labour Party campaign. It deepened the gloom in the party. Blair drove straight ahead with his reform agenda. On

13 July 2006 a paper issued by the Department of Health made clear that improvements were to be driven by 'contracting and contestability and service redesign'. The paper with its line of travel towards mixed service delivery on an unlimited scale was not part of a legislative process and therefore could not effectively be opposed. This was despite the fact that research by IpsosMORI for the Work Foundation had revealed that health-service workers were the most disillusioned and most critical in the public services.[92] Blair pressed on, now seeking to 'own the next generation of politics' by 'a great big argument' through which would come 'the next generation of ideas'.[93]

Registered supporters

Around the NEC, some minor procedural improvements, including provision of notes of the officers' group meetings, took place and the 'Party Report' quietly reverted to being the 'NEC Report'. The officers' meeting, which Prescott attended but not Blair, was as before always subject to the advisory managerial skills of the officials, especially in arguments over procedural defence of the Leader. However, the officers' meeting was now also increasingly defensive against proposals which could threaten the role of the party and damage the union-party relationship. The tensions showed themselves in attitudes to Blair's important organisational project to form an association of registered supporters.

As an addition to the party membership, still steadily sinking and now said to be 198,000, the registered supporters could add to the pool from which membership and activism and community penetration might grow. It was in principle widely acceptable as a means of extending the local dialogue, but it was neither new nor a panacea and it had dangers. Some experienced organisers challenged the No. 10 view that most electoral workers were not party members but were volunteers, supporters drawn in by the candidates. Further, the question was posed: Was there not a danger that paying members might transfer to become registered supporters?

Within a short space of time in 2005–6 party officials, encouraged from No. 10, claimed that there were 98,000 of these registered supporters but then, in classic managerial style, they were reluctant to hand over names to their CLPs. Once the names were revealed during the local elections the reluctance became much clearer. In a minority of CLPs there were some real registered supporters (Reading West was one prominent example) but a large number on the lists were already members of the party and many others just names taken from other lists that the party had. The crudity of all this now looked like fakery to cover for the failure to find a way of undercutting the members' voice.

In a significant political development in June 2006, an initiative from the Party Chair, Blears, to change the rulebook to include registered supporters was contested by Prescott, worried that the proposal was half-baked and would be understood as the first stage of undermining the rights of party members. His rejection of rulebook change was backed by the officers' meeting. Registered Supporters became just a reference in the preface of an NEC statement, without a rule change. Blair's ability to change the party into something more pliable had been blocked.

NEC elections and anti-control freakery

The NEC elections in June 2006 were, as usual, accompanied by a high number of complaints at the intervention of party officials, and all complaints rejected by the party officials. Experienced ex-*Tribune* columnist Barckley Sumner, who had closely monitored this election, was convinced that the interventions were extensive.[94] The contest was fought on two partially overlapping slates of Labour First and No. 10 against the Grassroots Alliance and it produced poor results for the Leader. The GRA took the first four places. Two Labour First-supported candidates, Peter Wheeler and Ellie Reeves, were elected but both were sympathetic to Brown and strongly linked to Amicus union positions. As with the Parliamentary Committee, no clear Blairites were elected. Loyalist Louise Baldock lost her place. In contrast, amongst the GRA successes was Walter Wolfgang. It was pointed out that only just over 20 per cent of the members participated and the 178,889 ballot papers issued was said to be 'the lowest on record'.[95]

Ingredients of a 'madness' and a very loyal revolt

Managerial obstacles

Athough the degeneration of Blair's managing capability had spread, he still appeared to have enough procedural control for his protection. When Labour formed a government, an election for the Leader and/or Deputy Leader could take place 'only if requested by a majority of party conference on a card vote'.[96] Where there was no vacancy, the nomination must be supported by 20 per cent of the Commons members of the PLP for an election promulgated by the party conference to go ahead. From the CLP left there had been two years of attempts to instigate resolutions calling for a leadership election, but they had met management opposition to the circulation of nomination forms in the PLP, and CAC objections to resolutions of this kind because of the absence of validly nominated candidates.

In July 2006 management attention had focused on a carefully drafted constitutional amendment from Erith and Thamesmead CLP and Weston-super-Mare CLP, which called for the automatic annual circulation of nomination forms for the Leader's election. These were an endorsement of the process used for Kinnock and Smith's elections and compatible with the rule which said that 'nominations shall be sought each year'.[97] But on the recommendation of the officials, on 11 July it was now judged by the officers' group (most of whom were NEC trade unionists not anxious to be seen as initiating a direct challenge to Blair) that nomination forms did not have to be supplied each year prior to the conference, as they could be requested and nominations be made any time. It was on its own a reasonable ruling but not one which had clearly and publicly been made before. The tactics over the forms appeared to have avoided an eviction attempt this year.

The unquiet summer

However, later that summer, disagreement over Blair's role in the new Israel–Lebanon conflict brought matters to a head. There was a responsible case for his refusal to support an immediate cease-fire; it would not solve the problem of Israel's vulnerability. But the lack of proportion in Israeli actions reignited simmering discontent about what was seen as Blair's subservient relationship with Bush. It did not help that on 18 July, during a lull in the G8 summit, a conversatiom between Blair and Bush had shown Blair in what appeared to be a demeaning junior role. This brought out the resentment carried over from Iraq focused again on the one-alone Leader who was not speaking for 'us'.

In August, an ICM/*Guardian* poll was showing Labour at a 19-year low and gave the Conservatives a nine-point lead, their best position for 14 years. Public trust in Blair had declined to its lowest level, minus 31 per cent.[98] But the cause of his downfall in this situation was not simply electoral adversity but something much more specific and personal to his leadership and party management. The years of his, at times, ostentatious lack of love for the Labour Party, lack of sentimentality about its history, frequent provocations and comfortable addiction to cross-dressing reinforced the importance of the question: was he much bothered whether the party thrived or even survivived after him? His record appeared to be drowning any contemporary reassuring words.

The well-informed columnist and Blair biographer John Rentoul had noted signs of a split between 'appeasers' and 'ultras' amongst Blair's advisers on whether a departure date should be specified. In Rentoul's view the ultras had the stronger case and the PLP agreement in May should not be binding on Blair, who was still in charge of events because it was already 'too late for the machinery of a leadership challenge to be cranked up at this year's conference'.[99] But it was a misunderstanding to imply that managerial control of the procedure for eviction was the end of it. It now meant that eviction would have to come in another way, an eventuality for which, crucially, there was no managerial preparation.

Prescott dealing with Blair

It was a mark of the search for that other way that John Prescott was amongst those who had now become increasingly concerned that Blair was primarily focused on himself and would not necessarily go when it was in the party's interest. At this stage he planned that if he himself resigned and urged a leadership election, Blair would be forced to go. Rawnsley later revealed that sometime in July, the Deputy Leader had a private conversation with Blair in the form of an ultimatum that Blair must make the announcement at the party conference that he would go by summer of 2007.[100] Prescott added that a private promise was no good because 'Gordon doesn't believe you and I don't fucking believe you'.[101] That view of Blair's promises was typical of growing numbers in the PLP.

It was becoming increasingly obvious to Labour MPs that only by Blair naming a date for his departure would there be enough reassurance. Blair, on the other hand, continued to see that as a recipe for government impotence and, on return from his holidays, he gave an interview to the *Times* journalists Philip Webster and Peter Riddell which emerged with the damaging heading 'Blair defies his party over departure date'.[102] The journalists described him as saying that he was 'not going to be intimidated by former ministers, trade unions or party members'. It was not a very sensitive view of the relationships.

Not only that, Blair accused 'a very significant number of MPs' who carried on about his leadership of doing so because they wanted 'a change of direction' away from 'New Labour' policies.[103] This was not totally inaccurate; distrust of his 'line of travel' over the public sector and his relations with George Bush were widespread. But insofar as away from 'New Labour' policies was often Blair's code for going back to 'old Labour', this became another provocation. The organised traditional left was not a rising force, whilst the policy revolts in the party were a broad-ranging phenomenon and the concern over his tenure was broader still. Blair's characterisation of this opposition to him suggested that they could not be trusted in their political objectives and was in Brownite eyes 'exactly what the Tories claimed'.[104] Blair appeared to be deliberately creating future difficulties for the next Leader.

Later it was said by Steve Richards[105] and by Patricia Hewitt[106] that in acting against Blair in the way that they now did, the party rebels were involved in a madness. Blair described it as 'irredeemably old-fashioned'.[107] Yet as Prescott's plan indicated, this situation had become an incentive for unconventional rebellious behaviour. The dissident action had a strong rational element in response to Blair's form of leadership and management, embodied particularly in the manipulated procedural constraints and compounded by a reasonable lack of trust in Blair, given his 'wily' reputation. Prescott's plan does not appear to have been revealed by Blair to his unsuspecting managers or, if it was, it was disregarded.

Blairites for Brown: the uprising

There was, by September, a discernible new movement of opinion taking place across the party, within the CLPs, the unions and around networks linked with the NEC and the PLP, focused on an early departure by Blair or a timetable for it. The large Amicus trade union group in the PLP began to discuss a possible draft letter to Blair but the collective view of the union leaders remained that they would not themselves initiate any eviction. However, if the PLP acted, they would then decide when and how to weigh in.

In spite of the fact that the House was not sitting at this time, from what was being said, there were signs that PLP members were involved in an urgent flurry of discussion and initatives. Even in the apparently loyalist 2005 intake of MPs, a circular letter to be sent to Blair gained some support, but did not get submitted before seventeen members of the 2001 intake took the lead with their own letter which had been partially drafted during the summer. As the final form of the letter emerged after a Midlands meeting, meal and social on Friday 1 September the tone was respectful and congratulatory, but it said bluntly that they no longer believed that Blair's remaining in office was in the interests of either the party or the country. It is possible to see some of this activity of the seventeen as a career-oriented show of advantageous loyalty to a potential new Leader. But where it existed, this was fused with a deeply emotional reaction to their perceptions that the party was in a rapidly deteriorating condition and that its future was threatened by a Leader who now had major problems of both public and party trust.

The most senior figure involved in the fifteen, Tom Watson, a junior minister in the defence department, was on the face of it an extraordinary person to appear at the front of such an uprising. Although he had become seen as part of the Brown camp he was also an impeccable trade union loyalist from the old AEEU (now Amicus) and he was also an ex-Millbank party organiser and conference manager who kept close links to party officials as well as to Labour First, the traditional loyalist right grouping. Watson had voted for the Iraq war, foundation hospitals, introducing student top-up fees, and anti-terrorism laws. In September 2006, he still prided himself that he had never let the Leader down. To that extent he was a model loyalist. The others were also seen as equally strong loyalists with a record of support in the House and outside it.

Watson and his rebellious allies agreed that the situation was urgent. The mood was described by one of them as 'If the Cabinet won't move, we'll have to do it'. Undoubtedly, Watson was a very gregarious man in regular touch with all Brown's aides and PLP allies, and Balls for some time had been an energetic figure in moves to seek a new Leader, as were many others. But in this first phase of revolt, it was Ian Austin, an MP who had been Brown's political adviser, who attended a limited Midlands meeting of rebels where the letter was agreed although no other collective decisions were taken. Austin felt especially strongly about what Blair was doing to the party, and also had a deepening frustration that Brown, admirable though he was, was so heavily constrained in acting decisively.

The full truth of this is uncertain and may remain so, but given Brown's caution over the years, it is very likely that, in the first phase, he was not fully aware of what was involved in this letter writing.[108] And as Boulton pointed out he certainly did not orchestrate it.[109] That was in spite of what Watson described later as a family visit from him and his wife to see Brown's child at Brown's home. Watson denied that any discussion took place there about a letter to Blair and if there had been 'he would have told me not to sign the letter'.[110] That was plausible given Brown's worries over future consequences, especially the media reaction. And if political planning was needed, there was little point in making a long trip; they could have done it on the phone.

The Chancellor's distance from the politics may also have been affected by the accident that Sue Nye, the most senior and cautious Brown aide, who had discreet links to No. 10, was away on holiday for part of the time. Khalid Mahmood, the only signatory that No. 10 had anticipated as a possible PPS resignation over Lebanon, indicated that it was not coordinated from the Brown camp but that they knew what was going on.[111] That fits the picture given by others. The signatories regarded this revolt as their own and it had an immediate expressive as much as tactical focus. As Watson reiterated many times in private later, it was more a spasm than a plan, more a riot than a coup. Also, the action speeded up into confrontation with No. 10 much faster than had been anticipated after the sending of the letter. The uncertainty about Brown's response and what would follow after the revolt had added to the mounting pressure for Blair to go or at least name a date, and left much to be put together ad hoc in messages on the mobiles.

Tactics and management

There was another history to Tom Watson relevant to the chosen tactics. He had never been fully committed to the Blair-Mandelson project over relations with the unions. His experience of being a party manager at headquarters and in the whips' office had made him very distrustful of Blair and critical of managerial attitudes. He thought that he knew what was to be expected from them now, given the proto-factional repoliticisation of the party machine as 'Blairite' and anti-Brown. Since 2001, under the militant Armstrong and in the face of Brown's obvious challenge, the whips' office had gradually become seen by critics, particularly and not exclusively Brownite critics, as over-influenced by a Leader's defensive sectarianism and failing to fulfill properly the two-way role which was their responsibility, especially in conditions of limited policy participation.

From some in the PLP it had encouraged a growing mood, familiar in reluctant armies, of 'why should we tell them anything?' The new Chief Whip, Jacqui Smith, was less aggressive and more receptive than Armstrong but thought of as likely to give Blair the kind of assessment of opinion in the party that he was favourable to receiving. As it turned out, that was a misreading, but the rebels' priority was that 'We needed to tell Blair what he needed to know and he needed to listen'. That view led to the judgement that discreet representations along the normal managerial route could not guarantee that the message would be properly conveyed with the right force and it would almost certainly move into a slower gear.

It was apparently agreed (it was said later) that because they did not want to appear as a threatening conspiracy, the number of signatories sought was to be restricted. In practice that limit gave No. 10 the ammunition that the letter was unrepresentative. From some in the PLP who were supportive of the revolt but not included in it, there was disappointment and frustration at the small scale of it and at their own sidelining. A common initial response included the view that, whatever it was, it had 'all gone off at half-cock'. Nevertheless, as it turned out, the impact was powerful, carried along within a PLP where amongst centre-ground opinion Blair's position had seriously deteriorated. Exposing that was the big success.

The managerial problems

Highlighted also but a generally unremarked feature by commentators was the acute weakness of the managerial response. There was plenty of evidence across the party that an unusual new burst of critical sentiment was building up, and the talk was of how a change might be forced. It had even become known within circles overlapping with the rebels that some of those who became signatories of the letter of revolt were now calling themselves privately 'Blairites for Brown'. In No. 10, party headquarters, the whips' office and the PLP office, they all failed to see this particular form of revolt coming and, when it happened, did not know what its support was. The shock to the managers was all the greater because of the range of unexpected rebels.

Why were these rebellious activities, which were not an absolutely tight secret, met by so much uncertainty by the managers? Years later, 'Good question' was an answer to that from a veteran of PLP management – after a silence and followed by admission that management relations with the PLP had 'slipped a bit'. The loss of contact at this point was partly the contingency of parliament being in recess and the difficulties of keeping track. It may also have been affected by the Blair observation that Brown now seemed less of a threat because he was even more fearful of pushing his policy oppositon too far.[112] But probably the most significant influence on PLP management was the confidence that headquarters managers had 'sewn up' the constitutional way of obtaining an eviction and therefore the Leader was untouchable, as Rentoul had concluded. It added an element of complacency to the managerial state of mind, a condition which had always been regarded by Blair as the cardinal political sin,[113] but one he and some of his advisers had begun to share.

As Mandelson noted, even the day after the *Times* article, key members of the No. 10 team 'were confident of weathering any immediate storm'.[114] The General Secretary was revealing on this later. Watt heard rumours of action by the Chancellor's allies with a sense that 'we'd heard it all before'.[115] Having met a group of key managers from No. 10 – McTernan, Turner and Wegg-Prosser – he was confident that they were 'ready for anything that Gordon and his allies might pull' at the September conference.[116] Although Blair's refusal to provide a public timetable for his departure, a position heavily backed by Mandelson,[117] had left No. 10 aides with not much room for pre-emptive managerial activity, they might have prepared more for what might happen before the conference.

Although a later account by Adam Boulton decribes the management as having begun a counter-attack immediately they heard reports from MPs who had been approached that weekend,[118] this is not entirely convincing. What became evident was that in this most heavily managed party in Labour history, the usual multiplicity of managerial ears and ad hoc friendly informers to be expected at such a time was strikingly limited, and failed to produce specific advance details for No. 10, the whips' office, or party headquarters. Rawnsley notes that the first that No. 10 heard of the signatories and the letter's contents was late on Monday morning.[119] The Chief of Staff Powell tells the same story.[120] In effect, they were out of touch.

The No. 10 response

In No. 10 after the letter had been revealed and with continuing rumours coming in of other letters in the pipeline supporting the rebels, there was a sense of not knowing what on earth was going on, as one of the managers, Wegg-Prosser, later candidly admitted to Seldon.[121] The first reaction of the managers, already a routine in fighting Brown, was to attribute the revolt directly to his machinations. It was labelled a 'Brown coup' and that message was then carried on by friendly journalists. To steady support in the centre of the PLP, No. 10 then organised a series of public intimations of Blair's intentions conveyed by chosen colleagues, without Blair having to give his own personal public commitment.

On Tuesday morning 5 September, Cabinet minister David Miliband came public tactically to offer the low-key view that the conventional wisdom saw the Prime Minister carrying on for another twelve months and 'It seems to me that conventional wisdom is reasonable'.[122] Later that day ex-Chief Whip Hilary Armstrong (not the best person to carry a centre-ground appeal) told the BBC that 'we expect that there will be a new Leader in place for the Conference of 2007'.[123] That evening, another Cabinet Minister, Hilary Benn, also put up by No. 10, gave a similar appeal but, in what turned into a more significant intervention, couched it in the questioning terms of 'Why don't they just trust him?'[124] On the face of it, this was a shrewd and potent appeal to his PLP colleagues by a respected middle-of-the-road figure for a bit of common sense and patience. But the greater impact, and what was left behind from Benn's contribution, was a reinforcement of what had become the most important question of all. The distrust that it located was too widely shared for Blair to be safe.

Athough the Parliamentary Committee, the executive authority of the PLP, did not normally meet outside a parliamentary session, there was provision in the rules for it to meet 'at such other times as may be determined'.[125] Its Chair, Clwyd, had publicly warned that the 'vast majority' of the PLP opposed the Lebanon strategy,[126] and this new situation in the PLP appeared to be one that demanded emergency deliberation by the managing committee. From that might have come an attempt at steering the PLP to consensual calm but, here again, another aspect of the management system failed to operate effectively. Ann Clwyd, still a greater admirer of Blair than most back-bench representatives on the committee, turned down a request to recall.

An acute problem now was that not only were the rebels known as loyalists rather than usual suspects, but Simon and Watson in particular had a reputation amongst managers as the kind of people who could be relied upon to be effective in assisting the management by mobilising others for crucial pro-government votes. Who might do that now? On the initative of No. 10, what was described as 'a loyalist letter' from Labour backbenchers was formally organised under the name of the Chair of the London group of the PLP, Karen Buck. It welcomed the statement by David Miliband. As Martin Bright pointed out in an article titled 'It's already over' this was not a commitment to loyalty.[127] It was known to parliamentary friends that Karen Buck herself had doubts about Blair's continuation. To them her role and the form of the appeal became a sign of Blair's weakness. An appeal for the party to 'keep calm' was the limited way that Mullin was approached to sign it.

After a ring round, described as 'panicky' by one leading figure in the PLP who received a call, over sixty signatures from Labour MPs was publicly reported by the morning of Wednesday 6 September.[128] This was not hugely impressive and it was later reported as 56, and only 28 of these were backbenchers.[129] Noted publicly was a 'conspicuous lack of Cabinet Ministers taking to the airwaves to defend the Prime Minister'.[130] To great aggravation from loyalists, these absent voices included Gordon Brown. That morning, in a new phase, Brown moved clearly into a front position, becoming involved in a tense combative meeting with Blair, which ended with no agreement.

The rebel signatories had no influence over the content of these discussions. The Blair-Brown meeting was followed by the resignation of Watson, who had refused a request from the Chief Whip that he retract and was pressurised by Powell to resign. Resignations from their PPS posts then came that day from seven other signatories. In the absence of a formal process, the developing balance of forces across the PLP remained uncertain. Although none of the other letters critical of Blair had made an appearance, and no further resignations took place, there was a growing sense amongst MPs that Blair had been found not to have as many defenders as he needed. Peter Watt, the General Secretary, later described a meeting with Blair who was looking 'old, grey and drained . . . shell shocked'.[131] Rawnsley tells us that the Chief Whip reported to Blair that she could no longer be confident that he had the support of a majority of MPs.[132] That crucial judgement put him in a weaker position for another meeting with Brown that Blair called for that afternoon, 6 September.

At the meeting they came to an understanding on his departure and the next day Blair publicly and reluctantly made the adjustment which a week earlier would have avoided the crisis. He announced to journalists, 'as for my timing and date of departure, I would have preferred to do this in my own way, but as has been pretty obvious from what many of my cabinet colleagues have said earlier in the week, the next party conference in a couple of weeks will be my last party conference as party leader, the TUC next week will be my last TUC, probably to the relief of both of us'. On the plus side, he had held on to power, and there was still no specific date of departure. Nevertheless he had become the first Leader in Labour Party history to be forced to give what amounted to a time-bound pledge to go.

Congress and Conference: the two goodbyes

Although Brown at last had a clear public boundary to Blair's occupancy, he had not gained any commitment that Blair would support him as the successor. The cautious man judged it politic not to push Blair any further in fear of further poisoning the atmosphere of his future leadership. As it was, the process of eviction, as he had feared for years, put him in the uncomfortable position of being accused of acting as a disloyal plotter against an elected Prime Minister.[133] When the furore appeared to be subsiding, there came a venomous personal attack on Brown from Charles Clarke, who talked of widespread fury in the Cabinet about Brown's failure to slap down the rebels.[134] The grievance, built up over years of Brown's failure to give full backing to Blair's agenda, was now followed by what was regarded as Brown's usurpation of power; what had happened to Blair, it was said, amounted to blackmail.[135]

Pessimists doubted whether the party could now pull itself into unity. The TUC Congress, which met from 11 to 14 September, added to the sense of unresolvable crisis. Cabinet ministers Hain, Johnson and Harman announced their Deputy Leadership candidatures even though it was probably a year before such a contest would take place. The backbencher Jon Cruddas, ex-Downing Street manager who had a distinctive analysis of the state of the party and the problems of its management, was persuaded by union leaders at the TUC to be a candidate. Blair's valedictory speech to the Congress was heckled and received with such a lack of favourable acknowledgement of his service that it became deeply embarrassing to union leaders. Reflecting on reports of the TUC reception, they sought to make amends and to try to hold things together. That contributed to the building of a unity mood in the lead-up to the party conference. In the CLPs there had been clear signs in the summer of a new acceptance that

Blair ought to go quickly, but now there was dismay at the public disunity, and fear of serial infighting between the national politicians. Here also the change of mood was to express thanks and hope for an end to conflict.

Drawing also from a deep reservoir of Labour Party sentimentality, across the board there was a conscious effort to give Blair a suitable collective farewell in recognition of his service. As even Tom Watson said on his website, 'More than anything, he deserved a good send off. And he got one.' The response was managed by headquarters' controllers, down to the last spontaneous placard. The audience was waiting, knowing its role, aware of history being made and genuinely wishing to show its heartfelt appreciation not only of his election victories but, as a survey of party members reported later, an appreciation of 'the often unsung achievements' and 'things happening below the parapet' which contrasted a Blair-led government with experience of the Tories in control.[136] Blair boosted the mood with a beautifully pitched speech, sharing his observations with an easy and comradely aplomb. A subtle and star showman to the last, he was rapturously acclaimed to a degree which surpassed any fantasy envisaged in No. 10. It could not eradicate the element of humiliation but it was read by Blair as the party giving him permission to stay on for some time before the next conference. As for the public, 69 per cent wanted him gone before the next spring,[137] but that could be ignored.

Party management problems

Dissent and sanctions

Meanwhile, some of the tensions over party management grew rather than being diminished by the time limit on Blair. In one final fling, Blairite disciplinarians again sought action for serious sanctions agaisnt PLP indiscipline. After Blair's response to the Israeli bombing of Lebanon, Clare Short had declared in July at the Hay literary festival that she was ashamed of the Labour Government and welcomed the possibility of a hung parliament. This aroused the ire of Labour loyalists and MPs in marginal seats. Disciplinary action was said to be imminent and possibly her expulsion from the party.

The normal procedure was that the Chief Whip reported to the Parliamentary Committee with her recommendation. If the committee approved, it went to the PLP for decision. Instead, after Short had refused to meet the Chief Whip, what appears to have happened is that Smith and Blears agreed another procedure ouside the rules. Short would be reported to the NEC. There followed much complicated toing and froing with the No. 10 Political Office supporting the Chief Whip's procedure but NEC managers telling them they did not want it. Eventually it was forced onto the agenda of the NEC pre-conference meeting where it was rejected as an improper procedure and redirected through the regular constitutional procedure. Meanwhile Short resigned out of acute alienation.

Conference decisions and indications

As for the rest of the conference there was no repeat of the Wolfgang incident, but otherwise little changed in the behaviour of the management except that some of it became harsher. Behind closed doors the CAC members now found not one official but a contingent of party officials to back the recommendations of the committee secretary Roy Kennedy. Of the 220 contemporary resolutions submitted, only 102 were found to be in order; previously a majority had always been ruled in. Resolutions on housing, the Middle East and the Single Equalities Act were forced on to the agenda only after strong representations from within the CAC. Its rejection of resolutions on Iraq – and, more contentiously, on the replacement of Trident – drew complaints from the ministers Benn, Hain and Harman, amongst others. In spite of that pressure, a conference debate and vote on the issue was denied, as it was to be on the NEC and at the NPF.

Composite motions on four topics on which the unions submitted resolutions were all included, covering corporate liability, health, pensions, and rights at work. Climate change and housing were accepted for debate through the ballot. Alongside the four union resolutions were also management-instigated resolutions more favourable to government policies and four draft NEC statements. At the NEC it was agreed that, as these statements were not in a condition to be agreed, they be put to consultation with those involved before the NEC decided its view. But on two of the issues, pensions and rights at work, there was no agreement reached in the consultations, and the NEC found itself in the same position as in the previous year – giving no recommendations.

Under pressure, a second NEC meeeting was held on the health service and on corporate manslaughter. At this meeting, Brown now led for the government and two NEC members were persuaded to change sides, with the result that the two decisions went narrowly with him 16–15. This appeared to be a sign of the new authority of a man considered already to be the next Leader. What then happened in the conference could be seen as a sign of its potential limitations especially in the unions. Critical resolutions on corporate management, employment rights, pensions and the health service were all carried against the platform although with only a minority support from the CLPs. Their highest support was over housing policy with 44.2 per cent of the CLP vote.

Rising tempers over the health service erupted after the speech of UNISON's General Secretary Dave Prentis, who had exceeded his time, was abruptly cut off; but anger increased when flyers appeared within the conference advocating support for the NEC statement on the health service – an intervention normally considered out of order. In a complex result the critical resolution was passed on a hand vote, the pro-leadership resolution was rejected on a hand vote and the NEC statement was defeated on a card vote. Again the vote showed a political difference in that 87.3 per cent of affiliated organisations voted for this defeat but only 34.76 per cent of the CLPs.

Management itself came under direct attack within the conference with an attempt from Beverley and Holderness CLP to institute a rule change which affirmed the obligation upon the staff to act impartially when carrying out their duties. This was rejected amidst calls for 'the hardworking staff' to be protected and on the grounds that there was already a code of conduct. In a later email circular on 2 October 2006 Ann Black noted, reasonably, that simply enforcing the codes of conduct covering party officials 'would protect the hard working majority who play by the rules'. As usual that voice was ignored. Was this conference politics the tail end of old Blairite management or a sign of its likely continuity?

NEC and party officials

At the NEC meanwhile, building on the reaction to their loss of control over finance, new NEC terms of reference had been pushed by Hayter, Beecham and Griffiths to find a means of bringing the NEC within proper procedures. The Hayter proposals relating to NEC governance ('*NEC terms of reference* 27 July 2007') were finally accepted, including that 'the NEC must be communicated with so that it knows what is taking place in its name'. Yet the fact was that there was still a strong strain of managerial independence. There was still also a lack of respect by managers for the NEC's authority, and still many on the NEC were inhibited from exercising too much supervision and getting into a war with the officials.

Nevertheless, the officers group in other respects continued at times to play an assertive and independent role in defence of the party and of the union-party relationship. There was a significant recommendation by the officers' meeting to drop the post of appointed Party Chair. It was a move more openly proposed by Jon Cruddas, a candidate for the Deputy Leadership, and was backed by Prescott. Both argued that a Party Chair should be elected by the conference.

Blair's freedom and the transition to Brown

Blair policy-making

Meanwhile Blair and his aides were making their own plans for the management of policy-making. Although Blair's political future was now circumscribed, and his influence over legislation which had to pass through the House was potentially limited, there was in effect a new realm of freedom for him. In relation to the party he could use what procedures he liked. Blair told the Progress conference of Blair sympathisers that 'we've got to be unashamed and unafraid of going out and making sure that when we have this internal debate, we're involving not just the cabinet, not just the party, but the people. And doing it, and making policy, in a different way. Not a sort of little policy commission where you know, we have a few trade union guys here and a few members of the Cabinet there, and a few sort of party people there, and we all put it together and do it on the basis basically of what you know the leadership has decided already.

Not that we ever did that all . . . well there were times when it got a little bit close to that and sometimes necessarily actually'.[138]

It did not take much experience and insight into Blair's politics to see this proposed process as a new management device to use the participation of the people, such as it was, as a cover for neutralising the party. On the eve of the party conference came the press release that there would be a Cabinet policy review, later named Pathways to the Future, to explore serious future problems and establish a wide range of policies. No public mention was made of Partnership in Power procedures or of a consultation with the PLP. Hearing of the plans, one disconsolate senior NEC figure – a strong advocate of partnership – commented that, 'They have stripped away the mask'. Later, the Leader's strategist Matthew Taylor, in an article for the *Observer*, revealed the priority. Blairism would not die if Blair pushed through the reforms he still felt passionate about.[139] Blair did suffer one major obstruction by Brown when Blair's Fundamental Savings Review which aimed to get to the point where 'we could focus on a smaller more strategic government', failed to get Treasury approval.[140] There was no party discussion of this objective either. There was no particular concern expressed that an IpsosMORI poll found that the Labour Party was 'much more liked' than Tony Blair.[141]

Whilst the new top-down Blairite push was operating over policy-making for the future, in briefings to the media it also focused on the electoral dangers from Brown. As political commentator Steve Richards noted, 'briefing anyone that would listen that Brown was unelectable . . . risked 'becoming a self-fulfilling prophecy'.[142] The warning also was that 'New Labour' was not safe in his hands; he would concede to the party and the unions. Put diplomatically by Matthew d'Ancona, a Conservative journalist with close links to the Blairites, the prediction was that 'Mr Brown will have to fight hard to avoid political imprisonment'.[143] In response, out of both habit and trepidation, the main thrust of Brown's post-conference activity was directed not to union policies but to the major powers of British political life in the media, and business. His activities were reported in the *Sunday Times* as 'Sucking up to the City' over taxation, regulation and red tape.[144]

At the same time, a consolidation of the move away from the personnel of Blairite PLP managers continued. On 5 December 2006, Tony Lloyd defeated Ann Clwyd in the election for chair of the Parliamentary Labour Party by 169 votes to 156. On 16 January 2007 Angela Eagle, Kevan Jones, Ann Cryer, Joan Ruddock and Martin Salter were re-elected and the sixth committee place was won by Don Touhig who had a similar political outlook.

Brown, Blair and leadership unity

Showing cooperation with Brown, in November Blair had jointly signed the Treasury's study of long-term opportunities and changes confronting the United Kingdom. But it was Blair who still had control over the non-Treasury policy process including the reviews that were undertaken. Through Pathways to the Future there was movement toward clearing away some of the differences between the two leaders, but Brown and his aides did not show much enthusiasm for documents which embedded the Blairite agenda and there was no way of guaranteeing Brown's future adherence. Matthew Taylor hailed a new openness and collegiality to the policy review,[145] but there were protests at the Parliamentary Committee about the lack of systematic involvement of the PLP departmental groups in the Pathways discussions. After similar protests to the JPC, the Pathways documents were reported to a poorly attended NPF in February 2007, but the documents varied in form and were not conducive to participation. They had no further party life.

When deemed necessary, the serious politics managerial approach extended to the wider political environment. Brown had joined with Blair in support of a new generation of nuclear power stations over which there was to be a national consultation of the people. But the democratic dialogue fell short in its standards. On 15 February 2007 the High Court found in favour of a Greenpeace application for judicial review. In the judgement Mr Justice Sullivan found the consultation 'misleading', 'seriously flawed' and 'procedurally unfair'.[146] A replacement consultation had to be held.

An ICM poll for the *Sunday Telegraph* found substantial majorities critical of City bonuses and the gap between rich and poor.[147] Although this was taken up by Hain and Labour backbenchers, there was no movement from either of the leading duo. Within the party, managerial controls continued to be operated so as to ensure that the extra-parliamentary party did not express its collective opinion before major issues went to votes in the House. This extended to the very divisive issue of Trident where Blair and Brown were again in agreement. In the House a rebel amendment tabled by a group of senior MPs calling for a more prolonged debate was supported by 95 rebels but ignored. It confirmed how limited was the Blairites versus Brownites framework in assessing dissent under Blair. It also confirmed, as Charles Clarke had pointed out, that Brown as well as Blair were both 'top-down' in their approach to policy-making.[148]

Hayden Phillips and party funding

Probably the most important development of substance that had happened at the party conference appeared at the time to be non-controversial. The party's submission to the Hayden Phillips enquiry had been the subject of both open debate at the NPF and a developing series of background meetings of party officers with TULO. In November 2006, the first draft of the Hayden Phillips report emerged. Its content came as a shock except to those who had been the most suspicious. It bore no relation to the policy that the party had evolved over the previous months, and raised serious issues over how far the party's policy had been pursued by No. 10

Downing Street. The report advocated a cap of £50,000 per union on donations which would include affiliations as donations. There would be not only a legal right to opt out from the political fund but also a right to opt out of Labour Party affiliation. Further, the union contributions of those who opted in would be passed straight to the Labour Party and would not enter the union's political fund. The Labour Party would be responsible for maintaining a relationship with these members and reminding them of the right to opt out.

This would be the end of the old collective institutional union-party relationship and a major undermining of the union political role. It would be the realisation of an age-old Conservative and Liberal dream, and achieve the aspirations of the Blairite radicals including Blair himself. The proposals were widely seen in the party as extreme and destructive; it pulled potential moderate reformers into the conservative camp. On 11 November there was a furious reaction from the PLP and especially the PLP trade union group. The moderate Jeremy Beecham described it as 'outrageous meddling in internal party affairs'.[149] On 14 December an emergency meeting of the NEC on political finance emphatically reaffirmed the party's position. Brown kept silent. Hayden Phillips then delayed his final report. There followed months of argument in which, by the time Blair left, his office tactics had made no headway but aroused further distrust in the unions.

Into Blair's backyard again

Growing union dissatisfaction with limited employment rights and the failure to implement all the Warwick Agreement led to the slow build-up of a new move 'into Blair's backyard'. It began with the submission of a Trade Union Freedom Bill backed on the left of the PLP but with limited union coordination from outside the House. More concerted union action came in February 2007, when a Private Members' Bill on agency and temporary workers was proposed by Paul Ferrelly and backed by the officials of the Trade Union Group, TULO, the TUC major unions and over 100 MPs. That was eventually talked out of time by the Employment Minister, Jim Fitzpatrick, and therefore not debated at all. But this avenue of representation had been renewed and voices raised.

Replacement

Departure

On 10 May 2007 Blair announced that he would stand down as Prime Minister on 27 June 2007. John Prescott also resigned. A historic settlement in Northern Ireland enabled Blair to go out on a high note. The reform of party funding had become a stalemate between the parties and later it was announced that the police had decided not to press charges over loans for honours. Polling in March 2007 indicated that he still had strong admirers in a large minority of those who remained members; 19 per cent had rated his performance as Prime Minister as outstanding and a further 37 per cent as good. Amongst union political levy-payers the ratings were much lower. Only 5 per cent judged him oustanding, only 21 per cent good.[150] Anthony King reported from other polling showing that amongst the electorate the 63 per cent who thought in 1997 that he was a man who could be trusted had became, ten years later, only 22 per cent.[151] It had become his biggest problem.

The Brown election and the deputy leadership campaign

Significantly, in spite of the decisions taken in 1995, after the last Leader's election, the party officials were adamant that there be no limits on expenditure in leadership or deputy leadership elections even though it was known that Brown had access to considerable finance. Watt's fear was of the problem that might occur if the victor was later found to have breached the regulations.[152] Yet as McCartney later complained, Watt had also built into the rules a 15 per cent levy on each candidate to go to party funds, thus encouraging a greater frenzy of finance chasing.[153]

As the only candidate with sufficient nominations to stand for Leader, Brown's election was uncontested. The lack of an opponent was an indication of both a weak and split left, a weakened alternative Blairite leadership and an energetic Brownite organisation manoeuvring to avoid a contest. As Watt disclosed later, he had turned down attempts by Brown to 'skew the process' for the leadership elections to make it more difficult for anybody else to run.[154] The absence of a contest meant that Brown did not give any major hostages to fortune in his commitments, but it also gave later critics of the Brown government an added sense of his illegitimacy. It also showed a lack of care for the procedures which would be a foretaste of things to come. There was even at this time an attempt by a group of Labour MPs, which received some support on the NEC, to get the election for the position of Deputy Leader abandoned in order, it was said, to save the expense and to curtail the public divisions which were increasing at Cabinet level.

But the election proceeded. The Ministers Benn, Blears, Hain, Harman and Johnson all stood, as did the backbencher and ex-Blair manager Jon Cruddas. This contest proved illuminating. Cruddas drove a new agenda of party renewal linked to a range of issues which to one degree or another all other candidates had to respond. This included movement against past leadership and managerial behaviour; Harman and Cruddas repudiated their own past support for the Iraq invasion and also the style of spin and leak. She and he also called for party renewal. The result of the exhaustive ballot announced on 24 June 2007 was indicative. Cruddas won the first round, taking a majority of the non-parliamentary vote. Blears the evangelical Blairite, in spite of the presentational opportunities of being Party Chair, came bottom of the poll. In the exhaustive ballot, Harriet Harman narrowly defeated Alan Johnson, who had been the favourite, with 50.43 per cent of the final redistributed vote.

Notes

1 In research for this chapter, by the autumn of 2005 my relations with No. 10 had largely broken down over various processes and issues including the management of the Warwick Agreement. In linking and interpreting the secondary sources cited, the chapter draws from participant observations of party meetings and some repeated interviews with ministers, MPs including Parliamentary Committee representatives, party officials and ex-officials, NEC managing representatives, trade union officials and CLP members.
2 Populus/*Financial Times*, 11 June 2008, data supplied by Populus.
3 Robert Worcester, Roger Mortimer and Paul Bains, *Explaining Labour's Landslip*, Politico's, London, 2005, p. 97.
4 Byron Criddle, 'MPs and Candidates', in Dennis Kavanagh and David Butler, *The General Election of 2005*, Palgrave Macmillan, Basingstoke, 2005, p. 166.
5 *Guardian*, 8 May 2008.
6 Populus/*Times*, 30 April 2005.
7 Worcester, Mortimer and Baines, *Explaining Labours' Landslip*, p. 96.
8 Peter Mandelson, *The Third Man: Life at the Heart of New Labour*, Harper, London, 2010, p. 407.
9 *Guardian*, 12 May 2007.
10 Jonathan Powell, *The New Machiavelli*, Bodley Head, London, 2010, p. 126.
11 Anthony Seldon, *Blair Unbound*, Simon and Schuster, London, 2007, pp. 346–7.
12 Chris Mullin, *Decline and Fall, Chris Mullin Diaries 2005–2010*, Profile Books, London, 2010, p. 41.
13 ICM/*Guardian*, 19 July 2005.
14 *Observer*, 18 December 2005.
15 *The Times*/Populus, 21 July 2005.
16 David Coates, *Prolonged Labour, the Slow Birth of New Labour Britain*, Palgrave Macmillan, Basingstoke, 2005, p. 124.
17 Peter Oborne, *The Triumph of the Political Class*, Simon & Schuster, London, 2007, p. 302.
18 *Independent*, editorial, 16 February 2006.
19 House of Commons Education and Skills Select Committee, March 2005.
20 *Business Information Centre E-Newsletter*, 17 May 2005.
21 *Daily Telegraph*, 5 June 2005.
22 *Independent*, 16 June 2005.
23 Patrick Seyd and Paul Whiteley, *New Labour's Grass Roots: The Transformation of the Labour Party Membership*, Palgrave Macmillan, Basingstoke, 2002, p. 73.
24 Ibid. p. 76.
25 Letter from Brendan Barber to Alan Johnson, Secretary of State for Trade and Industry, 9 September 2005.
26 *Guardian*, 15 September 2005.

27 Ann Black, email circular, 4 October 2005.
28 'NEC Report', *Socialist Campaign Group News*, November 2005.
29 Ann Black, email circular, 4 October 2005.
30 *Guardian*, 15 December 2005.
31 My verbatim notes.
32 *Guardian*, letters, 17 October 2005.
33 My verbatim notes.
34 IpsosMORI *Political Monitor*, November 2005.
35 Peter Watt, *Inside Out: My Story of Betrayal and Cowardice at the Heart of New Labour*, Biteback, London, 2010, p. 15.
36 *Independent*, 16 November 2005.
37 Jonathan Heywood, 'Class of 2005', *Fabian Review*, summer 2005.
38 *Guardian*, 11 November 2005.
39 *Tribune*, 27 January 2006.
40 Chris Mullin MP, an ex-Home Office Minister, Hansard, Column 162, 7 November 2007.
41 *Yorkshire Evening Post*, 17 November 2005.
42 Reported critically in the focus groups of Lab-OUR Commission, 'Renewal: a two-way process for the 21st century', 2007, p. 57.
43 Hansard, 6th series, Vol. 439, col. 302, 9 November 2005.
44 Peter Hyman, BBC *Newsnight*, 2 May 2008.
45 *Guardian* editorial, 11 November 2005.
46 *The Times*, 12 November 2005.
47 ICM/*Guardian*, 12 November 2005.
48 *Sunday Telegraph*, 4 December 2005.
49 Anthony King, YouGov/*Daily Telegraph*, 25 November 2005.
50 ICM/*Guardian* poll, 20 December 2005.
51 *The Times*, 12 November 2005.
52 *Independent*, 3 Febuary 2006.
53 Ann Black, email circular, 5 February 2006.
54 *Guardian*, 17 March 2006.
55 YouGov, Compass/*Guardian*, 13 March 2006.
56 BBC website, 15 March 2006.
57 'Delivery of the Warwick Agreement', Office of Hazel Blears, 24 July 2006, p. 1.
58 *The Times*, 14 November 2005.
59 David Coates, pamphlet, *Raising Lazarus*, Fabian Society, 2005, p. 52.
60 *Financial Times*, 3 March 2006.
61 *Tribune*, 3 March 2006.
62 *Morning Star*, 10 June 2006.
63 *Progress*, March/April 2006.
64 *Independent*, 13 March 2006.
65 Watt, *Inside Out*, p. 39.
66 Ibid. p. 47.
67 Tony Blair, *A Journey*, Hutchinson, London, 2010, p. 608.
68 Powell, *New Machiavelli*, p. 227.
69 John Rentoul, *Independent on Sunday*, 23 March 2006.
70 NEC Recommendations – agreed 21 March 2006.
71 Ann Black, personal NEC Report for 21 March 2006.

72 *Personnel Today*, 24 August 2006.

73 *Guardian*, 9 March 2007.

74 *Morning Star*, 5 June 2007.

75 Watt, *Inside Out*, p. 114.

76 Ibid.

77 *Guardian*, 6 July 2006.

78 IpsosMORI, for the Electoral Commission, 5 December 2006.

79 Powell, *New Machiavelli*, p. 233.

80 David Sanders and Paul Whiteley, 'The Blair Years, 1997–2007', *Observer*, 8 April 2007.

81 Survey of public attitudes by TNS BMRB through CAPI OmniBus, prepared for the Committee on Standards in Public Life, 2006, pp. 41–3.

82 'NEC Report', *Socialist Campaign Group News*, June 2006.

83 Office of Hazel Blears, 'Delivery of the Warwick Agreement', 24 July 2006.

84 Nick Assinder, BBC News website, 8 May 2006.

85 *The Times*, 8 May 2006.

86 Nick Robinson, BBC TV News, 8 May 2006.

87 Mullin, *Decline and Fall*, p. 98.

88 Ibid. p. 99.

89 YouGov/*Daily Telegraph*, 10 May 2006.

90 'NEC Report' *Socialist Campaign Group News*, June 2006.

91 Ibid.

92 IpsosMORI website, 23 June 2006.

93 *Guardian*, 15 July 2006.

94 Telephone interview with me.

95 Trevor Fisher, letter, *Tribune*, 25 August 2006.

96 Rulebook 2001, Rule 5 3C5.4(b).

97 Rulebook 2001, Rule 5 3C5.2(b).

98 IpsosMORI Trustworthiness of Politicians – Trends, 31 August to 6 September 2006.

99 *Independent on Sunday*, 27 August 2006.

100 Andrew Rawnsley, The *End of the Party, The Rise and Fall of New Labour*, Penguin, London, 2010, p. 388.

101 Ibid.

102 *The Times*, 1 September 2006.

103 Ibid.

104 Tom Watson in a letter to his local paper the *Express and Star*, 7 September 2006, said later that his course of action was affected by Blair's damaging *Times* claim.

105 *Independent*, 5 September 2006.

106 *Independent*, 7 September 2006.

107 Speech to Progress Conference, 9 September 2006.

108 This point is also part of Rawnsley's judgement in *End of the Party*, p. 398.

109 Adam Boulton, *Memories of the Blair Administration: Tony's Ten Years*, Simon and Schuster, London, 2008, p. 282.

110 Tom Watson, *Express and Star*, 7 September 2006.

111 Seldon, *Blair Unbound*, p. 486.

112 Blair, *Journey*, p. 574.

113 Mandelson, *Third Man*, p. 211.

114 Ibid. p. 423.
115 Watt, *Inside out*, pp. 140–1.
116 Ibid. p. 140.
117 Mandelson, *Third Man*, p. 418.
118 Boulton, *Memories of Blair Administration*, p. 284.
119 Rawnsley, *End of the Party*, p. 394.
120 Powell, *New Machiavelli*, p. 301.
121 Seldon, *Blair Unbound*, p. 486.
122 BBC Radio 4, *Today* programme, September 2006.
123 *Independent*, 5 September 2006.
124 BBC *Newsnight*, 5 September 2006.
125 Standing Orders F 13.
126 Watt, *Inside Out*, p. 140.
127 *New Statesman*, 11 September 2006.
128 *Guardian*, 6 September 2006.
129 Dennis Kavanagh and Philip Cowley, *The British General Election of 2010*, Palgrave Macmillan, Basingstoke, 2010, p. 48.
130 *Guardian*, editorial, 6 September 2006.
131 Watt, *Inside Out*, p. 144.
132 Rawnsley, *End of the Party*, p. 399.
133 Brown had a 23 per cent lead over Cameron as the man most likely to stab his colleagues in the back. ICM/*The Guardian*, 22 September 2006.
134 *Daily Telegraph*, 11 September 2006.
135 Comments of Wegg-Prosser reported in Lance Price, *Where Power Lies: Prime Ministers v the Media*, Simon & Schuster, London, 2010, p. 87.
136 Interim Report of the rank and file Labour Commission 2007, pp. 52–3.
137 YouGov/*Sunday Times*, 24 September 2006.
138 Verbatim report of 11 September *Progress Conference*, 2007.
139 *Observer*, 17 January 2007.
140 Blair, *Journey*, pp. 574–5.
141 IpsosMORI website, Attitude towards Leaders and Parties, 19 January 2007.
142 *Independent*, 5 October 2006.
143 *Sunday Telegraph*, 21 January 2007.
144 ICM/*Sunday Times*, 22 October 2006.
145 *Guardian*, 3 March 2007.
146 *London Evening Standard*, 15 February 2007.
147 *Sunday Telegraph*, 18 February 2007.
148 BBC Radio News, 3 September 2007.
149 *Guardian*, 13 December 2006.
150 YouGov/*New Statesman*, 1–4 March 2007.
151 Anthony King, comparing a contemporary YouGov poll with a past Gallup Poll, *Daily Telegraph*, 30 April 2007.
152 Watt, *Inside Out*, p. 152.
153 *Guardian*, 1 December 2007.
154 Watt, *Inside Out*, p. 153.

PART IV

Appraisal

19

Summary: analysis and characterisation

Section I summary: analysis

Leadership and party management

Behind the drive towards the Blair supremacy, was 'a love that dare not speak its name'. No public reference to party management ever emerged in Labour Party statements on procedures and process. It was regularly overlooked or only lightly touched on in insider commentaries. Yet managerial activity under Blair has been shown to be pervasive in, and between, all the major national venues, relationships and developments of the party. It was the crucial agency of the building of 'New Labour'. Blair had declared, as did others in his early days as Leader, that 'The Labour Party is more open and democratic than ever before'.[1] But governed by persistent subordination of procedural values to management, it was heavily driven and supervised by new arrangements seeking to guarantee that the important outcomes were ones favoured by the leadership.

Dynamo and distinctiveness

The dynamo of this managerial motivation was provided by a combination of influences. Blair, despite a huge victory in his election as Leader, had in practice only a narrow base of committed supporters of his full political project. Yet the scope of ambition of that project was huge: creating clear electability, and transforming what was deemed to be an inadequate party for government into one fit for purpose, including the capability of a new relationship with business. The battle was joined with what were regarded as recalcitrant intra-party opponents and, from the outside, ruthless Tories and their media allies. What was seen as the inadequacies of past management under both Kinnock and Smith had to be superseded by something more certain in its effectiveness. All this had to be achieved within a limited timeframe and integrated into what was represented as a 'members' party' and later a 'partnership in power' with the party.

The rolling coup

These objectives raised the motivation for a huge extension of management. It was not the case that Blair 'refused to be embroiled in party management',[2] but he made it appear that way. Blair was an eager initiator of its changing form and intervened directly in various managerial activities when the occasion demanded it. Central to the development of management was in effect a rolling coup which, either without party authorisation or covered by misleading rhetoric, strengthened the collective power of leadership within the party and, particularly, defended and protected the Leader.

Aggressive new management moved on from the subordination of the General Secretary, now removable at the Leader's call, through a redefinition of the role of party officials away from 'civil servants' to the sharper partisanship of 'political organisers'. The past multilayered loyalty of the party machine to the party, the movement and the Leader was now turned into a repoliticised loyalty to the Leader. This was a major coup, and with it a cross-departmental management task force was created within the party's head office to ensure control.

The rolling coup later involved covert virtual abolition of the NEC's policy role, an unannounced change in the practice of electing and removing the Leader, a special manifesto directed to business uncontrolled by the party, and a specially controlled managerial method of electing the CLP section of the National Policy Forum (NPF). More was to follow in the second term in a dual development in which insulation of the Leader was increased and his powers were expanded, whilst the policy role of the parliamentary party was more clearly curtailed. His ascendancy became even more of a managerial priority – even to the point, at the party conference, of secretly organised apparatchiki, leading the clapping to marked scripts – a presentational device but also a symbol of the managed democracy of 'New Labour'.

Management and leadership

Managing the party did involve some powerful persuasive statements of political purpose and policy by the political leaders, especially Blair and Brown, which moved party audiences in support of the idea of 'New Labour'. There was also a regular dialogue with the party's union allies and effective speeches to the party members by the front-bench spokespersons in the different forums. A series of campaigns enhanced the party's persuasion into 'New Labour' cultural and policy change. The Blairite policy amalgam, particularly in the first phase, involved some important areas of continuity in policy and areas of shared aims and values, with some controlled tactical concessions and adjustments. Blair's charisma, his diplomatic and communicational skills, his resilient determination, and his own crucial drive to secure effective control were continuous contributions to the management. Those abilities were enhanced in turn by favourably managed presentation and reception.

Two worlds of management

Party management conduct involved what can best be understood in terms of two behavioural worlds of activity. In the first world – the most time consuming – much of this management involved open roles, consensually attuned to the mainstream of the party, operating in harmony with wider party behavioural values. There was a non-partisan concern for applying the party's rules, the reasonable settlement of conflict, the preservation of trust and the facilitation of the party.

The second behavioural world was more covert and less neutral, focused on delivery of important policy and organisational objectives integrated within all-year-round management activities which were more extended, more intensive, more pre-emptive, and with fewer constraints than previously. It was affected by the claim of 'New Labour' leadership as having a special historical purpose, culture carriers of the party revolution which would become the basis for a new modernising revolution in Britain, and by their view of a party regarded as special in its degenerate character. That gave a new sense of legitimacy for management intervention to find special means of winning. Party reforms under 'New Labour' gave major new opportunities to the managers for these activities.

Historically, the politics of party management had been influenced by a majoritarian democratic perspective on the leadership's relations with the party and the party's relations with the electorate, with management acting on behalf of the working people and the majority of the party against an unrepresentative minority from the vanguardist or vanguardist-allied left. Now a vanguardism came from those who considered themselves to be '*the* modernisers', supported by an army of party officials acting as the instrument of the Leader's purposes, driving through his priorities.

Managerial officials worked closely with loyalist NEC representatives who took on special managerial responsibilities. Together, they underpinned the operation of the leading political core of 'New Labour' driven by a militant sense of moral justification for what needed to be done urgently to avoid going back to the failures of the past, and to keep up momentum towards electoral success, party transformation and 'New Labour' government support. Their behaviour was based on a heavy critique of the inadequacies of the existing processes, structures and character of the traditional Labour Party – weaknesses pronounced so severe that they amounted to moral failings which had to be counteracted.

Thus, as against the proclaimed importance of creating a 'new politics' which was 'purer than pure', behaviour in the second world involved another management reality. Practices were less guided by firm procedural values than under any previous generation of Labour's leaders and with counteracting forces now considerably weaker. Behaviour could include the fake and the deceitful, a cavalier attitude towards keeping agreements and to obeying rules. A covert code of behaviour gave permission to the creation of arrangements which were effective in producing 'a good result' for the Leader and management without the restraint of what was regarded as obsessive 'processology' and with an underdeveloped concern for collateral and consequential damage to the party. A power-oriented and partisan meaning was given to 'what works' in the management of reorganisation; the test of value was not simply practicability but 'what will deliver for Tony,' or 'for us' – the management. 'Serious politics' in this realm was playing to win in ways which involved at times pushing the boundaries of management conduct and seeking what could be got away with.

Control for delivery stretched also to managing the party's rules. The rulebook contents, undergoing regular change year by year, became regarded as a transitional arrangement. It lost reverence as a symbol of the party's history and identity. It became less understandable in form and less easily available to members. More than in the past, rules were regarded as flexible instruments of power, heavily attuned to the centrality of delivery. Pushing interpretations of rule to see how far they could be taken was supplemented by a much greater degree of managerial flexibility in rule-making interpreted under a constitutional change agreed at the 1995 party conference. The delegated powers of the managerial officials were extended and other opportunities emerged or were created, with the aid of an alliance with key NEC representatives who acted as managers, for rule-making outside what members thought were the formal conference constitutional arrangements, sometimes without announcement.

Sustaining the managers in their behaviour was a boldness regarded as admirable by a Leader who looked to free the 'can-do' personality from the constraints and discomfort of bureaucratic routines and whatever was intervening to slow down or obstruct delivery. With a variety of means but sharing the same values and code, the new party management linking to the media management was generally highly effective in achieving delivery of the immediate policy objectives, and constructing defence in depth. This managerial system, its scope and culture developed into the first and greatest organisational achievement of Blairism and arguably, in its implications, the most important facet of 'New Labour' newness, although unregistered in the literature which had that focus.[3]

New management and aspirations for the new party

Yet to a surprising degree it was an achievement which, compared with its ambitions, facilities and media presentation, always had failures, limitations and frustrations as well as major successes. Blair had sought he said, to 'rebuild this party from its foundations making sure that every stone is in its rightful place, every design crafted ... to a useful purpose'.[4] This conjoined initially with a loosely cohering vision which fused modernising democratic change with what was thought likely to be the facilitation of management objectives. Yet what has been shown here is that many of these objectives were in some form frustrated, or had adverse unanticipated consequences. That created further new exigencies which heightened the drive towards more command and control from headquarters and more use of management devices, albeit operating within limitations, some springing from past developments under Smith.

Rooted limitations and the OMOV victory that never was

On the face of it, Smith's famous 1993 'victory of OMOV' in candidate selection had been the beginning of a historic triumph for Blair and the modernisers proselytising for reform. But in encouraging the spin of separatism from the unions, and failing badly over that, Blair had tarnished the purpose of OMOV, and almost ruined the possibility of reform. The historic 1993 outcome of union-party reform was greatly misunderstood and often misrepresented. First, over the minority of contested areas it was still fought by the unions with flexibility and within restraint in accord with their past rule-governed behaviour noted in Minkin.[5] Had the unions not agreed in 1992 to redistribute some of the votes to the CLPs, that alone might have settled the OMOV battle against the leadership when it was fought in 1993. Second, the victory over candidate selection was attained by the managers through adroit procedural manoeuvres linking the rule change supporting OMOV in candidate selection with a levy-plus scheme and with all-women short lists. The only resolution which favoured pure OMOV, from the AEEU, was actually defeated overwhelmingly. In that sense, although the rule change was decisive and led to the adoption of OMOV for candidate selection, this was the victory that never was.

It was later accepted in practice only in the consensual terms defined by Prescott as defence of the union-party relationship. The way it was won in practice through complex agenda dexterity became a contribution to Blair's view of the managerial potentialities. Also, outside normal practice, party officials had been authorised into direct involvement in the mobilisation of CLP delegates' support. That may have developed differently later under Smith, or at least in more correct ways. But, with Smith gone, it became a bridge to extensive Blairite transformation of that aspect of the managerial operation also.

The rest of the 1993 outcomes also created important but little-noticed managerial repercussions, which have been shown to reverberate through the length of this study. The 'settlement' reinforced the unions' position in the leadership electoral college, fusing collective and individual representation. In a twist of history, Blair then turned out to be a major beneficiary; the procedure involving the union levy payers gave Blair a wide base of support (which initially, seeking removal of the unions, he did not want). The more inclusive procedures also involved extra time and costs, giving a Leader further security of tenure. The important decision of the review group in 1993 not to pursue an emergency method of changing a Leader indicated that though Blair would find it extremely difficult to get rid of collective union affiliation, the unions and the CLPs together would not find it easy to get rid of him.

Defeat in the spin-led war for separation from collective union affiliation waged by the modernisers illustrated the dangers of their Bolshevik impetuosity and their failure to evaluate consequences. Their sense of historical purpose and their confidence in spin misled themselves about the party. The episode produced a heritage of distrust of Blair's objectives in relations with the unions that he and 'New Labour' could never fully shed. The settlement in 1993 confirmed the view offered by Minkin in 1991 that this was not an immobile relationship but one that had the capacity for major reform within what was still recognisably a federal Labour Party.[6] Generally overlooked by commentators was also the longer-term significance of agreement over the creation of the National Trade Union and Labour Liaison Organisation (TULO).

Changing the foundations: successes and failure

Behind the spin-projected supremacy of Blair and in spite of the new management there continued to be a pattern of limitations and failures as well as major successes, even over 'the triumph' of changing Clause IV of the party's constitution in 1994–5. Amongst the important changes to the clause was a landmark replacement of the traditional commitment to common ownership and in its place the adoption of 'the enterprise of the market and the rigour of competition' and 'a thriving private sector'. That was the pivotal success.

But there was also an unpublicised limitation. The National Executive Committee, spun from the Leader's office as unimportant, was said to have been bypassed on the Clause IV issue,[7] and it was held that Blair's failure to discuss it with the NEC in 1994 demonstrated the committee's marginalisation.[8] Outstanding and comprehensive biographical studies of Blair in covering the change of Clause IV in 1995 made little mention of the influence of the committee on the new clause.[9] They all missed a protracted discussion in 1995 in which at least one crucially important change did take place. The famous assertion of collectivism, 'By their common endeavour', which later sat proudly in the front entrance of Labour Party headquarters as the essence of 'New Labour', was first left out, then pushed in the draft only after pressure by NEC trade union representatives associated with the party's traditional right. This became the prime example where the history of the operation of party management under Blair was also the history of a complex and varying set of union and institutional interactions. It was also a signal of the flexibility of 'New Labour values' as Blair then enthusiastically laid claim to the change.

There was also an example of something more mysterious but also indicative about 'New Labour'. Without it being noticed at the conference which agreed the new clause, an NEC amendment, which had affirmed the primacy of working with 'affiliated' unions, was lost from the document before the special conference. On the other hand there was a judicious retreat from direct mention of business organisations. Emphasis on individual aspirations and ambitions, which was later presented as the central theme of the Blairites, was nowhere explicit. In that respect, the great change was for the more militant 'New Labour' radicals a quietly frustrating outcome. The NEC role and the flexible values and tactics of 'New Labour' management politics have to be kept in mind when receiving the judgement that 'the new clause was an unalloyed triumph'.[10]

Triumph over the unions?

In spite of the fact that a majority of union votes went in favour of the change, the *Guardian* report by its specialist political correspondent Patrick Wintour came under the heading, 'Blair's rewrite sees off unions'.[11] The Clause IV result led some to believe it was 'pulling the rug from under the trade unions',[12] and that the unions had voted against the change.[13] The effect of the special conference victory, which united a majority in all sections, was almost ruined by an aggressive union-reform campaign encouraged by Blair accompanying and following the result. The spin got out of control in its anti-union rhetoric and specially aggravated those in the unions who had voted for the change. It also threatened to deepen the public perception of the party having a 'union problem', until the damaging spin was brought to a shuddering halt.

The remarkable feature here was that, though the continuing spinning onslaught on the unions was thought to pay off in electoral terms, each year in Opposition 1994–7, under Blair, as shown, on the question of which party had the best policies on the trade unions, those naming Labour actually dropped. And in 1997, the huge media furore over the party's proposed union recognition policy, causing Blair much anxiety, was found in the focus groups not to be hitting the party. That had no effect on the media strategy nor on the unprecedented abrogation by Blair of the largely unwritten 'rules' and protocols of relations with the unions and his refusal to negotiate new ones.

Changing affinity

Union responses

In driving the dynamic of management Blair comprehensively laid down that 'this is where we are going' and 'we are not doing that'. Yet in spite of this treatment, in great measure the rule-governed restraint of the unions with its differentiation of political and industrial roles survived, as did union willingness to play the role of management auxiliaries, encouraged by Blair in discreet meetings to consolidate a block vote of union support in ensuring 'a good conference'. Unions at this stage did react against anything seen as a fundamental attack on their own position in the party, and Blair's reduction in the affiliated organisations' vote at the conference of 1995 could not go beyond the Smith-union settlement of 1993. But unions also generally left policy initiation to be the right of the Leader, and they made no attempt to use financial sanctions in relation to policy, nor to use the party as an organisational instrument against the leadership as government.

The party of business?

An attempt to extend aspiring middle-class support and the pursuit of the wavering Tory voter in marginal constituencies dominated the electoral strategy and media-management concerns. That linked to a major break with the past, as the party was now moved into an unprecedented close relationship with business, described much later by Blair as 'a founding principle of New Labour'.[14] This development was driven by economic-ideological considerations and then, in addition, by what was seen as electoral benefits of business support in marginal constituencies and a sense of deepening social affinity encouraged by the regular close interaction moving 'New Labour' to a new receptivity to business outside of party influence.

The 'even-handed' approach to relations with business had no party-authorised legitimacy. And the political leadership moved behind the back of the TUC by operating through Europe in harmony with business to delay or circumvent British union policy. In 1997, in a discreet extension of the managerial coup, a separate manifesto for business was produced outside of party control. As the 1997 election approached, policy discussions with the unions were negligible, whilst those with business grew more intensive. Nevertheless, there was a constructive implicit if limited quid pro quo in the business acceptance of the adjusted minimum-wage procedure. Management of that issue showed Blair at his most determined, judicious and persuasive over adjusting party policy, which, coupled with agenda management, gave him more space for a change in the form of the policy. Background dialogue built the framework of a lasting agreement which brought the unions and the party in behind it, as well as the CBI and, in effect, the Conservative Party.

In spite of the importance attached to seeking business support and the considerable influence of business over the government, described rightly by Eric Shaw as 'a major modification of the role that Labour plays in the political system',[15] and although in effect Labour-business relations had been moved out of control of the party, the full potentiality of the change was never realised. Proposals for non-executive directors on the NEC were killed off and the regional reforms, which included 'liaising with business and affiliated organisations' (in that order),[16] were rejected in the regions. It proved not possible to bring business into the national party as an organisational, representational and constitutional entity nor to completely avoid discussion of issues which Blair thought might cause affront to the CBI. In all these ways, in spite of the developing public and academic impression, the party never did become what was described as Labour Party PLC.[17]

Hidden policy conflicts: government, employment dominance and pluralism

The complexities of building relations with business from what was still a labour-affiliated party was at its most intense in the politics of the legislative process over employment-relations legislation. It brought out contrasting facets of Blair's leadership. Blair at his most dominant attained a settlement with very limited new labour rights. Behind the apparent hierarchy and unity of what Kavanagh and Seldon described as *The Powers behind the Prime Minister*, Blair had established institutionalised liaison with both the unions and business though different managers in No. 10. In practice, that liaison operated by 'the powers' as an unusual duality working to different constituencies and pressures, the CBI and the unions. It also uniquely worked to contrasting documents of legitimacy, each produced by different managers. And working closely with the revived PLP trade union group, union-sympathetic managers were able to nudge and assist the role of that group and then to help protect much of the initial gains.

The industrial-relations arrangements which emerged from this policy-making has been described as a hybrid regime, a social democratic variant of neo-liberalism.[18] As illustrated here, it could also be described in this period as a party managerial variant of neo-liberalism, mainly controlling yet at times receptive. Polling indicated that over the terms of union recognition the electorate had more support for the TUC position than that of the CBI, but that was not allowed to be decisive. A freer flow of the collective PLP view and the unregistered collective Cabinet opinion responding to public opinion might well have produced another outcome. Also illuminated was the varied and complex role of the unions. They rebuilt an old form of PLP representation and their own unity. They were assertive but constrained in party behaviour. And in one crucial phase of policy-making over union recognition, the TUC moved to an accommodation.

Plebiscitarian party?

Although much of it has been lost to history, in pursuit of wider aspirations for transforming the party, the ballot on the Road to the Manifesto in 1996 had involved interlocked and potentially momentous agendas for changing party policy-making procedures to a plebiscitarian model and excluding the unions from the ballot. That led to major problems, omitted from Gould's idealised insider account.[19] Around the Leader they were faced with a dilemma unanticipated in months of advance strategic discussions before party officials were informed of the proposal. How could this process be a symbol of party unity if the unions were excluded against their

will? Retreat followed the union determination to stay in. Blair's aim
to seek approval from party members 'without the mediation of union
leaders or party institutions'[20] was also thwarted, although heavily managed. Over the form of a referendum Blair was initially opposed by the
NEC which wanted not a ballot but a pledge, more fitting to the yes or
no role that was being asked of members. Yet he bounced back (and them)
via the media spin that it was to be a ballot. That was his big success, but
in terms of reinforcing internal distrust it was very costly, now a common
duality of some of the party management.

The process, which Blair said would 'breathe new life and new hope
into our politics',[21] was also met by some media reaction that it resembled
a very old and potentially dangerous form of manipulative political life.
Even among a majority of the senior managers, in the end, the operation
was judged as deeply problematic because it was not a genuine consultation. Their unlikely and unprecedented reaction was that 'We don't want
it again'. As a result, this episode was not what was hoped for in Blair's
office and not the academically predicted future of 'the plebiscitarian
party'.[22] It was never tried again and could not act as 'a contagious model'.[23]

Partnership in Power and a dual heritage

Partnership in Power in 1997 was widely thought and presented to be an
ambitious attempt to make new arrangements which would secure a collective gain through a sharing approach to policy-making which avoided
the antagonism which had often marred government-party relations. Some
of the practices of Partnership in Power later turned out to be important
deviations from what was expected and sometimes promised in 1997. Yet
shown here also was that the problems over management of the process
went deeper, and also came earlier.

The misshapen character of the partnership became a product of the
management culture encouraged by Blair. Controls were already in gestation during the Party into Power discussions, reflecting directly the need
'to reassure Tony' of his control in 'getting a reasonable result'. As a result
of the governmentalised role of the party officials, the covert changes in
the policy role of the NEC, the prescription of the non-party role of the
special advisers and the changed role of the Joint Policy Committee, a
transformation had already taken place in the envisaged policy process
before the new NPF began to operate. 'Partnership' had already become
in great measure managed subordination.

One important exception to the control was that a negotiation over
contemporary resolutions did mark a break with the attempted 'no resolutions' edict from No. 10. This proved impervious to abolition although it
became a management-union joint device. Crucial distorting changes away
from what was expected in 1997 were then made in two stages. The first
was immediately after the conference authorisation but before any meetings
of the reconstituted National Policy Forum (NPF) had been held. An extension of the rolling coup included the deliberate failure to call meetings of

the NEC Policy Committee and, by edict, the NPF became advisory to the JPC not to the NEC. This was covered over by stressing the importance of the JPC as the policy-making body. But in practice, even the JPC was heavily limited in its policy deliberations, with the policy being made by government representatives working with No. 10 and carried through the policy commissions.

The JPC also became the arrangements committee of the NPF, and in practice a leadership-dominated management tool largely unaccountable to the NPF or to the NEC. The party officials operated with Nos. 10 and 11 Downing Street not to defend a party input but to defend the government. The role of special advisers in government made no concession to the concept of partnership with the party. Coordination with the government agenda was facilitated whilst a range of controls limited the role of the party. These included controlling the alternatives coming to the conference from the NPF by establishing just one process of registering policy preferences.

Throughout Blair's leadership, there continued to be contrasting faces to Partnership in Power. It enlarged the identities represented and expanded opportunities for dialogue, but it also enhanced Blair's support in the new composition of the NEC, insulated the Leader from the build-up of a challenge by rivals in NEC elections and reduced the opportunities to register dissenting votes at the party conference. Matthew Taylor, an influential manager of the new partnership, noted frankly later in a little-known pamphlet that in the three years after Labour's election victory, the principle of 'what matters is who wins' had seen 'political management being used to circumvent democracy and to marginalize dissent'.[24]

Overall, the delivery of Partnership in Power was a crucial test of short-term managerial skills, and in retaining their heavy managerial influence and creating defence mechanisms, they passed the test. It was also a test of trust and in this, as in other procedural areas, it failed, stimulating deep problems when agreements made and understandings thought to have been reached were not honoured in the practice. The traditional Labour Party process, it was said, had been 'dishonest', encouraging members to believe they had power that they did not have whilst failing to give them the role and influence to which they were entitled.[25] Yet in this new managed process, dishonesty of that kind had been laid deeply into the foundations and carried heavily into the forums. Each was signposted with misleading indicators, and external observation of each was often replete with misunderstandings.

Section II: managing the forums

National Policy Forum

Before Blair's leadership, the National Policy Forum had moved to greater significance as Labour's first national body to introduce an important element of deliberation and potentially mutual education between the leadership and the party in developing policy. The reality was that Blair never saw the NPF in terms of mutual education but as a controlled exercise in preparing the party for government and defending it. As early as 1995, Policy Director Roland Wales privately warned the NEC that the deliberative process had become accompanied by management practices. In a further development after his departure, at the NPF a CLP loyalist organisation was created by the managers, and NPF loyalists came through a guided election process assisted by the officials.

Two policy forums exhibited different mixtures of party management and their results. At Durham in 1999, victory was engineered by comprehensively managed defences. Crucially, a managerially encouraged pro-leadership block vote dominated the forum, involving the management-organised CLP loyalist group and with unions working to what was thought to be an agreement on a future welfare review and debate set up discreetly by Brown. Under managerial pressure all critical amendments on pensions were squashed. Embarrassingly, in spite of it being the big selling point to the party in 1997, no alternatives emerged for conference decisions. In an adjoining but linked managerial development, the first moves over employment conditions for NHS workers transferred to the private sector arose out of months of private dialogue between UNISON and the Secretary of State for Health. That then opened up more space for UNISON's loyalist officials to assist the leadership in preventing unwanted alternatives and to build a bridge to consolidation of the policy at the next NPF.

Facing deteriorating trust in the policy process, the management at the Exeter NPF in 2000 generally adopted a less combative but no less controlling style. From the unions there was an initial effort to achieve independent union policy-coordination through TULO but, in a responding managerial move which set a precedent, this union initiative was then turned into a package acceptable to Downing Street and used as a managerial device. There was a determined government attempt to prevent a new programme of labour-law policy which would have been unacceptable to the CBI. Exceptionally, an intra-government disagreement allowed NPF support for policies on transport workers' working time, and on the Agricultural Wages Board. Seven alternative positions on relatively minor issues did go through to the party conference. But the failure to deliver a promised welfare review in 1999 and the manipulation of the agenda over pensions at this forum stimulated a reaction that produced a crisis on the issue at the conference of 2000.

Conference

One typical loyalist refrain encouraged after 1995 was that at the party conference 'more and more power is being passed to constituency delegates'.[26] If focused purely on voting weight, by 1996 there was parity between the affiliated organisations and the CLPs. But power relations were very different from voting weight. Conference management was a high-priority preoccupation, not just because of its policy 'showcase' possibilities but also because of its rule-making importance and increasingly, later, because of ensuring the reception for the Leader's speech compared with that for Brown's. Through a hidden and expanded managerial structure, maintaining 'a vice-like grip around conference not just for next year but for 10 years' time', was the aim promised privately in a memo to Blair. It aimed 'to be conducted like a military operation to defuse, discount, and, eventually dismiss any vote against the leadership'.[27]

Regardless of the rise of the CLP vote and the growth of major tensions with the unions, it was the linkage to the unions which until 2000 continued to be the primary focus of managerial organisation, and was viewed as more likely to provide stability. The unions were not as has been suggested 'marginalised by replacing the block vote by OMOV at the party conference'.[28] Given the small number of union organisations in regular contact with No. 10, their cohesion, internal communication and political savvy meant that the managerial dialogue with the unions was always a priority.

Working arrangements were consolidated by union restraint, by advance and strictly limited management-union agreement on contemporary resolutions, and by a very discreet institutionalised annual pre-conference managerial meeting with union leaders called by Blair to achieve 'a good conference'. With some increasing strain from 1995 to 1999, the predisposition to assist Blair resulted in support for the platform from a majority of union votes at the party conferences on every policy issue. Management was also assisted at times by controlled and limited policy adjustments and deflections onto agendas with more agreement.

Because the CLP vote was judged unstable in terms of leadership support, CLP organisation achieved a new and lasting thoroughness. New procedures following the introduction of Partnership in Power were accompanied by a further mini-revolution in managed tactical communication at the conference. Drawing on a new loyalism and a receptive realism and aided by detailed political information on all CLP delegates, the managers were in the position to maximise the vote of supporters and persuade those noted to be persuadable. Openness to managerial delivery was facilitated by the managerially encouraged negative reference point of not assisting media enemies and by the ruling that there was no such thing as mandating.

New rules of gender representation meant that most delegates were new or relatively new to the conference. This facilitated management influence as did the fact that CLP delegates were also no longer rigorously encouraged to stay in the hall to listen to the debates. And there was no public instruction to visitors not to vote after being chosen to fill empty hall seats. There was a failure to implement the emphatic promises given by the leadership on presenting alternative proposals on organisational and campaigning issues in the NEC report and holding a more extensive debate.

The NEC liaison with the CAC over the conference agendas and its appeal role had been abandoned without advance information.

In 2000, on a contemporary resolution on pensions and earnings, the government lost majority union support and the overall vote but won the argument (for the moment) and the votes of a majority of the CLPs on this issue. This allowed the managers to make the general claim to 'the moral high ground' of support of 'the CLP membership' and that became the new emphasis of management taken into the second term. Nevertheless, in 2000 they avoided defeat only by procedural mechanisms on two unwanted alternative positions from the NPF.

National Executive Committee

Development of NEC management involved over time a curious two-step change between the Leader and the unions. With Labour in Opposition, the NEC trade union group, as of old, played its restrained supportive role in policy-making, whilst also, as in the past, defending the NEC's constitutional right of policy involvement. But unusually, outside policy decisions, in the initial phase union representatives mainly from the right of the party had, in effect, marked out a distinction between protecting the party's interests and accepting the leadership's preferences. This happened not only over preserving the party's collectivism in Clause IV but also over introducing the new liaison organisation TULO, and ensuring consultation on the Partnership in Power document. Over regulation of finance in leadership and NEC elections, and over opposition to plebiscitarian leadership, other attempts at control were pursued but later evaded or overcome by the Leader and management.

Coming up to and after the election year 1997, the NEC's traditional loyalty and subordination came more clearly into the ascendancy. The history of damaging past conflict between the NEC and the leadership was used as a management device reinforcing inhibition in not challenging the leadership, strengthening defences against what was judged to be oppositionists and consolidating the united loyalism of appointed and elected national managers. Following Partnership in Power, on the NEC an internal reorganisation and a changed composition reduced the NEC's effective collective role and increased that of the officials working with NEC loyalist representatives. A fusion of heavy management, adroit socialisation into a cooperative role, and concern for career opportunities bred a pervasive sense of loyal responsibility.

On administrative and organisational issues, the NEC worked to a loyalist managerial agenda sometimes made not directly by No. 10 but by the party officers and NEC loyalists as managerial allies. It had been argued consistently by the General Secretary, Sawyer, that reforms would improve the status of the NEC. The document Partnership in Power claimed that 'we propose a strengthened role for the National Executive Committee'.[29] Nothing of the kind occurred. In practice, it was undermined by a careful use of spin redirecting attention away from the committee, a change in the title of the NEC report, a disruption of liaison between the NEC and the Conference Arrangements Committee, and a new unregulated openness of NEC meetings to governmental representatives, all of which lowered the status of the NEC. Yet in the name of the NEC the control over rules and procedures exercised by party officials expanded their power.

As membership sank, so the party lost elements of potentially dissident forces including some of those who provided support for the left in elections, and at the conference. In that sense party management by alienation was proving to be a useful asset. Nevertheless, the heavy partisan attempt to influence CLP elections in 1998, the public as well as party reaction to what became known as 'control freakery' and the heavy hands of headquarters management did stimulate a shifting new middle ground of critical loyalist opposition on the committee. That strengthened the NEC's reluctance to support authoritarian constraints over its own operation, or abolition of the CLP General Committees. Most important was the trade union group reluctance to agree action on the Chief Whip's report on the record of MPs and an NEC-PLP alliance to prevent disciplinary sanctions in the PLP. The NEC did not, therefore, at this stage become 'nothing more than the administrative arm of the leadership'.[30] Its manipulated and loyal subservience retained some limits at this stage, and elements of its formal procedural role at the party conference continued to be protected.

PLP

The central thrust of PLP management intentions had been expressed in the view that 'troublemakers and extremist groups' would get 'short shrift'.[31] Yet this failed to happen. It was said later by Graham Allen, an ex-whip, that the PLP exhibited 'a new conformity and discipline'.[32] Yet this was true only insofar as the government's proposed legislation sustained no defeats. Regular voting dissent did take place, as Cowley's work copiously documents. And the Cowley analysis of House voting did not reveal the vital procedural war fought amongst the managers around the Parliamentary Committee and later the NEC. That was just one of several major indications of the limitations of examining party management purely in terms of votes in the House.

The PLP Secretary, PLP Chair and elected back-bench members did not share the headquarters' command and control agenda. The persistent conflict between the PLP officials and representatives and Millbank was reflected in the different managerial perspectives on the role of party 'civil servants' and 'political organisers'. The tension of what was recognised as 'a clash of two cultures' involved PLP resistance to 'control freakery' and disciplinary sanctions. And in the elections for PLP representatives on the NEC in 1998, heavy-handed action by the whips on behalf of favoured candidates provoked a reaction which facilitated, for the moment, a greater freedom in NEC elections, in spite of Blair's preferences.

The remarkable revolt in the Commons over lone parent benefit in 1997 was followed by the marked absence of PLP support for heavy sanctions.

There was strong opposition from the PLP officials and the Parliamentary Committee (with an important input from women MPs). It thereafter became a precedent in a long-term battle over sanctions on a terrain moving further against authoritarianism inside and outside the party. Replenishment of the PLP trade union group was established without prior No. 10 approval, but surprisingly with an element of sympathetic managerial minority support. It became geared up for dissent on labour-law issues, pre-empting constraints over authoritarian management, a significant development unregistered in Cowley's study of influences over the PLP.[33] The Leader's subsequent inhibition on the sanctions battleground facilitated second- and third-term pressures over policy.

The need for management by sanctions was also eased in practice at that time by the loyalty and self-discipline of MPs, limited but regular policy adjustments, satisfaction with much of the government first-term policy in accordance with the election manifesto, and the availability of numerous channels of communication. On that front, however, there was another low-key but important long battle over the Departmental Committees and the attempt by the 1996 PLP Review Group to produce an element of sharing in the policy-formulation process through agreed advance consultation. The attempt failed, held back by practical difficulties but mainly by the lack of active commitment and receptivity from Millbank, No. 10 and most ministers in spite of the promise Blair had made. That was a success in preserving the top-down non-inclusive style of the Leader's policy formulation, similar to what had happened behind the façade of Partnership in Power. There was also, with no information given to the NEC or the PLP, another extension of the rolling coup in the discreet procedural insulation against removal of the Leader by a failure to supply nomination forms.

Managerial spin and speeches

Party management of the public sector

Party management activity and distrust in relation to public sector policy problems became central to an intensifying conflict between the unions and the government within and outside the party. Trust had already been adversely affected by spin on increases in public expenditure on public services in 1998, which turned out to be a manipulation of the figures. Cooperation was also damaged by an unhelpful Blair 'scars on my back' speech in 1999 which appeared to affiliated unions to be unconnected with any failed dialogue with them.

Manifesto and management

The manifesto of 2001 which under Partnership in Power was thought to be the means by which the party shared ownership, in practice became subject to the misadventures of politics and the innovations of managerial control. In the Clause V meeting of 2001, by historic mischance, the PLP was unexpectedly more involved in manifesto-making under the name of the Parliamentary Committee, but with limited effect. Cabinet members not on the Parliamentary Committee were brought in, although with no formal voting rights. As in 1997, a business manifesto was produced outside party institutions. A bedrock major commitment of Partnership in Power had been that the party 'has the right to determine the framework of values and priorities for the next manifesto'.[34] In practice, the feed-in of party-influenced views was neutralised at all stages by the heavily managed process and the closure of party institutions in the manifesto-making period.

By close working relations which assisted management, between No. 10, ministers and loyalist union officials working for UNISON, including the later No. 10 liaison aide Nita Clarke, an important process of government movement towards eradication of a two-tier workforce did begin. But the most contentious policies that were to emerge under the 2001–5 government were either not in the manifesto or contradicted by it. The manifesto did not unite the party and the leadership on future policy nor did it create enthusiasm for the process. Most significant of all was the spin on the manifesto, launching what appeared to be a major private sector involvement in the public services without party discussion and without warning. That policy and that way of conducting politics undermined cooperation from the public sector unions, even when later there was a considerable new financing of health and education.

Resistances, pluralism and the paradox of party management

Management and underpinning

An appraisal of power relations in the party at the end of the first term in government confirms that Blair's charismatic driving leadership and Brown's economic management, together with important legislative achievement, had underpinned their appeal, allied to heavy practices in the management of the party. Brown was an aggravation to Blair, especially when seen as attempting to gain control over the party organisation, but otherwise he and Blair saw eye to eye on a party management which regularly, and often discreetly, facilitated, extended and protected the power of the leadership to an unprecedented degree. It was tempting, indeed common at this time, to see what was visible in the attempt to project and ensure Blair's supremacy and the impact of new controls, together with the regularity of conference and parliamentary victories, as not only the central but the whole story conveyed in the national press. This it was often said was 'total control . . . imposed on the party' by Blair.[35]

Pluralism

In reality, the unprecedented and growing strength of management, including the extensions of the rolling coup, existed with often unnoticed counter-tendencies and limitations. The Blair supremacy was never quite what it seemed, even in the seminal period from 1994 to 2001. Blair's aims still met frustrating party obstacles. Virtually unobserved from the outside, each institutional setting and culture did not fully replicate the central managerial style or the Leader's preference. This arose sometimes from variations in procedural values and priorities in different locations and sometimes variations in the roles played by different union representatives. Though the core managerial culture was a major influence operated through both managing officials and elected representatives acting as managers, lines of what was considered to be proper behaviour were sometimes drawn in different places.

It meant that the management was never as uniformly under Blair's command as commonly perceived. Most checks and balances had been undermined, but for the moment some were still partially effective even within the management itself. Included in these balances was the important and much misunderstood role of the deputy leader John Prescott. Steve Bell's *Guardian* cartoon image of the dog with the muzzle is wholly inappropriate here as was the No. 10 spin doctor Lance Price's later judgement on him as 'loyal but ineffectual'.[36] Understood by few but revealed here was his discreet self-ascribed role as party protector over some important procedural developments and non-developments in Opposition and during the first term in government. Prescott's party management was generally loyally supportive but his management was not the same as Blair's party management, and the post was not, as so often described in the media, something of a non-job.[37]

Chris Grey, in his short but illuminating study of organisation, alerts us to the general problems of securing persistent organisational control.[38] But there were particular weaknesses to the pursuit of Blair's version of strong leadership, vanguard minority politics and extensive control in a party with resilient alternative traditions. The paradox was that the most commanding and controlling expressions of management, or even the threat of it, at times stimulated a significant, if limited, counterpoint upon which later revolts could build.

Section III: crisis of control freakery and the search for supremacy

Candidate selection

That pattern of counterpoint became clearly important in critical voices over candidate selection and major public reactions. The Leader's assumption had been that unfiltered, uncontrolled party activity would be seen as a threat to the government and the people, and that the electorate would therefore reward control over the party by giving more trust to the strong, even domineering, Leader. 'Labour', Foley had diagnosed, 'had come to value and to promote leadership as a political instrument and even a programme in its own right'.[39] That was always doubtful as a view from the party as distinct from the Leader and management. The Falkirk result involved a rejection of control and it was specially contested after the London mayoral election controversy. Abandoning OMOV arrangements in London as in Wales and loading procedural arrangements involved denying the preference of the people.

'Control freakery', portrayed by managers as virtuous activity in defence of the people's best interests, became seen by increasing numbers of the public as a vice. Allied to this, strong leadership met some unexpectedly damaging criticism of arrogance and manipulation by misleading communicational spin and procedural control by the 'vote-fixing' party. By 2000 his style and party management was getting the Leader into acute difficulties. As 'control freakery' provoked increasing party and public resentment, his frustration at the limitations and potential obstacles in the party grew, adding to those springing from the problems of governing. It was an unexpected managerial predicament as Blair looked towards a new bold radicalism freer yet further away from the party's political centre of gravity.

Making room for the bold Leader

'The end of control freakery'

The proclaimed stance from No. 10 of 'the end of control freakery' did represent a new awareness of the counterproductive electoral consequences of obvious heavy control, especially if it affected public choice. In small measure there was an adjustment in managerial behaviour particularly in moving the control away from its public association with Blair. All this seemed to presage a new broad liberalisation of the party, a return to the initial spirit of Partnership in Power, and the drawing back of party management across the board. However, it is doubtful if that would have happened even if the terrorist attack on 11 September 2001 had not occurred. Some steps towards strengthening his freedom and control were already being drafted or in the pipeline. Whilst there was no master plan, just close managerial attention to 'what Tony needs', with great resourcefulness, the Leader and managers secured in 2001 a remarkable turnaround of the situation he had faced in 2000.

Extending the coup

Around the Leader with the greatest managerial powers in Labour history there was now an attempt to boldly further strengthen his party position, whilst presenting an image of diminished control freakery. Two critically important extensions to the managerial coup were involved. The first involved the Leader's imposition, outside of party rules, of a Party Chair. Discreetly Charles Clarke and his successors became the senior party manager delivering for the Leader whilst emphasising to the party that it was being given a voice at the Cabinet table.

It was also a mechanism for curtailing the threat of 'a party within the party' organisation by Brown (much of it myth but potentially very import-ant) and the interventions by Prescott in protection of the party (less hostile but much more of a reality). Numerous commentators made the mistake of judging that Blair did not act at this stage to stop his aggressive rival, Brown. Action through the governmental option was inhibited by reasoned consideration of the range of deep party problems it would cause including reviving accusations of control freakery. But Blair always had a strong sense of the importance of controlling the future. Bringing in a (Leader's) Party Chair had the advantage of building a defence of Blair's continuing and future management of the party. And in addition, the entirely unplanned formal exclusion of the cabinet from the authorising manifesto meeting, which now brought in the PLP, had cut off Brown's right to be there. Thus, though Brown was not weakened in his govern-mental role, his potential party role was now, for him, annoyingly limited.

The second extension to the coup in the period of the end of control freakery was even more covert and remarkable. It was a limitation of the potential role for the PLP in policy-formulation, which had been formally agreed in the PLP including the leadership in 1996. In 2001, with no publicity, no leakage and no information given to the PLP, the standing orders of the PLP were changed, curtailing the agreed aspiration and mechanics of sharing a role in policy-formulation which had been guided by the principle that 'except in exceptional circumstances, backbenchers will be consulted before major policy decisions are taken'.[40] Key to this were Blair's strong reassuring private signals around the Parliamentary Committee and to managerial officials that he recognised the pressure for an improved role for the PLP in policy-formulation. His signals led to nothing of substance.

At the same time, reinforcing the new management, there was also an evasion of the promised review of Partnership in Power which linked the leadership to the wider party. Also, without agreement from the General Secretary or announcement, there was a private declaration by Blair of his right to determine his staff salaries drawn from party funds. This was part of the attempt to keep the important No. 10 aide, Angie Hunter, whilst he rebuilt what he saw as a more effective and radical new No. 10 advisory team. His attempt to move her, a far from party-sensitive figure, to cover party relations had to be abandoned, but otherwise the pattern of change from 2001 involved a major extension to the managerial coup expanding Blair's powers in relation to the party, and further protecting him from what he regarded as frustrating interference.

The overall pattern of the managerial coup was largely missed by observers partly because whilst one face of the Leader's management was publicly ending 'control freakery', and giving 'a voice to the party' another masked face was using, even strengthening, the same managerial devices as in the past, protecting Blair from interference in his new pursuit of a bold radicalism in domestic and foreign policy, which in important features had not been jointly formulated with the party.

Managerial continuity and boldness

In some key respects, after an initial period of uncertainty, the controlling management in the wider party became more cocksure as the party managers became more clearly Blair's praetorian guard in the factional defence against Brown. The management was also seen as all the more necessary as Blair sought to safeguard the settlement with business and his domestic and foreign policies became more contentious. Epitomising the continuation of managerial arrangements was the continuing manipulative arrangements for elections by CLPs to the NPF and the failure to investigate and report on complaints against managing officials even after clear evidence of improper organisational communication from the General Secretary's office was publicly revealed. There was a pattern of taking no action against such managerial activities.

Most serious of all, in 2002 and 2003 the conference was not asked to authorise the constitutional change in union affiliation fees, and in 2003 there was no rulebook acknowledgement of this change although as in 2002 the increase was drawn from union resources. These were said later to be 'mistakes', but they were in harmony with a bold new managerial view that, under the rules, conference authorisation was not necessary. This position on affiliation was not rectified until forced by TULO four years later. The managers even succeeded in having various individual political rights of officials sanctioned in an Organisation Committee document of 17 March 2003. The party management system was the great unmentionable in that document, which appeared to even permit the officials to stand for election to national bodies. Although in practice that did not take place, the granting of permission was a potentially Stalinised development which would have been anathema to the past generations of Labour leaders.

Unanticipated consequences

Spinning and the lessons of management

Publicity for 'the end of control freakery' had been a considerable success in the media in spite of the reality of stronger and bolder party management. The problems of the composition of the Clause V meeting and the changes of the PLP Standing Orders had been successfully hidden by the managers from the wider party and the public. Much of the combined operations of media- and party management had been very adroit. Yet, once again, as had been shown in Opposition and in the first term of government, even for the smartest Leader and his aides things do not always turn out as planned. And the media-management which generally drove party management did not always proceed without damaging consequences to the latter. It had happened over the anti-union attack following the Clause IV result, over the politics of the Road to the Manifesto, over the purpose of the PLP Review, over what Partnership in Power involved and over the misleading spin on public sector finance. Now the intra-party politics post-2001 was heavily affected by angry reactions – over the manifesto spin on private sector involvement – which thereafter submerged reception for more favourable policies including the curtailment of the two-tier workforce.

Also a very surprising feature of Blair's second-term leadership was the tendency for collective ministerial responsibility to develop elements of break-down, in the form of signals and leaks about conflict. Both Norton citing a *Times* article by Alice Miles[41] and later Bennister[42] gave a plausible explanation that the limitations of Cabinet decision-making enhanced the propensity for disputes to spill out into the public arena. That case is strongest in the case of Clare Short's public belligerence over Iraq policy, but the party management role of the Party Chair in advocating the end of 'control freakery' was an often overlooked special case which influenced the Leader's options. The spin around that appointment added an extra inhibition on disciplinary action which might open up the damaging pos-sibilities of the media portraying a Labour split which had a martyr on the backbenches fighting 'the control freak' in No. 10. The limitations that Clarke's role placed on Brown's party involvement already gave the Chancellor an added incentive to send out semi-public signals of policy disagreement which had party appeal and to further nurse his difference from Blair in front of the party.

The party management of going to war

The managerial setting

An avowed readoption of the straight and narrow after 2001 was in permanent severe tension with the framework of managerial realism and Blair's own priorities. It also became clear that public problems with public distrust had not departed with the election victory. And the odium of Jo Moore's 9/11 'good day' to bury bad news was followed by an ini-tial failure to ask her to resign. It was also followed by what appeared to be an attempt to spin Blair into a leading role in a royal presentation, by accusations of sleaze and by complaints over the limitations on delivery.

The problem of public distrust had become deep-rooted. Before the Iraq invasion an anti-manipulative ethos had emerged amongst the highly crit-ical electorate, which was deeply disappointed by what was seen as Blair's duplicitous spinning performance, his performance as leader of 'the vote-fixing party' after the London mayor election and what was regarded as the insincerity of his promise of a change in political behaviour. Within the party management accompanying the claim of 'the end of control freakery', the manipulated private/public sector policy had consolidated distrust in the unions, as did the party management processes. Nevertheless, with regular acculturation into the successful management practices came a view that anything could be fixed, and successful manipulative initiatives against the odds could be admirable. The covert successes of party- and media-management in 2001–2 had reinforced the managerial confidence that innovative manipulative skills could help get the managers and politicians out of even the most acute difficulties. That lesson was taken into the politics of Iraq.

Party inside and outside the PLP

The analysis of Blair's success in taking Britain to war over Iraq generally focuses only on winning parliamentary approval through a well-organised parliamentary managerial operation, illuminated in Cowley's study.[43] But that narrow focus gives only part of the explanation for his victory in the House. The party management of Iraq began long before the final Commons decisions, with a control over party discussions and a structuring of party choices. There had been a remarkable avoidance of detailed party discussion of the path-laying Chicago speech of 1999. Party management outside the House was tightened in 2002 to ensure that the PLP was insulated in various party channels from an unambiguous authoritative voice of the party rejecting war without a second resolution involving specific UN approval. That also reduced the party's potential to reinforce the anti-war opinion of the electorate.

This management involved considerable pressure on the NEC and the party's policy commission to avoid the development of a distinctive party policy. Through managerial organisation to stimulate satisfactorily worded resolutions at the party conference, the conference was not allowed the choice a majority wanted. Then, there was an unprecedented withdrawal of the NEC's own policy statement without a committee vote, to avoid it being defeated at the conference. The choice of speakers was blatantly and overwhelmingly partisan, albeit possibly counterproductive. The favoured resolution was declared carried from the chair and a card vote refused. At the NPF neither discussion nor vote on Iraq was allowed and the withdrawn NEC statement on Iraq was initially reported to the party as having been endorsed.[44] Succeeding Party Chairs, Clarke and then Reid, worked hard to defend the government's position across the party and to portray the response of the party as supportive. In spite of the promise of 2001 they did not act as the genuine voice of the party in the Cabinet.

The unions are rarely even mentioned in accounts of the Iraq decision, but their varied activity and non-activity was a significant influence. Unions often acted not as a homogenous entity nor with consistency from proclaimed position to priority action. Although the TUC General Council debate on 8 March was impassioned, and some who normally were regarded as moderates were fiercely opposed to the war without a second resolution, more than appeared on the surface or has been registered in journalistic and academic accounts, management intervention over Iraq was in practice assisted by the complex union priorities in different sectors of activity and their restraint in the use of their potential power. That contrasted with the lack of restraint from pro-government union and managerial forces.

It was said that mandatory reselection was an influential procedure requiring 'PLP members to be more responsive to their local parties'.[45] Yet, as shown, this aspect of mandatory reselection had been procedurally undermined by management as the trigger mechanism became more dominated by union branches. They were not encouraged by union leaders to use it as an offensive influence on the Iraq loyalists. Also the Chief Whip, on the basis of territorial propriety, officially prohibited MPs from urging the deselection of their colleagues over Iraq. Although the PLP trade union group officials individually voted against the war, they made no attempt to engage the union groups in an anti-war campaign; that would have highlighted their divisions and damaged the groups' activities for other purposes. Pro-war NEC union loyalists, on the other hand, discreetly working to the No. 10 Political Office, used the phones to contact selected union-group members in order to build up the decisive supporting vote on 18 March 2003. By that date the extra-parliamentary party voice as a pressure on Labour MPs had been heavily filtered and in key respects neutralised.

In the PLP, a lack of cohesion amongst anti-war leaders, a divisive association of the wider anti-war leadership with the left and regime change in the party also eased the party management for the vote. Over this issue Prescott had become an important, perhaps crucial, loyalist influence. It was also significant that three big potential suspects as dissidents – Brown, Cook and Short, in different ways – eased the managers' task by limiting any adverse impact on the debate. Brown was closely shadowed by managers in his activities, and found to have been loyal and effective in his direct supportive lobbying. Cook resigned before the debate – not, as he originally intended, during it. Short was persuaded to stay in position to assist the UN post-war operation.

The vote for the invasion was an impressive triumph for Blair after a tour-de-force of a speech, which conveyed his case with considerable power and also gave the impression that Blair had strong grounds to be sure of what he was saying and that on this issue he ought to be trusted. It was not the case that as Polly Toynbee, searching with the best intentions to find anything good to say about Blair's Iraq venture, argued, 'there was nothing in it for him'.[46] In party management alone it was thought that there was much to be gained. It was envisaged that he could move nearer the supremacy which had eluded him, secure a greater degree of freedom from the party, and possibly extend the rolling coup. Within a wave of enthusiastic national fervour, Blair's electoral position would be strengthened and Brown and the repeated dissidents might be brought to heel.

Leadership factionalisation and PLP sanctions

The formidable persuasive power of the Blair speech became a cautionary tale. Failure to find weapons of mass destruction and the growing view that the country was misgoverned and misled into war reinforced the anti-manipulative ethos in the electorate and the doubts about Blair's political methods. This was shared by a growing section of the PLP especially incited by his one-alone control over policy-formulation. Those doubts continued over a range of issues, particularly foundation hospitals and top-up-fees legislation which were introduced without advance consultation of the PLP or support from the extra-parliamentary party and without an electoral mandate.

Armstrong, the Chief Whip, a natural pro-Leader militant, and personally closer to the Leader than previous holders of the position, became more obviously hostile in the face of what was seen as the disloyalty of the problem-making Brownites. The whips' office, like the party headquarters, was affected by a new factionalisation involving much of the time a more one-way definition of responsibilities with the PLP. Facing what was seen as the danger from Brown, across all the institutions, the party managers attempted to become, in effect, Blair's praetorian guard. Government measures were saved in the end by the scale of the Labour majority in the House, the constraints of party loyalty, some significant alterations and concession and, in a final twist over tuition fees, the role of Gordon Brown in support of the government.

Sanctions further constrained

In facing this degree of dissent against a background of still trying to avoid the public accusation of 'control freakery', and with a highly publicised element of indiscipline at leadership level, Blair's defensive sanctions against dissidents remained limited. The view that 'parties have generally succeeded in asserting greater control over . . . MPs'[47] did not take full account of this limitation. Now, the NEC did not even receive the Chief Whip's report on MPs' records. Managers did seek to put loyalist pressures on the MPs via the regional office to uphold party unity. But the major sanctions against dissident MPs had been fought off and MPs were in practice relatively free to dissent from local CLP opinion, providing that they handled it with sensitivity and were vigorous in their own local campaigning role. There was never enough support in the PLP nor on the Parliamentary Committee for new disciplinary sanctions to be introduced. Even the fierce and powerful open attack by Clare Short on Blair's form of governance could not be subject to such sanctions.

As for appealing to the people over the head of the party, thought to be Blair's potential presidential weapon in distancing from the party, that was heavily constrained given his loss of public trust and the lack of public enthusiasm for his more contentious policies. Crucially, there were acute dangers that more openly exhibiting fundamental divisions over policy would hand even more ammunition about a divided party to its growing media opponents. If they were further provoked by any attempt to go 'presidential' the now more cohesive and counter-managerial unions could have made their own public call and caused him and the government even greater trouble. So the limitations could not be removed.

Managing accountability and changing Blair

Even so, Blair, through his management process, in another important respect remained very strong, and the antagonistic Brown became, in effect, a managerial asset. The Partnership in Power document had laid down that the leadership would be accountable and responsive to the party in the country.[48] Blair's vision, he told the party in 1998, 'is of an unbroken line of accountability'.[49] But as shown here, at the same time, management planned and was operated so that accountability would not happen. The covert management system did not formally exist so it could not be made accountable. The NEC as a body had no control over it. There was also a managed fusion of procedural development and managerial encouragement to 'move on' rather than 'revisiting issues'.

That was accepted as a reasonable new responsibility, but its practice was at times far from reasonable. Procedural development reinforced restraint on accountability across the party. NEC elections, which under previous Labour governments acted as a barometer of party feelings, were changed in form, downgraded in significance and now made biennial. Policy forums on local, regional and national levels had no facilities for pursuing the accountability of those who were supposed to implement what happened in the discussions. There was a build-up of the significance of NPF reports to the party conference, but no reports back to the NPF on action taken on issues and no report back to the party conference on issues where the leadership had been defeated.

There was a failure to implement the heavy promise given by the leadership in 1997 on presenting alternative proposals on organisational and campaigning issues in the NEC report and having a more extensive debate on that report. Party conference verbatim reports became less available with no announcement that they even existed. At the conference, accountability of the CAC had been undermined on contemporary resolutions because of the new timetable of decisions already taken. The NEC appeal role over CAC decisions had been suppressed without consultation. The impressive question-and-answer session for the Leader at the 1998 party conference later disappeared without explanation.

It was particularly difficult to regularly challenge the leadership culture directly at senior reaches of the party. That found few openings and risked being labelled oppositionist or 'Brownite' if it did. Blair's managerial control was expressed in the failure of the NEC and, even more striking, of the Parliamentary Committee to hold a review of the problems stemming from Blair's style of leadership following the Hutton and Butler reports. It was emblematic that the post-Iraq pre-election 2004 NEC report did not go out in time for the CLPs to even read it.

In principle, accountability might, in extremity, have been signalled by the variable reception of the Prime Minister's conference speech. But that had not been the tradition for years, and a cultivated veneration management made the reception a celebration with organised social pressure to conform. Weak accountability, absence of review, and machine loyalty to the Leader cemented by the Brown-Blair wars became, in effect, a managed insulation which provided no springboard for change. That added to a frustration at the grassroots now in deep decline of membership and activity. At senior levels in the unions there was an increasing mood of scepticism and alienation.

New union assertiveness and its limitations

Unions, party finance, management and policy

'Will they threaten to withdraw their financial support unless more union-friendly noises start to emanate from Downing Street?', Sir Robert McRindle, ex-Conservative MP had asked in 1997, after discussing Labour's 'cosy relationship with the business community'.[50] The immediate answer was 'no'. After 2001 this appeared to develop into an affirmative, with the important albeit misleading example of the GMB's threat of financial sanctions over public sector policy, followed by the RMT political change of its sponsored-MP group.

Blair at this point did not favour an attempt at decisive confrontation with the unions. There were enough problems on the foreign horizon without going down a route which could only lead to impasse, implosion and ammunition for other parties. Yet, in a highly unusual development in party management, Clarke, the Party Chair, reacting to the GMB leader, moved spasmodically out of Blair's full control in relating to the unions. Clarke and Triesman, in effect, did lay the ground for a decisive battle. In doing so their behaviour affected relations between the GMB and UNISON unions which had tactically moved apart in 2001 over how to fight government policy on the public sector. Now they moved closer together in suspicion of and reaction to the managers.

Nevertheless, contrary to managerial expectations, in response to an urgent financial appeal that the party's future viability was at stake, all the unions (including the GMB which returned to its old solidarity role) pledged to come to the party's financial aid, without political conditions. That it took many months to activate, after an initial agreement to raise the affiliation fees for one year, had more to do with tardy and uncertain handling on the party side than with the resistance of union leaders. The main bulk of the new affiliation finance eventually came in the form of a further two-year deal in the middle of 2003, at a time when union dissatisfaction reached new political heights. Yet again the finance was unconditional.

Down below in the unions there was growing a different emphasis on the unions' transactional relationship with the party over 'our money'. But the loyalist outcome of the battle over finance, the union determination to deliver on supplying the increased income they had promised, and the recognition that the finance issue was still being used against the unions by some of the unions' opponents, all in practice had the effect of reinforcing 'the rules' prohibiting financial pressure by leaders in relation to policy outcomes.

In a study published in 2004 it was asserted that 'Union money no longer buys votes that make a difference so it is used by being made contingent on policy delivery'.[51] No evidence was given to substantiate this and the evidence here strongly indicates something much more qualified. At the edges, very occasionally and especially Edmonds in 2001, a union leader crossed the line of old propriety in reference to financial provision, but overall this was highly unusual, quietly repudiated by other unions, determinedly repulsed by the political leaders and broadly retreated from in 2002 to 2003.

The new anti-managerial mood

An often crude focus on union financial pressures and party financial vulnerability drew attention away from the real new assertiveness in relation to party management after 2003. The methods of party management were experienced by the unions as a perpetual danger to democratic representation within the party. By 2003 suspicion between No. 10 and the new union leaders was such that the normal discreet pre-conference management meeting of the Leader with the union leaders was called off. In another era both sides might have looked to tackle big problems by a replenishment of a committee linking TUC-government-party relationships, but this option was closed to them by the 'New Labour' media strategy of distancing from the unions.

On the NEC, critical pressures increased but the managerial hold was tenacious, albeit with some important exceptions. The right of the NEC to proclaim its attitude towards the policy resolutions at the conference became the site of a vote won only narrowly by Blair on foundation hospitals in 2003. That year also, restrictions on the right of public representatives to stand for the NEC as CLP representatives in the CLP section were now agreed by the NEC. And candidate selection by the CLP at Halifax involved a highly unusual challenge from the machine and an even more unusual defeat of these managers by the NEC majority. But in other respects the committee generally operated within the managerial constraints established from 1997.

Delivery by No. 10 of a proscription of the two-tier workforce in the NHS was expected by the managers to oblige the unions to move to a more solidaristic pattern of support at the conference. But grievance over other government policy and reaction to management behaviour had passed a point of no return. At the 2003 conference, extra policy seminars were arranged by the managers such that they clashed with the long-established time of union delegation meetings. Party staff were coming under increasing and acute criticism of their interventionist and manipulative behaviour. After twelve months of discussion the Organisation Committee document in March 2003 did express a prohibition on officials improperly using their position, party resources and time to intervene in party processes, but it had no discernible effect on managerial behaviour.

Conference management

Members' or managers' party: persuading or astroturfing?

The party conference, even in the era of 'the end of control freakery', was an institution where the managers could never see 'loosening a bit' as a possibility as they sought to defend the government. The managerial role of Ian McCartney, the new Party Chair in 2003, became even more important as a central figure of NEC and conference management. He played a two-way role consistent with his previous activity, although now with a greater need to prove his worth to the Leader. Delegates were further drawn away from the hall and even taken out of debates in groups to meet McCartney and ministers, for persuasion.

Although, in 2003, two hand votes did deviate from the government message over foundation hospitals and over pensions, and the government defeat on housing was overwhelming across the floor in 2004 and 2005, the platform generally managed support from a majority of the CLP representatives on card votes. This could again be regularly proclaimed as a moral victory of 'the party' contrasted with union-led conference defeats which were often attributed simply to the initiative and influence of union leaders. Particularly notable as a remarkable managerial success which raised suspicions in the unions was that in 2003 CLP representatives even voted against improving the allocation to CLPs of contemporary resolutions despite years of complaint against the limits.

Mandelson and Liddle had taken the view that 'the leadership must lead . . . persuading the party along every step of the way'.[52] And in 2002 Mandelson commented that 'it is now often easier to bring the constituency party delegates round to the leadership's point of view than it is the trade unions'.[53] This made no mention of the role of the extensive management system. Poll data of membership policy opinion indicates the importance of this system in sometimes turning the representatives in the face of CLP opinion including key policies on public sector reform.[54] These contrasts may be viewed as the product of skills of persuasion and the strength of the government and managerial case, but they could also be seen as derived from the creation of special conditions and influences to achieve what came to be known later in the wider political world as astroturfing (a reference to a brand of fake grass which is used all over the United States) creating an impression of grassroots support. It could also be argued that the pretence of 'a members' party' producing supportive CLP votes at the conference in this way contributed to losing in other dimensions, especially in the decline of membership and the weakening of participation at the grass roots.

TULO and counter-managerial organisation

Management, movement and the two wings

It was diagnosed reasonably by Chadwick and Heffernan that '[t]he divide between the supposed "political" and "industrial" wings of the old Labour movement was never as starkly pronounced as it is in this era of New Labour'.[55] In effect, there was an extraordinary and bold attempt by Blair to manage the union relationship in such a way as to make the unions simply outsider lobbyists in the party they had created. But union pressure through the PLP trade union group in 1997 to 1999 and the strengthening of TULO also ensured that the political and industrial differentiation under Blair was never quite as organisationally pronounced in the practice as it was in appearance.

In the unions, from 2003, as the old 'bond of mutual confidence'[56] with the leadership was heavily undermined, a majority of union leaders through TULO sought, as Taylor and Ludlam diagnosed, to reassert the position of the unions.[57] However, it came now not through finance nor over the co-ordinated seizure of positions. The major unions who created virtually all the contemporary policy submissions had not attempted and did not attempt now to prioritise constitutional changes that would have strengthened the union position or limited the leadership or made clearer or easier the process of eviction of the Leader. They did not in practice prioritise attempts urged from a minority on the left to 'reclaim the party'. When the first steps towards constitutional change affecting power relations was taken in 2003 it came from a single union – the UCW, not TULO – and it was to strengthen the CLPs over submission of contemporary resolutions, not to strengthen the unions.

The reassertion came through an unprecedented counter-management organisation that reflected union agendas and coordinated TULO unions, a linkage later interwoven through the extended TULO Contact Group, which included the TUC. A broadly shared union perspective on party managerial activities which had historically underpinned stable support for the leadership now began to underpin an institutionalised counter-management organisation. It sought to ensure that the union voice circumvented management controlling practices and that the conference was fed by the NPF in ways which did what had been expected from Partnership in Power – giving the conference a final say. The culminating point in this development was what became known as the Warwick Agreement.

Counter-management and the Warwick Agreement

Union pressure and managerial tactics

As the unions moved to increase coordinated policy pressure at the NPF before the 2004 party conference, so the managers, led by the Party Chair, moved to influence and take over union policy agreement on the basis of initiatives from No. 10, as had happened in 2000 at Exeter. At the same time, an attempt was made to change the rules of NPF voting in March 2004 without advance consultation and outside of the Joint Policy Committee procedures. Angry and united pressure from the unions forced them into retreat. In the face of united union coordination, the divide-and-rule managerial tactics of Exeter at this stage met many more difficulties. Extensive negotiations led to an agreement which covered between 56 and 110 items (depending on how the items were separated). Yet, as at Exeter, managers also laid down red-line limits on union proposals to amend labour law which – with just one exception: raising protection from dismissal for strikers from 8 to 12 weeks – they stuck to. And it was an important feature of the final agreement that no more than 40 of the 110 items came in proposals from the unions. The rest came from the managers.

Counter-management and not buying influence

The now routine accusation that the unions bought influence, this time at Warwick in 2004, in return for policy concessions[58] was not substantiated by credible evidence from participants, and consideration of finance was not raised as an influence in the many private post-mortems about what went on there. The view that the agreement was 'prompted in large part by the need for union financial support for the general election'[59] misses the crucial consideration that was in play at Warwick, as did judging the relative position of the NPF against the party conference to show the former to be arguably 'far more significant'.[60] Coordinated counter-management pressure at the NPF to produce alternative positions from the forum potentially made the unions more potent in the votes at the subsequent conference. It raised the acute concern of the Leader and his aides about an inability to produce a pre-election conference united in support of government policy. With the continuing decline in individual membership, the Leader also needed the enthusiastic use of the unions' organisational and communication resources during the election campaign.

The years of projecting the Leader's supremacy over the unions had given the government more confidence in facing a possible onslaught from the right-wing press over an agreement. Crude anti-union rhetoric had not been in use by the spin doctors since the fierce reaction to Blair's 'wreckers' speech of 2002. Significant also was the managerial attempt to use Warwick as an agreement with the unions to impose on them an obligatory role to act as managerial auxiliaries at the conference in outvoting critical CLPs' resolutions, including some over Iraq. That attempt was only a partial success, but it again indicated both the potential usefulness of the unions in a management role and the ease with which Blair and the managers changed their procedural values depending on 'what worked'.

Warwick Agreement and the manifesto

The discreet four-year battle over the composition of the next Clause V meeting was dealt with in the end by a degree of background policy accommodation of Blair and Brown and in procedural terms by agreed arrangements outside the constitutional rules. The PLP was still represented but now also the Cabinet was brought back with voting rights, ensuring senior ministerial supremacy. For the first time in Labour Party history the unions through TULO were represented as a distinct entity. To produce some measure of political balance there were also three representatives from the NPF – in practice agreed with the managers. Again there was no advance consultation of the NPF itself.

Following the Warwick Agreement, a manifesto commitment was made to its implementation. In accommodation with the strong and consistent tenor of party and union opinion, local authorities were to be given the ability to start building homes again. To keep unity over the Warwick agreement and to avoid opening Brown-Blair arguments, in the Clause V meeting union amendments to the draft manifesto were discouraged. The unions 'to solidify Warwick' at the prompting of the Party Chair agreed that votes for or against be on the whole document taken at the end of the manifesto meeting. No vote was taken on rail renationalisation, which a majority had supported at the party conference – aiding management once again. In an opportunist move a proposal for directly elected mayors suddenly reappeared and became part of the agreed manifesto. There was a commitment to the continuation of NHS reforms, but it excluded the limitations agreed in advance between UNISON and the minister. Independent of this process, the new business manifesto, again not controlled by any party institution, made commitments on light touch regulation. Significantly, the much publicised agreement with the unions had no adverse effect at the election.

Unions and the party: managing cohesion

There had always been forces pulling apart the unions and the party and forces holding it or moving it back together. Historically there had always been tensions of electoral strategy, social affinity, ideology and interests. But now, in each area large new problems were created under Blair's party management. Most problematic of all, the union-party relationship suffered long-lasting damage from the spin-driven modernising preference in 1992 for the end of union affiliation. This was followed under Blair by the rejection of any historical obligation to the unions together with a shedding of conventional 'rules' and protocols.

Union relations continued to be referred to from around the Leader with reservations and implications indicating that it was a transitional arrangement. A widespread expectation was engendered that these attitudes would lead to further tangible moves towards organisational separation; that was the issue which was seen to dominate the literature after 1997.[61] Blair's party management appeared to be creating grievances which would force it apart, and regularly spinning that the unions were a problem together with pushing various versions of 'Blair poised to loosen remaining union links'.[62] Yet, under the surface, something contrasting and startling was happening.

The party-union linkage continued to be supported by a majority of the membership active and inactive, including the new members.[63] More than that, not only was this relationship 'still enduring', confirming its rooted nature[64] at national level, relations between the unions and the party were being stabilised or pulled closer together. In the Blairite 1995 rulebook, obligations to be a member of a trade union ('if applicable') were doubly stated, for members and for those seeking nomination or selection as parliamentary candidates, as they had been in the 1993 rulebook. And now also for both there was an additional obligation to contribute to the political fund of their union. That cannot have had a major impact, but nevertheless by 1995 in Blair's 'New Labour' parliamentary party virtually all MPs were trade union members.

Three years later, maximising the drive to timesaving and stability, the trigger mechanism for candidate reselection was made the total of local nominations, giving power in many seats to the locally affiliated unions which normally had an overall majority of the nominating organisations and were traditionally supportive of the existing candidate. After 1999, with Blair now seeking to avoid the charge of control freakery, the union conservative role in reselections was seen as helpful to management in avoiding 'control freak' accusations.

In the Party into Power arrangements, in spite of intense Leader and managerial opposition, but because of pressure from some of the union representatives, and also because the manager concerned with union relations saw it as valuable, the procedure of contemporary resolutions became virtually a joint union-management operation at the conference. The long battle over the Employment Relations Act brought the unions and the party into closer organisation and accord.

In 2000, the role of TULO in policy coordination was accepted, albeit as a management device. By 2001, in recognition of the constructive role of the unions in campaigning, communication and joint electoral organisation, TULO's establishment became further integrated as part of the party's constitution.[65] In 2003, TULO representatives were brought on to the JPC to smooth organisational relations, and for similar reasons, as noted, in 2005, representatives of TULO joined the Clause V manifesto meeting. None of this had independent policy consequences and did not impede the role of the party managers who resolutely defended Blair's employment-relations settlement to the PLP trade union group and in discussions with TULO. But it raised the status of TULO and it added to the union-party coordination.

So, in spite of many predictions to the contrary, and in spite of the media spin undermining the unions, for varying reasons – which included at times a response to common campaigning activity of different kinds, encouraging organisational relations, and at times party management considerations – there had developed an increasing national integration, much as Minkin had found in the very different circumstances of the 1980s.[66] It was an extraordinary and virtually unnoticed outcome.

Approaching finale: leadership and management degeneration

It is a useful truism that, as Michael White pointed out as early as 1999, 'the long term trend is always against a sitting premier . . . ultimately (his colleagues) will turn against him'.[67] It has also been argued that there were always degenerative tendencies of long-serving governments.[68] Certainly, in the PLP, Blair was fighting the strains and stresses and thwarted ministerial ambitions generated by his length of time in office. And Brown was an unremitting, undermining pressure, albeit also an unrecognised asset useable by the managers in cementing loyalty to Blair in some critical internal discussions. What was described as the 'massive folly' of Iraq[69] did eat away at Blair's moral authority and became an impediment to the search for untrammelled supremacy rather than his hoped-for facilitating agency.

That points up the fact that Leaders have managers and allies and can create important elements of their own conditions and in that process make their own replenishment or undermine their strengths. Blair had by the third term been Prime Minister of a government creating very favourable elements of the political context which were sustained or further developed – economic success, a record public sector investment and defence of public safety. He had built enormous management resources and there was no degeneration of his communicational and presentational talents. The party's historic reluctance to seek eviction also gave him much to draw upon. The question is: why, with these defences, was he forced out at the stage that it happened, and with a highly unusual method?

The case made here is that to understand Blair's eviction we have to refocus on to the problem and consequences of his party management and that Blair's eventual downfall had deeper roots and broader interlinked causes in what was a more integrated party. The causes were specific to his leadership, including his long-term lack of respect, and the acute failure to involve the party in consultation on early policy-formulation. The management he had encouraged had tarnished Blair with the reputation for manipulation and duplicity, and that continued to generate distrust. Even the very perceptive admirer Rentoul described him in March 2006 as 'a politician of a ruthlessness and procedural amorality that is sometimes breathtaking'.[70]

On at least four occasions shown in this study, Blair gave indications that he was considering changing his leadership style or had changed it already. Significantly, that never transpired, and in the aftermath of a third election victory with new No. 10 staff nearer to his own inclinations, he sought means to keep his foot down on the accelerator of radical legacy-seeking leadership. Resistance to his form of leadership and management together with distrust of his behaviour and intentions contributed to the undermining of management effectiveness across all the different forums. The degeneration of the management that had so successfully protected him and advanced his causes became the crucial development of this third term.

Managerial degeneration

That degeneration began in conflicts with TULO in 2005 over limitations in the ministerial implementation of the Warwick Agreement, which had been seen as a new unifying arrangement. At the party conference, Blair's plans for local party reform ignored the party consultations and NEC decisions, but on that he had to retreat. On the annual NEC away day, held in November, a session on 'making the NEC work better' became the setting for a powerful reaction to the aggravations of the management of the past eight years. Following the conference and the sudden resignation of the General Secretary, the No. 10 staff became split over the new appointment. The Leader's preference remained for Ray Collins but another party official, Peter Watt, was elected. He appeared to some who voted for him to be returning to the role of party officials as civil servant but he proved to be operating within a Blair-like framework.

In the Commons, two defeats on counter-terrorism proposals were especially significant because they were on Blair's chosen and strongest terrain and raised major doubts about his judgement. Two further defeats, one the Racial and Religious Hatred Bill, were attributed by some MPs to sinking morale and failure to keep contact with the rebels and party opinion; a pattern of growing non-cooperation with the whips was detected, including hiding voting intentions. Proposals to impose more discipline with sanctions against dissent in the House failed to gain Parliamentary Committee support in the remaining period of his leadership.

What became the Education and Inspections Bill was carried into law but only after major amendment and a revolt which involved a public policy dissent by Prescott and what appeared to opposition across the party. Blair's vulnerability increased when it was publicly acknowledged on 16 March 2006 that in the use of loans to the party he had evaded the rules on British political finance that he had himself initiated. The form of it led to the charge of acting like a party within a party, and it led also to an attempted reassertion of the NEC role in finance management. However, Blair used it as an opportunity to seek major reform of the union-party financial relationship as part of his legacy, with managers operating covertly behind the scenes through the Hayden Phillips inquiry. After a protracted argument, this Downing Street position was thwarted. There was a formal return to the agreed party policy on finance and another sign of the deterioration of Blair's managerial position.

In a particularly important but barely noticed development, the strains of Blair's leadership style and legacy radicalism caused increasing intra-managerial tensions. As with the PLP managers, the NEC managers now became more divided between the managerial officials and the managerial representatives. There was new linkage amongst representatives across the party, independent of the officials. On the NEC, representatives in the officers' meeting, significantly including Prescott, became increasingly concerned over Blair's governing style and management. Although still going along with the procedural defence erected against party assault on the Leader's tenancy, they protected what they regarded as the party's interest and resisted proposals they regarded as potentially damaging to the union-party relationship.

The end of the rolling coup?

Very significant around this time was an unnoticed double non-event. In June 2006 Blair's initiative to change the party rules to include proposals for registered supporters was contested and halted by Prescott and the party's officers' meeting after much of the list of such supporters was judged to be invalid. It indicated that Blair's major party management project was in serious trouble, and that following the public argument over education policy, his understanding with Prescott about loyalty was now in question. Also indicated and also unnoticed was that given the potential reaction at a senior level of the party, a further extension of the managerial rolling coup would, unless it was so thoroughly hidden as to be useless, cause more trouble than it avoided. As events were to show, the coup had ceased to roll.

Notice of termination and the paradox of Blair's management

In the literature much attention is rightly focused on the 'Brownite' role in Blair's eviction but crucial failures of management received little or no attention. Strong management can generate major weaknesses. The self-protective and uncertain time limit that Blair had instituted to protect his reign created increasing demands for more clarification and increasing frustration amongst those around his unremitting rival, Brown. Crucially, the first major weakness was that there had emerged a growing concern about Blair's self-preoccupation rather than a concern for the future viability of the party, and there was growing scepticism about the importance he attached to departing when it was in the party's interest rather than in his own.

The form of revolt which Blair later described as 'irredeemably old-fashioned' behaviour was shaped by the irredeemably Blairite management failure to accept a modern workable procedure for removal of a Leader who might be judged *in extremis* as undesirable. There was a managerial interpretation of the rules to impede the initiation of the procedure, so that the revolt had to go outside formal processes. It may even have been more effective in the surprise of that happening, and in practice it also highlighted a centre-ground reluctance to commit to Blair's defence. The reaction to Blair's style of leadership and the proto-factional reputation of the whips had also resulted in the growth of non-cooperation, the usual multiplicity of managerial ears and friendly informers to be expected at such a time becoming very limited in producing specific advance details for No. 10, the whips' office, the PLP office or party headquarters.

Dissidents directly involved in the revolt unexpectedly came mainly from those thought to be serial loyalists with little recent record of dissent and with strong regular links to management. They had come to see the whips' office management as, like headquarters, heavily Blairite factionalised and operating a one-directional partisanship which was ineffective in conveying the party view. That led the rebels to believe that they had to go round the whips' office in order to guarantee prompt action.

Finally but perhaps the most important, Blair and the managers had a confident sense of the apparently entrenched procedural power of their defensive position created in headquarters to avoid a challenge to Blair. This led to a complacency that any immediate danger to the Leader had been thwarted and also to a failure of imagination about what alternative form rebellion might take. A reasonable encapsulation of the immediate causes of the eviction would be that in this, the most heavily managed and integrated party in Labour history, a feature which initially appeared to be strengthening managed unity under more central control, had become an agency for the spread of revolt. Blair was brought down when, as he later acknowledged, he did not want to go, by a combination of deep personal distrust linked to a crisis of his party management.

Section IV: characterisations: politics and power

Overall, how is this experience of Blair's party management to be characterised in terms of the form of politics and the relations of power? The striking feature was the combination of skilful, audacious leadership with flexible procedural values in tandem with an enhanced managerial machine based on a major change in organisation and culture, including political obligations. This creation, the Leader's vanguard organisation, was the first move in an unprecedented covert managerial coup, subject to rolling extensions, creating the capacity to extend the collective resources of the leadership and particularly to enlarge and defend the Leader's personal influence. So pervasive was much of this management in the extra-parliamentary party and so pre-eminent was it over procedural values that the party is best understood (if clumsily expressed) as a managerised party, and the democracy as a managed democracy. The public claim by party officials that Blair 'won the argument for change within the party'[71] obscures the evidence provided here of the scope and extent of other managerial methods. It is also misleading to portray 'New Labour' change as, in Meg Russell's description, resulting from 'negotiation'.[72] The rolling coup and managerial use of extensive manipulative practice were the negation of negotiation.

Management and its relations with the unions exhibited an asymmetrical normative order with two generally contrasting patterns of behaviour affecting the form of politics and the exercise of effective power. Party officials, as 'political organisers', performed their role according to a code which gave them room for the exercise of more influence, even a liberation from control, in securing the Leader's objectives. The trade union leaders and supporting union officials, in contrast, as party affiliates or through the TUC, generally performed according to a role definition and 'rules' which created inhibitions and constraints in relation to party activity, policy-making, and party regime change. With a degree of exceptional friendly management support, however, they did achieve limited representational extensions to their party role.

Once in government, the ways of communication management could be encapsulated, as it was by Ivor Gabor, as a 'Millbankisation' of government,[73] as managerial attitudes and practices were transferred from one area to another. It also has to be said that the management transfer went much wider and that also under the guise of a partnership in power a 'governmentalisation' took place of the party's communication machinery, policy and decision-making processes to ensure compliance. There was a mutually reinforcing education here in values, priorities and the use of power, advantageous to the leadership.

The overall resulting power relations corresponded in great measure with what Thomson described as a Leader-centred party[74] and much of the time with what Quinn described as a leadership-dominated structure.[75] It also involved enough to justify describing it as Heffernan put it, 'the strongest, most centralised, leadership Labour has known; more powerful than the "social democratic centralism", of 1930–70',[76] described by Shaw in his seminal study of 1988. Shaw himself later gave a more qualified version but still encapsulated a new democratic centralism in which there was 'a much more solidly implanted centripetal pattern of power'.[77] All of that unsurprisingly confirms the main thrust of the diagnosis of the concentration of power forecastable from both Michels and McKenzie.[78] But those statements of tendency can be strengthened or counteracted by other local contextual forces. Here they have to be coupled with the extraordinary culture, organisation, scope, intensity, facilities and methods of management. And they were driven by the attempts to influence the business alliance and the expansion of political marketing; these entwined and intensified the pressures for control.

However, previous studies also suggest a limited understanding can be derived from an assumption of inevitabilities drawn from Michels and McKenzie and the seductive polarised model of power. Under Wilson, the modernising Leader of the 1960s, it had been found that 'no simple categorisation of the distribution of power' did justice 'to its subtlety and variability'.[79] Despite striking appearances to the contrary, and even with the extraordinary extra powers created through Blair's managerised party, this same insight retained its force. In different locations over time, the evidence did not fit as easily into a one-dimensional one-directional characterisation. Power relations around and arising from party management were not the static condition often assumed to be the case by the descriptions of 'command and control'. Relations were changeable either in ethos or mechanisms or new organisational initiatives, subject to movement and counter-movement in both directions with extensions of control but also regular contestation and sometimes revolt against overbearing or threatening management.

Spin doctors and some journalistic rhetoric helped perpetuate a myth of supremacy. 'Total control', it was said, was 'imposed on the party' by Blair,[80] or by Blair and Brown together.[81] Yet the evidence here, and the warnings from Labour culture and archaeology, indicate that it could not be. A view of the NEC and the party conference as 'mere shells'[82] misses their spheres of continuing importance, including reactions to Blairite management, even within their diminished role. Prescott was generally a unifying loyalist figure working with management, but the characterisation of his muzzled subordination to Blair is far off the mark. His self-ascribed role as 'protector of the party' was in evidence both at the beginning and at the end of Blair's leadership. A PLP showing what was described as 'a new conformity'[83] in House votes, and revealed here, the covert curtailment by the leadership of agreed procedures for shared policy formulation, suggests an unusual degree of ascendancy. Yet behind that, PLP representatives were involved in a prolonged and generally successful private battle of PLP self-defence against the central managing officials and at times against the Leader and Chief Whip. In this arena the supremacy model never existed.

Shaw's terminology is useful in emphasising the centrifugal features, but it must also register the centripetal resistance and its far-reaching consequences in preserving, even replenishing, alternative procedural traditions and protecting a non-Blairite version of the party. This resistance came not just from the left as Mair suggested,[84] but at times involved the party mainstream and in Opposition, the traditional right. It was remarkable that some dissenting expressions were even transposed into management itself, before the party attained governmental power and especially in the first and third terms of government. Amongst the managers, appointed and elected, including the Deputy Leader, there were at times significant differences over the form of the party, the methods of achieving discipline, and relations between the members, activists and leadership.

Blair's procedural first preference involved a plebiscitarian party working with a plebiscitary government. Yet the extent of opposition, the practical difficulties, the reputational damage from the Road to the Manifesto experience, and a managerial revolt caused the demise of that dream – at least for this Leader. Reforms carried though in Bennister's description as 'subjugation to a charismatic Leader',[85] were limited in scope and in authoritative completion. In terms of his purposes he had not, as Barber and so many others concluded, 'successfully transformed a political party'[86] nor fully, as Seldon concluded, 'succeeded in remodelling his party'.[87]

After the gains made under the cleverly misleading managerial guise of 'the end of control freakery', a counter-management operation was created and strengthened by the TULO unions building on the legitimisation provided by managerial tactics at the NPF in 2000, operating now in a form which led to the Warwick Agreement of 2004. Even with the new limitations placed on the unions under Blair, this was still more a 'labour party' than the party of Blairite preference. The Gould characterisation of unions as a 'conservative' force[88] was true of their protection of their right to remain affiliated and to collectively advance and defend the interests of labour. But the union role in relations with the party, whilst it became more frustrated with the managers, remained flexible and capable of renewal and adaptation. Through the PLP trade union group and through TULO, a still significant 'dialectical element'[89] in action-reaction relations with the managing political leadership was replenished, despite many modern descriptions and predictions to the contrary and without resort to financial sanctions.

In the third term, the 'solidly implanted' pattern of power was undermined as in the more integrated party the whole interlinked management structure degenerated, with Prescott moving back to his role as party protector. The new-legacy radicalism of Blair's staff became matched by a new managerial deviance when elected representatives in the PLP and NEC were brought into conflict with managerial officials. In their role at the apex of the two 'bureaucracies', appointed and elected, they ceased to be simply, in Panebianco's language, unified 'tools of the party's dominant coalition'.[90] Blair was unable to extend the rolling coup in a way which removed limitations on his leadership and management. The notice to quit confirmed in the party sphere Hennessy's diagnosis in examining British government that 'Command models, Napoleonic or otherwise, have a habit of ending in tears'.[91] And, as will be shown in Chapter 20, by 2007 the tears to be shed also extended to a range of dangerous new problems for the Labour

Party bequeathed by Blair's leadership and party management values. In that sense, whatever history makes of the rest of his record, in its political behaviour, the Blair dynamo had driven a significant and very damaging legacy.

Notes

1 *Observer*, 28 July 1996.
2 Michael Foley, *The British Presidency: Tony Blair and the Politics of Public Leadership*, Manchester University Press, Manchester, 2000, p. 110.
3 Paul Allender, 'What's New about 'New Labour?', *Politics* 21(1), February 2001, pp. 56–62.
4 *Guardian*, 6 July 1995.
5 Minkin, *Contentious Alliance*, especially Chapter 2, pp. 26–48.
6 Ibid. p. 386 and p. 658.
7 Foley, *British Presidency*, p. 101.
8 Meg Russell, *Building New Labour: the Politics of Party Organisation*, Palgrave Macmillan, Basingstoke, 2005, p. 183.
9 John Rentoul, *Tony Blair: Prime Minister*, Little Brown, London, 2001; Anthony Seldon, *The Blair Effect: The Blair Government 1997–2001*, Brown, London, 2001.
10 Donald Macintyre, *Mandelson: the Biography*, HarperCollins, London 1999, p. 278.
11 *Guardian*, 10 June 1995.
12 David Mitchie, *The Invisible Persuaders*, Bantam, London, 1998, p. 292.
13 David Coates, pamphlet *Raising Lazarus*, Fabian Society, 2005, p. 25.
14 *Daily Telegraph*, 16 November 2001.
15 Eric Shaw, *Losing Labour's Soul: New Labour and the Blair Government 1997–2007*, Routledge, London, 2007, p. 141.
16 Do 3/10/97, NEC minutes, 29 October 1997.
17 David Osler, *Labour Party PLC: New Labour as a Party of Business*, Mainstream Publishing, Edinburgh, 2002.
18 Stuart Hall, 'New Labour's Double Shuffle', *Soundings* 24, 2003, pp. 10–24.
19 Philip Gould, *The Unfinished Revolution: How the Modernisers saved the Labour Party*, Little Brown, London, 1998, pp. 262–7.
20 Dennis Kavanagh and Anthony Seldon, *The Powers Behind the Prime Minister: the Hidden Influence of Number Ten*, HarperCollins, London, 2000, p. 287.
21 Labour Party Press Release, 29 March 1996.
22 Patrick Seyd, 'New Parties/New Politics? A Case Study of the British Labour Party', *Party Politics* 15(3), July 1999, pp. 383–405.
23 Ibid.
24 Matthew Taylor, *Political Exclusion: Changing the Political Culture*, firstthoughts pamphlet, Local Government Association, 2000, p. 11.
25 Jon Cruddas and Matthew Taylor, 'New Labour New Links', Unions 21 seminar paper 1998.
26 Paul Richards, *Progress*, Autumn 1996, p. 20.
27 Macintyre, *Mandelson*, p. 315.
28 Kenneth O. Morgan, 'New Labour in Historical Perspective', in Seldon, *The Blair Effect*, 2001, p. 584.

29 *Partnership in Power*, p. 7.
30 Patrick Seyd, 'Labour Government-Party Relationships: Maturity or Marginalisation?', in Anthony King (ed.), *Britain at the Polls 2001*, Chatham House, New York, 2002, p. 101.
31 Peter Mandelson and Roger Liddle, *The Blair Revolution: Can New Labour Deliver?*, Faber & Faber, London, 1996, p. 231.
32 Graham Allen, MP, *The Last Prime Minister: Being Honest about the UK Presidency*, Graham Allen, House of Commons, 2001, p. 31.
33 Ibid.
34 Cruddas and Taylor, 'New Labour New Links' Unions 21 seminar paper 1998.
35 Simon Jenkins, *Thatcher and Sons: a Revolution in Three Acts*, Penguin, London, 2006, p. 232. Also, Henry Porter, *Independent*, 31 December 2006.
36 *Guardian*, 29 August 2007.
37 'The Coffee House', *Spectator*, 23 September 2008.
38 Chris Grey, *A Very Short Fairly Interesting and Reasonably Cheap Book about Studying Organisations*, Sage, London, 2005.
39 Michael Foley, *John Major, Tony Blair and a Conflict of Leadership: Collision Course*, Manchester University Press, Manchester, 2002, p. 162.
40 Report of PLP Review Committee, 1996, p. 2.
41 Philip Norton (Lord Norton of Louth), 'Governing Alone', *Parliamentary Affairs*, 56(4), October 2003, p. 557, citing a *Times* article by Miles.
42 Mark Bennister, 'Blair and Howard: Comparative Predominance and "Institutional stretch" in the UK and Australia', *British Journal of International Relations* 9(3), August 2007, p. 334.
43 Philip Cowley, *The Rebels: How Blair Mislaid his Majority*, Politico's, London, 2005, Chapter 5, pp. 106–34.
44 Ann Black, National Policy Forum Report, 29/30 November 2002, dated 12 December 2002.
45 Russell, *Building New Labour*, p. 279.
46 *Guardian*, 29 May 2012.
47 Parliament First, *Parliament's Last Chance*, 2003, p. 26.
48 *Partnership in Power*, p. 2.
49 LPCR 1998, p. 13.
50 *House Magazine*, 8 September 1997.
51 Thomas Quinn, *Modernising the Labour Party: Organisational Change since 1983*, Palgrave Macmillan, Basingstoke, 2004, p. 189.
52 Mandelson and Liddle, *Blair Revolution*, p. 215.
53 Peter Mandelson, *The Blair Revolution Revisited*, Politico's, London, 2002, p. xxv.
54 ICM/ *Guardian*, 24 July 2004.
55 Andrew Chadwick and Richard Heffernan (eds), *The New Labour Reader*, Polity Press, London, 2003, p. 5.
56 Robert McKenzie, *British Political Parties: the Distribution of Power within the Conservative and Labour Parties*, Mercury Books, London, 1955, p. 505.
57 Steve Ludlam and Andrew Taylor, 'Political Representation of the Labour Interest', *British Journal of Industrial Relations* 41(4), 2003, p. 734.
58 *Sunday Telegraph*, 20 November 2005.
59 Dennis Kavanagh and David Butler, *The General Election of 2005*, Palgrave Macmillan, Basingstoke, 2005, p. 25.

60 Lewis Baston and Simon Henig, 'The Labour Party', in Anthony Seldon and Dennis Kavanagh (eds), *The Blair Effect 2001–5*, Cambridge University Press, 2005, p. 115.

61 John McIlroy, 'Under Stress But Still Enduring', in Gary Daniels and John McIlroy, *Trade Unions in a Neo-Liberal World: British Trade Unions under New Labour*, Routledge, London, 2009, p. 166.

62 *Sunday Times*, 4 August 1996.

63 Patrick Seyd, 'New Parties/New Politics?', *Party Politics* 5(3), 1999, p. 307. Also unpublished data on new members supplied by Patrick Seyd from the Seyd and Whiteley study of New Labour's Grassroots: 2002, covering the period 1990–1999.

64 John McIlroy, 'The Enduring Alliance? Trade Unions and the Making of New Labour 1994–7', *British Journal of Industrial Relations* 36(4), 1998, pp. 537–64.

65 NEC Minutes decision, 24 July 2001. Rulebook 2002, Clause II 2(i), National Trade Union and Labour Party Liaison Organisation.

66 Minkin, *Contentious Alliance*, pp. 651–3.

67 *Guardian*, 21 January 1999, quoted in Foley, *British Presidency*, p. 327.

68 Timothy Heppel, 'The Degenerative Tendencies of Long-serving Governments', *Parliamentary Affairs* 61(4), October 2008, pp. 578–96.

69 Chris Mullin, *Decline and Fall*, Profile Books, London, 2010, p. 174.

70 *Independent*, 26 March 2006.

71 Letter from twelve officials and advisers to the *Guardian*, 17 May 2008.

72 Russell, *Building New Labour*, p. 251.

73 *New Statesman*, 19 June 1998.

74 Stuart Thomson, 'The Changing Structure of the Labour Party: A Leader-centred Party'. Unpublished paper, Political Studies Association conference 1999.

75 Quinn, *Modernising the Labour Party*, p. 179.

76 Richard Heffernan, 'Politics of the Parliamentary Labour Party', in Brian Brivati and Richard Heffernan, *The Labour Party: a Centenary History*, Macmillan, London, 2000, p. 254.

77 Eric Shaw, 'New Labour in Britain: New Democratic Centralism?', *West European Politics* 25(3), 2002, p. 166.

78 Robert McKenzie, *British Political Parties: the Distribution of Power within the Conservative and Labour Parties*, Mercury Books, London, 1955; Robert Michels, *Political Parties: A Sociological Study of the Oligarchical Tendencies of Modern Democracy*, Hearst's International Library Co., 1915.

79 Minkin, *Labour Party Conference*, p. 317.

80 Henry Porter, *Independent*, 31 December 2006. See also Jenkins, *Thatcher and Sons*, p. 232.

81 Steve Richards, *Whatever it Takes: The Real Story of Gordon Brown and New Labour*, Fourth Estate, London, 2010, p. 123.

82 Ross McKibbin, 'The Destruction of the Public Sphere', *London Review of Books* 28(1), 5 January 2006.

83 Allen, *The Last Prime Minister*, p. 31.

84 Peter Mair, 'Partyless Democracy', *New Left Review* 2, March/April 2000, pp. 21–9.

85 Bennister, *Blair and Howard*, p. 327.

86 Michael Barber, *Instructions to Deliver: Tony Blair, Public Services and the Challenge of Achieving Targets*, Politico's, London, 2007, p. 305.
87 Anthony Seldon, 'The Second Blair Government: the Verdict', in Anthony Seldon and Dennis Kavanagh (eds), *The Blair Effect 2001–5*, Cambridge University Press, Cambridge, 2005, p. 410.
88 Philip Gould, *The Unfinished Revolution: How the Modernisers saved the Labour Party*, Little Brown, London, 1998, p. 25.
89 Minkin, *Labour Party Conference*, 1978, p. 317.
90 Angelo Panebianco, *Political Parties: Organisation and Power*, Cambridge University Press, Cambridge, 1988, p. 224.
91 Peter Hennessy, *The Blair Centre: a Question of Command and Control*, Public Management Foundation, London, 1999, p. 18.

20

Evaluation and perspectives

The managerial success story

An important evaluation of the legacy of that managerial experience has
to begin by engaging with the perspective of what may be called the supportive realist. A composite of comments heard often in the privacy of
dialogue with party officials and politicians goes as follows: 'OK, perhaps
this is near how things happened, and the power tactics involved in management. Management is difficult. This shows that managers were doing
a good job and a smart job, contributing to the election of a three-term
Labour government. Important progressive changes were carried through
in the party; the party was prepared for power and the 'New Labour'
governments were protected. There were many policy achievements. The
wilder party forces were kept in check and the unions were no longer seen
as commanding ogres standing over Labour's leaders. Management has
always tried to carry out that helpful function; it was absolutely necessary.
You can't take the politics out of management. What matters is what works.
This is a success story; end of story'.

Those views have an immediate plausibility, and in Chapter 4 the reasons
for the form of this management and the influences which brought it about
are fully acknowledged. At the heart of it was an understandable eagerness
about advancing the party's electoral chances and safeguarding a Labour
government. Chapter 19 can be read in great measure as a summary of
considerable, although not total, success. There is no denying the skills,
commitment and, at times, audacity of those who led and managed the
party. In different ways, the managerial 'good job', with different balances
of methods and tactical ingredients, involved sophisticated expertise. And
as shown, the management's most striking and important feature was its
pervasive impositional and particularly manipulative successes.

The most important accomplishment was the covert creation of the
new organisation and culture of the management. Then there was a 'rolling coup', which periodically changed the conditions of political conflict
in ways that strengthened Blair's leadership. Party officials moved to a
different definition of their role. And the operative version of Partnership
in Power turned it into a mechanism of Blair's influence and insulation
with the NEC policy role taken away. There was also the creation of
a stable loyalist block at the NPF via partisan officials and a heavily

managed electoral process. Removal of the Leader was made more difficult. The manipulative skills proved to be particularly effective in one key period in 2001 by imposing the hidden role of the new Party Chair and particularly the covert changes in the rules of the PLP. More and bolder management became hidden behind the façade of 'the end of control freakery'. Perhaps the greatest individual policy success was the filtering and suppression of the view of the party in the country over Iraq, followed by Blair at his most impressive presenting his case in the Commons and then the absence of accountability here as over other developments. From a narrow perspective, all this could be evaluated as the epitome of successful political artistry.

It also has to be accepted that, regrettable though it is to a pure view of democracy, party management in some form is probably a universal function within political parties. Sat in the Leader's chair, there is always a case for adding to authority and rhetorical skills by advance regular managed understandings, consultative networks, favourable agenda settings and tactical devices seen as necessary to make relationships and institutions work towards the best outcomes. Nevertheless, the defence of management is not the defence of every form in every forum. Still less is the claim of exceptionality and unusual circumstances a reasonable justification for all actions all the time.

'New Labour' management was often portrayed by its defenders in terms of a giant dichotomy with the virtues of 'now' contrasted with the worst of 'then'. Yet management can involve diverse combinations of encouragement and trust, persuasion and alliance, receptivity, and facilitation, as well as imposition and manipulation. It can embrace the roles of political organiser and civil servant in different proportions and varying sensitivities. In encouraging self-discipline it can also extend opportunities for early participation as well as attempting to curtail them. Every style and balance in management has its potentialities, including its capacity to create greater difficulties. As pointed out earlier, it was not unrealistic to visualise a modern politics under Smith, managed through mutual education with diminished manipulation and encouraging the growth of trust, and yet also achieving electoral victory.

It is probably right that the art of leadership invariably has a dark side, as N.G. Bailey asserted,[1] but it is just as important to proclaim that it can be limited by inhibitions and constraints, thus becoming less free to operate. The dark actions can vary from the trivial, spasmodic and minimal to the fundamental, regular and comprehensive – the form that it approached in management under Blair. Only time will tell what measure of greater good in Blair government policy achievement may be viewed as justifying some of the behaviour revealed here. At the moment, the policy record evokes a very mixed policy judgement, best summed up perhaps in Toynbee and Walker's *The Verdict*.[2] That judgement is complicated by the fact that the contemporary Conservative-dominated coalition shows how far 'New Labour' had created space and established precedent for the Conservative policy agenda, and yet also illustrates what the differences were. But if we now bring an analytical examination to bear on party management and the conduct of politics under Blair, it shows that the realist's perspective is not the end of the story. It reveals the many problems that were created and raises huge danger signs for the party, for British politics and for Blair himself from his methods.

Management, misjudgement and the creation of problems

Warnings and blinkered realism

A basic feature of 'New Labour' party management was the strong sense of what had to be avoided in the behaviour of others but that they themselves had to be free to operate. This, together with the urgency of the managerial operation, the self-confidence about their diagnosis and skills in assisting the special mission, and the constantly guided media presentation of their success, adversely affected the ability of Blair and the managers to observe problems of their own behaviour and to listen to warnings about it. It became at times a wilful blindness in which the failure to change in the face of early warnings was striking. There had already been a forerunner, before he became Leader, in the early refusal of Blair and his allies in 1989–1993 to heed warnings that union reaction to separationist spin could create major obstacles in the way of candidate-selection reform – as it did, leaving a damaging and lasting legacy of distrust.

The fact was that, as outlined in Chapter 15, by 2000 virtually every major axiom and assumption of the confident new Labour management culture, as it emerged after 1994, proved to be faulty, unbalanced or highly problematic. In spite of warnings, the Blair methods became embedded in mindset and practice, and also eventually in party and public consciousness, with damage done in both spheres. There were particular warnings about the essential qualifications which needed to be made to claims of the benefits of strong leadership, for both party and electoral reasons. Blair's insightful biographer and supporter John Rentoul judged that 'He and Clinton appear to sense shifts in public opinion before they happen'.[3] Perhaps so, but many of Blair's anticipations of the attitudes and behaviour of the electorate which touched on leadership and party management turned out to be insensitive and faulty, and when such misunderstandings were finally detected it took time for him to adjust in the light of his absolute confidence in his instincts and judgement and his version of strong bold leadership.

Years later, as Blair became a hero to a section of Conservative opinion under Cameron, the normally very sophisticated columnist Matthew D'Ancona made the judgment, in giving advice to the Tory Prime Minister Cameron, that 'no party leader was ever punished electorally for taking a firm grip on his or her party'.[4] That was simply wrong. In practice, the electoral response depended on what the grip involved and the public's views on the leader's judgement. What happened over the London Mayor indicated very clearly that criticism of the processes adopted by politicians to take a firm grip could get in the way of judgements of policies and objectives. Blair was punished (as was the party) by losing the London contest as he had done in Uxbridge and Falkirk, and losing the Wales Assembly elections, following the mismanagement of the Wales leadership election, causing him to go 'f-ing and blinding'.[5]

There was a strikingly mistaken prediction about the likely pattern of future alignment. Amongst the managers there had been an initial assumption that the people would always be on the Leader's side in the tactics he used to battle against old Labour opponents in the party. Yet the manipulative treatment of Livingstone, following what had happened in Wales over Rhodri Morgan, made 'control freakery' unpopular, and it produced a conflict of party and people versus the strong leader and his managers. That same alignment happened again in the second-term policy over Iraq, and to some extent over the form of public sector reform. It was not that these or other problems of management were hard to discern. It was that, facing them, the 'New Labour' special people psyche, Blair's in particular, found it difficult to cope with their own errors and shortcomings. Warnings were not given due consideration until the damage became publicly obvious and especially destructive. This was blinkered realism and at times a wilful blindness. It was a condition which placed a giant question mark over the value of such a heavily controlling management.

Attachment of the Leader and managers to the axioms of 'New Labour' party management forged in one era made it difficult to consistently challenge their own beliefs in the next, when the situation – including party and public opinion – had significantly changed. The culture and strategy developed after 1994, heavily influenced by perceptions of the 1970s and 1980s, was an inadequate grounding for what needed to be done about a declining, devitalised and devalued party, losing both manual working-class support and a section of the radical middle class. The central management frequently urged others to 'move on' from their past behaviour but, as some of them tardily and grimly acknowledged, they found 'moving on' themselves very uncomfortable.

Of the greatest significance was that Blair's professed objectives had been accompanied by an extraordinary honeymoon with the electorate which had raised hopes of a new politics and a new politician who was straight and trustworthy. Privately however, as shown here, they were also accompanied by an approving 'New Labour' view of the professional skills of manipulation as a way of getting things done effectively. Intra-party resentment over this eventually became allied to the strength of the rebellious tradition in British politics, and that further contributed towards a developing anti-manipulative ethos.

Management and self-deceit

Further, a confidence in the benefits of strong and bold leadership and heavy management, when reinforced by the spin-declaring supremacy and success, acted at times as a form of self-deceit and contributed to some significant specific failures. Over lone parent benefit in 1997, the manipulated avoidance of a conference debate hindered understanding of and advance preparation for the first major PLP revolt that shook the leadership. Manipulated victory over pensions and the welfare review at the NPF in 1999 created the assumption that it could be easily driven through in 2000. It could not, and the public row was all the greater. The past manipulation of the NEC, including unauthorised abolition of its policy committee, gave a misplaced confidence about further subversion of its role at the 2005 Conference, and miscalculated the reaction that it then provoked. The managerially organised enthusiasm for Blair's policy on the 90-day detention vote in 2006 led to a misreading of PLP support, encouraging Blair in the headlong charge to a damaging defeat that impressed neither the PLP nor the electorate. In 2006, confidence over the 'sewing up' of the procedure for evicting the Leader misled Blair's managers about the security of his position, contributing to a complacency which left them significantly unprepared for an alternative form of attack which, without formal warning, pushed him to a date of departure.

'New Labour' reform, manipulation and conservatism

Aspiration, manipulation and conservatism

There was another self-defeating reason why attitudes towards this form of managed democracy and its excesses created special difficulties. An aspiration for a modernised party democracy was a feature of the early ideals of 'the modernisers', especially in the early battle over OMOV. They often argued that the problem of reforming the Labour Party was its conservatism. This was Gould's case in *The Unfinished Revolution*. The case was overstated, but also what could increasingly be seen after 1997, although not by all Blair's managers, was the problem created for the aspiration of party reform by the practices of 'New Labour' management. The vice of 'an apparent willingness to go outside the spirit of the democratic rules', Matthew Taylor's later description,[6] undermined the moral authority of the 'New Labour' reformers. Management was specially discredited by the obsessive search to maximise control and by the inconsistency of procedural values in pursuit of 'a good result'. Mandelson and Liddle declared that 'like any group of people who are given democratic rights, Labour Party members are not going to allow them to be taken away'.[7] In practice, by adroit controlling devices, that was exactly what was managed to happen, undermining morale and trust.

In elections for the NPF, one-member-one-vote (OMOV), which had been the focus of the original Blairite crusade for members' power, was for managerial reasons rejected, and the elections later became loaded by the partisan behaviour of officials and the abolition of open hustings. Members' representation was disadvantaged also in the reduced composition of the CLPs on the NEC. They lost the ability to vote for national politicians on the NEC, yet it was managerially convenient for members of the House of Lords to be judged to be 'rank and file'. OMOV was abandoned when it failed to satisfy the needs of party management over European selections and over the Wales and London selections. As a principle it was not fully 're-established', as Russell appears to suggest.[8] In the face of the hostility of Blair's managers, it was not brought in either for candidate reselection or in elections to the National Constitutional Committee. A party victory over the Leader and the managers concerning OMOV for representation at the NPF did not happen until 2009, when there was an accumulation of pressure from all sections of the party (see Chapter 21, pp. 754–5).

Stringing them along and distrust

We make ourselves as we make our history. Blair became adept at, and psychologically unable to move away from, the tactic of stringing people along about their future role, suspected by one of his closest allies Mandelson[9] and patently obvious about Brown.[10] It was also, as illustrated in this study, integral to his repeated treatment of the party through apparent acceptances, hints and declarations of change over the process of policy-formulation. All of this added to deepening distrust and deteriorating relations. In Powell's analysis of the eviction of Blair in 2006, the ex-chief of staff's observations showed a remarkable distortion of perception. Although he emphasised the importance of encouraging trust between Northern Ireland politicians in arriving at an agreement,[11] and warned that a minister seeking his own ends was not to be trusted,[12] he made no mention at all of Blair's loss of trust as a factor in his self-generated problems and his downfall.

Much later, Mandelson lamented that serious efforts at party reform ended the day after the election victory of 1997.[13] As shown here, this was not the case: Partnership in Power was implemented after the election, but in a control-distorted trust-destroying form. Proposals coming from the leadership for abolition of the General Committee in the local parties met some traditional conservatism, and were damaged by practical weaknesses in the managerial case, but primarily they were destroyed by heightened distrust of the behaviour of the party centre and the spin, including from Mandelson, which appeared to be a likely cover for other objectives. Similarly, distrust contaminated the next major Blairite reform proposals, for registered supporters. Suspicion over controversial leadership proposals became the offspring of Blair's management. That was the penalty for mis-leading.

Strong leadership, policy-formulation and disunity

'I have no reverse gear', Blair proclaimed in 2003 as an expression of virtue and pride, rerunning, some thought, a 'New Labour' version of Thatcher's strength. Yet their strong leadership was not as popular as was often assumed in the parliamentary arena. Confirming and refining the Joseph Rowntree/ICM 1996 findings noted in Chapter 15, which had received little attention from commentators, the Committee on Standards in Public life came up with some startling survey evidence in 2004 and 2006. In judging the preferred influence on an MP's vote on national issues, the general public tended to favour first what would benefit the people of the country as a whole; second, what the election manifesto promised; third, what would benefit the people living in the constituency; fourth, what the MP personally believed to be right; and fifth, what local party members would want.[14] All of these were ranked with greater favour than how the party leadership thought that the MP should vote, and public rejection of leadership dictation over MPs grew during Blair's third-term radicalism.

Mishandling the public sector

And although leadership boldness has an attractive and sometimes imperative place in politics, it has to be combined with wisdom and judgement. Blair had at times much of both but there were acute dangers in the regular 'go for it' approach to policy-formulation; what the ex-No. 10 adviser Peter Hyman later described as the 'shit or bust' style that he appeared to judge admirable in Blair.[15] It involved a contradiction in purpose. Avoiding party disunity and its media vulnerability had been a major goal of the management urged on the PLP. Yet, under Blair, the regular vanguardism and strong leadership involved increasingly positioning in relation to business and the right-wing press. They became an institutionalised form of 'the bounce' challenging the party to defeat him and damage the government. As Robin Cook complained in relation to the advocacy of large-scale private sector involvement in the health service, it was 'not a sensible way of proceeding'.[16]

Too much rested on the Leader's judgement. Tony Wright MP, chairing the Parliamentary Liaison Committee and questioning Blair, noted of the public sector policy, 'If I said to you where is the Government document that sets out the intellectual case for these propositions, where is the evidence amassed, where is the international examples assembled? I would suggest to you that there is not such a document'.[17]

The political management of public-services policy which dominated various rows in the second term, might have been started with an extensive party partnership enquiry into problems and potential solutions. Instead, it was foisted on the PLP, the party at large, and the public in repeated government initiatives which became a provocation to new dissent and reinforced a reluctance to cooperate. It is regarded as a fact of commercial life that the best marketing of a company product is done by enthusiatic staff, yet staff in the health service were the most disgruntled in the public sector. Some of that can be put down to the problem of repetitive large-scale reorganisation, undermining morale. But it was also influenced by the health service unions' political experience of imposed reforms and their deteriorating relations with the party managers which led union officials into passing downwards their resentment.

Blair's reasoning on policy-formulation was later revealed to be that 'nothing gets done unless it's driven from the top',[18] and that 'people expected governments to take unpopular decisions, expected to complain about them and expected leadership to overcome complaint'.[19] That would have been a reassurance to any thoughtful aspirant autocrat throughout history and, for Blair, it was a useful justification of whatever he wanted to do. The downside, as Alastair Campbell noted much later, was that it was 'hard to drive though change without not just the mandate of the electorate but also its consent'.[20] Another downside of that perception was that the view of Blair as having sound judgement sank sharply from 27 per cent in October 1997 to 6 per cent in April 2004, rising to only 9 per cent in the pre-election poll of April 2005.[21] For 18 per cent of 'maybe Labour' voters it was Blair who was keeping them from Labour commitment.[22]

Damaged opportunities

Management, manipulation and the flaws of leadership

The Leader and his management were so intensely focused on control and narrowly focused delivery within the party that the lost opportunities of other forms of management were not given the attention they needed. This was particularly true of the management of Partnership in Power which had involved the most serious attempt in Labour's history to reconcile the traditions and justifications for intra-party democracy with the responsibilities and practicalities of government. The arrangements offered a sharing of problem identification and solution, with the possibility of a policy-formulation which heightened cooperation and enhanced unity, morale and party activity. From that perspective, it was in the interests of the party and its leading politicians to see that Partnership in Power became widely respected.

Yet, practical difficulties aside, the greatest problems of the partnership, as with the agreed relations with the PLP over departmental committees, arose from the failure of the Leader and the managers to abide by the sharing spirit and the ideal of mutual education. The old policy-making was said by Blair in 1998 to have been 'not an honest form of policymaking'.[23] Yet both the new PIP process and the role of the PLP departmental committees were subverted or hampered into dishonesty with his encouragement before they ever went into operation, and partnership was subject to the heavy hand of the Leader's managing police force. And far from the election manifesto being a prelude to a new party consensus and more trust, because it was not a genuine partnership product, it could not create for the party a sense of ownership.

As time went by, the managerial operation lived with huge inconsistencies at the heart of its behaviour arising from manipulation. Bold Blairism developed a passionate concern for choice in the public services even though consumer demand was not behind that priority in all the different aspects of public services. Yet time and again, Blairite politicians and managers were insensitive to increasing public and party reactions against a manipulation that loaded or threatened to impede political choice. Overall, this experience of leading the party and government confirms that even a talented and presentable Leader ought not to be left with inadequate checks and balances, especially when the Leader is working closely with a secret managerial system.

One profound historic warning on this might be taken from Dilbert: 'Life is just too complicated to be smart all the time'.[24] Another might be derived, in broadened form, probably from an original by Alastair Campbell: 'We are all psychologically flawed'. These were reasons why the undermining of a viable party process of accountability was so damaging. In addition, the consequence of this style of leadership and management policing was the nurturing of a fatalism-realism amongst members and MPs. This was true, as Powell noted, of the constraining effect on government departments,[25] and true of the PLP input and the wider party process. The concentration of power around the Leader and the policing management had its short-term advantages to him in terms of limiting obstacles to his action, but it also contributed to the devitalisation of other potentially creative innovators and decision-makers. Within the party Blair and his managers could never bring themselves to build upon the British quality of inventiveness which he had lauded appropriately in the 1997 manifesto.

Party concerns and misconceptions

The party abode of the unreasonable and the dangerous?
In justification of the form of leadership and the scale and character of managerial practices, the party, especially its conference, was often portrayed by managers and their supporters as it had been viewed in the 1970s, as an abode of the unreasonable who could not be guaranteed to fill an attractive electoral shop window. It was assumed that the party members and the unions were likely to go dangerously adrift of electoral opinion and to attempt to anchor the leadership to their suicidal electoral extremism. Management also took the view not only that the government must be allowed to govern, but that managerial qualifications for disrespect of

the party had special features. They had the authority, the information, and the electoral sensitivity of past occupants of the role and they also saw themselves as having the finely tuned judgement and rectitude of culture carriers of the future. The 'New Labour' cognoscenti always knew best. Yet as the argument has developed in this chapter, that view is very questionable.

True, conference delegates and the PLP, like everybody else, were not always knowledgeable or wise. And conference decisions could not all have the same claim to obligatory action regardless of the scale of party and public opinion. Many considerations came into play, and rejection of that absolute obligation was a strength of the realist's case. But not only had the leadership disposition to disrespect the conference many weaknesses arising from collateral and consequential damage but, as well, attention can be drawn to important ministerial and managerial examples in the period 1997 to 2007 which illuminate the fact that leadership and managerial responses to the conference were very mixed in quality, and key instances point to the wisdom of the party not the government.

The party policy of public ownership of railways was backed in 1995 by 57 per cent of voters,[26] but public ownership of railways was never implemented and it is doubtful whether it was ever intended to be. Nevertheless by 2009 the transport minister, Lord Adonis, was arguing that the government should have pulled the plug on privatisation.[27] The most controversial conference decision of the first term of government, the pensions link to earnings, rejected by Blair and Brown, had by 2009 become a policy orthodoxy. The NPF diagnosis of the social problem of predatory lending, and its prescription of personal culpability and sanctions over environmental pollution by business, were so hidden after the decisions of the 2000 conference that they were not able to be used to build up a public momentum. Both were innovative and the predatory-lending concern particularly is increasingly relevant.

In the second term, in 2002, a proposed review of the highly important public sector policy, PFI, supported by the conference majority and with solid majority public support across the political spectrum,[28] began a series of conference conflicts between the government and the unions. The review was not an unreasonable move given the problems being stored up; as the *Guardian* editorial declared, the unions were 'right to want a review and ministers wrong to deny them'.[29] By August 2011 PFI was judged by the Commons Treasury select committee as poor value for money and no more efficient than any other form of borrowing. In the second term also, the response to the social housing crisis was desperately slow in spite of overwhelming party support at the party conference and amongst the membership.[30] Government failure over this policy then became a particularly significant electoral problem related to the growth of anti-immigrant sentiment.

Voice and votes

Party managers often strongly argued for a shift from vote to voice in party procedures. Others, seeking a better quality of process, have also argued this case for a voice politics of mutual education. However, as attractive as that appeared, experience of the 'New Labour' years confirms that an interplay between voice politics and vote politics to register majority opinion at key stages is often essential. Whilst the sound of voices can be disputed in their accuracy, votes cannot. Horton and Katwala argued that the role of the party is just to exercise pressure though the voice.[31] Even if that was the limit, pressure is all the sharper if the voice is registered in a vote and especially if this vote is in advance of the government decision.

More than that, proponents of voice politics have to take account of the extensive management system which used 'voice politics' as a means of avoiding commitment. Indeed, what was most striking was not just the disjunction between some conference decisions and some leadership behaviour, it was the way that the party voice at the conference was managed into complete silence on some key issues. There was a case for renewing and improving the relationship with business, but its form and status was never thoroughly discussed nor therefore were the majority of the party and unions persuaded. As attendance at party meetings clearly indicated, privatisation was unpopular all the way through but it was never fully debated, let alone authorised. The party-wide welfare-state review after 1999 never happened. The role of the private sector in public sector policy was never fully debated in the party. Later, Trident was renewed without a party debate although as Blair later admitted, there were common sense and practical arguments against Trident.[32] What was decisive was the leadership's view of the national status of having a big weapon.

Over the most important policy issue, the Iraq war, an impressive Chicago speech by Blair, with a philosophy of international intervention, accompanied by an exploration of five important tests of justification, might have been taken into the party in 1999 for a sustained debate, and from there out to the people. That discussion might have carried the case although it might also have detected various problematic consequences unintended in the Blair focus. Blair and his managers carefully failed to share the speech. From all the indications, over Iraq, the extra-parliamentary party had in 2002–3 the same judgement as that of the public majority; there should not be military action against Iraq outside of second and specific UN authorisation. The management never allowed that choice to be voted on. Iraq management suppressed the ability of the party to convey – to the party's parliamentary representatives and to the public – the strength of its support for an alternative party position. Later, Iraq policy became increasingly recognised as catastrophic. A defence of strict and heavy management in the future, which is justified by reference to the dangers from the party, has to note also the dangers from this kind of leadership and management, and at least to face the crucial question of how it would prevent a rerun of something like the Iraq disaster.

The heavily managed party conference never gained from the leadership the disposition to respect it that would have changed the internal atmosphere, enhanced receptivity to leadership proposals for reform after 1997, encouraged cooperative policy inventiveness and contributed towards party revitalisation. An examination of the issues evaded and the decisions ignored shows that there could have been a greater possibility of more constructive and advantageous harmonisation of the governmental voice and the people's voice with that emanating from the party if partnership and the party policy voice had been more respected in a dialogue of mutual education. And it would have been healthier if reasonable relations of accountability had been allowed to operate.

The price worth paying?

For the managers, a central assumption was that their methods and any distrust generated in the party by management and manipulation was a price worth paying if it meant that the management could deliver the electoral appeal they judged appropriate. In this, much emphasis was placed on the primacy of the immediate media effect on the electorate at the cost of denying or distorting members' influence. Yet a growing body of evidence indicated also the importance of local party campaigning which could significantly affect electoral turnout levels and levels of party support.

There was also a rediscovery of the potentially crucial factor of interpersonal communication. The IpsosMORI excellence model on brand loyalty registered the often under-emphasised importance of old-fashioned word-of-mouth in politics. With the decline in membership, by 2005 the ex-party critical ambassadorial message about the party and its leadership had grown, especially over Iraq. It was calculated that between 1997 and 2006 around 50,000 members left the party because of a real or perceived lack of influence.[33] Between the election of 1997 and April 2005 the number of encouragers of Labour voting dropped from 31 per cent to 21 per cent whilst discouragers of Labour voting rose from 14 per cent to 30 per cent.[34] As explained in Chapter 16, respondents to advertising at this time were taking up word-of-mouth recommendation as a safeguard against manipulation. The findings raised the importance of traditional doorstep and workplace message-carrying by advocates who were strong in their command of the case and persuasively sincere in their own convictions that the leadership, particularly the Leader, was trustworthy.

Instead, a diminished organisational vitality undermined the party's level of potential effectiveness in campaigning. There was disdain for the activist culture and, as Helen Jackson MP – an elected internal representative on the NEC from the PLP, seeking a more active party – pointed out, little effort was made by the leadership to encourage some countervailing powers and build up the resources from below. 'In practice the opposite was the case.'[35] Party officials who could have been more employed in the electoral organisation spent considerable time in internal policing activities. Watching government policy and behaviour and experiencing the consequences of party management, increasing numbers of party members became either limited in their willingness to spread the messages of trust or disillusioned to the point of leaving the party after which they could develop into the opposite – ambassadors of disillusionment and distrust.

Overlooked often was the porous quality of the party in its reactions to developing internal distrust of features of 'New Labour' managerial behaviour. It came as ex-Labour members shared perceptions with neighbours, families with each other, friends likewise. Disgruntled MPs talked to the media. Sometimes, as over the London Mayor, this fused with an external campaign. An early warning conveyed privately to Blair in October 1994, as part of a broader critique of trust-undermining party management, had been implicitly: would a future Leader want to increase a core of knowledgeable testifiers to his untrustworthiness?[36] That electoral imperative was acknowledged by Blair in what came over as a passionate passage on mutual trust at the conference in 1998: 'One thing is for sure: if we don't trust each other we will never connect that to the rest of the country'.[37]

Yet as shown, this view was not fully operationalised in managerial behaviour that year, and was not followed subsequently. Blair, after the Iraq invasion, facing unusually frank and critical contributions from some of his colleagues in 2003 (covered in Chapter 17) did not want to hear about it. In the election campaign of 2005 the decline of trust because of the circumstances leading to Britain's involvement in the war over Iraq became more central to evaluations of Blair's character as the campaign unfolded.[38] There was also a special revelation of the consequences of undermining party members' public enthusiasm about Blair in that they noticeably failed to come to the aid of Blair when he was personally under acute media attack. Managers also confessed privately that an upsurge of personal responses from party members could not be organised by them for fear that it would be exposed as artificial, further reinforcing the 'New Labour' reputation for manipulation.

Gaining through trustworthy behaviour

That was an indication of at least temporary managerial recognition that public attitudes to the party were likely to have been adversely affected by imposing policy on the electorate sometimes via the manipulative behaviour associated with the increasing stage management and treatment of politics as 'a set of tricks and a dark art'.[39] From Peter Kellner's polling analysis he had judged that 'The party string-pullers land them in the frying pan of glib insincerity that alienates more voters than it attracts'.[40] In countering that, it was important to change the string-pulling and cut some of the strings.

Of course, the party and its members have to emphasise listening to the public; as focus-group specialist Frank Luntz pointed out, 'we've lost our voice' was a common public complaint about government.[41] However, this did not point simply to the value of imposing the heaviest management. Open intra-party debate, even an occasional revolt against the leadership, could show the integrity of the party in defining political problems and predicaments from its own experience, advocating its values and policies and seeking to persuade the electorate in such a way as to influence and re-prioritise the centre ground. It would also be in tune with what the public wanted as they reacted to their own powerlessness, the leadership's 'arrogance' and the stage management of politics. The operation of manipulation was an albatross as much on the back of the people as on that of the party. There was a lot to be gained by the party developing a more favourable reputation as the transformed agency through which important public concerns were more openly and authentically registered, genuine controversy occurred, and more independent party voices were freer to be registered.

What this pointed to was not the abolition of management but the potential advantage of a sensitive rebalancing of considerations in a health-ier more consensual process. In that rebalancing it had to be recognised that the party was not always as adrift of the public as the managerial myth indicated, whilst heavy management produced its own problems both in terms of diminished activism and in public reaction to the style of man-aged and manipulated politics. Conference authority had varied historically not directly by changes in rules but because of a changing attitude towards respect for it, most notably in the move by the leadership generation after 1931. There could be much more of a predisposition to respect the party view replacing the knee-jerk 'New Labour' predisposition to repudiate it.

Further, signs of internal party dissent from this form of leadership were not as invariably publicly unwelcome as the Leader and his management often suggested. Public hostility to intra-party revolts against the Leader depended on the issue and the reason for revolt. Thus, there is no evidence that the crucial PLP dissidence on lone parent benefit in 1997 caused an adverse electoral reaction against the party over disunity. There was a sign at one stage in 2000 that the party's recovery in the polls was assisted by the public response to its passionate concern over the pensions issues, regardless of the specifics of the conference vote. After 2005, disunity did have a marked detrimental effect on the party's standing although much of this appears to have been a by-product of what was seen as the conflicts at government level between Brown and Blair, rather than because the party was in disagreement with the Leader.

Management and 'the union problem'

There were many aspects to the arguments both for and against the union-party relationship,[42] and many factors were involved in the development of changing attitudes to managing 'the problem'. But one increasingly relevant and influential inhibition over pushing for a separation under Blair's leadership was the greater realisation that, as Minkin noted in 1991,[43] an enforced divorce was unlikely to be a clean one-dimensional affair, even though the language of the separate entities – government and unions, party and unions – suggested this.

Divorce was made even more difficult under Blair because, as noted in Chapter 19, for varying organisational reasons party management was actually strengthening integration between the unions and the party. Around the Leader during the Hayden Phillips inquiry there were still a few sharing the ideal of pushing the party towards organisational separation using allies in the media. It was a project which, handled crudely, had created years of intensified distrust following the failed project of 1992–3, and it continued to act as a conservative blockage. As for a union departure, minority demands in the unions that affiliation money be redirected were also repulsed after the exit of the RMT and the FBU. Keith Ewing showed that alongside the policy conflicts, access for and representation from the unions into government had increased considerably under Blair.[44] This consolidated political stability here also. Union leaders and most officials saw new political frustration and new costs coming through disaffiliation, and therefore as in the past did not see such a move as realistic. In any case, most still thought of the party as 'ours'.

In spite of years of media criticism of the unions as a problem for the party, there was consistent majority support for the relationship in every major forum of the party. As Seyd had found, there was support for the relationship from members old and new, with some differences in the degree of commitment amongst meeting attenders and non-attenders, but even here the majority of both were in favour of union affiliation.[45] What this confirmed was that a managerial war over affiliation and separation would not be a conflict with a few recalcitrant 'union bosses'. It would be a disaster for party unity and management, producing a damaging split running all the way down within the Labour Party, with very uncertain outcomes.[46] Blair reluctantly learned that lesson, if rather late for the trusting engagement that could have facilitated both invigoration and possibly consensual reform.

An important element of the case for radical reform of union representation, short of separation, had been linked – at least rhetorically – to giving individual party members more of a vote and an influence. But that case suffered from the experience, and the evidence accumulated here that managerial commitment to members' influence only came to life when it could be used by the managers as an asset in the battle with the unions, portraying them as 'riding roughshod over constituency activists'.[47] The overriding concern of the leadership and management was that uncontrolled rank-and-file-activity could make leadership problems more difficult. Hence the evidence here that the Leader and managers were never reluctant to forge a union block vote against the CLPs and in effect 'the members' party' when it suited them.

This management made internal democrats and disillusioned supporters more aware of the value of the unions as a check on the extensive power of the Leader and the managers. The evidence here points up that the absence, or severe weakening, of the unions within the party would further diminish pluralism in policy-making. In contrast, one feature of the Warwick NPF of July 2004 was that the union push made the government at least verbally more sensitive to other groups in the party who were encouraged by the assertive role of the unions. In 2005–7 the inability of legacy-seeking No. 10 managers to initiate wider support within the party for a reform which would weaken the union position was striking, as was the absence of a burst of new knowledgeable academic argument in favour of separation.

The party discussions over the Hayden Phillips report and party financing did indicate that to further legitimise the relationship there had to be a reform which brought closer concurrence between individual levy-paying and union totals of affiliated members. Historically, deviation from the norm of concurrence had been enhanced by the party's need for finance, not the unions' need for influence. The last 25 years has shown that trade union opinion on some major issues of reform was not intractable but persuadable; the union support for a huge reduction of their conference votes leading up to the agreement in 1993 has few parallels in modern politics. But an element of trust about the trajectory of party policy and a willingness to abide by agreements was essential. Yet true to Blair's style of leadership, the government pulled further away from the party's centre of gravity, and the implementation of Partnership in Power and of the Warwick Agreement involved significant changes in procedure away from that agreed, and left significant policy dissatisfactions. As for the Hayden Phillips report, this was tarnished and compromised by suspicions of back-door manipulative dealings involving No. 10, which helped produce the extreme content of aspects of the report's conclusions.

The approach to the unions might have been more productive if it had involved an interactive three-dimensional process. There needed to be a patient rebuilding of trust between the unions and the party, counteracting the damaging managerial attitudes and practices noted above. There also needed to be a new attempt at an across-the-board party revitalisation in which the union levy-payers and party members would play an invigorated part in the internal policy process. It would have specially helped also if there had been an attempt to agree new unwritten 'rules' and protocols implying a restoration of transparency, mutuality, restraint and a sense of permanence. At crucial times, there were opportunities to rebuild such a framework; each time the opportunity was ignored or rejected. This created and sustained the impasse and also added to the case for another kind of political leadership and management.

Party management and social affinity

There was a special prudential reason why there now had to be other changes in the culture of party management. 'New Labour' party management had been impressively successful in building its middle-class base of support, and middle-class members and public representatives in the party. But there was a social downside discernible in the undermining of manual workers support, the falling proportion of trade unionists amongst party members and the problem of under-representation of the ex-manual working class in the party, acutely expressed in the PLP.

By 2005, ex-manual working-class representation in the Commons had sunk to 38: It meant that one-third of British people were being represented, in social terms by only 6 per cent of MPs.[48] Yet there was no practical managerial move to boost manual worker parliamentary representation. Between 1990 and 1999 there was a sharp drop in the number of the party's members who thought that it looked after the interests of the working class and trade unionists and a large rise in those who felt that it looked after the interests of big business and 'the very rich'.[49] This made the union contribution to the party all the more significant as a redress of under-representation, going some way to adjust the public perception of the 'all sound alike' middle-class politicians and to rectify the inequities of social power and representation within British politics as whole.

The leadership and managerial priority defensive guidance was still heavily affected by managerial concern over avoiding damage from what was seen as the unions' electoral unpopularity and their association with unpopular industrial actions. Yet recent evidence suggests that under Blair after the Smith reforms of 1993 this was exaggerated. As noted in this study private research conducted in 1994 for the Conservatives had indicated that raising the union bogey was no longer an effective political tactic. The focus-group responses to the media-led row over recognition in 1997 indicated that it had 'not yet' become an electoral problem. In the 2001 election campaign the union problem was not a live issue. The well-publicised Warwick Agreement with the unions in 2004 and the manifesto defence of modern trade unionism did not stir up an electoral problem in the 2005 election. This could be read as a triumph of Gould's emphasis on 'New Labour' reassurance, but there were other factors at work. The rise in the power of the Prime Minister, of business and of wealth, had changed perceptions of and reduced concern about the unions, whatever it had been initially. Yet the 'New Labour' mindset could not adjust.

At the same time there was the beginning of a new, albeit reluctant, awareness of the case for using unions to reach out to parts of the electorate that were not being reached by the party, utilising union communications more effectively as potential linkage into networks of families with a history of Labour voting. By 2004, this was also being linked to the signs that the party's ancillary organisations were less distrusted by the public than were the government and party politicians.[50] Trade union leaders were

more trusted by trade unionists than were politicians but also trade unions
as institutions were more trusted than politicians in terms of telling the
truth by 33 per cent to 18 per cent.[51] In this context, TULO had become
potentially a more significant coordinating organisational and communicational asset, because by the end of Blair's reign the party was in virtually
all-round decline.

'New Labour' and business

There was another series of problems which pressed the claim for protection of intra-party democracy and union representation against managerial
excess. The party's movement away from being 'anti-business' had been a
constructive attempt to broaden the party's public representation and to
build a basis of new economic cooperation. With that was conjoined a
tactical goal in securing business electoral support in the marginal seats.
But the dynamic of building and sustaining new arrangements and perpetually concerned with reassuring business created a range of other socio-
psychological influences. That sensitivity meant avoiding the problematic
issue of relations between democracy and the power of multinational
organisations which was raised but then ignored in the 1995 Clause IV
discussions. Similarly, the special problem of the likely pressures from
powerful socio-economic forces, pointed out by *Daily Express* owner Clive
Hollick in the Party into Power process in 1996, was not taken further in
the partnership discussions. A view that there might be problems for the
democratic political system of a socio-economic power elite was repudiated
by the No. 10 Policy Unit.

Yet even Stephen Byers, a past critic of the unions, came to view the
union role in the party as a necessary counterweight to the power of business lobbying, a point that was even made privately and occasionally by
No. 10, when it suited them. Byers had experienced this business power
himself in 2001 over his proposal, supported by the unions, designed to
strengthen the link between directors' pay and their performance. It was
buried. Action against greed, pressed from the unions in the first term
of government, was always ignored. In 2007, as Blair prepared to depart,
35 per cent of party members thought that the party was under 'a great
deal of' influence from large companies' but only 2 per cent thought that
this was right.[52] Amongst the public, Blair was judged by 59 per cent to
have been 'too influenced by the rich and powerful'.[53] At the very least,
the relationship ought to have been more transparent and opened up to
the watchful gaze of the party members and their institutions. As events
were to show in 2007 as an economic crisis emerged, this was a relationship which needed to be reassessed if the party's purposes and values were
to be defended. The political tendencies of the party's leaders towards what
Kettle had once termed their political 'crouching position' proved to be a
desperate economic as well as political weakness.

Cohesion and procedural management

There was potentially also a huge problem arising from less-recognised management attitudes. Shaw's description of the managerial role in his path-breaking 1982 study of party management, as it was then, was that it was concerned with 'the safeguarding of rules' and 'the maintaining of cohesion'.[54] What has been found here has approached the opposite. Although systematic party management appeared to be an obsessive new stabilising force and at times Blair was privately concerned with holding the party coalition, at no time has cohesion been a central subject of internal inquiry, or even an initiative from the Leader or others at the centre to alert the party to the dangers. Nor was it a subject for discussion in Party into Power meetings. That would have been at odds with the glorification of change within a continuous revolution of Blairite modernisation.

As for the safeguarding of rules, adverse consequences were embedded in the rolling coup, imposing or manipulating change without party agreement. Cohesion requires endorsement of the collective ownership and integrity of the decision-making process. Under Blair, rules became more flexible and uncertain in their consensuality. The danger grew that a bitter dispute over rules for which there was no obvious solution could turn into lack of cooperation and even degenerate from conflict into civil war.

There was also a managerial failure to appreciate the wider significance of abandoning the framework of conventional 'rules' and protocols which covered the union-party relationship. That had been an important and long-standing element of Labour's stabilisation capital. The loss, and the failure to renovate, removed important symbols of continuity, rule obedience, mutuality and collective endeavour, all of which contributed to cohesion. Manual working-class trade unionists, a declining breed in the PLP, were important historical carriers of this tradition. With their decline had come a weakening of instinctive self-disciplined collectivism in the face of a new individualism and an assertive localism. This also caused potential damage to cohesion.

Overall, 'New Labour' managers had a weak appreciation of the potentially dangerous consequences of their behaviour. The argument over the procedures for eviction of the Leader epitomised the damage caused by this managerial short-sightedness. The mechanism for eviction, already weak, was deliberately further weakened and made unclear. The would-be evictors of Blair, thwarted by his rule management, were then forced to move outside official processes creating a potentially dangerous clash over the legitimacy of the curtailment of Blair's term in office. That in turn left behind simmering resentment by Blairites that they and the party had been cheated, again with potentially damaging consequences for cohesion.

Open decisions on rules by the conference was still an obligation held in the wider party to be supreme, and it is doubtful whether much of the party was aware of this alternative managerial interpretation of the proprieties, and even more doubtful that it would have been agreed. The 'mistakes' in 2002 and 2003 (though rectified later on TULO insistence), in failing to properly authorise new affiliation fees coincided with a new managerial interpretation that it was not necessary to do so. Whether or not it was a genuine mistake, when revealed it gave out a warning of potentially destabilising behaviour. By hampering union grassroots' awareness of what was happening to their levy payments, it could have opened an unprecedented vulnerability to public criticism and from that a potential threat to the future consensual basis of union financing of the party. Failure to issue a verbatim conference report to the party within a year made it harder to exercise membership vigilance and secure accountability over such matters.

This problem of cohesion was also exacerbated by the dismissive shedding of a neutral civil service tradition of party officials, and the adoption of a role definition as the Leader's political organisers. They could not now fully play a neutral stabilising role, and within their code felt much less inhibition about intervening in an election for Leader in order to secure the desired outcome. By the end of Blair's regime, a major covert problem was that, as many in the machine did not share the wisdom of that eviction, could future party relations with the Leader work properly? More generally, because the 'New Labour' managers were insensitive to problems of party cohesion, as Blair left the scene, he and they together had severely weakened some of the invisible bonds which held the Labour Party together.

Manipulation and its legacy

New Machiavellianism and the anti-manipulative ethos

Overcoming public distrust of politicians was initially handled deftly in 1994, and it is possible to see the Blair early years as an unusual interlude before the distrust of politicians picked up again at the beginning of the next decade. But this distrust was not a simple continuation. The condition of politics had changed for good. The difference now was an anti-manipulative ethos, arising from the factors analysed in Chapter 16, producing a particularly acute awareness of, and a harsh public attitude towards, the behaviour of politicians. Whereas 'New Labour' practitioners of political manipulation had developed more resources, techniques and freedom in their operations, the public's socio-psychological reception had become more sceptical and resistant. Politics became identified not with the hopes raised by Blair for a new cleaner and more trustworthy politics but with a new machiavellianism of 'New Labour' professionalism.

Outside as well as inside the party, detoxification of distrust generated by manipulation was now more difficult. It remained an open question how far Blair fooled himself or was misled by the evidence, or misled the party and the people over various features of the government case on Iraq.

What can reasonably be said is that in the light not only of some of the evidence available but also of the deception and devious practices in party management revealed here, it is difficult not to give the worst interpretation to some of Blair's actions in pursuit of – in Mandelson's imagery – his tunnel vision over Iraq policy.[55]

And that conduct of politics had longer-term effects. Research on advertising deception by Darke and Richie pointed to the wider effect of making consumers defensive towards all marketing messages – distrusting advertising in general, minimising the possibility of being fooled again.[56] In politics, as noted, a reputation for manipulation can, with varying intensity, contaminate all facets of trust. Manipulation once diagnosed could produce the most bitter and resentful of responses. It was no surprise therefore that in 2005 Gavyn Davies, in an article headed 'Watch out Tony, he's hell bent on vengeance', should write of 'the fetid pools' of politics and 'the short-term chicanery' which had 'poisoned serious debate'.[57]

That sense of chicanery affected the awareness of a significant number of voters in the 2005 election, and became a special problem for those 'New Labour' politicians who had come to understand manipulation as a sophisticated, effective and modern way for the politician to behave. Manipulation even became a regular publicised irresponsibility in terms of the conflicts between 'New Labour's' leading politicians and their aides. This became particularly on show in the corrosive Blair-Mandelson-Brown-Whelan interplay, and especially over their relations of aggressive personal critical spin. The cognoscenti of 'New Labour' grew to distrust intensely the standards of their own carefully honed and trained style of party management politics when applied to their personal relations, leading to a bitter disunity and enmity that became increasingly part of public awareness.

Generating distrust: an overview

There is a final overview point to be made about the party management and the generation of distrust. Although the lack of trust between the Labour Party and its leaders had remnants of traditional attitudes and suspicions, to place the emphasis there is to understate the important impact of the managerial culture and practices examined in this study. A leading international analyst and theorist of trust, Piotr Sztompka, gives us the framework for another perspective.[58] His synthesis was that cultural resources conducive to the emergence of a trust culture were these: normative coherence, stability of the social order, transparency, accountability.

What has been registered here is that the nature of Blair's leadership and management was just the opposite: normative incoherence, permanent revolution, pervasive secrecy of the managing order, undermining of accountability. To managers, in pursuit of short-term imposed and particularly manipulative measures, all that appeared to be 'what worked'. Yet the heritage of this management was that all of the damaging consequences

were coalescing in the direction of internal distrust. A distanced view of
Blair and his party management might reasonably conclude that generation
of distrust was their supreme aptitude. Thus, it was poetically fitting that
distrust played such a significant part in the groundswell of party reaction
which ensured the date of the end of the Leader's tenure.

Ethics, politics and party management

The irony and tragedy of Blair's time as Leader was that initially it was
Blair's widely believed view that he would contribute a new ethical dimension to political life and that he saw political activity as an extension of
morality.[59] Yet it is hard to survey the pattern of practices of the Leader
and his managers in this study and find there a convincing exemplification
of what Blair described as 'our sense of fair play' and the importance of
'playing by the rules', let alone seeking 'the highest standards of honesty
and propriety in public life', as the Queen's Speech of 1997 prescribed the
objective. One influential private realist view from a leading ex-manager,
who outlasted Blair, was that 'you can't apply morality to party management'. It might be pointed out that, at the very least there was something
wrong with a situation where managerial party activities were paid for by
members who had little knowledge of most of what the managers did for
and to them. And the party management practices were not the healthiest
offerings for emulation in social relations to be bequeathed as an education
in political engagement. Much of the 'New Labour' record offered a socially
damaging model of how to behave.

The harshest public flavour of the discomfort all this produced came
from the columnist Robert Harris. He was a close friend of Mandelson,
and had admiringly first given the spin doctor the title of the 'Machiavelli
of Walworth Road'.[60] In 1997 Harris had predicted, with no apparent
concern, that Blair was 'going to exert more power over his party than all
his predecessors put together'.[61] By 2001, after seeing the master of the
political arts, Mandelson, become the victim of a removal for an offence
of which he thought himself innocent, Harris gave a devastating portrait
of the character of 'New Labour' and 'its cold hearted ways'. 'Something
has got lost', he wrote, 'some quality . . . some sense that there was a line
that could not be crossed. It is a dream come true. It is a nightmare'.[62]
Divorced from the reference to the Mandelson case, that sentiment about
something 'getting lost' and 'lines being crossed' could be found in the
views of an increasing minority of disconsolate, disillusioned party and
ex-party officials. They had developed an unusual degree of private disassociation from their managerial experience.[63]

The chief of staff, Powell, was of course right that politics under Blair's
leadership was not 'just about cynical manoeuvring and manipulation'.[64]
But as shown in this study, 'New Labour' leadership and party management were heavily, extensively and persistently influenced by them. Powell's
study gives a classic replication of the failure of defenders of the Leader

to admit publicly the existence of the elephant which was Blair's party management, the methods it employed, and the damaging legacy of distrust, destabilisation and debilitation it incurred. Machiavelli was portrayed by Powell as, like Blair, an exponent of the wisdom of 'what worked'.[65] Yet from the evidence offered here, the Blair version of 'what works' constituted a warning of what does not work in terms of collateral and consequential dangers. It tells what to attempt to avoid. Blair's party management could only be said to have 'worked' if eyes are shut to a great deal of damage. As the No. 10 adviser Mulgan recognised, 'we expect leaders to be able to think through the full implications of what they do'.[66] With that in mind, the most significant feature of the study here is the uncovering of a litany of the operative fallacies, inadequacies, dangers and encumbrances of the British machiavellian in politics.

And the answer to the realists' view that 'you can't take the politics out of it' is that here, as in so many other places, in respect of an excess of manipulative politics you have to, or you are likely to create bigger problems. One end-product of Blair's conduct of politics was that the Blair persona, so attractive in 1994 and so celebrated in 1997, became loaded with odium. A Luntz focus-group analysis for *Newsnight*, in December 2006, showed that he had come to be seen by the electorate as a manipulator of public opinion.[67] At a time when, largely in response to the Blair regime, the anti-manipulative ethos had been strengthened, Blair was out of tune with the times and 'New Labour' party management was seriously outmoded. In a poll in June 2007, whilst 45 per cent of people thought that being heir to Blair was a bad thing, only 14 per cent thought that it was a plus.[68]

The mode of governing

Blair and his team of close associates were a team inexperienced about the processes of governing the country. But they had a hinterland of governing the party, and brought with them a strong sense of worldly wisdom about the serious conduct of politics in struggle with obstacles and enemies. That wisdom had been educated and finessed through the experience revealed here, including the covert rolling coup of unilateral changes in the terms of engagement. The manifesto mantra in 1997 that they had 'won as "New Labour"' and would govern as "New Labour"' was more than a statement of distinctive identity. It was a claim to the ways of 'getting the job done effectively'.

It would have been difficult for Blair, a man who had some difficulties in changing his political behaviour patterns, not to draw from lessons learned facing what he viewed as limiting attitudes and procedural constraints similar to those which he, his allies, aides and managing officials confronted and were still managing in the party. A rose-tinted perception of that party experience which saw him having 'conquered with ease',[69] now nurtured and prized the creative attempt to ask 'why not some other way?' in facilitating delivery, and in dealing with what Blair saw as old-fashioned governing methods and institutions and the inertia of a conservative and risk-averse civil-service culture.

Having shied away from attempting a comprehensive Whitehall and civil-service reform through agreed procedures, he found, as he had in the party, ad hoc extra means to 'get the job done', by various forms of radical change outside of formal institutional authorisation. This included his limited version of cabinet government, especially the failure to adequately consult the cabinet collectively over Iraq and, as explored here, as he had failed over the Employment Relations Act. In both cases, in 'reducing the scope for informed collective political judgment', as the Butler report put it over Iraq, Blair changed power relations and, through that, brought the policy outcomes he wanted. With the unwavering confidence that his own judgement was the best, 'defying and transcending established ways of getting things done', Blair fitted comfortably the N.G. Bailey categorisation of 'heroic leadership'.[70]

In doing so, however, he also created a range of political vulnerabilities and a broad front of critics of his way of governing, including Conservative parliamentarians who took advantage of the opportunity to contrast Blair with his favoured model, Margaret Thatcher, said to be 'tempered not least by her instinctive appreciation of the basic norms and structures of our constitutional arrangements'.[71] More damaging to Blair, in commentaries which replicated or approximated what was being said within the party about its management, Blair, an apostle of centre-ground-focused politics grew to be judged adversely on this by an informed and influential middle ground of government watchers.

Riddell noted the often cavalier exercise of power[72] and that Blair failed to 'understand or have an interest in proper boundaries between ministers, special advisers and civil servants'.[73] He had a 'blind spot over standards in public life'.[74] A lack of respect for due process, as in the much-criticised arbitrary setting up of the Supreme Court, was judged to be characteristic. These were all features familiar to the observer of his party management and they reinforced the image of tainted governing methods. In his final conference speech in 2006, his message to the delegates had included the sentiment that 'Whatever you do, I am always with you'. But there was danger in that promise. The party got the worst of his reputation as well as the best. The ex-Chairman of the Committee of Standards in Public Life, Sir Alastair Graham, gave the view that Blair had 'degraded British politics'.[75]

In the years that followed his departure from No. 10, Blair continued to be a hugely divisive figure damaged by the memory of his governing methods. This contributed to a lack of support in the UK for his attempt to secure the EU presidency. He had, as an *Observer* editorial put it, 'a proven record of ignoring constitutional niceties'.[76] That record and the loss of trust in government had strengthened the case for urgent re-examination and reform not only of government but of the party management influences that directly and indirectly fed into it.

Notes

1 N.G. Bailey, *Humbuggery and Manipulation: The Art of Leadership*, Cornell University Press, Ithaca and London, 1988, p. xiii.
2 Polly Toynbee and David Walker, *The Verdict, Did Labour Change Britain?* Granta, London, 2010.
3 *Independent on Sunday*, 4 September 2005.
4 *Sunday Telegraph*, 28 May 2010.
5 Lance Price, *The Spin Doctor's Diary: Inside No. 10 with New Labour*, Hodder & Stoughton, London, 2005, entry 7 May 1999, p. 105.
6 Matthew Taylor, *Changing Political Culture: First Thoughts on Political Exclusion*, first thoughts pamphlet, Local Government Association, 2000, p. 10.
7 Peter Mandelson and Roger Liddle, *The Blair Revolution: Can New Labour Deliver?* Faber & Faber, London, 1996, p. 217.
8 Meg Russell, *Building New Labour: the Politics of Party Organisation*, Palgrave Macmillan, Basingstoke, 2005, p. 6.
9 Peter Mandelson, *The Third Man: Life at the Heart of New Labour*, Harper, London, 2010, p. 322.
10 Ibid. p. 372, and Jonathan Powell, *The New Machiavelli*, Bodley Head, London, 2010, p. 108.
11 Powell, *New Machiavelli*, p. 54.
12 Ibid. p. 70.
13 Mandelson, *Third Man*, p. 561.
14 'Survey of public attitudes towards conduct of public life'. BMPB international for the Committee on Standards in Public Life, 2006. Table on results for 2004 and 2006, p. 42.
15 BBC *Newsnight*, discussion of leadership, 2 May 2008.
16 Robin Cook, *The Point of Departure: Diaries from the Front Bench*, Simon & Schuster, London, 2003, p. 23.
17 Minutes of the Parliamentary Liaison Committee, 22 November 2005.
18 Tony Blair, *A Journey*, Hutchinson, London, 2010, p. 337.
19 Ibid. p. 486.
20 *New Statesman*, 21 January 2011.
21 IpsosMORI, 'Labour Leader image', October 2006.
22 Worcester's Weblog, 28 April 2005.
23 LPCR 1998, p. 9.
24 Scott Adams, *The Dilbert Principle*, Macmillan, London, 1997, pp. 2–3.
25 Powell, *New Machiavelli*, pp. 79–80.
26 ICM/*Observer*, 1 October 1995.
27 *New Statesman*, 9 July 2009.
28 ICM/*Guardian*, 26 September 2002.
29 *Guardian*, 1 October 2002.
30 YouGov for Cruddas found 82 per cent of members believing that funding should be available to local councils to build low-cost council housing on the same basis as housing associations. *Guardian*, 9 May 2007.

31 Tim Horton and Sunder Katwala, *The Future of Party Democracy*, Fabian Society pamphlet and submission to the NEC in 2007.

32 Blair, *Journey*, p. 636.

33 TULO submission to the review of the policy-making process 2010, drawing from the YouGov/Save the Labour Party data, 2006.

34 IpsosMORI website, 'Advocacy of Political Parties: the Word-of-Mouth Effect', April 2005.

35 Helen Jackson MP, private memo circulated to PLP colleagues in 2003.

36 My letter of 10 October 1994 to Blair, sent via Murray Elder, then Head of Blair's Office, at Elder's suggestion after discussing with him the sources of internal distrust of Blair.

37 LPCR 1998, p. 14.

38 Daniel Stevens and Jeffrey A. Karp, 'Leadership Traits and Media Influence in Britain, *Political Studies* 60(4), December 2012, p. 802.

39 Ben Page, MORI. 'The Future of Political Parties', *Progress Magazine*, September 2005.

40 Peter Kellner, 'Mo Mowlem and the Campaign for Real Politics – the Kellner/Saunders Index', YouGov, September 2000.

41 *Sunday Times*, 3 December 2006.

42 Minkin, *Contentious Alliance*, Chapter 21, pp. 646–58, concluding in favour of the relationship.

43 Ibid. p. 650.

44 Keith Ewing, 'Rethinking the Law of Work: The Continuing Role of Trade Unions in Labour Law', unpublished appraisal, circa 2003, pp. 4–8.

45 Patrick Seyd, 'New Parties/New Politics? A Case Study of the British Labour Party', *Party Politics* l5(3), July 1999, p. 397.

46 Ibid.

47 *Guardian*, 2 October 2003.

48 'Skipper' Bill Jones, letter, *Guardian*, 18 November 2009.

49 Patrick Seyd and Paul Whiteley, *New Labour's Grass Roots: The Transformation of the Labour Party Membership*, Palgrave Macmillan, Basingstoke, 2002, p. 144.

50 My verbatim notes of a speech by Douglas Alexander, NPF, Warwick, March 2004.

51 Robert Worcester, MORI, Veracity Index cited in Anthony Sampson, *Who Runs this Place?* John Murray, London, 2005, pp. 12–13.

52 Peter Kellner, YouGov/*New Statesman*, 19 March 2007.

53 You Gov/*Telegraph*, 3 April 2007.

54 Eric Shaw, *Discipline and Discord in the Labour Party*, Manchester University Press, Manchester, 1988, p. vii.

55 Mandelson, *Third Man*, p. 353.

56 Peter R. Darke and Robin J.B. Ritchie, 'The Defensive Consumer: Advertising Deception, Defensive Processing and Distrust', *Journal of Marketing Research*, 44(1), February 2007, pp. 114–27.

57 *The Sunday Times*, 11 July 2005.

58 Piotr Sztompka, University of Krakow, 'Trust: a Cultural Resource', Background paper for the project *Honesty and Trust*, 1999, pp. 4–5.

59 A.J. Davies, *To Build a New Jerusalem: The British Labour Party from Keir Hardie to Tony Blair*, Abacus, London, 1996, p. 438.

60 Mandelson, *Third Man*, p. 103.
61 *Sunday Times*, 9 February 1997.
62 *Sunday Times*, 16 May 2001.
63 Interviewing ex-managers met a revulsion about management from some officials which I had not previously come across in forty years of interviewing managers and ex-managers of the party.
64 Ibid.
65 Powell, *New Machiavelli*, p. 10.
66 Geoff Mulgan, *Good and Bad Power: The Ideals and Betrayals of Government*, Allen Lane, London, 2006, p. 212.
67 Luntz focus-group report, BBC *Newsnight*, 3 December 2006.
68 YouGov for *Sky News*, reported by Wells, UK Polling, 27 June 2007.
69 Blair, *Journey*, p. 4.
70 Bailey, *Humbuggery and Manipulation*, pp. 7, 51 and 166.
71 Philip Norton (Lord Norton of Louth), 'Governing Alone', *Parliamentary Affairs*, 56(4), October 2003, pp. 543–59.
72 Peter Riddell, *The Unfulfilled Prime Minister; Tony Blair's Quest for a Legacy*, Politico's, London, 2005, p. ix.
73 Ibid. p. 159.
74 Riddell, *The Times*, 23 February 2004, quoted in Peter Oborne and Simon Walters, *Alastair Campbell*, Aurum, London, 2004, p. 296.
75 *Daily Telegraph*, 19 March 2007.
76 *Observer*, 25 October 2009.

21

Epilogue: Brown, management inheritance and new moves to reform

Section 1: the impetus for management reform

New pressures towards a reform of party management had built up in the course of the election for Deputy Leader in 2007. The pamphlet on managerial activities by Jon Cruddas and John Harris declared that, 'The general strategy of circumventing the party . . . delivered through an informal cross-departmental task force within the party's head office' . . . has 'cultivated a new culture of cynical management'.[1] Coming from Cruddas, a front-rank ex-party official and ex-prime ministerial aide, this was authoritative and unprecedented as a critique of the hitherto unmentionable character of 'New Labour' management. True to form, there was no reply from party officials. There was no reaction either to the publication in 2007 of the interim report of the rank-and-file Labour Commission, supported financially by several unions and chaired by the PLP Deputy Chair Angela Eagle. Her introduction was magisterial: 'Underlying the loss of votes, seats and members is a profound cultural crisis arising from the side-lining of party democracy by centralised command and control . . . It has bred cynicism and stifled activism.'[2]

Accompanying that report was survey evidence and focus-group reports of grassroots opinion summarised as 'the Party hierarchy had a condescending and contemptuous attitude towards the party members, seeking to manipulate them rather than consult and work with them as equals'.[3] The report advocated a 10-point plan for Labour renewal, including OMOV for the election of NPF constituency representatives, a transparent separation of functions between the party in government and party headquarters, and abolition of the post of the Leader's appointed Party Chair. In a special challenge to the methods of management, it also called for the establishment of a charter of Labour Party members' rights, together with a new post of ombudsman and a code of ethics, including a whistle-blowing policy.

Moving past Blair: the opportunity

It appeared possible that this movement might gain some support from Brown, if only because it provided an opportunity to be seen to be the agent of across-the-board renewal. He could implicitly but firmly differentiate himself from Blair without publicly disrupting party unity. Brown's history of manipulative activities had not caught much public attention and had not detracted from his reputation in the way that Blair's had. This opportunity was all the greater because Cameron, in his attempt to replay the electoral rise of 'New Labour' and push a modernising agenda for his party, had developed a style and presentation which were recognisably early Blairish. That produced, as the Luntz focus groups indicated, an 'underlying fear of Cameron's spin' giving a concern that he might turn into the Blair of 2006.[4] Brown was expected by Sir Alastair Graham to set a 'new tone of seriousness about ethical standards'.[5] Accepting the nomination for Leader of the party, Brown repeatedly referred to 'listening and learning' in earning and rebuilding trust in democracy. It would be 'a different type of politics'.[6] Building on the emphasis of his 'seriousness' in politics might also have been a prelude to some difference from the 'serious politics' which legitimised manipulation. Having learned from the acute degeneration of Blair's reputation and perhaps having taken on board Jack Straw's warning that 'Fancy tactics . . . always catch you in the end',[7] he might have made that difference a new trade mark.

Boosting optimism about public trust

In implied criticism of what had gone before, Brown announced his support for constitutional change and was seen to be 'putting civil servants and civil service due process back at the heart of Whitehall'.[8] Brown's early governmental initiatives included removing the right of the two 10 Downing Street special advisers to give instructions to civil servants, and the abolition of the post of chief of staff. An 'independent adviser' was appointed to judge alleged breaches of a new ministerial code. The media operation appeared downgraded, cabinet government did became more collective and inclusive in form, parliament's right to declare war was legally confirmed and Brown even indicated moving towards a consensual written constitution. A positive sign of change away from manipulation occurred with the announcement on 26 November that the Office of National Statistics would be freed from government control, and on 1 April 2008 the UK Statistics Authority was established.

Encouraging union and party trust

In relation to the unions and the party, advance discussions with the NEC and the TUC were congenial, leading to some optimism there also. The NEC was told that he had talked to the unions before the employers and sought from union leaders a new cooperation. One TUC official reflected later, 'He knew how to talk the union talk'. Union leaders could not see any great policy difference between Brown and his predecessor but, as with party members generally, they wanted to believe that there was a difference. They thought constructively in terms of wiping the slate clean, and starting afresh in the relationship with the Leader, even without receiving any firm advance specific commitments.

As for the internal party management, David Gardner, an ex-Assistant General Secretary who had grown very critical of the methods of party management, hoped that the Leader would be 'extending the spirit of reform in the country to reform of the Labour Party'.[9] The private message from the new Leader's inner circle of advisers and close parliamentary supporters was that the reform agenda included party management. Although very wary of publicly differentiating himself from Blair,[10] privately, in intra party discussions there was an important repeated tactical insistence from his aides that Brown is 'not like him' (Blair) and 'we are not like them the Blairite aides. You can trust us'. Pessimists, especially on the left, saw this as more Blair-like flannel. Some Blairites saw Brown as congenitally incapable of what he appeared to be offering.

Negative signs and negative developments

Confirming that, it transpired that in October, the document offered by Brown about future management, titled *Extending and Renewing Party Democracy*, did not move away from the Blairite arrangements other than to restrict voting on contemporary issues, which had been Blair's original aim. What were now referred to as 'contemporary motions' would not be voted on in the year of their submission. Instead they would go into another process of dialogue. The procedures of Partnership in Power were reactivated without any focus on the reasons for the internal party grievances.

The Road to the Manifesto plebiscite, which even Blairite managers in 2001 had recognised as discredited, was now to be reintroduced. There were other indications that change was not to be carried out as democratic optimists hoped. The Deputy Leader Harriet Harman was made the Party Chair, again with no constitutional amendment to authorise it. Now, there were also six Deputy Party Chairs appointed by Brown, where there had been none before, also with no rule amendment. This was in spite of his election declaration in 2007 that this was a party that 'values people who play by the rules'. As with Blair, that did not apply to the behaviour of the Leader. There might have been a problem for Brown from Harman acting as the voice of party reform, but she was also made Leader of the House and Minister for Women so that her voice was often otherwise engaged.

The early promise and the election that never was

Brown as crisis manager

What the party and public saw of him as he faced major problems virtually silenced his critics and alarmed the Conservatives. Attempted bombings, floods and cattle disease were met with reassurance and determination. Through it all, his behaviour conveyed a move away from the dazzle of spin and celebrity. To the surprise of many, this Brown proved publicly very attractive, even his awkwardness conveying a sense of the genuine. The slogan 'Not flash just Gordon' became, it seemed, the appropriate and appealing watchword of a straight politician. The result of all this, added to his newness, was a rise in public support for him and a poll lead for his party leaping up to double-digit figures.

The opportunity emerged for an attempt to further destabilise the weakening Conservative Party position. Briefing the media on the forthcoming election prospects became ever more confident, with the signals moving from going early to going now. In spite of the emphasis on trust as a major theme of Brown's new regime, these signals appeared remarkably free of any focus on the public interest, and oblivious to an underlying public suspicion of self-interested and cynical politicians. This failure to prioritise gaining the trust in practice that was rhetorically being emphasised became a trademark of Brown's management, as it had become with Blair.

The likelihood of an early election also opened up the possibility of justifying heavy management in the extra-parliamentary party behind the call for unity and urgent preparation. With the Leader heavily involved overall and working with generally accommodating unions, it became the opportunity to manage candidate selection so as to parachute in 20–30 preferences. Brown's activities showed no inhibitions about this intervention in selections as the managers continued with their methods of protecting the 'New Labour' brand.

Calling it off

Against all his implied promises about spin, Brown, whilst in Iraq during the Conservative Party conference, announced new troop withdrawals, with statements not strictly accurate. It was seen as a cringe-making crude and calculating use of British service personnel for party political advantage. At that Conservative conference, promises of limiting inheritance tax from the Shadow Chancellor George Osborne were followed by a cleverly performed speech by Cameron producing a poll boost for them in the marginals. Having delayed, Brown now judged from the private polling that it was unsafe to hold a snap election.[11] Without any Cabinet discussion it was called off. One and a half million pounds of Labour Party funds had been wasted.

The whole episode was sadly acknowledged in the party to be a fiasco exposing him to a range of charges including dithering and incompetence. His claim not to have been influenced by the polls was widely ridiculed as blatantly dishonest. This and his record of small-print budget deviousness became another sustained Conservative focus of criticism. In another development that took account of public opinion but muddied the image of Brown as a conviction politician with clear Labour values, Brown and Darling also moved towards Tory policy on inheritance tax.

By 10 October Brown's impressive trustworthy rating had dropped from 54 per cent on 10 August to just 48 per cent, whilst in the same period

Cameron's trust rating increased from 36 per cent to 44 per cent.[12] The huge poll lead disappeared and Brown never recovered his August ascendancy in trust. The public reaction involved a disappointed sense of being let down about the character of the man. Within the party, the handling of this non-election created deep dismay mitigated by the hope that something else would emerge from a man still thought to have his loyalties and his heart in the right place. But his closest supporters were aware of a now deeply defensive man who had lost dynamism, especially after the misfortune of the loss of computer disks with private information on millions of child-benefit claimants. There were private reports of internal disorganisation and discord among his closest aides especially over spinning about who was to blame for the non-election. Staggering from one firefight to another, operating with an insecure form of micro managing, and the postponing of decisions until the last minute made him difficult to work with and affected activities in various dimensions, including the positive management of his relations with the party and the unions.

Changing affinity

Appointments reassurance and the TUC

But though better relations with the unions might indirectly have changed the atmosphere of party management, Brown's plans had already put that relationship in dificulties. In a speech to the Bankers and Merchants dinner at Mansion House on 20 June 2007, Brown had congratulated the City on entering 'an era that history will record as the beginning of a new golden age for the City of London'. As Prime Minister he created a Business Council for Britain, yet nothing was said about a new liaison arrangement with the unions via the party or outside it. The highly capable ultra-Blairite John Hutton was appointed the Secretary of State for a renamed Department of Trade and Industry. It became the Department of Business Enterprise and Regulatory Reform (BERR). Another capable Blairite, Pat McFadden, was made Minister of State for Employment Relations and Postal Affairs at BERR and Chair of the party's National Policy Forum.

Brown's appointments also included some from outside the Labour Party – a move thought to be publicly appealing about politicians working together. The TUC had not been forewarned about any of this and initially did not see it as closing the possibility of more fruitful relations with them, particularly after very friendly discussions in which positive markers were laid down in what appeared to be a shared perspective. Those hopes soon received a setback. His appointment of the ex-CBI leader Digby Jones as a minister at BERR signalled an even greater emphasis on the needs of business, and Jones anounced immediately that Labour would 'increasingly' become 'less in thrall' to the unions.

The closest of Brown's allies, Balls, later offered the insight that Brown worried at being seen as 'too much the Labour figure'.[13] His move towards business and his admiration of the role of the City of London was combined with an element of fearfulness about their reactions. And it was also now a condition of fearfulness-plus, springing from constant anxiety about what angry and in some cases mischief-making Blairites could make of any changes in the party which could be portrayed as 'opening the door to Old Labour'. Although Brown was said by biographer Steve Richards to be sceptical about most of the Blair reforms,[14] generally he did not attempt to undo them inside or outside the party.

In spite of anxieties over what his critics and business might make of the policy, facing the severe Northern Rock bank crisis in February 2008, Brown initiated a measure of nationalisation to create new financial stability. The policy was publicly recognised as a necessary measure and gained strong support in a party ever-hopeful of its Leader recovering his harmony with members' instincts. In contrast, Brown began to come under some sharp criticism from business following tax changes. He was aware that it was being said in financial circles that he needed to rekindle Labour's love of 'the filthy rich'.[15]

Managers, trepidation and defensive skills

The pessimists who had argued that the personality of Brown was never going to be comfortable with a cultural change that potentially energised a more party-assertive membership proved to be right. There also remained the complicating and unprecedented problem left by Blair that the ex-Leader's redefinition of the primary loyalty of party officials was to Blair personally. Many of them retained that covert allegiance. They also had a deep-seated pride in protecting their high-status managerial skills and a strong inclination to keep them in play. For those reasons alone, forcing any change in their position or behaviour away from the old code and practices had to be handled with care, and preferably not handled at all.

Blair wrote later in his autobiography that he had feared that Brown would rehabilitate 'old style trade union fixing and activist stitch-ups'.[16] Yet that behaviour had, as shown, always been a part of the ways and means of Blair's own management. Instead of extending democracy as promised, Brown repeated the heavy Blair management performance whilst even looking to extend it to those few areas where past concessions had been forced on Blair. Tactics and machinations resumed as before, paying little attention to Brown's emphatic declaration that 'fair play' was one of the core values of Britishness.[17] Whilst he talked in terms of extending democracy, in practice he developed a vision of how to add to his own defences. And whereas Brown's tactical skills on the offensive often involved miscalculation, his skills in protecting himself within the party was much more surefooted.

This was quietly achieved in building new influences in the largest union, titled 'Unite – the Union', formed on 1 May 2007 by the merger of Amicus and the TGWU, with two General Secretaries, Derek Simpson and Tony

Woodley. Both were keen to make a new start working closely with Brown. His old spin doctor Charlie Whelan could be recommended as a man with the ear and trust of the Leader and he emerged as head of what became the Unite political unit. Simpson was especially amicable to the new arrangements but Woodley, on the TGWU side, had little understanding of Whelan's past role, and did not appreciate how far he would be his Downing Street master's protector, acting as an adroit tactical spoiler in one forum after another.

Whelan's influence over Unite representatives significantly weakened the TULO collective union role on Labour's NEC, and further strengthened support for the Leader there. Brown's authority was also strengthened on that body by the role of government representatives. Eagle came back on the NEC but now as the government's representative, together with Pat McFadden and Tom Watson. As runner-up to Eagle in the PLP elections, Janet Anderson went on to the NEC as PLP replacement. All moved solidly in tune behind Brown. Ellie Reeves and Peter Wheeler, strong union-sympathisers but also loyalists associated with the traditional right, were re-elected as CLP representatives. The retiring Wolfgang was replaced by a left-wing critic of the managers, Peter Kenyon, although the signs were that left organisation was being further weakened at the base and in the PLP.

Donorgate and the Blair managerial culture

Finance and problems of the culture

Unfortunately for Brown, he could not prepare a defence for everything about the party that had happened under Blair. In November 2007 it emerged that the law on funding drawn up by the government in 2000 had been circumvented by using third parties as conduit of donations from a businessman, David Abrahams. Public attention on what became labelled the Donorgate scandal traversed over possible explanations with one question at the heart of it: what was it about the culture of 'New Labour' which produced deviance from commitment to propriety? Watt explained later that in party finance 'there was a culture in the parties that you play the rules right to the edge'.[18] It must be noted that officials, including Watt himself, also saw that mode of politics as an expression of the normality of internal party management at the boldest edge of the managerial codes. Some rules were pushed to the far end of possible interpretation to see what could be achieved without provoking too heavy an internal reaction. Thus, this crisis of finance management could reasonably be judged an extension of Blair's party management.

Brown had been determined not to get associated with sleaze. Seeking to escape what Watt described as the 'smell of corruption'[19] now surrounding the fundraising operation meant forcing Watt to resign after he had announced his acceptance of full responsibility.[20] Watt later denied that he had made that acceptance and let it be known that he had been scapegoated by a 'brutal' Prime Minister.[21] Dianne Hayter, the Chair of the NEC, stuck by her account of his acceptance.[22] That still left open the more important questions of how and why this had happened without NEC knowledge, and after the committee was thought to have moved back into financial control following the 'loans for honours' affair. Brown immediately requested an independent report from ex-general secretary Larry Whitty. After a discreet party inquiry which was limited because it covered the territory of a police investigation, Whitty's report, which was never published, drew attention to a range of continuing problems.

He reported that what followed from the loans-for-honours affair in 2006 'ought to have been a welcome, if belated, clarification of legal, financial and political responsibilities under the aegis of the NEC'.[23] In practice, what Whitty found was that the NEC and the party officers had not discharged their responsibilities effectively. Detailed reporting of financial activity did not pass to any NEC committee and neither the Treasurer nor the Audit Committee were kept in the loop. In effect, once again the officials had taken over much of the committee's role. Most disturbing was the information that the minutes of the meeting at which the Abraham's decision had been taken were unavailable, with no explanation offered to Whitty.[24] His private warning about the procedures and relationships was that what emerged in the Abraham case 'could have been a lot worse in the damage caused to the party'.[25]

The report made some important recommendations for a new system of governance and financial accountability of the NEC which, together with proposals from Dianne Hayter, was partially implemented by the new General Secretary, Ray Collins. But Brown followed Blair in not disturbing the controlling culture of the management and the subordination of the NEC. The Whitty report was never made available to the committee and the NEC majority continued its sometimes frustrated loyalism. Much later, after the police had investigated, the eventual decision of the Crown Prosecution Service was that there was insufficient evidence for any charges to be made.

Distrust of politicians

Meanwhile, Brown's early ambition to raise the trust of politicians crumbled. Relevant here in revealing Brown's failure and confirming the focus of the distrust was a particularly informative poll and analysis in January 2008.[26] In response to the question whether they agreed or disagreed that in general they tended to trust politicians, only 16 per cent did and 83 per cent did not. In giving open answers on why they did not trust, a majority gave a series which indicated primary concerns over manipulative behaviour. Responses of 31 per cent gave as the reason 'lie/mislead/don't tell the truth'; another 12 per cent gave 'Say what they want people to hear (to get votes)', and a further 10 per cent gave 'evasive/don't give straight answers/ two-faced'. To this 53 per cent could be added 22 per cent who gave 'don't keep promises/don't do what they say they will do', which could be attributed to lack of competence or, in an increasingly anti-manipulative climate, more likely to be attributed to insincerity over some of the promises.

Tactics, tax and party values

Donorgate produced some unfair public criticism of Brown, but a tactical move which was nobody's fault but his own now caused him huge damage. The abolition of the 10p tax rate had been linked to the 2p tactical reduction of income tax, made in the budget of 2007. By spring 2008 it was uncovered that this abolition was going to affect five million of the lowest-paid. Brown's initial refusal to even acknowledge the scale of the problem added to the aggravation and revolt which now embraced a wide spectrum of Labour MPs, party members and voters.

On 2 April 2008 Brown limited the immediate PLP revolt with cash payments for pensioners and childless people, which still left over a million worse off. It had been an astonishing performance by a man with an honourable if discreet redistributive record. The party sentiment that he was 'ours' was now complicated by a growing sense of a man who had lost his political compass through what appeared to be his obsession with tactical gimmicks at the expense of principle. Whilst Blair had created new management problems in the party by finding new purpose that pulled him further away from the party, Brown now created new party problems by apparently losing a major purpose. Hostile public reactions were reflected in a range of adverse electoral results. In the party, alongside a diminishing residue of hope a sorrowful question came to the fore: what did the government now stand for?

New General Secretary

Following the resignation of Watt, his post went to David Pitt-Watson, an administration and financial specialist who had been a strong candidate before the Clarke-Triesman appointments in 2001. Within weeks, on 3 May 2008, Pitt-Watson had resigned over concerns about the personal financial obligations arising from the post. In a battle over the next new appointment, the Leader's candidate became Ray Collins, an official on secondment from the transport workers' section of Unite. This was the very appointment that Blair's office, seeking major changes in union influence, had attempted but failed to secure in 2005. With the procedural desperation that was beginning to accompany all No. 10 activity under Brown, there was no hitch this time as the party officers produced a new initiative, a shortlist of one. Collins, now deeply loyal to Brown, was appointed on 13 June 2008.

Shortly afterwards, following the very bad result in the Crewe and Nantwich by-election, the post of Director of Governmental relations passed from Fiona Gordon, the original Brown appointment, to Joe Irvine, an official from Unite who, with Jonathan Ashworth, was made responsible for trade union liaison. Discussions with Irvine in 2007 had left an impression with some of the union leaders that he would attempt to play a role like that of Cruddas under Blair, working an interactive management to mutual benefit. In practice, under the Brown regime there was not the same room for delegation and there appeared to be a higher level of inhibition in attempting it. After he left the office of Chancellor, Darling later publicly reported that 'advisers were afraid to tell Mr Brown anything he did not want to hear.'[27]

To the outsider, on the face of it the links between Irvine as Political Secretary, the General Secretary Collins and the Treasurer Dromey looked publicly like an extension of the influence of Unite ex-TGWU officials into the party and government. In practice, in the main, the reverse was the case. Brown's tactical vision and domineering character ensured protection for him through these links, with the ex-TGWU managerial voices generally working cooperatively with Whelan, and overall influencing Woodley in support of Brown and his objectives. Woodley and Simpson occasionally made protests but they were both drawn into cooperative if at times fretful relations.

The unions as financial stability

Party funding

Collins now faced a huge financial task as the party's high-value donors were further frightened away by the Donorgate affair and the party was in danger of being declared bankrupt. Though some donations continued and Collins in the next two years rebuilt some of the finances, soliciting was hard going. The agenda of seeking again a cross-party agreement on state funding had collapsed after the failure of negotiations with the Conservatives. In June 2008, a white paper on party funding from Straw at the Ministry of Justice (referred to privately in the party as 'Hayden Phillips-lite') recognised the need to ensure that reform would not damage union political activity or their relations with the party.

PLP and union reactions

From the outset, there was a heavy continuity in PLP dissent under the new Leader and the same problems of management as those faced by Blair. But now, also heavy and increasing concern in the unions over the growing problem of unprotected agency and temporary workers led to a new initiative in which frustrated unions attempted to move 'into Brown's backyard' through private members' legislation. In the second reading on 22 February 2008, two-fifths of Labour MPs voted to support a Temporary and Agency Workers (equal treatment) Bill introduced by Labour MP Andrew Miller which would give rights to these workers equal with those of permanent workers.[28]

That strengthened the momentum behind the union's campaign and fed into the negotiations taking place through the TUC. What emerged in the Agency and Temporary Workers Agreement on 21 May 2008 was a compromise regarded by Brown as 'the right balance between fairness and flexibility', by the CBI as the least worst available solution, and by the TUC as 'the best we could get'. For the first time, 70 per cent of agency workers were now being offered equal treatment, though only after twelve weeks in the job. Later, in the light of worsening economic problems, implementation was postponed and did not come into effect until October 2011.

Brown had believed that he would be able to build more broad-based party support than Blair had. Yet now dissatisfaction with the government's performance grew in the unions as it did amongst other hitherto loyal Labour supporters in the period immediately after the 10p tax blow. Private polls for the unions that summer produced some startling results. One private poll found more than half of those who had 'always or more often than not voted Labour' declared themselves less likely to vote Labour than they did in 2005.[29] In July 2008, another private poll found that a sample of trade union voters who had voted Labour in 2005 by a margin of 16 per cent now leaned to the Tories by 16 per cent, with the greatest lead amongst working-class voters (C2 D and E) of 18 per cent.[30] Indicative also was the big drop in those in the electorate willing to define themselves as 'New Labour' in IpsosMORI polls. In June 2001 it had been 29 per cent, but by March 2006 it had dropped to 18 per cent. By June 2008 it was down to 14 per cent. That mood was also feeding into and from the party and that summer there was a flurry of angry responses from within the unions including more internal pressures to disaffiliate.

The disappearing Warwick agreements

Warwick 1 Agreement tidying up
At the time that Brown took over, it had been hoped that he might follow through on a further implementation of the Warwick Agreement, looking to recover the cooperative atmosphere that the agreement had initially encouraged. Instead there was a long delay in returning to the discussion of the remaining elements and this was followed by an attempt by No. 10 to close down that discussion. Attention shifted to Warwick 2 preparations. There had been one school of thought around Blair that the policy role of TULO ought to be curtailed. Now Collins, as Brown's voice, let it be known to TULO officials that he favoured TULO returning to simply organisational support. In relations with the unions, managers sought to work tactically to that end.

Yet that aim was undermined by the newly aggressive pro-business agenda of BERR and the sense of how far Brown appeared to be moving away from Labour values. Within TULO, in order to avoid divide and rule from the managers, attempts were made to bring large and small unions working together during Warwick 2 discussions. But, as it happened, when the time came for NPF policy-making on Warwick 2 in July 2008, this unity was made virtually irrelevant in securing policy commitments by a combination of the misjudgement of union leaders and the tactics of the managers.

Warwick 2, NPF and union restraint

In one dimension Partnership in Power was a more open process with broad circulation of documents compared with 2004. Three thousand amendments from CLPs were allowed direct submission although only if taken into the final process through NPF members. It was chaotic and heavily pressurised in the light of Brown's electoral adversity. Amendments acceptable to the party were tabled en bloc twenty minutes prior to voting, and considerable efforts were made by managers to persuade the unions to vote down any CLP amendments deemed by the managers as unacceptable. The unions did decide to abstain on controversial political issues which were not their priority. They saw the draft document section on industrial and labour-related policy as mundane and inadequate, but did not immediately regard this as of pressing significance because the NPF opened on 25 July, the day that a big by-election defeat at Glasgow East was declared. Brown's speech to the NPF was deeply unimpressive and the consensus in the unions and elsewhere was that he would probably be gone shortly. Unions were also reassured that a second NPF would be held to follow up the limitations of this one. That never happened either.

The unions' failure to move against the Leader was also part of a general historical pattern already noted. They did not consider it to be their function and were aware of what hostile media forces would make of it. They had not supported giving clearer power to evict the Leader in the 1993 review and did not attempt it now. They had not led a move against Blair whom they generally distrusted and found more alien than Brown. 'Gordon' was seen as, at least, not obsessed with making money. At times he verbally refreshed the perception that in his heart he was still Labour.

Conference resolutions and management

The 2008 party conference was the first to which affiliated organisations and local parties did not have the right to submit motions on contemporary issues. Only one resolution on votes at 16 had been agreed at the NPF in the face of ministerial misgivings, and only two amendments had secured enough CLP support to go though to the party conference. At the conference, the local government representative Jeremy Beecham, who was to move the two amendments to the policy document from the NPF, was absent because of family illness and each amendment was then managed so as to avoid commitment. One, on legal aid, was withdrawn on the promise of a further review (which eventually proved unsatisfactory to the movers) and another, on direct election to police authorities, was unpopular and not put to the vote on the understanding there would be meetings to consider the proposal further. These came to nothing and there was a vigorous campaign, led later by Beecham, which resulted in the plan being dropped.

Unusually, an emergency resolution opposing the European working time opt-out by Britain was not discussed by the NEC which met only briefly. Nevertheless the managerial mobilisation against the resolution continued, pushed by Brown's aides led by McFadden on the basis that the words 'maintaining flexibility' in an NPF document already defined policy. Despite the fact that in the conference only around 16 hand votes were raised against the emergency resolution, the decision was ignored and, when the issue was picked up and supported in the European Parliament later, it was fought to an impasse by the British government.

PLP: a win is a win is a lose

Changes in managerial personnel

Under Brown the bringing in of backbenchers into governmental positions expanded further, including, as Mullin noted, a record number of ministers and parliamentary private secretaries.[31] On the Parliamentary Committee, from 2007 to 2010 there was a turnover of personnel beginning with Eagle and Ruddock moving into ministerial roles. Although Ann Cryer remained in the Socialist Campaign Group she was not seen as an ultra and she topped the polls for two years becoming Deputy Chair. It was not as cohesive a back-bench group since Blair's departure, yet it was still at times a significant voice representing PLP opinion, in particular articulating doubts over the Brown proposals in the new Terrorism Bill. There were more early detailed discussions than under Blair but they still arrived at a predetermined outcome of allowing terrorist suspects to be detained by police for up to 42 days before being charged.

Victory in the House on 11 June 2008, by a majority of only nine votes, was influenced by desperate offers and promises on the part of the weakened Brown and with the whips reportedly securing a series of deals which included an understanding with the nine Democratic Unionists. Challenged on the ethics of some of this, one response in the whips' office was 'A win is a win is a win'. That made sense in terms of saving Brown from the immediate consequences of a defeat. And it was also an implicit classic proclamation of 'serious politics'. But as this study has amply demonstrated, in party management a win is not always a win. The proclamation was emblematic of a deeper-rooted problem of 'New Labour' party management. Under pressure, there was an insensitivity to collateral damage and adverse consequences. In this case, the manner of victory was not judged to have strengthened him,[32] there was no clear sense that the government had won the argument and there was no net poll lift for Brown from the victory.[33] As it turned out, predictably, the bill was so overwhelmingly rejected by the Lords, and this Commons decision had been so concocted with unrepeatable deals, that in October a crucial section had to be dropped.

From 'New Labour' managerial assumptions, it might have been thought that Brown's weakened position would have led to multiple public calls for a stronger leader. Yet the experience of Blair and Brown appears to have influenced another view. When asked, 64 per cent of electors said that they would 'prefer a Prime Minister who mainly acts on the views and opinions of the general public to make decisions', as opposed to a Prime Minister who 'mainly trusts [his/her] own experience and judgement to make decisions'.[34]

The challenge of eviction and the problem of cohesion

Cohesion, the rules and protection of Brown

Brown's acceptance of Blairites in his government and his unwillingness to attempt to undo Blair's policy work did not bring him closer to most of the aggrieved Blairites. Their criticism took on a leftist tinge with an attack on his move away from Labour values over the 10p tax abolition. David Miliband was not an orthodox Blairite, and published only a restrained article arguing that 'against all odds we can still win, on a platform for change'. He called for humility 'about our shortcomings' but also being 'more compelling about our achievements'.[35] Brownites took this (or used this) as a warning of impending attack on the Prime Minister from the Blair stable.

On 12 September 2008 Siobhan McDonagh, sister of ex-General Secretary Margaret McDonagh, became the first Labour MP to call for a leadership election. The failure of party officials to routinely supply nomination forms to all the PLP, hitherto a Blairite defence mechanism by headquarters, now became subject to a Blairite critique. Eventually there were said to be twelve MPs making the personal request for nomination forms but, led by Collins, the NEC agreed that nomination forms should not be routinely sent out annually to the whole of the PLP when the party was in government. This it was said had been 'the convention for the past 11 years' and the NEC had a responsibility to follow these 'longstanding procedures'.[36] That pronouncement added further to the dangerous and fractious situation of lack of agreed rules.

Some of the Blairites who had been hitherto uninterested in the machine and its manipulations found this experience of 'Brownite tactics', including the anonymous attacks on Miliband, an eye-opener. However, a poll of members showed a majority did not want a leadership election.[37] In any case, there had been no clear sign of an immediate Labour bounce in the polls if any of the possible candidates replaced him. Reinforcing Brown's party position was also a fear of continuing internal war and a reluctance, played upon from No. 10, to give victory to 'the Blairites'. Brown was also bolstered by his own improved performance at the party conference, which included the punishing comment against Cameron (and Miliband) that 'This is no time for a novice'.

New managed protection: reshuffle

Brown's tactical preoccupation now again found its greatest skill in self-protection. The reshuffle of government places on 3 October 2008 involved a series of clever tactical moves. He promoted Nick Brown from Deputy to Chief Whip after Jacqui Smith resigned, with Tommy McAvoy as Deputy and John Spellar as pairing whip, strengthening the managerial operation in the House. Most significant was that Peter Mandelson was suddenly brought back on completion of his role in the European Commission. He was given a peerage, became Secretary of State for Business, Innovation and Skills in a renamed department and given the title of Lord President of the Council.

This was accompanied by new ministerial appointments for some of the disenchanted and the beginning of a healing relationship between Brownites and some of the Blairites. Geoff Norris moved to become special adviser to Mandelson. Together with McFadden they made a powerful new business-sympathetic alliance and were a trio of skilful party managers. Mandelson, who had always been a better organisational manager than Blair or Brown, was seen to make improvements in the government's competence in ways which impressed commentators.

An important economic initiative also gave a boost to Brown's party support. In October 2008, as the international financial crisis spread across the world, Brown led a bold operation to commit the necessary amounts of public money to defend the financial system by recapitalising British banks. It was a policy that was paid the compliment of being followed later by every major country. In December Brown received a poll lift as the man most likely to get the economy back on track.[38] In the party the new economic measures gave his supporters more confidence and a reinforced justification that he should not be replaced, although his poll bounce petered out amongst the wider electorate.

Unions, government and distrust

Some limited policy changes encouraged a little more party support. An increase in statutory redundancy pay had been followed by an increase in the minimum-wage rate from October 2008 with the adult rate applying to 21-year-olds from 2010. A new issue emerged involving the government banning the inclusion of tips in employers' calculation of the national minimum wage. Public support especially in the London activity of community action groups had pushed that, and it became a good issue to be publicly associated with. On an old issue of legal action over the blacklisting of trade unionists, in March 2009 new government regulations were finally introduced making it a criminal offence, but it fell short of union expectations. There was no promise of further delivery from the leftovers of Warwick 1.

PLP dissent, discipline and defence

Almost immediately after he took up his new office, Mandelson with Brown's backing led a move towards part-privatisation of the Post Office. This was another binding-up of wounds from an old conflict between them. But it opened up other wounds. Over a hundred Labour MPs expresssed opposition and two-thirds of party members were opposed.[39] To Mandelson this oppposition was union negativity allied to party traditionalism refusing to face economic realities. To his opponents, privatisation was a dogmatic ideological attack. Crucially, the conflict also revolved around resentment at the government's initating new policies regardless of what the party had said in the manifesto, the decisions of the conference and the Warwick 1 agreement. It was also done, as was learned later, without a Cabinet decision,[40] and it fed into a growing procedural crisis in the party (see below). In another political twist some of the PLP Blairites worried that Mandelson was being managed to carry all the fault of this joint decision with Brown.

In spite of the reshuffle and strengthening of the whips' office, maintaining PLP discipline and constraining absenteeism did not improve and there was little constructively that the returning chief whip, Nick Brown, could do about it. When he proposed a new sanction that anybody who had voted against the government in the past year would not be appointed to select committees, that met a sharp reaction at the PLP on 10 November 2008. In effect it was referred back to the Parliamentary Committee and rejected there because, as a member reported, 'We don't have enough MPs willing to be representatives anyway'. The issue of strengthening sanctions against regular dissidents from the PLP still came up on occasions at the Parliamentary Committee but, facing a view that the proposed action would make the situation worse, it made no headway.

An attempt by TULO to again move into parliamentary action against the government was made by a coalition of ten unions and 146 supporters for an increase in redundancy payments through a Statutory Redundancy Payment (Amendment) Private Member's Bill sponsored by Lindsay Hoyle on 3 March 2009. It was fiercely opposed by the government but had enough support for it to become an influence on the 2009 Budget. Payment rose from £350 to £380 per week, far short of the £500 that unions were asking for. Meanwhile tension built up between No. 10, the headquarters management and Byron Taylor in the TULO office over the latter's support for this organised intra-party opposition.

As under Blair, there were regular minor amendments to legislation to take the edge off opposition. And the government suffered three Commons defeats in the period from April to July 2009: over Ghurka veteran settlement, the venue of the East Midlands regional committee and the scope of parliamentary privilege in relation to investigations of MPs. But none of these were central issues. Largely unobserved by commentators, a significant new parliamentary defence for the Leader had come about not through the formal PLP managers but via a management control which began to be exercised in 2008–9 through Whelan, the Unite Political Office and the huge PLP Unite union group of over 160 MPs. Whelan attempted here, as in other party spheres, to thwart and break down centres of critical opposition to the Leader. Group meetings became irregular and sparsely attended. This had costs. Whelan's activities within Unite led to a big clash over accusations of 'bullying' between him and members of the Unite headquarters Political Office,[41] and later to a new media focus on Whelan's methods.[42] On the transport side of the union and in other unions there was a growing frustration at Whelan's role.

Candidate selection

In candidate selection Whelan encouraged union support for strongly expressed No. 10 preferences and targeted favourites. A priority was the avoidance of candidates who might later cause Brown trouble. In this it was highly successful. It was unusual that left-wing union candidates John Cryer in Leyton and Wanstead and Ian Lavery in Wansbeck did later come though this system in safe seats, but Cryer only did so after an attempt from No. 10 to stop him met internal opposition from Tom Watson, and Lavery, an ex-union official, secured the support of the GMB. Late on, a very lively leftish Asian woman, Lisa Nandy, gained the selection in the all-women short-listed seat at Wigan.

Towards the end of the parliamentary term there was also an adjustment of union behaviour in ending the stabilising blanket defence of sitting MPs. Veteran left MPs Bob Wareing in Liverpool West Derby and Frank Cook in Stockton North had been subject to such a strong and lengthy pressure from their constituencies that the unions did not intervene to save them. In a third case, a long dispute over former UNISON President Anne Moffat (previously Picking) in East Lothian went to the NEC in 2010. They assented to the constituency beginning reselection with a decisive vote of 24 to 4, with two abstentions. These cases were each pressed locally and were also supported from party headquarters.

'Smeargate' and the dark management forces

Meanwhile, another aspect of management was moving into difficulties. The rise of blogging on the net had strengthened a proliferation of centre-right and right-wing Conservative commentators. A new website, *Labour-Home*, helped generate a recognition in the senior ranks of the Labour Party that in the new media the days of command and control were over. Those developments led to the launch of LabourList backed by Whelan and assisted by Unite political funds. Collins appointed Derek Draper as editor. It was a constructive development linked informally to Brown's media adviser in No. 10, Damian McBride.

But in April 2009, uncovered by the Guido Fawkes website, was a covert operation initiated from No. 10 in cooperation with Draper. This played with the idea of smearing individual Conservatives in the most crude and offensive form. It led to McBride's resignation and that stimulated a new public examination of Brown's methods. As an arm of Brown's party management, McBride had long been suspected of organising briefing of the media in a way that could assist individual favourites and damage those considered troublesome.[43] That had included establishing Douglas Alexander and Ed Miliband as being to blame for the briefing which pushed towards the election fiasco,[44] and unleashing what Darling called 'the forces of hell'[45] in the summer of 2008 after Darling had made public his judgement that the economic crisis was the worst in 60 years.

Charles Clarke was bold enough to make the accusation that 'Damian McBride . . . was part of a poisonous team' and they should be 'removed from their positions'.[46] Draper did eventually go, but nobody else. Brown privately justified the initial failure to move McBride by reference to Cameron's employment of the former *News of the World* editor Andy Coulson,[47] a man with a past association with phone-hacking. His appointment was taken by Brown as yet another indicator of the dark ruthlessness of Conservative politics which had to be matched by Labour politics.

Brown aides privately had been emphatic when Blair was Leader that the Blair 'side of the family' had been especially manipulative, and their own behaviour was not to be confused with that experience. Blair's strategist and experienced party manager Matthew Taylor, when he was briefly out of managerial employment, had himself referred to the apparent willingness of the Blair management 'to demonise those who express doubt or dissent'.[48] The 'Little Hitlers' of 1994 may have set a bullying example followed by some other conference managers when word got out amongst managers about that approved behaviour. But generally both camps, though convinced, found it difficult amidst all the covert spinners and misleading informants, to prove absolutely who was the source of what behaviour and who was the worst.

Some indication of what was a significant difference was that Blair was more tolerant of disagreement around him and was never accused of personally intimidatory behaviour. Brown was, and sympathetic biographer Steve Richards described him as having 'an habitual ugly side' in his serious political fights.[49] The media preoccupation with Smeargate was thought by Mandelson to have reduced media focus on Brown's success in influencing international economic policy at the G20 conference, held in London in April 2009.[50] But the smallness of the electoral boost he received may also have been affected by the substance of the complaints over Brown and their contrast with his 'new politics' promises of summer 2007. Of wider significance was that, after 'Smeargate', so low had politicians sunk in public opprobrium that Ben Page of IpsosMORI diagnosed that this was now 'how people expected politicians to behave'.[51]

Eviction revisited

In May 2009, new efforts began seeking to topple Brown but Alan Johnson, potentially the strongest candidate, did not offer himself and there was a fragmented opposition to Brown. One veteran Blairite noted privately 'we are all fighting each other'. Still constraining a removal was the problem of the lack of an easy procedure and the difficulties of avoiding a long internal war. Anonymous former Labour party officials offered the public view that party election of the Leader need not be a lengthy process, but their advice hinged on avoiding full participation by affiliated union levy payers.[52] That solution had no constitutional validity and its source was again seen as 'Blairite'. To this was added warnings from No. 10 that if Brown was forced from office, a new prime minister would not be able to withstand the demands to hold an immediate general election that would lead to a Labour wipeout.[53] The unions were determined that they would stay in the procedure although they refused either to openly come out in support of Brown or to attack him.

Mandelson swung his influence towards managing party unity by arguing that an apparently Blairite putsch was 'not the way to go'.[54] That helped raise his low level of popularity in the party and further strengthened his position in relation to Brown. He was now given the honorific title of First Secretary of State and seemed to have enhanced his status as, in effect, the Deputy Prime Minister. In spite of his intervention there were still a series of Blairite ministerial resignations from government with the most pointed, Hazel Blears, Caroline Flint and James Purnell on 4 and 5 June. Purnell directly urged Brown to resign. Blears's resignation, her comments and personal demeanour were seen as specially damaging to an already faltering local election campaign. Those elections results and the European elections were generally agreed to be disastrous; the loss of councillors was a further blow to the party's grassroots organisation.

On 1 July 2009, still facing huge party opposition, Mandelson announced a step back from a huge potential confrontation over the Post Office. The explanation – that part-priviatisation was being put on hold until market conditions improved – was read in the party as an accommodation with critics. There was even talk (possibly instigated) of him being a potential Leader, but his old reputation still stood in the way; as veteran political correspondent Michael White had pointed out in May, the question 'I wonder what he is up to' was 'the price for being thought devious'.[55] Nevertheless, in a speech to the 2009 Conference, Mandelson received a standing ovation for a very clever speech which subtly conjoined the personal and party lesson that 'you can work your passage back'.

The degeneration of party procedures

The vibrancy of the rank-and-file organisation in the victorious Obama campaign in the USA brought a new focus on the possibility of Labour's own renewal and a new awareness of the oppressive and debilitating atmosphere produced by its management. On LabourList on 20 June 2009, Jessica Asato, acting Director of Progress, lamented that the Partnership in Power structures were 'probably accurately seen as a way of silencing the grassroots of the party'. That silencing became more chronic as across-the-board agreed party procedures now in various ways further degenerated or were deliberately undermined. Although, when he was a critic of Blair's leadership, Brown was seen by some fellow critics as more likely to respect the party and its procedures and to revive its vitality, the opposite had proved to be the case.

The most contentious development concerned the selection campaign in Erith and Thamesmead, in the period leading up to 17 May 2009 in which, following claims of postal vote irregularities, a ballot box was found to have been interfered with whilst at party headquarters. After the selection, efforts by the NEC to secure from officials a written report on this failed and continued to fail in the years that followed, in spite of the damaging account that emerged in the public domain as 'Labour party abandons ballot-tampering inquiry'.[56]

Building Britain's Future, a white paper introduced by Brown in the House of Commons on 29 June 2009, was mainly a re-assembling of previous positions, but it was not made the subject of prior discussion by any partnership institutions. In the PLP the departmental committees became moribund with a couple of spasmodic exceptions. PLP meetings reverted to what appeared to be choreographed support for the Leader.[57] Under pressure from critics following the local election defeats, Brown told the PLP on 7 June that he wanted to act in a more collective way.[58] That failed to happen, and Brown's attendances at the Parliamentary Committee deteriorated without any attempt to reschedule for his absences.

Under the reform of NEC meeting times brought in by the Sawyer changes of 1997, that committee was not due to discuss the local government and European poll wipe-out in elections on 4–7 June until its meeting on 21 July. A *Tribune* editorial on 26 June looking for any Labour Party national activity complained of 'a void'. The JPC, which was held to have been a strengthened body under the policy of extending and developing democracy, did meet but ministers often failed to attend. In July 2009 it might have discussed *Building Britain's Future* even after the public event but was only attended by one Minister for 10 minutes. That led to much bad temper.

Because of the shortage of finance and because it was not prioritised by managers, the NPF did not meet before the 2009 conference. A new Road to the Manifesto ballot remained in the Brown plans, but without funding; and in the absence of a party welcome for a procedure which had a top-down manipulative history, it was, as one senior NEC member described it, 'a dead parrot'. The change in managing contemporary issues under Brown had led not to extending democracy but to a frustrating managerial procedure where issues were referred back to policy commissions and emerged without new outcomes.

The party membership and level of activity continued to sink. CLP representation at the party conference declined each year: 501 in 2007, 465 in 2008, 444 in 2009 and 412 in 2010. Given the management of the conference in policy-making, as BBC political editor Nick Robinson pointed out in a message directed at spin doctors, 'speeches that are delivered to empty halls and ignored by your own party workers, let alone large parts of the media, is not serving them well, let alone everyone else'.[59]

Brown continued to receive regular national support from Unite and often from two traditionally loyal unions from the Labour right, USDAW and Community. But in many of the unions and the TULO office the degeneration of national procedures and the pattern of manipulative man-agement produced a permanent sense of truculence and unease in national relationships. There was an increasing demand that everything agreed in discussions be tied down. That took more time and effort from the man-agers. As a result of the weakening of trust, and sense of loss of direction, insiders noted a lack of energetic enthusiasm from the unions in mobilising the grass roots for pro-Labour electoral campaigning.

The revolt

Privately, signs also began to emerge in the unions of a low-key disagree-ment about how the unions and party members in the future might respond to this decay. One view was that the original spirit of partnership must be replenished. Another view was that there should be a rejection of the whole paraphenalia of 'partnership' and the re-establishment of a resolution-based conference. Both were accompanied by a realism that no reform would work if the behaviour of the management did not change. And it was realised in the unions that if they were to carry a broad measure of CLP support for renovation they had to escape the managerial stereotype that they were the force stopping the CLPs from democratic expression, a characterisation often used as part of the managerial armoury of divide and rule.

Now, what had appeared to be a deepening atmosphere of demoralised disengagement within the party proved to be a revolt awaiting an opportune moment and an appropriate issue. The TULO unions had hitherto refrained from proposing any constitutional changes but now, following an initiative from Byron Taylor and the TULO organisation, the majority of unions moved behind a constitutional amendment from Islington CLP at the 2009 party conference. That called not for an improved position for the unions but for the introduction of one-member-one-vote in the CLP elections to the NPF which had operated as the most corrupted part of the implementation of Partnership in Power under Blair and then Brown. The Islington proposal was backed by the CLPD organisation but it ignited a much wider support.

There was considerable alarm and pressure from No. 10 and the General Secretary's office to kill off the OMOV proposal, and much tension and suspicion as a result. The outcome, a surprise even to the delighted organisers, was 67 per cent in favour, with a majority in both sections on a card vote. CLPs were 55 per cent in favour and affiliates 79 per cent in favour. In the minority vote within the unions were those of USDAW and Community. It was an expression still, as on the NEC, of the instinctive response of some on the traditional right to appeals for defence of what the Leader needed, even if over a procedural reform which years before had given them a principled procedural purpose.

But the result was a significant advance for campaigners for a less corrupted intra-party political process, an advance for the members and a step forward by the unions. It was also the biggest defeat for the General Secretary and the managerial regime under 'New Labour'. A striking feature was that Whelan and his ex-TGWU managerial allies Collins and Irvine were unable to prevent Unite delegates from voting for the change, even though those arguing for it found themselves facing the argument that it was not 'our' (i.e. a union) issue. This defeat was therefore a particularly damaging blow to Brown's greatest managerial defence mechanism; Unite now appeared unsafe.

It was a little-noticed but major development, and not the end of the story. In the months that followed and before the publication of the 2010 rulebook, a rule change was brought in by the General Secretary, covering union representation on the NEC. This was done without consultation with the unions, the NEC or its Chair and without any announcement. The change involved in effect an undermining of the representation of the largest unions, including Unite, whilst strengthening Brown's position through the now better-represented smaller loyalist unions. The episode was to lead later to a battle over party management after the general election (see below).

The expenses scandal and party management

MPs, trust and independence

Meanwhile, the parliamentary-expenses scandal emerging in 2009 provoked a public revulsion around two entwined sources of distrust. First, the extent to which MPs had focused on their own financial interests confirmed the worst fears that some in the electorate had held about greedy and self-oriented MPs and now provided evidence that made more think the same.

Second, the existence of what was in practice a hidden system of allowances whereby 'indecent rules were exploited in a way that is indecent',[60] and an attempt made to cover up the practice against investigation, fitted into the huge concern over manipulative politics. The Hansard Audit of Political Engagement in 2010 showed that those who did not trust MPs 'very much or not at at all' had risen from the already high level of 70 per cent in their previous study to 73 per cent. Within that there was also now a significant increase in the minority who did not trust politicians at all, from 19 to 25 per cent.

Amongst Labour Party members, many of whom automatically assumed that financial behaviour like this was to be expected of Conservatives, the sense of anger was palpable. The behaviour fitted too closely with the tolerance of people getting 'filthy rich'. There was a public and party demand for the purge of deviant MPs. In the PLP, dismay was deepened by Brown's apparent reluctance to defend the honour of the majority of MPs as they now became subject to a new independent external regulation of MPs' expenses.

Amongst some NEC members, Brown's response was considered tardy and, unlike Cameron, unable to pull his colleagues together on reform in a way which helped the party electorally. An attempt was made to push for an independent NEC statement on the expenses scandal, but Brown was not happy with that and as usual the NEC meeting on 19 May 2009 was cross-pressured between unwillingness to damage the Leader and a desire to articulate their own deep concerns. In the end there was a compromise agreement that a three-person NEC committee would interview any Labour MPs where there appeared to be evidence against them.

But this procedure was managed so that it depended on who was referred to it by the Chief Whip and the General Secretary. Three of four MPs referred were refused permission to stand as Labour candidates although they had already taken the decision to go. The fourth refused was Ian Gibson, who admitted using his parliamentary expenses to pay for his daughter's London home before selling it to her for half its market value. It was not one of the worst cases and Gibson had a long record as an independent-minded and principled critic of the government. He immediately resigned as an MP thereby losing a substantial resettlement grant and forcing a by-election.

That by-election on 24 July was especially noteworthy in that all parties claimed to continue Gibson's integrity. Labour lost the seat. Out of this experience came a new awareness of the electoral value to the party of having independent-minded MPs, a feature barely registered within the old managerial mindset but, as shown, indicated for some time in surveys. An extensive *Guardian* survey on 3 June 2009, analysed by Tom Clark, confirmed the hardening public mood over party management shown in the 2006 Standards in Public Life survey. There was 'concern over the inability of parliament to control the government and the way that the party line strangles independent thought'; it was significant that proposals to weaken the grip of the party machines and strengthen the role of back-bench MPs were 'highly popular'. The expenses scandal enabled this already strengthening public opinion to be registered, whilst the crisis disoriented the party machines.[61]

One of the consequences of these developments was to give a new opportunity for back-bench critics of executive dominance over MPs to take the initiative. Tony Wright had been one of the first parliamentary supporters of Blair but was also one of the first friendly critics of the controllers of 'New Labour'. He had looked towards the political project as 'an enterprise of advocacy and persuasion and example'.[62] But quickly and often since 1995 he had pointed out that in practice they had a managerial politics which 'simply does not work anymore'.[63] As Chair of the Public Administration Select Committee, he was able to lead a radical report on changing the balance between MPs and the government and eventually, in the next parliament, able to establish a cross-party back-bench Business Committee, operating in public, to hear representations with the power to schedule debates and votes in the House. Chairs and members of select committees were to be elected by MPs, and not chosen by the whips. That marked a significant, if untested, move away from executive and management influence over back-bench MPs.[64]

A broken politics?

In the public dialogue that followed the expenses scandal, not all of the reform proposals were clearly moored to the origins of the crisis. Electoral reform had a stronger case regardless of the expenses scandal, given the way that the present system had concentrated political sensitivity on a relatively small number of voters in the marginal seats. But the electoral system was exaggerated as the cause of deviant expenses behaviour. Reform had a place in producing additional formal safeguards against unacceptable behaviour, but it was not the solution to some deeper problems of political culture and the behaviour of politicians, some of it trained in a particular mode of public influence and party management.

What Cameron called 'broken politics' could not usefully be equated simply with an 'anti-politics' sentiment, given that two-thirds of the public valued politics and did not think it was a waste of time.[65] However, a more reasonable meaning of broken politics, if that concept has to be used, would be the many instances of the dislocation between the behaviour of politicians and the behaviour regarded by electors as appropriate for sincere politicians. As against the many contributions which talked past the big problem in the year following the expenses scandal, there was a salutary offering by Daniel Finkelstein, commensurate with the analysis here, that 'what the people mean by political reform is politicians talking straight'.[66]

Mattinson's focus-group analysis suggested to her at this time that there was less anger about politicians than had been expected because 'cynicism

had led to total disengagement'.[67] This proved pessimistic. In what at the
general election became labelled Cleggmania, the huge reception for Clegg's
contribution to the Leaders' Debate showed strong indications of the anti-
manipulative ethos and the desire for a more trustworthy politics.[68] Later,
there was a huge critical reaction to what was regarded as Clegg's deceitful behaviour. Both phenomena involved an engaged and assertive public
expression.

Final attempt at eviction

A few months ahead of the 2010 general election Brown's continued poor
public ratings brought a new attempt to seek his eviction as Leader. On
6 January the ex-ministers Geoff Hoon and Patricia Hewitt proposed that
the PLP decide whether they wanted an election for Leader. Quite properly,
this was declared by officials to be illegitimate under the rules. As before,
those thought to be Cabinet supporters of change failed to move, although
the obvious tardiness of most of them in coming out in public support of
Brown indicated no great enthusiasm for him. Yet in the PLP and the wider
party, the majority view was that highly publicised moves to evict Brown
did his standing no good and continued to project an image of a divided
leadership.[69] Stopping the challenges was the dominant inclination.

Managing the manifesto

Leading up to the manifesto discussions, the economic crisis and its association with neo-liberal economics, and the undermining of the mythology
of the endemic superiority of the private sector, created space for new
policy developments in the Labour Party and, from that, a more consensual
basis of management. At the same time, new evidence was available of the
social effects of inequality affecting everybody.[70] However, there was no
new movement towards a new social democratic radicalism which might
involve extra spending. The raising of taxation on the wealthy from 40p
to 45 p and then to 50p had been welcomed in the party and popular with
the public but it was defended only apologetically by Brown, Darling and
Mandelson as a pragmatic and temporary move. A rise in national insurance contributions which drew criticism from Conservative business supporters made the reception for Labour's business manifesto more difficult.
   The preparation of the general election manifesto, 'A Future Fair for
All', was done by Ed Miliband from the Brown camp with assistance from
the more Blairite Patrick Diamond. Both were a little to the left of their
political leaders but could not fully operate in that way. The manifesto
was in the end a mixed bag which, as Douglas Alexander admitted later,
bore little relationship to the Partnership in Power process.[71] An effort
had been made to sustain the new Blairite-Brownite rapprochement with

commitment on public sector reforms towards local service delivery, with failing services taken over by successful ones and all hospitals becoming foundation trusts. A united 'New Labour' offering also included making it easier to create John Lewis-style mutuals – a policy also broadly acceptable even to the Conservatives providing it was not focused on reform of the private sector. There was a more activist industrial strategy, influenced by Mandelson and welcomed by both the CBI and the TUC, which saw it as in line with Congress House longer-term thinking. Once again, there was commitment to a Blairite procedure unasked for by the party and not a product of public clamour – directly elected mayors, this time in new city regions.

Covering new ground, there were living-wage proposals for government employees, an input from citizens' action organisations concerned with poverty, particularly in London, and pushed from some in the PLP including Jon Cruddas and Ed Miliband. There was also a move to local investment funds to deal with the intensifying loan-sharks issue. In three discussions with TULO leaders in 2010 and in the continuing dialogue with the TUC, the unions had hoped for something more radical in countering restrictive employment rights; but that faded in the face of determined opposition from Brown and absence of a proper Warwick 2-style process. However, some inclusions and omissions were potentially consoling.

The rejection of part privatisation of the Royal Mail was firmed up, in spite of Mandelson's indication that it could be brought back in the future. There was a critical reference to the bogus self-employment designation which avoided legal rights for workers; minimum-wage changes were to be linked to earnings; there was the promise of legislation covering gangmasters in construction and there was support for a law to restrict the takeover of British firms on public-interest grounds, a campaign led by the Unite union.

The slowing down of the pro-market reorganisation policy in the NHS had also left health service workers in a better mood to talk up an NHS that had received years of substantial rises in funding. Those together probably contributed to what was found to be new levels of public satisfaction with the NHS. In the manifesto pre-meeting there was a warm welcome when Andy Burnham, the Secretary of State for Health, made clear that they had no plans for another major restructuring. Brown had always seen the problems of permanent revolution.

Over the Hayden Phillips proposals on party funding no further discussion had taken place in the party. Brown had let it be known in December 2007 that he favoured starting from there. TULO had rejected that as unwelcome and untimely. Nevertheless, without any discussion at the pre-election meetings the draft manifesto did contain the commitment to Brown's position. The TULO office and some senior union leaders did not find out about it until 18 May.

Distrust and word-of-mouth campaigning

The party had by October 2009 lost the support of Rupert Murdoch's News International group of newspapers. Together with a shortage of finance, it led to a new emphasis on a word-of-mouth election strategy. Announced in February 2010, it cited the Obama campaign example and the use by party members of all social networks and new media to extend this word-of-mouth operation. That potentially fitted the new communication wisdom that in facing pervasive suspicion of manipulation the 'best trust agents' were through 'people like me'.[72] Headquarters introduced a running tally of campaign contacts made in each constituency.

The results are difficult to assess but some of the limitations are clear. It did not help that a poll in January 2010 had found that under half of natural Labour supporters believed that a Labour Government would deliver on a new manifesto compared with three-quarters of Liberal and Conservative supporters about their parties.[73] As for the party's message conveyors, membership was down to 153,141 at September 2009 and still sinking. Brown's version of 'extending and renewing' party democracy had done neither, and his form of management of policy-making appeared to give a low priority to preparing the members' role as ambassadors of policy and trust. The degeneration of the policy-making infrastructure was not conducive to passing enthusiastic commitment outwards.

It had been argued from US experience that 'new mobilising techniques will not prove a magic bullet unless there is an inspiring mission and message'.[74] Missing from Brown's leadership until the final days when he addressed the community organisers of Citizens UK was a clear assertion of identity and values. Too late he also gave then a passionate and impressive personal statement that 'life is about more than self-interest, work is about more than self-advancement, that service is about more than self-service, that happiness is about more than you earn and own'.[75]

Within an often chaotically led national campaign in 2010, the party did best against the tide through incumbents who were seen as trusted local champions and where the local party was involved in a regular dialogue with community concerns.[76] In some areas the determination of the local party partially made up for the depleted and often disillusioned membership. Responding to the party's warning that Cameron was fronting a Tory party whose instincts could not be trusted on jobs and the public sector, the last phase of the 2010 campaign was marked by an anti-Tory resurgence of activity through both some 're-awakened' members and also volunteers.[77] Significantly, the latter were not involved as much as party members in the dialogue work of telephoning and canvassing.[78] Yet if the word-of-mouth strategy was to work fully, a substantial and continually engaged membership was still to be sought as a major asset.

As with the individual membership, Labour's affiliated union membership had further declined. From 3.3 million in 1997 it was down to 2.6 million in 2010. That was still a potentially considerable supportive constituency, especially if subject to committed union and party mobilisation. Yet, informal communication networks in the unions added to the disillusionment and dissatisfaction expressed in the unions over the Brown years, and it complicated the official pro-Labour election campaigning message down the organisational chain to the grass roots. There, membership in most unions was not growing, the appeal to potential new members to join the union was weak,[79] and as the polls had shown, commitment to the Labour Party had declined significantly.

Whelan in Unite had drawn media attention to the unions' effort in providing considerable resources, introducing online phone banks, and urging union members to contact others. Opinions on its effectiveness sharply diverge, probably because Whelan and the atmosphere around him in the unions was so controversial. Because of the failure to hold a Warwick-style forum, the campaign was de-linked from the kind of policy agreement which had been managed with the unions a year before the 2005 election. As a result, there was no agreed union-party agenda putting out a broad message before the election campaign, and there was a limited commitment on future Labour policy which had industrial resonance. For reasons of political control, TULO coordination was barely used by the party in this campaigning, leaving it to the individual unions working with campaign officials in support of party policy.

Economic trust and party management

Brown's electoral advantage over economic management after 2008 had become his vulnerability as the man in charge who, in spite of his boasts, had not 'ended boom and bust'. That passed into folklore as a misleading and unrectified spin which was found out by events. The reaction of around three-quarters of the electorate in 2008–9 had been that Brown had some responsibility for allowing lending and borrowing to get out of hand in the first place.[80] All this provided ammunition for the Conservatives to use and misuse and Brown was not helped by the lack of trust in his narrative and the sincerity of his promises. In the summer of 2009, Labour had been considered by non-aligned voters as the least honest of the main parties on their future tax and spending plans.[81]

Despite the instinctive Labour opposition to cuts 'caused by the bankers', at different levels in the party and in the leadership, doubts developed over the honesty of Brown's portrayal of the choice as simply investment versus cuts. Eventually, Brown was forced by these internal party pressures into a highly publicised adjustment in which the Chancellor, Darling, promised halving the budget deficit in four years whilst protecting front-line services and the most vulnerable. In the election campaign itself in 2010 there was a limited anti-Tory recovery in Labour support. But the IpsosMORI analysis of the election found that 'few of the voters were enthusiastically endorsing either of the parties' economic policies'.[82]

The defeat of 'New Labour'

The election result was the worst for Labour since the disaster of 1983. In fear of Conservative cuts, people in the public sector remained relatively loyal[83] but Labour lost ground particularly in seats where there were many working-class voters and a large increase in unemployment.[84] These had been centres of Labour strength. By election day, support for Labour from the C2 category had dropped by 11 points since 2005, and amongst the DE category by 8 points. In contrast the AB category had dropped by only 2 points and the C1 category by 4 points.[85] The controverial issue of immigration was damagingly integrated with bread-and-butter dissatisfactions over housing, jobs and wages.

Fighting an electoral campaign which included a supportive role for veteran Blairites, especially Mandelson, but also Campbell, Gould and Blunkett, and on one occasion Blair himself, this defeat was a 'New Labour' not a specifically Brown phenomenon. In 1997, 'New Labour' had secured 13,518,167 votes on an anti-Tory wave. In stages, by 2010 the vote had dropped to 8,609,527 votes. Around the time of the argument over Clause IV, which had been followed by an anti-union spin barrage, the proportion of those in the manual working-class who identified with Labour fell and continued to fall as the leadership managers failed to emphasise its appeal to traditional supporters, and the image of the party and its social affinity changed.[86] That management contributed to an acute problem that 'New Labour' was not judged by that quarter of the electorate who still identified themselves as working-class to be on the side of 'people like us'. Also, Labour MPs were now seen to be all from the same middle-class background, with the same income and property as Conservative MPs, too similar with not enough equality and diversity.[87]

In the aftermath of this defeat, discussions (which did not involve the PLP) were led by Brown to see if a new arrangement could be reached with the Liberal Democrats; but a coalition arrangement of Conservatives and Liberals emerged. Brown resigned as Prime Minister. During the inter-party political vacuum, the Conservatives and their press allies focused ruthlessly and cleverly on 'Labour's financial crisis'. This was in spite of the fact that it arose in the US, that Cameron and Osborne had earlier pledged to match Labour spending and increase it year on year and that they had opposed stronger regulation. This barrage of spin left for any new Labour leadership a deeply problematic context. Meanwhile, Cameron and Clegg as Prime Minister and Deputy initiated what was portrayed as a 'new politics' based on politicians working cooperatively together in the national interest.

Section 2: Miliband and the end of 'New Labour' management?

Adversity and the party's task

With some differences of focus, it was broadly agreed in the party that this defeat marked the end of the era of 'New Labour',[88] although Blair later portrayed the end as dating from his own departure.[89] Following Brown's resignation, a discussion about the future of the party began to emerge with a new willingness to acknowledge shortcomings and mistakes, albeit still with the usual reticence in referring publicly to the detail of the managerial system. Five candidates for Leader, Andy Burnham, Ed Miliband, Ed Balls and Diane Abbott (who was nominated with the support of some of those backing the expected winner David Miliband, because he wanted to ensure a more open and pluralistic contest) all distanced themselves from some of the processes and practices of 'New Labour'. They appeared to be moving towards a degree of consensus on the aim of opening up and revitalising the party, and giving the members a stronger voice.

One important procedural problem was cleared up. Responding to Harman's decision not to resign as Deputy Leader after a new Leader was elected, on 20 July 2010 the NEC clarified the rule on future leadership challenges that had caused so much trouble under Blair's managerial control. The onus in seeking a contest would be on the challenger to obtain the nomination of MPs, rather than the party inviting nominations every year. That was, in effect, a rulebook authorisation of the managerial conduct since 1997 and it was now a clear rule with an NEC consensus behind it.

Moving on: the three trajectories

The new Leader, Ed Miliband, was elected with only a narrow majority of just over 1 per cent in the electoral college, and though he had won a majority of the individual levy-payers voting in the affiliated organisations section he did not have a majority in the MPs/MEPs section nor the CLP members section. The victory of a man backed by most union leaders including the leader of the largest union, Unite, and given union organisational and financial support, was easily criticised as 'the party members supported David and the unions supported Ed'. For some supporters of the defeated candidates and also some academic commentators,[90] Ed Miliband's occupancy was judged not legitimate. The defeated brother David Miliband behaved with dignity and restraint, but from some others there was persistent carping in and to the media that the wrong man was in position and Ed was not up to the job. That did not assist the build-up of his public support, but he was also organisationally relatively unprepared and did not seek to immediately cultivate a prominent public profile.

The union role as problem

Three different trajectories for party reform marked the distinctive management politics of this new period in Opposition, and their development and conflicts appeared likely to be a feature of the immediate future, with the alliances and perspectives sometimes overlapping and sometimes diverging. The union role in the party was one focus. It had not been as electorally damaging as often presented to be the case. In 2010, out of the well-publicised Whelan and Unite role, and its connection with the British Airways strike, the Conservative Party with the aid of press allies had attempted again to turn the union link with Labour into an adverse election issue. It had failed yet again. It did not register on the election issues index of IpsosMORI[91] and was not mentioned in the thorough Kavanagh and Cowley contribution to the Nuffield series of general election studies.[92]

However, with 1,030,100 votes, Unite had a considerable chunk although still a minority, 39.3 per cent, of the voting weight of the 14 unions in the affiliated organisations' sections of the electoral college. There was also in that section, as in the past, an openness to multiple votes for individuals with multiple membership in the different organisations. These features made that flank of the union role a prominent target for those advocating major reforms of the union position in the party.

And it made the victorious Leader himself all the more sensitive to the need to show public independence from the unions, although he did it with more balance and less enthusiasm than the early Blair, and still preserving a sense of mutual respect. At different stages later, Miliband spoke out against public sector strikes and he and Balls made clear their support for the continuation of a public sector wage freeze as part of the attempt to reduce the public sector deficit. But his strong public support for the continuation of the union-party relationship conveyed to the unions that they were valued in a way that they had not been under 'New Labour'. He also broke eventually with 'New Labour' distancing by supporting a TUC rally against government economic policy, and in 2012 attended the traditional Durham miners gala, to a very warm welcome. Yet hovering behind the anti-cuts unity and once coming uneasily to the fore, was the problem of what Labour itself would do in office, and how the unions would respond, about the debt and public expenditure.

Management and control

A second major focus arose from the momentum of party complaint about management control. What remained in place after Blair went and had been sustained by Brown was the distinctive culture, conduct and organisation of party management. Ed Miliband's first conference speech was bold and potentially far-reaching in his diagnosis that 'we have to leave quite a lot of what the "New Labour" establishment did, behind us, particularly in its methods'.[93] He disassociated himself from the Iraq invasion over which, as shown here, there had been a ruthlessly effective manipulated distortion of the party's voice. The Leader summarised past failings later, in a speech to the 2011 NPF, that 'the leadership believed its role was to protect the public from the party' and yet it 'lost touch with both party members and the people'. Here was an outlook clearly different from that of Blair and Brown, establishing the project of securing electability without producing the kind of damaging problems 'New Labour' management left behind.

Whilst Miliband remained handicapped by not being able to shake off association with all dissatisfactions about elements of 'New Labour' government policy and behaviour, Blair had forecast that he always knew that 'we were going to be in trouble' if there was a departure 'by even one millimetre from New Labour'.[94] This potentially disastrous dogmatism from the ex-Leader was wisely ignored by many of his admirers, but Blair's stance was still an encouragement to the old managerial loyalties. There was initially a very poor relationship between some of the new Leader's staff and ex-Blairite senior managers who had actively supported the other brother. This was not simply a fit of pique over the defeat of a preference. It had been built into the managerial obligations from 1995 that their primary loyalty was to him and his cause.

Revolt against the management

A major problem of management behaviour came into sudden sharp focus in Februrary 2011 when the rule change over NEC representation produced by Collins after the 2009 conference was discovered. That led to a revolt around the NEC and an outraged response from union leaders. Collins's explanation that a rule change had been agreed at some time in the past but missed out by oversight until 2009 was regarded as unconvincing. The episode confirmed a growing view that 'a culture has arisen that does not feel itself bound by the rules, or the checks and balances of party democracy'.[95] It suggested the danger of a management-engendered crisis of rules and rulemaking.

Facing potential NEC repudiation, Collins accepted the closure of his term of office. At the March NEC, a timetable for appointment of a new General Secretary was proposed by the Leader, and a resolution to remove the Collins rule from the rulebook was accepted. In response to Ed Miliband's first conference speech as Leader, Neil Kinnock had reported a trade union delegate saying to him that 'we have got our party back'. In practice, led by a broad TULO-CLP alliance, operating in defiance of the managerial organisation, the 2009 conference decision on OMOV for CLP voting had been the first step towards that goal; and Collins's departure was a further step in the same direction. This potential turning point contrasted sharply with Blair's first steps towards new party management in 1994, which had been prepared by pressure on Whitty to resign as General Secretary whilst the NEC was on holiday.

In 2011 a different kind of managerial problem grew over *Progress*, initially a Blairite publication. That arose not from the content which, though still within the Blair orbit was generally relevant and reasonable, still steadfastly ignored the problems caused by 'New Labour' party management. There was special concern over the extent of its huge financial resources and that its political loyalties were being used now in discreetly enhanced internal factional activities including candidate selection. In response, some of the unions, including Unite, began to organise more systematically in support of their favoured candidates. Critics of the unions feared that 'union bullying' against *Progress*, including what was reported as a 'kick the Blairites out' comment from 'Labour's biggest financial backer, Len McCluskey', could lead to a prohibition of the journal and an inhibition upon party pluralism. Miliband made public his own opposition to any such development. Perhaps, given Blair's long hostility to union affiliation, some reciprocal unwise and unacceptable outburst of this kind could be expected, but McCluskey denied making the prohibition call. The rule-changing proposal from the unions involved an attempt to reassert some rules over external influence on internal party organisation and to return to the spirit of the NEC decision over controlling finance in internal elections, made in 1994. That had never been consistently operated by the managers.

Competence, strength and leadership

The third trajectory of intra-party reform concerned the powers of and support for the Leader, seeking now to lead Labour back into power after a huge election defeat and with a much lower base of strong identifiers. Ed Miliband had the authority of the post and some traditional conventions of policy process and appointments. But initially he was accompanied in the Shadow Cabinet by only five people who had voted for him, and there were many MPs and their aides who felt thwarted by his surprise emergence and aggrieved at the internal electoral politics that had produced it. Forecasts that the party would collapse into squabbling groups proved to be wrong. Miliband sought to encourage an atmosphere of party unity, a focus all the more necessary in the light of the fragility diagnosed here as inherited from 'New Labour'. And making a significant contribution to the possibility of cohesion, consensual change and a new party management culture was that the main grassroots mood amongst members and affiliates in 2010 was to achieve an authentic partnership in policy formulation, and not to pursue more constitutional control over the party and its representatives. TULO unions were anxious to avoid an internal implosion. The party as a whole had learned from the lessons of the conflicts of the 1980s as it had learned also from the subversion of Partnership in Power. There was new hope now for more constructive development returning to the spirit of what the conference of 1997 thought that it had voted for, and with it more leadership respect for the party's rules, traditions and centre of political gravity.

In adversity, the new Leader remained calm, patient and seriously concerned about improving the conduct of politics. Even outside the party he was regarded by Conservative commentator Peter Oborne as trying to 'move away from the manipulation and cynicism of the modernising era'.[96] That was not a widespread understanding but it was potentially an external encouragement to a less manipulative management of the party and it was in harmony with the anti-manipulative public ethos. Nevertheless, unlike the early Blair, Miliband had very few media supporters whilst Cameron had many. Until opening an attack on Cameron's handling of the News International phone-hacking scandal in July 2011, he found commanding public attention difficult to achieve. Even after his impressive role in that scandal, although the party under his leadership took a consistent lead in the polls, he was widely judged not to look the part of a competent future Prime Minister. In polling, the Conservative Leader was ahead of Miliband on most leadership attributes.

For the moment, the initial presentation of the coalition as 'new politics', and a major shift in the focus of public trust towards the priority of economic competence helped quell some of the public doubt about the cynicism and dishonesty of governing politicians who had no mandate for some of their major policies. On the other hand, Labour's ex-Brownite leaders were on the defensive in seeking to regain public trust in the party's economic competence at a time when overcoming the electorate's economic fear was the major challenge. They had not only been in charge when the crisis began, but Brown and Balls, supported by Blair, had created what turned out to be a failed regulatory system and had spun without qualification 'the end of boom and bust' as the distinctive character of the economic management. On this, as on other features, Labour under Miliband was fighting not only Cameron but the 'New Labour' record and method.

In reponse to his polling adversity and suspicion of 'Blairite' moves against him, Miliband and his advisory team sought procedural means to strengthen his position at senior levels of the party. He had asked Nick Brown not to stand for the post of Chief Whip and later secured support from the PLP and eventually from the party conference for the abolition of Shadow Cabinet elections. He had refrained from recreating the appointed Party Chair but had not moved to an elected position either. He openly turned the elected Chair of the National Policy Forum into what it had informally become in effect, a Leader's appointment from senior MPs, first under Peter Hain and then Angela Eagle. He also eventually created a position of Deputy Party Chair for the new campaign coordinator Tom Watson, and later still a special post for Jon Cruddas in charge of the policy review at Shadow Cabinet level.

Whilst these strengthened his management, there were indications of uncertain purpose and of uncertain processes in the redevelopment of a range of policy positions. Around thirty Shadow Cabinet review groups were established, but their membership details were not available to the wider party, there was no systematic feed-in from the PLP and no clear procedure for the emerging policy statements to link with the party's views. Within the PLP, departmental policy groups functioned, but not consistently. The Joint Policy Committee was still badly attended by departmental shadow ministers. The messy form of the policy process and the influence of some of the old managers raised the question of whether the responsibilities and immediate pressures on Miliband would drive an underlying thrust of policy development through an elite arrangement which could, in the end, bypass the party.

Refounding and reforming the party

There was hope that changes in the behaviour of managers would emerge through the new General Secretary whose appointment would come into effect after the party conference. The choice on 19 July was between Chris Lennie, a Deputy General Secretary, long-serving party official and before that a union official, and Iain McNichol, a GMB official and before that a party official. On the surface there was not much to choose between them. The Leader and his office favoured Lennie but the NEC went 17–14 for McNichol before a unanimous vote of acceptance. The most significant feature of the result was that all six NEC CLP representatives from right and left regarded themselves now, as before, as 'Ed's supporters' but had supported McNichol's appointment. It was a decision heavily influenced by the priority of seeking a healthier and more satisfactory management of the party and its rules.

This priority was accompanied by a developing view that in working towards a constructive accommodation rather than factional victories, there had to be a move away from the dated analysis and faulty assumptions that had underpinned 'New Labour' management. It was hoped that reform of management and a rebalancing of management considerations would lead to a more publicly attractive organisation, the creation of more vitality, greater community campaigning energy and the stimulation of more knowledgeable ambassadors of trust in the trajectory of purpose and the honesty of method. In potentially strengthening these ambassadors of trust it was helpful that by the end of 2010 the membership had grown by 31,000 to 187,000 and to 193,300 at 31 December 2011. Some local union political activity had also begun to improve, as had participation by party members in internal elections.

Crucially, McNichol, both in declaring his plans to the NEC and in answering questions from LabourList on 20 July, pledged to end the command and control systems of the past. From the Leader's office the defeat of Lennie was blamed on the unions and caused a lasting aggrava-tion amongst the Leader's aides. That began to create a new working relationship between some of the old managers and some in and around the Leader's office. McNichol was unafraid of stating his union credentials, but the reality was that his and the TULO objective was not simply a pursuit of union interest. The TULO perspective involved a concern to reassert propriety and the freeing of party democracy from the worst features of the 'New Labour' *ancien régime*.

Although Ed Miliband shared much of the reinvigoration and reform outlook, his media critics, including some remaining Blairites, and elements of headquarters' and the Leader's staff were concerned that the TULO and McNichol perspective was likely to limit the Leader's options. Some man-agers and MPs were still attracted to the ideal of a commanding leader building his image of strength, if necessary by confronting his own party with an alternative imposed reform agenda. It was indicative that the document *Refounding Labour: a Party for a New Generation* which set the priority to repair, restore and reform a more open, community-based, grassroots party reaching outwards saw no connection between this aim and the avoidance of the managerial problems bequeathed in 2010.

Indicative also was that for a period the developing media spin on *Refounding Labour* concentrated attention on changes which would broadly weaken the unions. Like some similar exercises under Blair, that spin attack was widely resented in the party, regarded as a damaging mistake in caus-ing internal conflict and weakening campaigning attention on the priorities. To the unions, showing that the Leader was not in hock to them was not a convincing argument for constitutional change. Financial leverage over policy, as shown here, had always been greatly exaggerated if present at all. The orchestrated and often ruthless media prejudice against the unions and the union-party relationship made the financial linkage immune from plentiful evidence about union restraint, mounted in *The Contentious Alliance* and in this study. As it happened, the scale of union financial input was about to change with donations from companies and individuals increasing and the union annual percentage (as at April 2013 according to the General Secretary) dropping to 23 per cent.

For his part, Miliband gave the NEC in September 2011 the clear non-Blairite message that he was not interested in picking fights with part of the movement.[97] That said, under pressure from him a reform of procedures for the election of the Leader and Deputy Leader to avoid multiple voting was agreed in principle. Agreement was also reached over the major inno-vation of giving registered supporters a party place: they would be enlisted around constituency parties and only when they passed a minimum thresh-old allowed to participate in elections for the Leader/Deputy. Their votes would be taken equally from the existing three sections and not involve a specific weakening of the union position. Later, Miliband emerged with radical new proposals to deal with the funding of political parties without upheaval largely because he encouraged union cooperation and public support by emphasising the value to the party of the affiliation of millions of levy payers.

Party management reform and the way ahead

In the media there was an increasing questioning of the usefulness of heavily controlled party conferences. Martin Kettle saw them as 'demeaning rituals' with little impact on the polls, and suggested that they be abandoned.[98] An alternative view from the new General Secretary, the TULO office and various reformers was that the broader corrupting of politics under 'New Labour' management needed other, more constructive solutions which liberated the members' representation, changed the demeaning features and allowed party voices to be heard with more authenticity.

It was crucial in assisting future consensual party management that Miliband was at ease in drawing from Labour's own traditions and perspective on socio-political power. He also showed more interest than Blair and Brown in rectifying the gross parliamentary under-representation of those from working-class backgrounds, and eventually that was built into party rules, albeit still within a search for diversity and a broad winning coalition which included 'the squeezed middle'. The broad coalition, and more consensual party management, might be helped by the fact that the number of people who saw themselves as working-class rose from 24 per cent in 2010 to 57 per cent by the end of 2012.[99]

Significant in shaping a new management was that Miliband's innovative speech to the conference in 2011 became the inception of a series of movements away from 'New Labour' positions. His differentiation between productive and predatory capitalism was appealing to the party as it changed the focus on problematic vested interests to include those elements of business with publicly damaging values. The analysis also broadened the category of productive wealth creators from its narrow entrepreneurial focus, and presented all this on an ethical base of fairness and mutuality. He initially received little credit for the speech in much of the press and from some Blairite sources, but it later became widely accepted and admired. This was a Leader able to revisit issues such as corporate greed and major disparities of wealth and concentrations of financial power where public and party opinion had been virtually ignored by the previous leadership and policy aides. He was also free to begin a critique of inappropriate markets, and to move towards a new interventionism. All this enabled Miliband to create more consensus underpinning important elements of party management.

On the procedural aspects of management, the General Secretary-designate McNichol frankly focused on the need for fundamental cultural change and a new emphasis on regaining trust. His role was seen in veteran national circles as a return more to the operating behaviour of Larry Whitty than to that of any subsequent General Secretary. In the party organisational restructuring, McNichol began to secure some changes in personnel and later, in order to create 'a fair open and transparent party', to warn all party officials against interfering in internal elections and selections.[100]

Conservative retoxification, Miliband's opportunity

From March 2012, Labour's position was strengthened by a range of developments which retoxified the Conservatives, brought the coalition new vulnerabilities and began to fortify Miliband's internal party situation. A budget which advantaged the well-off, the revelation of hidden Conservative fundraising from the wealthy and the party's close relations with the discredited News International executives, drew attention to what Miliband characterised as 'a government of the wealthy for the wealthy'. The government claim that 'we are all in it together' in facing austerity began to be seen more clearly as a manipulative cloak. It was significant also that in April 2012 many of the public, acting in effect as impromptu petrol-station forecourt analysts, saw and repudiated the government deliberately attempting to turn an industrial-relations problem over tanker petrol supply into a political crisis for which unions were to be given the blame.

The projected image of governmental competence turned into the image of an 'omnishambles' in 2012, as one blunder followed another against a background of increasing challenge to the government's management of an economy moving into a second downturn. The polls showed a major shift away from the Conservatives and a gain to Labour in party support. Cameron, whose internal party support was weakening, also slumped in public support, whilst columnist Rawnsley reported that Miliband's net approval rating on the YouGov tracker, though still negative, had improved 31 points since mid-January.[101]

Assisting this development and building his party support, Miliband had become more consistently impressive in his performances. In September 2012 one poll showed that he had moved ahead of Cameron as trust-worthy by 26 per cent to 23 per cent, although with 43 per cent don't knows.[102] By November 2012, the percentage of people who said that they 'tend to trust' the government had sunk to 21 per cent from the 32 per cent a year before.[103] Clegg's extraordinary loss of personal support since Cleggmania, following his failure to implement his promises, was a reminder to all politicians about the dangers of underestimating the potential long-term damage of distrust linked to what had become seen as manipulative politics. It now began to look potentially much more damaging to the Conservative future that, as Peter Oborne commented, with a sideswipe at 'New Labour', 'from such people as Mandelson and Blair', Cameron and Osborne had picked up '. . . a certain cynicism and moral corruption'.[104]

Further ingredients of a more consensual party management

At the Labour conference of 2012, in a hugely successful speech, Miliband had the confidence to draw from the Tory 'one nation' tradition in the search for Southern voters as Blair once had done. Yet Miliband was also now capable of evoking within the party the trust that he would implement a left-of-centre version, developing in harmony with both the party traditions and the movement of public opinion, and providing a potent critique of the Conservative government's record. Miliband could feed from and into a wider and growing consensus on the unacceptability of a huge inequality of wealth and power. Polling by Stan Greenberg showed that 68 per cent of the people believed that the British economy was too harsh for ordinary working people and 70 per cent thought it too generous to upper-class families.[105] All this provided the basis potentially for further new departures away from 'New Labour's' past managerial assumptions.

The Leader also took the opportunity to advance his own early call to rebuild and maintain trust in politics and politicians.[106] At a time when, linked to critical public attitudes towards the coalition government, there was an alienated public move away from engagement in national politics,[107] he made the striking promise that he would seek to show the sceptical public that politics could work and that not all politicians were alike. Blair had made fairly similar early commitments in the past and Miliband's will be tested in the years ahead, both inside and outside the party, but this was an important and necessary covenant in forging new trust and new management.

It also became clear at the conference that the move away from 'New Labour' was already becoming a change in party management. There was no comprehensive covert-management sytem run from headquarters. Party management had become a plurality of forms, forces and procedural purposes, responding to different priorities as the party moved towards a new consensual equipoise in reconciling the old management with the new. Running alongside a more rigorous focus on the members' engagement with community activism was a new concern for freeing the members' voices in internal politics and freeing officials from an excess of heavy policing duties. Noteworthy in reporting at the conference of 2012 was Jackie Ashley's expression of delight at watching a Labour Leader 'sans bullying spin doctors'.[108] That also played a part in creating a new atmosphere where delegates could be liberated from an excess of managerial muscle. The word from headquarters and some erstwhile critics of managerial behaviour was that 'the bullying' by officials had ceased, although spasmodic complaints continued to come from the Campaign for Labour Party Democracy about partisan behaviour by some officials and at times the CAC.

Outside and inside the party there was a growing acceptance of the need for clear alternative policies to be advocated. However, around the Leader extensive policy-making in some areas at this distance from the general election was deemed to be injudicious. Although the restrictions over policy-making did give some immediate protection from focused media attacks, they provided an open target for accusations of opposing without responsible alternatives. And, inside the party, there was a danger of such restrictions becoming seen yet again as partisan policy control. Also stimulating suspicion was that Cruddas's difficult role in charge of the cohesion of policy-development operated outside internal party procedures.

The way ahead

The yearning in the party to move away from the managerial politics of 'New Labour' was recognised at the 2012 conference in the contribution of Angela Eagle, Shadow Leader of the House and now also the Chair of the NPF, who acknowledged that the conference shared the view that in policy-making 'we have been too controlling and too top-down'.[109] Cruddas, Eagle and Watson, with different role responsibilities, were committed to integrating the party – including its affiliates – into policy-making. Nevertheless, the contemporary reality was that Miliband and those around him had become determined that the new version of Partnership in Power would not be, and could not be, presented as an imposition from the unions in the form of TULO proposals.

With strong managerial support, which included the PLP figures brought into leading party positions, it was the Leader's approved version of the future policy process which was adopted by the NEC. The union response to this was significant and in line with the traditional pattern of behaviour noted here, and before that in *The Contentious Alliance*, holding to the differentiation of industrial and political roles and conventional restraining rules, and acting in the light of priorities. In the end, the TULO proposals were withdrawn rather than promulgating a public confrontation with the Leader on his overall party reform. That was helped by the agreement that the new policy process would preserve the present allocation of conference votes, as well as the procedure for contemporary resolutions.

The new policy process had some uncertainties but it was proclaimed as laying heavy emphasis on giving members more of a say, being more transparent, meaningful and easy to engage with by members and public alike. It was impressive that party members would in future have the new facility of an 'on-line hub' where they could gain access to the papers and ideas that the shadow cabinet groups were discussing and could join in the debate. With the new technology and a new managerial approach to the reinvigoration of effective intra-party dialogue, it was emphasised that NPF representatives could more easily be able to communicate with each other and stimulate both input from the grass roots and accountability to those below. However, the process was to change its name and not now be described as a partnership process between the party and the leadership.

That could be said to be a reflection of the party's scepticism about their experience of partnership under Blair and Brown. It was also a practical reflection of the limited ambitions envisaged for the members and affiliates, a limitation which, however honest, was losing something important about the sharing process in policy-formulation which was likely in practice to create the problem in government of falling short of giving members a sense of future policy ownership. Especially would this be a problem if the Labour leadership became involved in a form of governmental partnership with the Liberal Democrats.

In the future process it was envisaged that conference delegates would also be able to vote to choose a small proportion of priority topics for policy-making consideration by the NPF. Yet that choice would be subject to an element of collective central steering though JPC filters. For the moment, the JPC was sensitively adjusting in accommodating to the commencement of a range of important party-policy discussions. But those with experience of the old Partnership in Power knew that much would depend on the developing culture of the party management. On the face of it there was the potential outline here of a receptive workable relationship but also, alternatively, of a new centralised managerial system. Under pressure to deliver, and with a different judgement of policy and priorities, respect for the members' voice could become as it was under 'New Labour', mainly rhetoric, with a manipulated agenda control becoming revitalised, rather than the party organisation.

'Reclaiming the party' for a fairer more transparent and more consensual process, giving members and affiliates a more genuine voice, may well be regarded by some managerial realists as an unwelcome wager with the future and a distracting irritation from other leadership concerns. Some still looked to the 'New Labour' model of leadership and management and noted that Miliband did not have the public approval won by the early Blair. The latter was seen by his diminishing band of admirers as the epitome of the strong and successful election-winning Leader in spite of the strong move from positive to negative in public judgements on him during his time as Prime Minister. Blair himself reappeared, sensitively making clear his availability for some new party role and offering public advice in international intervention. There was even a warning in October 2012 by the Miliband-friendly and normally discerning commentator Mary Riddell that 'Labour's worst enemy' was 'the Labour Party itself' and Ed was 'about to give Labour the shock of its life'.[110] This was a very severe old-Blairista-style attack on the party, particularly dangerous in the light of the evidence here of the acute problems that Blair's leadership and 'New Labour' party management created and left behind. Miliband had shown a determination to ensure that there should be a strong party sensitivity to his developing project, but was still mindful of his own learning of the lesson that 'New Labour' under Blair and Brown had 'lost touch with both party members and the people'.

In that purpose, it was an asset that Miliband has none of the 'New Labour' fetish about control over and distance from the dangerous party. The new appreciation was that, if the party members were to be strengthened, enthused and made more trustful as knowledgeable ambassadors, the behaviour of the Leader and party management needed to change from the 'New Labour' legacy. Before and during a future Labour government an important feature of an effective relationship with the party will be the extent of building a more consensual partnership over the values, methods and power of management. Nevertheless, there will still be questions that are provoked by the past behaviour of 'New Labour' management, especially if it appears that more of the old management style is creeping back.

Agreement will be helped by the fact that under Miliband the party was winning back ex-Labour voters, winning over Liberal Democrats and enthusing stay-at-home voters in such a way as to strengthen an election-winning centre-left coalition.[111] In developing that coalition, the party stands the strongest chance of election victory and sustained public support if it strengthens the role of grassroots activity and local representation in campaigning organisation. That indicated that the party was likely to consolidate the steps towards the rehabilitation of a healthier form of internal management than that practised under 'New Labour'. The future active role of the party members will be very important in what may well be a narrowly contested election.

Death throes or revival of the old politics?

But there were other forces at work. By July 2013, Miliband was not making much headway in public assessments of his political strength in spite of changes to the party's welfare policies and a pledge of responsibility to match the Conservatives' spending limits involving no reversal of the cuts. The three trajectories of reform suddenly came together as the party did receive 'the shock of its life'. A controversy over the role of the union Unite in a candidate selection in the Falkirk constituency involved a public dispute between Miliband and the Unite General Secretary, McCluskey. It followed a leaked report by a party official which found, apparently, an irregularity that some members enlisted through Unite were unaware of joining the local party prior to a candidate selection. There was a huge surge of aggressive agitation in the media, including from Blairite commentators, urging major reform. This became also a campaign to counter a rise of the union left. Headquarters' response here was to hand the report over to the police, a measure which media critics took as the opportunity to label what had happened 'a scandal', although the police decided there was insufficient evidence to proceed. The union denied that it had broken either party rules or the law. The report was judged by them to be essentially political in character, but disciplinary action began.

The shock was that Miliband made an attack on Falkirk the centrepiece of a major programme of fundamental reform. It advocated a shift away from the traditional block affiliation of union members towards a process of registering individual assent by union members to joining the party – in effect a new contracting-in.

He did this with a forceful affirmation of what was described as a strengthening of the relationship with the unions, but the individualisation could be construed as a major step towards severing the collective link. Indications were also that the contracting-in was bound to threaten Labour's financial support from the unions and possibly leave the party open to a new entryism of the wealthy who had none of the union traditions of political restraint. It would also involve changes in the internal party role and influence of the unions, a plan now given to Lord Collins, the controversial ex-General Secretary, after first choice Lord Whitty had rejected the proposals as unworkable.

Although the old forces which sought to pull the Labour movement together were still in operation, there were some signs that the media assault and the unanticipated proposals emanating from an unexpected source, following years of 'New Labour' disrespect, had created an exceptional sense of injury. This was beginning to discourage their traditional sense of restraining conventions and encourage forces within the unions pursuing a new transactionalism in the provision of finance and alternative political identities.

It was also deeply problematic that Miliband's attack on what happened in Falkirk had been based on a report which was never released to the party and that the action taken by the Leader had been subject to only limited advance consultation. The heavy leadership on the issue was welcomed as impressive, even 'awesome', by Blair and Blairites who saw it as a move towards their own long-lost territory and style. Yet it did not immediately change public perceptions of Miliband on an issue which raised little public interest; the unions had for some time created a diminished sense of threat. The proposal also raised concerns in the party* about the way that this had been handled and where it was going. For those persuaded to become individual party members, how would the promised 'real voice inside the party' operate if this was to be the form of leadership behaviour? How would their commitment to membership be maintained?

However, another uncertainty pointed in a different direction. Over Falkirk he had spoken strongly about seeing there 'the death throes of the old politics ... the machine politics that people hate'. 'There is', he said, 'no place in our party for bad practices wherever they come from.' That would have been widely agreed and it fitted well into the new perspective

---

* Later, on 6 September, the party in another unpublished report accepted that Unite had not breached the rules and rescinded disciplinary action.

which had been forged from a critique of 'New Labour' managerial behaviour. In the near future, having taken a highly publicised castigatory position on all bad practices, Miliband's managers are likely to find themselves closely monitored and bound by that pledge, especially as the new perspective is more suited for coming to terms with the anti-manipulative ethos and for overcoming the growing public withdrawal from politics.

All the emphasis placed on building individual membership means that the new generation of Labour members will have the responsibility to act as ambassadors of trust of the party in all manifestations of that feature. To be effective in this requires the leadership and party management to generate the trust. Machiavellian realism has limited value here. The party has to become an admired, attractive and obvious example of fairness and transparency. Establishing the integrity of the internal political process and the dialogue in and from the party can go some way towards laying the groundwork to realise the ambitious consensual goal of creating a broad-based movement as well as producing a thriving party. It can contribute to engendering new public interest as it seeks to produce an infectious combination of enthusiasm, respect, trust and commitment linking community and party. There is much to be gained by setting a new reassuring public example of authentic voices and honest behaviour.

24 July 2013

Notes

1 Jon Cruddas and John Harris, *Fit for Purpose: a Programme for Labour Party Renewal*, Compass, London 2007, p. 12.
2 Angela Eagle, 'Introduction', Renewal: a Two Way Process for the 21st Century, Labour Commission, 2007, p. 3.
3 Labour Commission, p. 11.
4 Luntz, BBC *Newsnight*, 3 December 2006.
5 *Independent*, 28 March 2007.
6 BBC Website, 18 May 2007.
7 Chris Mullin, *A View from the Foothills*, Profile Books, London, 2009, p. 86.
8 *Guardian*, editorial, 7 June 2007.
9 *Tribune*, 13 July 2007.
10 Deborah Mattinson, *Talking to a Brick Wall*, Backbite, London, 2010, p. 175.
11 Ibid. p. 182.
12 Robert Worcester, Roger Mortimer, Paul Baines and Mark Gill, *Explaining Cameron's Coalition: How it came about, An Analysis of the 2010 British General Election*, Bite back, London, 2011, p. 84.
13 Steve Richards, *The Brown Years, No. 1*, BBC Radio 4, September, 2010.
14 Steve Richards, *Whatever it Takes: The Real Story of Gordon Brown and New Labour*, Fourth Estate, London 2010, p. 252.
15 *Financial Times*, 15 February 2008.
16 Tony Blair, *A Journey*, Hutchinson, London, 2010, p. 620.
17 *Guardian*, 8 July 2004.
18 Andrew Marr programme, BBC 1, 17 January 2010.

19 Peter Watt, *Inside Out: My Story of Betrayal and Cowardice at the Heart of New Labour*, Biteback, London, 2010, p. 167.
20 Ibid. p. 186.
21 *Sunday Times*, 10 May 2009.
22 Interview December 2007, confirmed again 19 January 2010.
23 Interim report from Larry Whitty, 'Issues arising for Labour Party Fundraising Procedures and Accountability from the David Abrahams Case', 2009, section 4.18.
24 Interview with Larry Whitty.
25 Ibid.
26 IpsosMORI/BBC, 22 January 2008.
27 *Sunday Telegraph*, 4 September 2011.
28 *Guardian*, 25 June 2011.
29 IpsosMORI/UNISON, 19 June 2008.
30 YouGov/TULO, Field work, 9 to 14 July 2008.
31 Chris Mullin, *Decline and Fall, Chris Mullin Diaries 2005–2010*, Profile Books, London, 2010, p. 191.
32 PoliticsHome 100 panel, 12 June 2008, 51 per cent thought him weakened by it.
33 YouGov/*Sunday Times*, 15 June 2008.
34 IpsosMORI/*Political Monitor*, September 2008.
35 *Guardian*, 29 July 2008.
36 NEC statement on nominations by Dianne Hayter, NEC chair.
37 YouGov/*Sunday Times*, 20 September 2008.
38 ICM/*Guardian*, 16 December 2008.
39 Anthony Wells, UK Polling, reporting YouGov website data, 7 March 2009.
40 Mullin, *Decline and Fall*, p. 315.
41 *The Times*, 10 November 2008.
42 Fraser Nelson and Ed Howker, 'How New Labour Met its Nemesis', *Spectator*, 17 April 2010.
43 This came out publicly and most forcefully in interviews with Barry Sheerman MP and a resigning minister, Jane Kennedy, BBC *Newsnight*, 9 May 2009.
44 Richards, *Whatever it Takes*, p. 304.
45 Sky News, 23 February 2010.
46 *Mail on Sunday*, 3 May 2009.
47 Peter Mandelson, *The Third Man: Life at the Heart of New Labour*, Harper, London, 2010, p. 462.
48 Matthew Taylor, *Changing Political Culture*, first thoughts pamphlet, Local Government Association, 2000, p. 10.
49 Richards, *Whatever it Takes*, p. 95.
50 Mandelson, *Third Man*, pp. 451–62.
51 BBC1 News, 12 May 2009.
52 *Guardian*, 3 June 2009.
53 *Guardian*, 6 June 2009.
54 Mandelson, *Third Man*, p. 472.
55 *Guardian*, 18 May 2009.
56 *Guardian*, 29 September 2010.
57 Paul Flynn blog, 14 June 2009.
58 *Guardian*, 8 June 2009.

59 Nick Robinson's Newslog, 8 October 2009.
60 *Guardian*, Editorial, 9 May 2009.
61 Tony Wright, *Doing Politics*, Biteback, London, 2012, p. 45.
62 Ibid. p. 94.
63 *Guardian*, 29 May 1995.
64 The parliamentary developments are covered in Meg Russell 'Never Allow a Crisis to go to Waste: The Wright Committee Reforms to strengthen the House of Commons', *Parliamentary Affairs* 64, 4 October 2011, pp. 612–33.
65 Survey data and analysis by IpsosMORI, Hansard Society, Audit of Political Engagement, The 2010 Report, London, 2010, p. 45.
66 BBC *Newsnight*, 8 July 2010.
67 Mattinson, *Brick Wall*, p. 222.
68 The polls indicated that the extraordinary reception for Clegg was not just approval for a new voice which differentiated Clegg from the other party leaders but that he was by far the most unwilling to be evasive in answering questions. YouGov/*Sun*, 16 April 2010, he was more substance than spin, and more honest than Brown or Cameron, ICM/*Guardian*, 20 April 2010.
69 Comres found 60 per cent of the electorate thinking the Labour Party divided, reported on UK Polling website, 8 January 2010.
70 Richard Wilkinson and Kate Pickett, *The Spirit Level: Why More Equal Societies Almost Always Do Better*, Penguin, London, 2008.
71 *Tribune*, 1 October 2010.
72 Phillips-Edelman, 'The Role of PR in the New Media Landscape', Sally Falkow website, 31 August 2009.
73 PoliticsHome polls, 18 January 2010.
74 Nick Anstead and Will Straw, 'What British Politics Can learn from Obama', Fabian Society, *Next Left*, 20 March 2009.
75 Extracted from passage quoted in Paul Richards, *Labour's Revival: The Modernisers' Manifesto*, Biteback, London, 2010, p. 30.
76 Dennis Kavanagh and Philip Cowley, *The British General Election of 2010*, Palgrave Macmillan, Basingstoke, 2010, p. 239.
77 J. Fisher, D. Cutts and E. Fieldhouse, 'The Electoral Effectiveness of Constituency Campaigning in the 2010 General Election: The Triumph of Labour?', *Electoral Studies* 30(4), 2011, pp. 816–28.
78 Ibid., tabular data.
79 Alex Bryson, 'New Labour, New Unions', in *British Social Attitudes 2006–2007: 23rd Report*, Sage Publications, London, 2007, pp. 198–202.
80 YouGov/*Daily Telegraph*, 15 March 2009, covering October 2008 and January 2009.
81 PoliticsHome research, 20 June 2009.
82 Worcester et al., *Explaining Cameron's Coalition*, p. 185.
83 Kavanagh and Cowley, *General Election 2010*, p. 390.
84 Ibid.
85 IpsosMORI, 'How Britain voted', Ipsos MORI website 21 May 2010.
86 John Curtice and Justin Fisher, 'The Power to Persuade; a Tale of Two Prime Ministers', in Park, Curtice, Thompson, Jarvis, and Bromley, *British Social Attitudes 2003–2004: Continuity and Change over Two Decades*, Sage Publications, 2004, p. 241.
87 Mattinson, *Brick Wall*, p. 250 and p. 309.

88 Giles Radice, *Trio: Inside the Blair, Brown, Mandelson Project*, Tauris, London, 2010, p. 237.
89 *Daily Telegraph*, 9 July 2011.
90 Richard Jobson and Mark Wickham-Jones, 'Reinventing the Block Vote? Trade Unions and the 2010 Labour Party Leadership Election', University of Bristol, 2011.
91 Worcester et al., *Explaining Cameron's Coalition*, pp. 172–6.
92 Kavanagh and Cowley, *General Election 2010*.
93 *Labour Uncut*, 21 July 2010.
94 Interviewed by Andrew Marr, BBC1, 1 September 2010.
95 The terms of a letter sent from TULO officers to Ed Miliband, 2 February 2011.
96 *Daily Telegraph*, 29 December 2011.
97 Luke Akehurst, NEC Report 21, September 2011.
98 *Guardian*, 7 October 2010.
99 *State of the Nation: Where is Bittersweet Britain Heading?* British Future 2013.
100 Circular to staff from Iain McNichol, 1 June 2012.
101 *Observer*, 30 September 2012.
102 YouGov/*Sunday Times*, 23 September 2012.
103 Report from the Office for National Statistics, cited *Daily Telegraph*, 1 November 2012.
104 *Daily Telegraph*, 6 February 2013.
105 *Guardian*, 11 September 2012.
106 *Guardian*, 21 September 2011, and Foreword to David Blunkett's pamphlet *In Defence of Politics Revisited*, 2012.
107 Hansard Society, Audit of Political Engagement 9, Part One, 2012.
108 *Guardian*, 1 October 2012.
109 My verbatim notes.
110 *Daily Telegraph*, 17 October 2012.
111 Andrew Harrop, 'Stay-at-home voters are the key to Labour victory', Fabian Essays, drawing from Fabian Society research conducted by YouGov, 3 February 2013.

Index

21st Century Party 395, 476, 528–9, 619

Abbott, Diane 179, 193, 763
Abrahams, David 740, 741
accountability 14, 156, 157, 316, 366, 512–13, 633, 688–9, 726, 741
Adonis, Lord 488, 716
affiliated organisations 16, 87, 103, 182, 188, 189, 260–1, 262, 335, 529, 603, 670, 761
Afghanistan 493, 495, 503, 523
Agency and Temporary Workers Agreement 744
Agricultural Wages Board 326, 674
Aitken, Jonathan 141, 340
Alexander, Douglas 172, 395, 602, 751, 758
Allaun, Frank 31, 34
Allen, Graham 559, 677
Amalgamated Engineering and Electrical Union (AEEU) 32, 55, 87, 90, 99, 103, 161, 185, 192, 224, 237, 240, 245, 246, 254, 260, 274, 308, 326, 336, 379, 381, 392, 397, 445, 447, 454, 478, 550, 551, 667
AMICUS 274, 478, 508, 550, 563, 583, 589, 603, 622, 640, 642, 739
Anderson, Janet 613, 638, 740
anti-manipulative ethos 509–13, 684, 710, 726–7, 729, 742, 767, 777
Approved List, the 25, 29
Archer, Geoffrey 141
Arms-to-Iraq Affair 140–1
Armstrong, Hilary 100, 223, 236, 326, 328, 491, 522–3, 579–80, 614, 628, 636, 644, 646, 687
Ashdown, Paddy 382
Ashley, Jackie 429, 772
Ashworth, Jonathan 743
Association of Locomotive Engineers and Firemen (ASLEF) 275, 343, 392, 478, 564

asylum issues 349, 365, 494–5
Attlee, Clement 23
Austin, Ian 643

Bailey, N. G. 708, 730
Bain, George 294
Baldock, Louise 583, 638, 640
Bale, Tim 417
Balls, Ed 286, 520, 625, 738–9, 763, 764, 767
Barber, Brendan 290, 504, 545
Barker, Sara 25–6, 28, 31
Barlow, Frank 417
Barnes, Harry 402
Basset, Phil 440
Beckett, Margaret 74, 82, 89, 110, 111, 213, 294, 410, 430, 437, 440, 441, 442, 449, 451, 636
Beecham, Jeremy 256–7, 321, 328, 620, 631, 654, 745–6
Benn, Hilary 377, 646, 650, 655–6
Benn, Tony 31, 35, 38, 43, 48–9, 51, 53, 69, 71, 109, 209
Best, Harold 410
Bevan, Andy 37
Bevan, Aneurin 19, 20, 21, 23, 27
Bevanites 20, 22, 23
Bevin, Ernest 18
Bickerstaffe, Rodney 93, 95–6, 97, 100, 212, 246–7, 275, 284, 337, 363–4, 392, 478
Big Conversation, the 570, 576, 592, 602
Bish, Geoff 44
Black, Ann 235, 242, 243, 249, 531, 531–2, 539, 544–5, 584, 598, 618, 621, 651
Blair, Tony 38, 82, 120, 133, 223, 468
  accountability 688–9
  advisers split 641
  announces departure date 599–600
  announces departure timing 648

Blair, Tony (*cont'd*)
  backing 118
  and Brown 395, 466, 612, 637, 696, 739
  business links 266–7, 268–9, 299–300,
    447, 458, 477, 498, 506, 670–1, 724
  and candidate selection 369, 371–2, 374,
    376, 377, 385, 394–5, 396–8, 585,
    680–1
  Chicago speech 329–30, 475, 495, 685,
    717
  Clause IV campaign 176–84, 184–5,
    185–6
  conflict with Brown 5, 172, 520–2, 573–6
  creation of 'New Labour' 117
  criticism of FSA 616
  de-selection 384
  election as leader 112, 117, 161
  Employment Relations Act negotiations
    441, 442, 445, 446–9, 454, 456–7
  eviction 107, 654–5, 696–7, 698–9, 725
  frustration 472–8
  general election, 1997 214–15
  general election, 2005 7, 609–10, 610
  and the General Secretary 151
  handling of industrial disputes 282–3
  and the Iraq War 503, 540–1, 542,
    545–6, 548, 557–61, 570, 696, 717,
    726–7
  and the Joint Policy Committee 109
  and Kinnock 61–2
  leadership 1, 118–21, 503, 576–7, 602,
    614–15, 640, 679, 681, 696–8,
    713–18, 729–31
  leadership reassertion 636–9
  leadership threatened 580–3
  limitations 468–9
  and Livingstone 387–94
  loans for peerages scandal 631–2
  loss of trust 509–20, 558, 558–9, 560, 609,
    636–7, 641, 684, 712, 718–19, 726–9
  management priorities 126
  managerial coup 485–9
  meeting with Brown, Sept 2006 647–8
  and Miliband 774
  motivations 132–3, 134–5, 663
  and the NEC 615–16, 673
  and the NPF 312, 673–4
  objectives 106–7, 128–30, 132–3, 187,
    475–6, 666, 668, 710
  and OMOV 91, 667
  and party conference 333, 337, 353–5
  party conference speech, 2003 570–2
  and Party into Power 200, 201, 204–5,
    209, 210, 213, 220

party management 2–4, 88–9, 121–4,
    162–4, 468–70, 472–8, 497, 560,
    610–12, 663–8, 680, 681–3, 696–9,
    709–10, 712, 727–31, 740, 751
  party managers 165
  pensions policy defeat 364–5
  and the PLP 401–2, 408–9, 409–10,
    419, 423–4, 428–31, 445, 472, 492–3,
    495, 522, 523–5, 573, 577, 582,
    623–7, 687–8, 696
  and policy implementation 441
  Policy Unit staff 292–3
  and policy-making 601–2, 651–2,
    713–14
  power relations 699–703
  Prescott's ultimatum to 641–42
  procedural management 725–6
  public sector reform speech 298
  relations with Cabinet 120–1
  relationship with Brown 69, 121, 171–2,
    472, 485, 487, 520–2, 581, 599–600,
    604–5, 611–12, 652–3
  relationship with Campbell 167
  relationship with Prescott 122, 173, 487
  reputation for manipulation 512–20
  rise of 109
  role 5–6
  and the rulebook 157, 158–9
  satisfaction rate 509
  Sedgefield constituency 83
  self-characterisation 262
  send off 648–9
  and the September coup 640, 645–8,
    698–9
  and Smith 84, 85, 92
  speeches 353–5
  and the spin campaign 85–6
  staff 148–50, 394–5, 397, 488, 610
  supremacy 213, 267, 273, 281, 353–5,
    550, 679, 680, 693
  Terrorism Bill defeat 626–7
  and the Trade Union Review Group 89,
    102–3, 106–7, 108, 118, 119, 129
  and the traditional right 160–1
  transition to Brown 651–4
  and the TUC 441
  and the unions 65–6, 75, 77, 108, 186,
    186–7, 190–1, 193, 272–3, 276,
    286–7, 324, 435–9, 442, 446–9, 533,
    667–8, 669–70, 671–2, 689, 693–4,
    694–5, 721
  and the Warwick Agreement 597–8, 603,
    629, 637
  and women's representation 72

Blairites for Brown 642–5, 645
Blears, Hazel 615, 636–7, 639–40, 655–6, 752
Blevin, John 214
Blunkett, David 213, 277, 282, 283, 315, 328–9, 329, 352–3, 353, 375, 414, 419, 436, 488, 494–5
Bok, Sissela 511–12
Boulton, Adam 646
Boyle, David 511
Bright, Martin 647
Brown, George 28–9
Brown, Gordon 1, 7–8, 38, 82, 89, 97, 108, 110, 284, 307, 352, 518, 582–3, 601, 735, 739
    and Blair 395, 466, 612, 637, 696, 739
    business links 266–7, 738–9
    and candidate selection 374, 737, 750, 753
    CBI speech, 2005 616
    as Chancellor 121, 292
    conflict with Blair 5, 172, 520–2, 573–6
    creation of 'New Labour' 117
    crisis management 736–7
    and Donorgate 740–2
    economic management 297–8, 359, 679, 761–2
    elected leader 655–6
    general election, 1997 287–8
    general election, 2005 609
    general election, 2010 760–3
    health-service spin 467
    ice-cream-sharing unity 605
    and the Iraq War 549, 686, 737
    and Kinnock 61–2
    leadership 748
    leadership bid 172
    leadership challenges 747–8, 752, 758
    and Livingstone 391
    and loans for peerages scandal 631
    lone parent benefit policy 357
    loss of trust 737–8, 741–2, 760–1
    and manifesto, 2001 480
    and mass membership 129
    media management 735, 750–2
    meeting with Blair, Sept 2006 647–8
    minimum wage 294
    and the NEC 573–4, 735, 740, 753
    NEC resignation 238
    and the NPF 745, 753–4
    on OMOV 129
    and the parliamentary-expenses scandal 756
    party management 573–6, 682, 736–7, 753–4
    party management inheritance 734–6, 739–40, 740
    pensions policy 327, 343, 364–5, 624
    and the PLP 412, 522, 574–6, 613, 625, 740, 742, 746–7, 749–50, 753
    and policy-making 574
    and privatisation 361
    public support 605, 627
    relationship with Blair 69, 121, 171–2, 472, 485, 487, 520–2, 581, 599–600, 604–5, 611–12, 652–3
    resignation 762
    and the September coup 643–4, 647, 647–8, 648, 698
    Smeargate 750–2
    and Smith 84
    tax policy 742
    transition to 651–4
    and the unions 187, 276, 319, 735–6, 738, 739–40, 743–4, 748–9, 754–5, 761
    and the Warwick Agreement 744–5
Brown, Nick 69, 172, 326, 379, 381, 406–7, 412–13, 424, 425, 426, 448–9, 575, 576, 748, 749, 767
Bruce, Luke 592, 618
Building Britain's Future white paper 753
Building Prosperity, Flexibility, Efficiency and Fairness at Work 277, 278–9, 281
Burlison, Tom 62, 89, 180, 244
Burnham, Andy 759, 763
Burton, John 204
Bush, George 503, 641, 642
Business Liaison Unit 269–70, 270
business links 76, 125–6, 181–2, 210, 257–8, 266–71, 284, 287–8, 299–300, 447, 458, 477, 498, 506, 670–1, 724, 738–9
Butler enquiry, the 558, 597, 689, 730
by-elections, candidate selection 374–5, 396, 397, 529, 585–7
Byers, Stephen 283, 285, 307, 438, 447, 456, 459, 481, 484, 494, 517, 577–8, 602, 630, 724
Byrne, Liam 333

Callaghan, Jim 35, 36, 38, 42–3, 45, 47, 51–2, 420
Calman, Sir Kenneth 329
Cameron, David 627, 709–10, 735, 737, 738, 756, 757, 760, 762–3, 767, 771
Campaign for Democratic Socialism (CDS) 25–6

Campaign for Labour Party Democracy
    (CLPD) 34, 42–3, 43, 49–50, 54, 74,
    100, 157, 238, 342, 362, 380, 772
Campaign Group of Labour MPs 69–70
Campaign Strategy Committee 53, 61
Campaigns and Elections Committee 235
Campbell, Alastair 95, 117, 133, 150,
    167–9, 171, 177, 186, 283, 299, 390,
    402, 440, 450, 465, 466, 469, 473,
    475, 476, 484, 488, 491, 492, 503,
    514, 515, 516–17, 517–18, 542, 559,
    605, 714, 715, 762
Canavan, Denis 384–5, 418, 423
candidate selection 24–6, 86, 87, 92,
    99–101, 108, 251, 370, 476, 584–7,
    695
  all-women short lists 375–6, 586, 750
  and Blair 369, 371–2, 374, 376, 377,
    385, 394–5, 396–8, 585, 680–1
  and Brown 737, 750, 753
  by-elections 374–5, 396, 397, 529,
    585–7
  campaign expenditure 392–3
  and CLP 24–6, 93, 380
  European Parliamentary Labour Party
    382–3
  fixing 467–8
  general election, 2001 396
  levy-plus 93, 94, 97, 98, 101
  London Mayor elections 387–94, 467,
    468
  managerial control 370–1, 373, 381–2,
    528–9, 680–1
  mandatory re-selection 44, 78, 380–1
  National Parliamentary Panel 377–8
  NEC and 32, 376–7, 381, 585
  OMOV 369, 373, 380–1, 386, 476,
    528–9, 681
  parachuting 376–7, 476, 595–6
  positive discrimination 375–6, 377
  procedure and management 369–74
  reform 78, 189–91, 395–6
  re-selection contests 78
  rule change 101–2
  sanitisation 394–5, 398
  Scotland 383–5
  and Smith 96–7
  targets 372–4
  union membership requirement 378–81
  and the unions 372, 378–81, 381, 750
  vetting 377–8
  Wales 385–7
  women's representation 375–6, 377, 378,
    385

Carter, Matt 528, 530–1, 561, 618, 622
Castle, Barbara 20, 343, 357
Cattermole, Jim 25–6, 155, 160
Chater, Alicia (later Kennedy) 526, 527, 623
Chief Whip 404, 406, 406–7, 412–13,
    424–5, 523, 572, 579–80, 626, 628–9,
    649, 677, 686, 687
Chief Whip's report, 1999 252–3
Clark, Katy 585, 627
Clarke, Charles 53, 65, 75, 77–8, 282,
    371–2, 375, 486, 487, 489–92, 494,
    497, 498, 504, 521, 525–6, 526, 530,
    531, 532, 533–4, 539, 542, 543, 575,
    595–6, 615, 626, 636, 648, 681–2,
    684, 685, 689, 751
Clarke, Eric 50–1, 73
Clarke, Ken 297
Clarke, Nita 318, 325, 337, 478, 480–1,
    481, 504, 507, 527, 539, 565, 594,
    610
Clarke, Tony 89
class de-alignment 33, 723–4
Clause IV 23, 126, 150, 151, 153, 155,
    176–87, 316, 401, 418, 463, 465,
    570, 668–9, 676, 684
Clegg, Nick 758, 762, 771
Clements, Barrie 617
Clinton, Bill 124, 125, 260, 709
Clwyd, Ann 407, 408, 492, 546, 612, 614,
    647
Coates, David 604, 630
code of conduct 136–8, 256–7, 257–8, 539
Cohen, Nick 386
Coleman, Peter 89, 149–50, 195, 334, 382
collective responsibility 580, 684, 730
Colling, Gordon 65, 89, 91, 103, 105–6,
    161, 180, 244
Collins, Ray 622–3, 697, 741, 742–3, 743,
    750, 765, 776
Commission of Enquiry into Party
    Organisation 45
Committee of Standards in Public Life 261
Communication Workers Union (CWU)
    247, 261, 282, 296, 299, 319, 336,
    339, 478, 508, 534, 563, 565, 567,
    591, 593
Community 564, 621, 754, 755
Comprehensive Spending Review 298,
    482–3
Confederation of British Industry (CBI) 5,
    182, 266–7, 267–8, 285, 295, 324,
    328, 438–9, 442–3, 446, 448, 449,
    452, 454–5, 455, 458, 477, 480,
    492–3, 498, 504, 596, 670–1, 744

Conference Arrangements Committee
(CAC) 15, 43, 45–6, 62, 99, 166, 177,
225, 245, 249, 334, 338–42, 362,
493–4, 537, 567, 623, 650, 688
Connor, Bill 535
Conservative Party, as model 140–2
constituency parties (CLPs) 12, 16, 18, 19,
21, 24, 43, 54, 62, 70, 71, 73, 326,
381, 618, 677
  amendments 745
  and Brown 754–5
  and candidate selection 24–6, 93, 100–1,
102, 373, 380
  Chief Whip's report, 1999 253
  and Clause IV 179–80
  ideology 139
  and the Iraq War 542, 543, 547–8
  leadership election votes 104
  local organisation 129
  loyalist network 312–13
  managerial control 536–8
  membership 188
  NEC section 218–20, 236, 237–8, 567,
583, 690
  NPF representatives 312–13, 321–2,
330
  opposition 313–14
  party conference delegates 344–5,
618–19, 675–6
  and party conference management 334,
335, 342, 344–7, 348–9, 355–7,
674–5
  and Party into Power 209, 215–16
  pensions policy victory 365
  and PFI 538
  reapportionment of votes 188, 189
  reform 254–5
  registered supporters 639
  Road to the Manifesto ballot, 1996
195–6
  and the rulebook 157
  and the September coup 642, 648–9
  and the trade unions 103
  trust 138–9
  and the Warwick Agreement 595
  and the Warwick meetings 594
Constitution 54–5, 86, 567
  Clause 3 189
  Clause IV 3, 23, 126, 150, 151, 153,
155, 176–84, 316, 401, 418, 463,
465, 570, 668–9, 676, 684
  Clause V 16, 47, 216, 403, 479–80,
481–2, 574, 600, 679, 694
Constitutional Officer 159

contemporary resolutions 220–1, 223,
360–6, 494, 537–8, 567, 599, 650,
736
Cook, Greg 356, 410, 543, 567
Cook, Robin 89, 110, 121, 122, 177, 213,
304, 311, 317, 322–3, 329, 352, 355,
480, 491, 498, 546, 549, 578, 686,
713
Cooper, Yvette 340, 377, 573–4
Corston, Jean 68, 407, 421, 491, 546, 611
Cousins, Frank 27, 29, 32
Cowley, Philip 4, 412, 413, 415, 427, 428,
431, 548, 625, 677, 678, 685, 764
Cranfield School of Management 200–1,
232, 233
Craven, Mike 256
Crewe, Ivor 468
Criddle, Byron 378, 398, 584
Crossman, Richard 20, 29–30, 31, 32, 36
Crouch, Colin 270
Crow, Bob 508, 590
Cruddas, Jon 89, 148, 149, 153, 164, 177,
188, 192, 202, 211, 212, 219, 220,
221, 224, 241, 276, 284, 293, 296,
311, 318, 323, 334, 343, 361, 379,
389, 397, 437, 439, 442, 444, 445,
449, 452–3, 455, 457, 472, 478, 587,
648, 651, 655–6, 734, 759, 767, 773
Cryer, Anne 371, 612–13, 652, 746
Curran, Kevin 550, 565, 566–7
Curtice, John 468

D'Ancona, Matthew 652, 709–10
Darling, Alastair 319, 353, 355, 737, 743,
751, 761–2
David, Wayne 382–3
Davidson, Ian 384–5, 423, 443
Davies, Garfield 178, 336
Davies, Gavyn 727
Davies, Liz 239–40, 242, 248–9, 252, 334,
375, 377
Davies, Ron 385, 386
Deakin, Arthur 22–3, 27
defence policy 20, 27
deliberative culture 111–12
democracy 11–12, 88, 129, 446, 464, 473,
708
Departmental Committees 419–21, 577–8,
678, 714–15, 753
Deputy General Secretary 151–3, 623
Deputy Leader 44, 44–5, 680, 734, 763
deselection 32, 36, 252–3, 381, 384, 426,
547, 686
Desmond, Richard 519

devolution 383–7
Dewar, Donald 384, 417, 418, 442–3, 529
discipline 4, 67, 249–50, 416
  Parliamentary Labour Party (PLP) 407,
  412–13, 415–16, 425–7, 578–80, 626,
  628–9, 638, 649, 678, 687–8, 749–50
Dobson, Frank 122, 307, 343, 388, 390–4,
  420, 469
Domestic Policy Committee 207, 593
Donorgate 632, 740–2, 743
donors 259, 261–3, 477, 518–19
Doran, Frank 445, 457, 505
Draper, Derek 473, 750–1
Dromey, Jack 272, 619, 631–2, 743
Drucker, Henry 160
Dubbins, Tony 65, 192, 443, 588–9, 591,
  595–6, 617, 619
Duffy, Dan 189
Durham NPF meeting 315–22, 323, 326,
  330, 674

Eagle, Angela 592, 612, 614, 623, 637,
  638, 652, 734, 746, 767, 773
economic policy 125, 277, 359
Economic Policy Commission 364
Edmonds, John 65, 71, 77, 77–8, 93, 96,
  107–8, 184, 192, 212, 219, 225–6,
  274–5, 287–8, 317, 318, 321, 336,
  442, 443, 447, 451, 494, 508, 533,
  534, 547, 563, 690
education top-up fees 560, 567, 567–8,
  574–6
Egan, Jon 207, 322
Elder, Murray 90, 99, 100, 101, 150, 384
electoral positioning 124–5, 131
electoral trust 126–8, 139
Electrical, Electronic, Telecommunications
  and Plumbing Union (EEPTU) 108,
  274
Elliot, Larry 450, 609
Employment Relations Act, 1999 293, 296,
  323, 324, 435–59, 477, 504, 505,
  562–3, 695, 730
Engel, Natasha 271, 323
Equipping Britain for the Future 287–8
Ethics Committee 519, 632
European elections, 1999 383, 409–10
European Parliamentary Labour Party
  382–3
European Social Chapter 288, 289
European Social Charter 66
European Union 120
Evans, John 89, 91–2
Ewing, Keith 257, 503–4, 635, 721

Exeter NPF meeting 299, 317, 322–30,
  507, 591, 674, 693
expulsions 395, 579, 615
Extending and Renewing Party Democracy
  736

Fairness at Work white paper 442, 444,
  449–55, 458
Falconer, Charles 323, 377, 452, 457,
  599
Falkirk 385, 395, 470, 681, 710, 775–6
Fatchett, Derek 156, 209, 220
Financial Services Authority 616
Finkelstein, Daniel 757
Fire Brigades Union (FBU) 275, 299, 506,
  590, 591, 721
Fitzpatrick, Jim 636, 654
Flanders, Allan 27, 272
Foot, Michael 27, 34, 35, 36, 48–9, 51,
  51–2, 417
Framework of Working Principles, Themes
  and Values 108
Fryer, Bob 202, 203, 212, 219, 220
Fundamental Savings Review 652
Funding Committee 519

Gabor, Ivor 141–2, 700
Gail, Gregor 563
Gaitskell, Hugh 23, 27, 28, 178, 354
Galloway, George 579
Gardner, David 100, 150, 214, 215, 218,
  334, 372, 382, 386, 426, 736
general election, 1983 51–2, 58
general election, 1987 60, 75
general election, 1992 68, 82, 85–6, 86
general election, 1997 123, 142, 152,
  214–15, 252, 287–8, 288, 401, 670,
  712, 762
general election, 2001 153, 173, 396, 422,
  483, 483–5, 510, 512
general election, 2005 7, 581, 609–10,
  610, 727, 761
general election, 2010 760–3
General Election Fund 259, 262
General Management Committee 24
General Secretary 146–50, 154, 156, 159,
  165, 194, 234, 244–5, 525, 526, 527,
  561–2, 622–3, 664, 683, 697, 742–3,
  755, 768–9, 770, 770–1
  party conference management
  organisation 333–4, 352
  and Party into Power 202–3, 209–10
Gibson, Ann 101, 318
Gibson, Ian 575, 756

GMB 74, 91–2, 94–5, 97, 108, 166, 178, 213, 318–19, 321, 324, 336, 337, 494, 508, 532, 532–3, 550, 566–7, 569, 619, 622, 689
Gordon, Fiona 523, 611, 742
Gould, Brian 69, 89
Gould, Joyce 26, 64, 68, 89, 242–3
Gould, Philip 1, 57, 61–2, 64, 70, 82, 84, 85, 86, 117, 119, 123, 124, 160–1, 176, 194–5, 280, 281, 334, 389, 464–5, 469, 471, 473, 509, 605, 671, 702, 711, 723, 762
government, separation from party role 29
government advisers 306
Graham, Alastair 730, 735
Grassroots Alliance 220, 238–43, 245, 248–9, 255, 257–8, 313–14, 320, 349, 351, 519, 542, 583, 593, 594, 597, 640
Graphical, Paper and Media Union (GPMU) 89, 178, 192, 221, 224, 245, 247, 324, 336, 342, 343, 439, 443, 478, 589
Grayling, Tony 213–14, 214, 218, 230
Greater London Authority 387
Greenberg, Stan 298, 468, 518, 592, 772
Grey, Chris 680
Grice, Andrew 486
Griffiths, Jim 20
Griffiths, Mike 245, 247, 306, 538–9, 567, 571, 586, 589, 623
Grocott, Bruce 445

Hain, Peter 156, 209, 220, 580, 648, 650, 655–6, 767
Hakim, Faz 149, 219, 311, 334
Hannett, John 247, 563
Harman, Harriet 109, 238, 261, 284–5, 358, 441, 648, 650, 655–6, 736, 763
Harris, John 734
Harris, Nigel 89, 91, 153, 587
Harris, Robert 728
Hastings Agreement, 1933 18, 190
Hattersley, Roy 52, 69, 70, 352–3, 356
Haworth, Alan 164, 376, 405, 417, 418, 421, 479–80, 495, 546, 577, 611
Hayes, Billy 508, 563, 565, 633
Hayter, Dianne 236, 251, 631, 651, 741
Hayward, Ron 26, 31–2, 42, 68
Healey, Denis 35, 51–2
Healey, John 279, 443
Healthy Party Project 162
Heath, Edward 32, 34, 34–5
Heffer Eric 43, 48, 51, 56, 69

Hewitt, Patricia 53, 61–2, 70, 82, 441, 592, 595–6, 620, 623, 636, 642, 758
Higher Standards, Better Schools for All White Paper 624, 625, 627–8, 629
Hill, David 559, 610
Hill, Robert 495, 525, 539
Hince, Vernon 247–8, 255, 258, 366
Hobsbawm, Eric 55
Hodgson, Derek 245, 247, 261, 317, 336, 361–2
Hoggart, Simon 353
Holland, Diana 231, 246, 251, 528, 544–5
Hollick, Clive 70, 210, 724
Hoon, Geoff 613–14, 624, 758
Horam Report, 1976 417
House of Lords 328, 416
Howard, Anthony 132, 376
Hughes-Hayward inquiry 51
Hunter, Angie 149, 150, 488, 682
Hutton, John 738
Hutton enquiry, the 557, 689
Hyman, Peter 467, 713

immigration 348–9, 513, 762
Implementing the New Policymaking Process 358–9
In Place of Strife White Paper 33
Ingham, Bernard 57, 140
Inside Labour 170
Institute for Public Policy Research 70
internal communication, weakness of 169–71
Iraq War, the 6, 133, 329–30, 487, 503, 522, 537, 565, 684, 696, 717–18, 730
    and the Big Conversation 592
    and Blair 503, 540–1, 542, 545–6, 548, 557–61, 570, 717, 726–7
    and Brown 549, 737
    build up to 540–50
    consequences 557–61, 570, 580, 587, 609, 614–15, 617, 719
    and de-selection 547, 686
    military victory 550
    and NEC 542–5, 546, 685
    opposition 543, 545, 546, 549–50, 563, 686
    and party conference 598–9
    and PLP 545–6, 547, 548–9, 685–6
    September dossier, the 557–8
    troop withdrawal announced 737
    and the unions 542, 543, 545, 547, 598–9, 685–6
    weapons of mass destruction 557–8

Iron and Steel Trades Confederation (ISTC)
    178, 195, 336, 343, 376, 564
Irvine, Derry 180
Irvine, Joe 193, 203, 212, 325, 742–3
issue management 436–7

Jackson, Catherine 577
Jackson, Glenda 388, 393
Jackson, Helen 425, 492, 496, 531, 570–1,
    576, 588, 718–19
Jackson, Ken 178, 192, 222, 254, 274,
    282–3, 336, 379, 391, 546, 550, 584,
    600
Jeuda, Diana 74, 89, 94, 180, 192–3, 202,
    212, 214, 215, 218, 220–1, 247, 306,
    386
Johnson, Alan 178, 194, 247, 336, 551,
    575, 595–6, 648, 655–6, 752
Johnson, Gerry 201
Joint Policy Committee (JPC) 4, 74, 109–10,
    205, 207, 229–30, 230–1, 243, 249,
    277, 306–8, 310, 314–15, 316–17,
    530, 672, 673, 693, 753, 768, 774
Jones, Digby 738
Jones, Jack 32, 34, 35, 343, 534–5
Jones, Maggie 101, 147, 153, 201, 202–3,
    204, 209, 212, 218, 222, 233, 234,
    244, 245, 247, 255–6, 306, 318, 325,
    337, 489, 588
Jones, Michael 375
Jones, Nick 517
Jordan, Bill 178, 336

Kampfner, John 518, 544, 558
Kaufman, Gerald 52, 71
Kavanagh, Dennis 154, 597, 671, 764
Kellner, Peter 85, 429, 472, 719
Kelly, Dr David 557
Kennedy, Roy 650
Kenny, Paul 619, 622
Kettle, Martin 118, 333, 468, 581, 770
King, Anthony 109, 654
King, Oona 374, 390
Kinnock, Neil 2, 6–7, 38, 49, 52, 53–4,
    54, 56, 57, 58, 59, 59–63, 63–7, 67,
    68–72, 73–8, 82, 85, 88, 107, 108,
    117, 121, 123, 131, 168, 239, 369,
    445, 625, 765
Knapp, Jimmy 100, 337
Kosovo, campaign, 1999 429, 475, 541

Labour Against the War Group 547
Labour Coordinating Committee 70, 71,
    76, 77, 161–2, 186, 216, 220

Labour Finance and Industry Group 76,
    110
Labour First 161, 178, 237, 239, 349, 379
Labour into Power: a Framework for
    Partnership 201, 205, 210, 215, 305
Labour Party see Parliamentary Labour
    Party
Labour Peers Group 406, 416
Labour Representation Committee 591
Labour Women's Action Committee
    (LWAC) 72
Labour Women's Conference, 1988 103
labour-market policy 291–2
Laird, Gavin 178, 336
Larkin, Isobel 445, 457
Law, Peter 586–7
leadership 12, 276, 580–1, 714–15
    accountability 688–9
    challenges 107
    elections 44, 44–5, 69–70, 104–5, 161,
        763, 769
    loss of trust 718–20
    Miliband 766–8
    and party management 664
    patronage 119
    strong 468–9, 614–15, 636, 680, 711,
        713
    transition to Brown 651–4
leaks 92, 256, 275, 465, 473
Liaison Committee 34, 35, 35–6, 38, 64,
    438, 479–80, 551, 713
Liberal Democrats 60, 123, 274, 279, 382,
    457, 492, 570, 609, 626, 654, 760,
    762, 774, 775
Liddle, Roger 135, 197, 281, 402, 474,
    691, 711
Lincoln, Deborah 592, 595–6
Livingstone, Ken 186, 238, 253, 258, 381,
    387–94, 468, 585, 615, 710
Lloyd, John 446–7, 512
Lloyd, Tony 430, 491, 492, 546, 612
loans for peerages scandal 631–2, 635, 741
local government re-selection 250
local party reform 254–5
London Mayor elections 153, 253, 254,
    258, 270–1, 387–94, 467, 468, 469,
    481, 510, 684, 710, 719
lone-parent benefit 357–8, 409, 410–13,
    414, 677–8, 711, 720
Lucas, Ann 313
Ludlam, Steve 484, 692
Luntz, Frank 720, 729, 735
Lyons, Roger 178, 222, 246, 274, 276,
    564

McBride, Damian 751
McCartney, Ian 150, 173, 218, 219, 236, 254, 285, 294, 311, 314, 318, 323, 389, 437, 439, 440, 440–1, 442, 444, 445, 449, 450, 452, 453, 454–5, 456–7, 490, 498, 505, 525, 561–2, 588, 591, 592, 593, 595–6, 614, 617–18, 619, 623, 636, 655–6, 691
McCluskey, Len 766, 775
McDonagh, Margaret 149, 151, 151–3, 154, 166, 172, 173, 195, 239, 242, 245, 251, 252, 254, 257–8, 262, 311, 360, 362, 390, 391, 392, 395–6, 410, 421–2, 424, 488, 507, 525
McDonagh, Siobhan 747
MacDonald, Ramsay 12, 18
McFadden, Pat 149, 173, 177, 276, 284, 334, 374, 395, 488, 539, 565, 585, 594, 625, 740, 746, 748
Macintyre, Donald 299–300, 451, 535
McKenzie, Ian 389, 425, 700–1
Mackenzie, Robert 12, 521
McKibbin, Ross 582
MacKinlay, Andrew 407, 408, 430, 492, 546
McNichol, Iain 768, 770–1
Macpherson, Hugh 185
McSmith, Andy 334
McTiernan, John 594, 610, 635
Maguire, Kevin 455
Mainwaring, Tony 89, 102–3
Major, John 121, 140–1, 190, 280, 406, 415
Malik, Shahid 242, 243
managerial vulnerability 5–6
Mandelson, Peter 1, 7, 57–8, 58–9, 59, 61–2, 69, 82, 84, 92, 117, 121, 135, 148, 167, 169, 171–2, 181–2, 186, 197, 201, 238, 239, 254, 261–2, 307, 333, 347, 361, 398, 402, 440, 450–5, 456, 466, 473–4, 487, 509, 513–14, 515, 516, 518, 534–5, 605, 610, 645, 646, 691, 711, 712, 728, 748, 752, 762
manifesto, 1992 76
manifesto, 1997 382, 670, 715, 729
manifesto, 2001 479–84, 678–9, 694
manifesto, 2005 600–1
manifesto, 2010 758–9
manifesto, NEC responsibility for 45
Manifesto Plan for an Efficient Party 30–1
manipulation 5, 112, 121, 135, 138–90, 163, 215, 241–3, 256, 298, 328, 386, 388, 393, 425, 464, 467, 470, 472, 509, 510, 512–18, 539, 559, 609–10, 613, 615, 626, 674, 678, 681, 696, 708, 710–11, 714–15, 718–19, 735, 747, 760, 767
Mann, John 271, 443
Manufacturing, Science and Finance Union (MSF) 94, 100–1, 178, 231, 237, 274, 317–19, 342, 392, 441, 478, 564
Marjoram, Annie 358, 411
Marr, Andrew 428, 467
Marsden, Paul 523
Marshall-Andrews, Robert 628
Mattinson, Deborah 57, 84, 558
Meacher, Michael 61, 360
media management 58–9, 141–2, 167–9, 465–7, 683–4, 685, 700, 735, 750–2
Mellish, Bob 30
Memorandum on the Selection of Candidates 18
Michels, Robert 12, 700–1
Milburn, Alan 307, 318–19, 484, 561, 573, 605, 630
Miliband, David 292, 397, 476, 479, 621, 646, 647, 747, 759, 763
Miliband, Ed 7–8, 585, 625, 751, 758, 763–77
Militant Tendency 37, 42, 51, 56, 67, 550
Millbank Tendency, the 153
Milne, Seamus 280
miners' strike, 1984 54, 55, 64, 282
Minimum Income Guarantee 364
minimum wage 266–7, 267–8, 284–5, 294, 297, 440, 454, 463, 670, 748
Minkin, Lewis 13, 74, 78, 90, 102–3, 107, 202, 203–4, 211, 212, 214, 219, 667, 668, 696, 721
modernising tendency 82–5, 88–9, 92–3, 117
Moffat, Anne (formerly Picking) 247, 318, 750
Monks, John 65, 200, 279–80, 280, 282, 283, 283–4, 285, 289, 290, 291–2, 295, 296, 299, 442, 443, 444, 445, 446, 447, 447–8, 448, 449, 450, 453, 457, 504, 505, 517, 532
Moore, Jo 516–17, 517, 684
Moraes, Claude 374, 391
Morgan, Rhodri 385–7, 391, 454, 529, 586, 710
Morgan, Sally 99, 100–1, 148–9, 151, 181, 189, 193, 203, 204, 207, 212, 219, 245, 251, 323, 334, 360, 389, 413, 472, 488, 503, 543, 550, 581

Morris, Bill 93, 100–1, 107, 185, 246,
    260, 271, 272–3, 274–5, 319, 323,
    336, 343, 365, 391, 443, 447, 449–50,
    504, 535, 588, 630
Morris, Estelle 484, 521, 625
Morrison, Herbert 20, 135, 398
Mortimer, Jim 51, 56–7
Mowlem, Mo 201, 202, 202–3, 204, 206,
    212, 226, 236, 238, 305, 353, 388,
    417, 466
Mudie, George 172, 406–7, 575, 576, 626
Mulgan, Geoff 601–2, 729
Mullin, Chris 394, 407, 408, 492, 493,
    495, 524, 546, 576, 746
Murdoch, Rupert 141, 436, 440, 455–6,
    576, 760
Murray, Len 35

National Agents Department 372
National Constitutional Committee 67,
    249–50, 529, 579, 712
National Council for Creative and Cultural
    Education 328
National Council of Labour 46
National Executive Committee (NEC) 3, 4,
    20, 43, 45, 46–7, 49, 122, 166, 486,
    711
  accountability 14
  balloting powers 187
  and Blair 180, 213, 615–16, 673
  and Brown 573, 735, 740, 753
  and candidate selection 32, 376–7, 381,
    585
  Chief Whip's report, 1999 252–3
  and Clause IV 179, 180–1, 182, 184,
    668–9, 676
  CLP section 219–20, 236, 237–9, 567,
    583, 690
  code of conduct 257–8
  and the Conference Arrangements
    Committee (CAC) 340
  disciplinary role 249–50
  dispute resolution 159, 249–50
  Domestic and International Policy
    Committee 110
  and Donorgate 741
  election management 161, 236
  elections 238–43, 258, 423–4, 527, 528,
    583–4, 640, 676, 688, 702
  expulsions 615
  financial scrutiny 262–3
  and the General Secretary 146, 147
  governance 651
  and the Iraq War 542–5, 546, 685

  and the Joint Policy Committee 109–10
  and Kinnock 53, 54, 60
  Late Retirement Panel 586
  and Livingstone 389–90, 391
  loans for peerages scandal 632, 741
  managerial control 15, 248–9, 527–8,
    615, 619–20, 676–7
  members and union obligations 245–8
  membership 14–15, 209
  and Miliband 765–6, 768–70
  non-executive directors 210, 270, 670
  Organisation Committee 234, 235
  and the parliamentary-expenses scandal
    756
  and Partnership in Power 230–3, 249,
    497–8, 676–7
  and Party Chair 489–90, 525
  and party conference management 338,
    340, 351–52
  and Party into Power 200–1, 202, 206,
    207, 212–13, 218, 222–3
  Party into Power reforms 208–10, 224–5
  party management 14–15, 44, 46
  party organisation report 362–3
  and the PLP 403, 423–4
  Policy Committee 315, 673
  policy role 23, 38, 74, 229–32, 244,
    307–8, 490, 528, 574, 664, 672, 707
  reform 62, 71–2, 187–8, 233–5, 251–6
  relations with 35–6
  report 639, 689
  revolts 42–3, 622, 697, 765–6
  Road to the Manifesto ballot, 1996 193,
    193–4, 196
  seats 12
  separation from government role 29
  shift to the left 31, 36–7, 43–4
  trade union group 21, 88, 161, 188, 191,
    209–10, 222, 222–3, 229, 236, 243–4,
    251, 253, 258
  trade union review group 603
  undermining 249–51
  and the unions 50–1, 75–6, 88, 583–4,
    690
  and women's representation 72
  women's section 212–13, 223, 234
  Youth Section 236, 236–7
National Health Service 127, 309, 475,
    482–3, 512, 519–20, 522, 531,
    539–40, 560, 566, 567, 567–8, 573–4,
    593, 596, 599, 600–1, 620–1, 623,
    636, 639, 651, 674, 690–1, 713, 759
National Joint Council 18
National Parliamentary Panel 377–8

National Policy Forum 4, 74, 110–11,
    111–12, 149, 159, 169, 170, 200,
    204, 205, 207, 215–16, 216, 217,
    222, 223, 229, 230, 258, 293, 303–5,
    307, 310–13, 314, 316–17, 351,
    359–60, 403, 425, 480–1, 490, 498,
    527, 529–32, 544, 587–8, 618, 623,
    672–3, 673–4, 688, 711, 745, 753–4,
    765, 774
    see also Durham NPF meeting; Exeter
    NPF meeting; Warwick NPF meeting
National Policy Forum Report, 2000 330
National Union of Mineworkers (NUM)
    21, 32, 51, 104, 275, 444
National Union of Public Employees
    (NUPE) 49, 55, 91, 94–102, 150, 336
National Union of Railwaymen (NUR) 51,
    55
National Union of Rail, Maritime and
    Transport Workers (RMT) 96, 98–102,
    178, 221, 247, 282, 299, 328, 336,
    343, 360, 366, 392, 478, 506, 508,
    534, 536, 565, 590, 591, 689
NATO 120
neo-liberalism 562–3, 671, 758
'New Labour' 1, 57, 61, 70, 118, 131–2,
    142–3
    code of conduct 136–8
    defeat of 762–3
    electoral trust 126–8
    end of 763
    fear of the past 130–1
    leadership 117, 118–21, 134
    legitimacy 134
    mass membership 129–30
    motivations 134–5
    move away from 772–5
    objectives 126, 128–30
    rights of the party 105
New Labour: a Stakeholder's Party 216
New Labour, New Life for Britain 194,
    277
Newcastle NPF meeting 531–2, 544
News International 440, 455–6, 458, 760,
    767, 771
Nolan Inquiry, the 141, 190
Norris, Geoffrey 150, 284, 290, 292–3,
    323, 324, 439–40, 442, 478, 480,
    595–6, 610, 748
Norris, Steven 394
Northcott, Jim 30–1
Northern Rock bank crisis 739
Norton, Jon 76
Norton, Philip 36, 401, 417

nuclear disarmament 63
Nye, Sue 583, 644

Oborne, Peter 141, 167, 767, 771
one-member-one-vote (OMOV) 2, 54–5,
    66–7, 70, 71, 77–8, 83, 87, 90–1, 93,
    94, 97, 98, 101–2, 107, 119, 129,
    215–16, 238, 369, 373, 380–1, 386,
    476, 528–9, 667, 681, 711–12, 754–5
O'Regan, John 443, 589
Organisation Committee 243, 538–9, 589,
    623, 632, 683, 691
Organising for Recovery conference 93
Osborne, George 737

Page, Ben 559, 752
Parliamentary Labour Party (PLP) 4–5, 12,
    46–8, 126, 164, 206, 403–4, 424–5,
    465, 584–7, 614, 716
    autonomy 15–16, 18, 405, 406
    and Blair 401–2, 408–9, 409–10, 419,
        423–4, 428–31, 445, 472, 492–3, 495,
        522, 523–5, 573, 577, 582, 623–7,
        687–8, 696
    and Brown 522, 574–6, 613, 625, 740,
        742, 746–7, 749–50, 753
    Chair 405–6, 430
    code of conduct 414, 418
    communication 415
    Departmental Committees 419–21,
        577–8, 678, 714–15, 753
    discipline 407, 412–13, 415–16, 425–7,
        578–80, 626, 628–9, 638, 649, 678,
        687–8, 749–50
    elections 612–14, 702, 740
    Employment Relations Act negotiations
        443–5, 446, 447, 448–9, 452, 453
    general election, 2005 609
    and the Iraq War 545–6, 547, 548–9,
        685–6
    lone-parent benefit revolt 409, 410–13,
        414, 677–8, 711, 720
    management 403–4, 404, 421–3, 427–9,
        431, 522–5, 572–3, 614, 652, 677–8
    and manifesto, 2001 479–80
    and Miliband 768, 773
    and NEC elections 423–4
    Parliamentary Committee 406, 407,
        407–10, 413, 422, 423, 426, 431,
        479–80, 491–2, 493, 547, 572, 612,
        628–9, 647, 653, 679, 746
    and Party Chair 491–2
    and party management 68–9
    and policy-making 495–6, 682

Parliamentary Labour Party (PLP) (cont'd)
  Preparing for Government 417, 418,
    419, 429
  review 684
  Review Committee 416–17, 418
  revolts 4, 20, 36, 358, 524–5, 572–3,
    624–7, 628–9, 638, 677–8, 711, 720,
    742, 749
  and the Schools White Paper 624, 625
  Secretary 405
  and the September coup 625, 642–5,
    647
  staff 419–20, 611
  trade union group 21, 30, 33, 34, 275,
    413–14, 443–5, 448, 452, 453, 505,
    671, 692, 696, 702
  union membership requirement 379–80
  and the Warwick meetings 594
  whips 404, 406–7, 415–16, 523,
    579–80, 628–9, 687
parliamentary-expenses scandal 755–7
Partnership Fund 297
Partnership in Power 73, 156, 214, 250,
    303, 306, 311, 314, 320, 327, 335,
    351, 362–3, 420–1, 422, 490, 493,
    496, 591, 620, 688, 707–8, 736, 745
  assessment 672–3, 712, 714–15
  Conference Arrangements Committee
    (CAC) 339–40
  managerial controls 232
  and members' representation 321–2
  and NEC 230–3, 233–5, 249, 676–7
  and party conference 358–9
  and policy-making 310, 529–32
  review 497–8, 617–18, 682
  and the unions 273, 722
Party Chair 153, 485–6, 487, 489–92, 521,
    525–6, 526–7, 539, 561–2, 617–18,
    636, 651, 681–2, 684, 685, 693, 708,
    767
party conference 12, 14, 716, 717
  1989 76–7
  2001 493–4
  2002 536–8
  2003 563–4, 565–8, 570–2, 574, 691
  2004 591, 598–9, 691
  2005 602, 618–22, 691, 697
  2006 649, 650–1
  2008 745–6
  2011 770
  2012 772
  accountability 366
  agenda 334, 338–42
  and Blair 337, 353–5

  and CLPs 334, 335, 342, 344–7, 348–9,
    355–7, 618–19, 674–6
  communication 349–51
  and contemporary resolutions 360–6,
    494, 537–8, 599, 650
  floor contributions 355–7
  fringe meetings 349
  and the Iraq War 598–9
  lone parent benefit debate, 1997 357–8
  management 333–5, 691–2
  NPF elections 351
  and Partnership in Power 358–9
  Party into Power reforms 207–8
  and policy-making 217, 358–60
  regional liaison teams 347–8, 350–1
  speeches 351–3, 675
  and the unions 335–7, 338, 340, 342–4,
    675
  voting 357, 691
party distrust 538–9
party employees 156
party finance
  accountability 633, 741
  crisis and debt 506–7, 540, 632–3
  Donorgate 632, 740–2, 743
  donors 259, 261–3, 477, 518–19
  loans for peerages scandal 631–2
  management 258–63
  and Miliband 769–70
  Phillips report 653–4, 721, 722, 759
  reform 633–5, 698
  and the unions 6, 12, 258–61, 507–9,
    532–6, 568–9, 597, 632–3, 653–4,
    689–90, 721, 726, 743
  and the Warwick Agreement 597
Party into Power, The 4, 126, 151, 170,
    193, 194, 196, 201, 226, 268, 305,
    463, 467, 695, 724, 725
  Bishop's Stortford meeting 218–21
  conference reforms 207–8
  and consensus 205
  consultation 210–14, 224
  and contemporary resolutions 220–1,
    223
  convenors' group 214, 218–21
  Cranfield School of Management
    discussions 200–1
  creation 200–26
  discussions 216–18
  draft document 204, 206–7, 213–14
  final document 211–12, 216, 219
  interim document 214
  and the manifesto 479
  NEC reforms 208–10, 224–5

NEC support 222–3
and OMOV 215–16
partnership proposals 203–7, 212, 217,
    221–2
significance 225–6
steering group 202–3, 207, 211–12,
    214
and the unions 212, 213, 217–18,
    221–2, 224, 695
vote 223–5
party management 1–2, 2, 19–20, 34–9,
    142–3, 476
appraisal 463–4, 707–12, 715–20
behavioural worlds 665–6
and Blair 2–4, 88–9, 118–24, 162–4,
    468–70, 472–8, 497, 560, 610–12,
    663–8, 680, 681–3, 696–9, 709–10,
    712, 727–31, 740, 751
and Blair/Brown conflict 520–2
bottom-up pressure 70–1
and Brown 573–6, 682, 736–7, 753–4
Brown's inheritance 734–6, 739–40,
    740
candidate selection 24–6
code of conduct 136–8, 256–7, 539
control 154, 256–8, 526–9
crisis 463–80
democracy 33–4, 446, 464, 473, 708
destabilization, 1960s 26–9
ethics 726–9
expansion 153–4
Gould's advisory memos 464–5
heritage 11–12
and the Iraq War 560
and issue management 436–7
Kinnock 68–72
and leadership 664
managerial framework 23–6
managerial interventionism 15–16,
    38–42, 305–6
Manifesto Plan for an Efficient Party
    30–1
and media management 168, 465–6
and Miliband 764–6, 772–5
modernising tendency 88–9
and the NEC 44, 46
'New Labour' 2–4, 117, 126, 133–6
Party Chair 525–6, 617–18
and the PLP 68–9
pluralism 679–80
and policy-making 276
power relations 699–703
procedural management 725–6
reappraisal 470–2

reform 83–5, 665, 720, 734, 768–71,
    772–5
reorganisation, 1985 56–8
repoliticisation 155–6, 158
rules and rulebook 241, 57–60
Smith and 105–7
staff 154, 478, 538–9
top-down 71–2
tradition 11, 61–4
and the TUC 279–80
and the unions 13–14, 45–6, 62–3,
    317–20, 532–6, 588–91, 690–1,
    720–2
vanguardists 122–3
party managers 164–7, 233, 538–9, 561–2,
    597, 665–6, 715–20, 725–6, 777
party membership 19, 21, 470, 587, 598,
    639–40, 677, 693, 718, 723–4, 754,
    760, 777
party referendums 187
Party Secretary 15
party staff 36–7, 156
Pathways to the Future 652, 653
peers 376, 377, 396, 416, 476
pensions policy 327, 343, 353, 356–7,
    363–5, 595, 621, 624, 711
Peston, Robert 172, 574, 600, 627
Phillips, Hayden 633–5, 653–4, 698, 721,
    722, 759
Pickering, Steve 245, 248, 547
Picking, Anne see Moffat, Anne
Pilger, John 196
Pimlott, Ben 45
Pinder, Phil 237
Pitt Watson, David 262, 263, 269, 742
plebiscitary leadership 106–7
policy commissions 308–9
policy cycle 310, 531–2
Policy Director 307, 314, 360, 674
Policy Directorate 488
policy documents 310
policy implementation 435–9
policy staff 148
policy statements 229
policy supervision 305–6
Policy Unit 154, 292–3, 295, 296, 304,
    307, 397, 437, 457, 479
policy-making 38, 61–2, 276–9
alternative positions 314–15, 359–60
amendments 316–17, 320–1
and Blair 601–2, 651–2, 713–14
and Brown 574
commissions 530
contemporary resolutions 360–6

policy-making (*cont'd*)
  controlling 286–7
  JPC role diminished 306–8
  Kinnock 59–63
  and Miliband 773, 773–4
  NEC role 230–2, 244, 307–8, 490, 528,
    574, 664, 672, 707
  NPF role 531
  and Partnership in Power 529–32
  and party conference 217, 339–40,
    358–60
  and Party into Power 205
  party role 216–17
  and PLP 495–6, 682
  process 229–30
  union role 16, 273–5, 317–20, 693
political engagement audit, 2004 559
Political Office 154, 172–3, 323–4, 388,
    420, 426, 427, 430–1, 473, 488, 504,
    506, 527, 581, 649
political reform, broken politics 757–8
political-education programme 170
Porter, Henry 614
positive discrimination 72
Post Office privatisation campaign 184,
    247, 282, 296, 319, 361–2, 481, 600,
    620, 633, 749, 752
Powell, Jonathan 150, 167, 298, 488, 503,
    605, 610, 631, 646, 712, 715, 728–9
power relations 12, 75, 157–60, 699–703
Prentice, Bridget 417, 546
Prentice, Gordon 492, 546
Prentis, Dave 478, 494, 534, 565, 601,
    650
Preparing for Government 417, 418, 419,
    429
Prescott, John 78, 97, 101, 109, 110, 112,
    117, 121, 122, 147, 161, 173, 176–7,
    179, 192, 195, 231, 234, 241, 252,
    282, 326, 343, 352, 386, 391, 417,
    418, 425, 487, 506, 586, 590, 601,
    625, 629, 636, 639–40, 641–2, 651,
    654, 680, 682, 698, 701, 702
presidentialism 84, 472, 559, 580–1,
    687–8
Price, Lance 123, 172, 173, 340, 469, 473,
    514–15, 680
Prime Ministerial Government 120
Prime Minister's Department 120
Private Finance Initiative 110, 318–19,
    519–20, 537–8, 540, 566, 685, 713,
    716
privatisation 346, 361–2, 482–3, 600, 749,
    752, 759

proscribed list 28
Prosser, Margaret 89, 147, 153, 192, 211,
    213, 222, 234, 244, 245, 246, 253,
    261, 262, 306, 318, 319, 325, 327,
    389, 496
public distrust 466–8, 471, 509–20, 558,
    558–9, 560, 609, 636–7, 641, 684,
    712, 720, 726–8, 737–8, 741–2,
    760–1
public expenditure 297–8
public sector reform 298, 516–17, 519–20,
    602–3, 678, 685, 713–14, 715, 759

Queen's speech, 1997 128, 289, 728

Rank and File Mobilising Committee
    (RFMC) 42–3, 46
Ranney, Austen 25
Rathbone, Jenny 358
Rawnsley, Andrew 142, 172, 196, 298,
    428, 578, 642, 771
Raynsford, Nick 388, 625
Reeves, Ellie 640, 740
*Refounding Labour: a Party for a New
    Generation* 769
Regional Liaison Teams 311, 347–8,
    350–1
Registered Supporters 91, 95, 102, 639–40
Reid, John 139, 519, 521, 525, 526–7,
    539, 544, 561, 587, 601, 636, 685
Renewing Democracy: Rebuilding
    Communities 271
Rentoul, John 119, 126, 133, 137, 277,
    632, 641, 645, 697, 709
Richards, Steve 451, 492–3, 642, 652, 739
Riddell, Mary 774
Riddell, Peter 394–5, 504, 642, 730
Rix, Mick 564
Road to the Manifesto ballot, 1996 163,
    191–7, 201, 203, 216, 267, 278, 401,
    465, 671–2, 684, 702, 736
Road to the Manifesto, The 3, 276–9, 287,
    305
Robinson, Geoffrey 172, 456
Robinson, Nick 637, 754
Robinson, Tony 242, 243, 583, 587–8, 631
rolling coup 118, 136, 156, 431, 464, 486,
    663–6, 672, 678, 679, 686, 698–702,
    707, 725, 729
Rosser, Richard 71, 147, 180, 244, 245,
    247, 564
Ruddock, Joan 652, 746
rulebook, the 157–60, 187, 231, 378–9,
    486, 526, 569, 639–40, 666, 695

'rules', conventional 3, 12–16, 27, 50–1,
160, 272–3, 694–700, 725
financial and organisational sanctions 15,
18, 508–9
Russell, Bertrand 5, 28, 234, 317, 322,
526, 547, 711
Russell, Meg 700

St. Ermin's Group 50–1, 54
Sampson, Anthony 293
Sawyer, Tom 53, 56, 61, 74, 88, 89, 95,
95–6, 97, 100, 110, 147–8, 150–2,
177, 178, 180, 200–1, 202–3, 204,
206, 209–10, 218, 229, 239, 242,
244, 333, 360, 525, 584, 676
Scanlon, Hugh 32, 34
Scargill, Arthur 54, 184
Schools White Paper 624, 625, 627–8, 629
Scotland 383–5
Seddon, Mark 242, 243, 248–9, 257,
257–8, 528, 529, 542, 544–5, 646
September coup 625, 640–8, 698–9
Seyd, Patrick 25–6, 184, 346, 470, 721
Shadow Communications Agency (SCA)
57–8, 60, 64, 76, 84, 119
Sharp, Andrew 356, 529
Shaw, Eric 22, 24–5, 28, 30, 32, 68, 370,
384, 670, 700, 701, 725
Shawcross, Christine 242, 243, 250
Short, Clare 74, 89, 102–3, 122, 179,
182–3, 209, 220–1, 223, 241, 300,
329, 339, 466, 522, 549–50, 559–60,
579, 649, 684, 686, 687
Simon, Sion 396, 647
Simpson, Derek 508, 550, 563, 565, 589,
619, 633, 739–40
Single Equalities Act 592
Skinner, Dennis 53, 71, 89, 179, 193, 201,
212, 213, 223, 251, 287, 389, 408,
423, 425
Slaughter, Andrew 374–5
sleaze 127, 141, 190, 376, 518–19, 631–2,
740–2
Smeargate 750–2
Smith, Jackie 374, 636, 644, 748
Smith, John 2, 82, 83–5, 90, 92, 93,
94–102, 104–5, 105–7, 107–9,
109–12, 111, 117, 122, 131, 135,
142, 165, 176, 269, 369
Snelgrove, Ann 313, 531–2, 587, 594, 622,
623
social change, and public distrust 510–12
Social Democratic Party 48, 52, 60
social justice 286

social partnership 294–5, 295–6
social policy 297
Socialist Campaign Group 49
social-partnership 285
Society of Graphical and Allied Trades
(SOGAT) 105, 443
Soley, Clive 253, 405–6, 408, 410, 421,
423, 425, 430, 480, 491
Special Advisors 306, 308, 309, 672–3
Special Conference, 1995 126
Spellar, John 63, 91, 161, 551, 748
spin 58–9, 85–6, 297–8, 463, 464, 465,
466–7, 484, 510, 538, 559, 667–8,
678–9, 683–4, 711, 769
spin-doctors 167–9, 517–18, 701, 728
sponsorship 189–91, 257–8, 261–3
standing order K12 495–6
standing orders 404
Stephens, Philip 132
Stewart, Ian 595–6
Stewart, Neil 67–8, 73
Strategic Communications Unit 293
Strategy Unit 488
Straw, Jack 182–3, 238, 298, 315, 348,
382, 480, 542, 546, 570, 593, 636
Stuart, Mark 86
subordination 305–8
Sullivan, Willie 242–3
Sumner, Barclay 527, 640
Sutcliffe, Gerry 443, 445, 456, 539, 595–6,
636
Sztompka, Piotr 727

tax credits 297
taxation 285–6, 477, 567–8, 574–5, 601,
742, 758
Taylor, Ann 110, 424–5, 426, 491
Taylor, Byron 271, 507, 569, 589, 591,
617, 749
Taylor, Matthew 129, 149, 214, 218, 223,
231, 235, 304, 311, 314–15, 483,
532, 581, 592, 600–1, 610, 635, 652,
653, 673, 692, 711, 751
terrorism 476, 485, 493, 495, 497, 503,
516, 540, 614–15, 626–7, 681, 684
Thatcher, Margaret, and Thatcherism 38,
42, 51–3, 57, 120, 125, 570, 610,
730
Third Way, the 473
Toynbee, Polly 119, 609, 686, 708–9
Trade Union and Labour Party Liaison
Organisation (TULO) 106, 210, 218,
271–2, 323–4, 330, 336, 443, 454,
484, 507, 534, 535–6, 565, 568–9,

588–9, 590, 593, 597, 600, 602–3, 617, 629–30, 668, 674, 683, 692, 695–6, 697, 702, 724, 740, 744–5, 749, 754–5, 759, 769, 773
Trade Union Freedom Bill 654
Trade Union Review Group 88, 89–92, 102–3, 105–6, 106–7, 108, 118, 119, 129, 379
Trade Unionists for Labour (TUFL) 64, 95, 106
trade unions 3, 16, 87
  and Blair 65–6, 108, 186, 186–7, 190–1, 193, 272–3, 276, 286–7, 324, 435–9, 442, 446–9, 533, 667–8, 669–70, 671–2, 689, 693–4, 694–5, 721
  block vote reform 188–9, 616–17, 630–1
  block votes 12, 17, 21, 23, 62, 72–3, 83, 86, 87, 94–5, 102–3, 336, 566, 572, 604, 669, 722, 764
  and Brown 187, 276, 319, 735–6, 738, 739–40, 743–4, 748–9, 754–5, 761
  and candidate selection 24–5, 93, 372, 378–81, 381, 750
  and Clarke 525
  and Clause IV 182–3, 184, 185, 669
  dissatisfaction 505–6
  electoral role 34–5
  Exeter NPF meeting 323–6
  and the Iraq War 542, 543, 545, 547, 598–9, 685–6
  and Kinnock 60, 62–3, 63–7, 73–8
  leadership 6, 45–6, 272–5, 550–1, 563–70, 589–90
  leadership election votes 104
  and Livingstone 391–2
  management 17
  manifesto, 2001, contributions 481, 679
  membership decline 604, 761
  and Miliband 764, 766, 768, 769, 773, 775–6
  modernisers critique of 90–2
  and the NEC 14, 245–8, 583–4, 690
  and neo-liberalism 562–3
  and 'New Labour' 126, 164
  and the NPF 317–20
  organisational separation 83
  and Partnership in Power 73, 273, 722
  and party conference management 335–7, 338, 340, 342–4, 675
  and party finance 6, 12, 258–61, 507–9, 532–6, 568–9, 597, 632–3, 653–4, 689–90, 721, 726, 743
and Party into Power 209–10, 212, 213, 217–18, 221–2, 224, 695
  and party management 13–14, 62–3, 317–20, 532–6, 588–91, 690–1, 720–2
  and the PLP 413–14, 443–5
trade unions (cont'd)
  and policy commissions 308–9
  policy-making 16, 273–5, 317–20, 323–6, 693
  Political Fund ballots 63–4
  problem 82–3
  reapportionment of votes 188–9
  recognition see Employment Relations Act, 1999
  relationship with 12–14, 17–19, 19, 24, 32–3, 34, 35, 50–1, 63–7, 73–8, 85–8, 105–6, 107–9, 177–8, 271–3, 288–91, 299, 361, 463, 477–8, 494–5, 503–9, 563–70, 602–4, 667–8, 683, 692, 694–6, 720–2, 723–4
  representation reforms 603–4, 604
  restraint 94–5
  rights of the party 105
  Road to the Manifesto ballot, 1996 192, 193
  role 6, 12–14, 17, 23, 73–5, 94, 283–4, 568–9, 700, 702, 764
  sanctions 95, 187, 259, 633, 670, 689, 702
  and the September coup 642–3
  Smith and 83, 92, 93, 94, 96–8, 107–9
  the spin campaign 85–6
  sponsorship reform 189–91
  and the Warwick Agreement 602, 603, 629–31, 654, 722
  and the Warwick meetings 595–6
Trade Unions for a Labour Victory (TULV) 37, 45–6, 50–1, 64
Trades Union Congress (TUC) 3, 13, 17, 21, 29, 64–6, 275, 279–84, 286, 436, 459, 505, 633
  and Blair 441
  and Brown 735–6, 738
  Employment Relations Act negotiations 438–9, 442–3, 446, 447–8, 452–5
  Fairness at Work white paper 450
  handling of industrial disputes 282–3
  and the Iraq War 543, 545, 685–6
  labour-market policy 291–2
  management problem 281–2
  and Mandelson 451, 452–5
  manifesto, 2001, contributions 481

minimum wage 294
and neo-liberalism 562–3
and party finance 533–4
and party management 279–80
policy coordination 324
relationship with 289–91, 295–6,
  589–90
role 283–4, 503–4, 700
and the September coup 648
social partnership 294–5
Transport and General Workers Union
  (TGWU) 21, 23, 27–8, 31, 32, 54, 74,
  95, 97, 102, 107, 108, 185, 213, 246,
  260–1, 272, 318–19, 325–6, 336, 365,
  494, 543, 550, 619
Transport Salaried Staffs' Association
  (TSSA) 178, 245, 247, 328, 336, 343,
  564
tribalism 123–4
Tribune Group 22–3, 49, 69
Triesman, David 489, 490, 494, 519, 525,
  526, 532, 533–4, 535, 543, 561–2,
  565–6, 689
trust, loss of 466–8, 471, 509–20, 558,
  558–9, 560, 609, 636–7, 641, 684,
  712, 718–20, 726–9, 737–8, 741–2,
  760–1
Turner, Mary 211, 248, 255
Turner, Muriel 251
Turner, Ruth 243, 610, 638, 646
Tyrie, Andrew 635

Underhill, Reg 26, 32, 37, 155
Underhill Report, the 155
Union of Communication Workers (UCW)
  89, 94, 96, 98, 100, 178, 184, 185,
  245, 336, 342, 633, 692
Union of Construction, Allied Trades and
  Technicians (UCATT) 104
Union of Shop, Distributive and Allied
  Workers (USDAW) 48, 55, 89, 94, 98,
  100, 178, 185, 245, 247, 274, 319,
  336, 381, 391, 441, 535, 563, 593,
  621, 754, 755
Unions 21 589–90
UNISON 97, 147, 150, 153, 185, 190,
  201, 213, 224, 246–7, 274, 275, 284,
  294, 299, 317–19, 325, 336–8, 343–4,
  348, 357, 362–4, 392, 441, 445, 478,
  494, 506, 532, 537–8, 540, 543, 550,
  656, 583, 588, 593, 598, 601, 620,
  633, 650, 674, 679, 689, 694
Unite the Union 604, 619, 739–40, 742,
  750, 755, 759, 763–4, 775

vanguardists 122–3
voice politics 717–18

Wadey, Clare 359
Wales 383, 385–7, 586, 710
Wales, Roland 111, 149, 303–4, 305, 674
Walker, David 708–9
Wall, Margaret 147, 153, 201, 203, 211,
  212, 218, 222, 231, 234, 244, 245,
  246, 306, 311, 318, 489, 497, 543
Warwick Agreement, 2004 6, 330, 593–8,
  599, 600, 601, 602, 603, 616–18,
  629–31, 633, 637, 654, 692, 693,
  694, 697, 702, 722, 723, 744–5
Warwick NPF meeting 578, 590–9, 722
Watson, Tom 379, 380, 643–5, 647, 649,
  740, 750, 767, 773
Watt, Peter 571, 597, 622, 631, 645–6,
  647–8, 655, 697, 740–1, 742
Webster, Philip 642
Wegg-Prosser, Benjamin 610, 646
Welfare and Pensions Bill 319
welfare state 132, 319
Wertheimer analysis, 1929 13
What Next for the Unions? 589–90
Wheatcroft, Geoffrey 133
Wheeler, Margaret 245, 318, 338, 340,
  359, 361
Wheeler, Peter 379, 583, 640, 740
Whelan, Charlie 171, 361, 740, 750, 755,
  761, 764
whips 47, 404, 406–7, 415–16, 523,
  579–80, 687
White, Michael 201, 276–9, 483, 696, 752
Whitty, Larry 61, 66, 68, 73–5, 84–5, 89,
  89–90, 99, 100, 107, 108, 146–7,
  154, 156, 226, 325, 382, 525, 741,
  771, 776
Wicks, Sir Nigel 512
Wilby, Peter 395
Wilkinson, Frank 338, 340
Williams, David 374–5
Willsman, Pete 240, 248–9, 257–8, 349,
  619
Wilson, Harold 20, 25, 29–34, 33, 35,
  701
Wilson, Phil 129, 149, 162, 195, 214, 219,
  220, 311, 313, 334, 350
Wilson, Tom 67
Winstone, Maurice 317
Wintour, Patrick 92, 482, 490, 543, 577,
  669
Wise, Audrey 340, 358, 411
Wolfgang, Walter 621, 640, 650, 740

Women at Work Commission 602
women's representation 72, 158–9, 375–6,
    377, 378, 385, 586
Woodley, Tony 550, 563, 565, 619,
    739–40
Woodward, Shaun 397, 476, 525
Wootton, Barbara 28
Worcester, Bob 558–9, 605

work groups 111–12
Wright, Tony 408, 560, 713, 757

Young, Hugo 140, 429, 469, 475, 517
Your Voice at Work 439
youth organisation 236–7

Zeichner, Daniel 588